KU-573-323

Processing of Sensory Information in the Superficial Dorsal Horn of the Spinal Cord

NATO ASI Series

Advanced Science Institutes Series

A series presenting the results of activities sponsored by the NATO Science Committee, which aims at the dissemination of advanced scientific and technological knowledge, with a view to strengthening links between scientific communities.

The series is published by an international board of publishers in conjunction with the NATO Scientific Affairs Division

A	**Life Sciences**	Plenum Publishing Corporation
B	**Physics**	New York and London
C	**Mathematical**	Kluwer Academic Publishers
	and Physical Sciences	Dordrecht, Boston, and London
D	**Behavioral and Social Sciences**	
E	**Applied Sciences**	
F	**Computer and Systems Sciences**	Springer-Verlag
G	**Ecological Sciences**	Berlin, Heidelberg, New York, London,
H	**Cell Biology**	Paris, and Tokyo

Recent Volumes in this Series

Volume 170—ras Oncogenes
   edited by Demetrios Spandidos

Volume 171—Dietary ω3 and ω6 Fatty Acids: Biological Effects
   and Nutritional Essentiality
   edited by Claudio Galli and Artemis P. Simopoulos

Volume 172—Recent Trends in Regeneration Research
   edited by V. Kiortsis, S. Koussoulakos, and H. Wallace

Volume 173—Physiology of Cold Adaptation in Birds
   edited by Claus Bech and Randi Eidsmo Reinertsen

Volume 174—Cell and Molecular Biology of Artemia Development
   edited by Alden H. Warner, Thomas H. MacRae,
   and Joseph C. Bagshaw

Volume 175—Vascular Endothelium: Receptors and Transduction Mechanisms
   edited by John D. Catravas, C. Norman Gillis, and Una S. Ryan

Volume 176—Processing of Sensory Information in the
   Superficial Dorsal Horn of the Spinal Cord
   edited by F. Cervero, G. J. Bennett, and P. M. Headley

Series A: Life Sciences

Processing of Sensory Information in the Superficial Dorsal Horn of the Spinal Cord

Edited by

F. Cervero
University of Bristol Medical School
Bristol, United Kingdom

G. J. Bennett
National Institute of Dental Research
National Institutes of Health
Bethesda, Maryland

and

P. M. Headley
University of Bristol Medical School
Bristol, United Kingdom

Plenum Press
New York and London
Published in cooperation with NATO Scientific Affairs Division

Proceedings of a NATO Advanced Research Workshop on
Processing of Sensory Information in the
Superficial Dorsal Horn of the Spinal Cord,
held May 22–27, 1988,
in El Escorial, Spain

Library of Congress Cataloging in Publication Data

NATO Advanced Research Workshop on Processing of Sensory Information in
the Superficial Dorsal Horn of the Spinal Cord (1988: San Lorenzo del Escorial,
Spain)
    Processing of sensory information in the superficial dorsal horn of the spinal
cord / edited by F. Cervero, G. J. Bennett, and P. M. Headley.
        p.   cm.—(NATO ASI series. Series A, Life sciences; v. 176)
    "Proceedings of a NATO Advanced Research Workshop on Processing of Sen-
sory Information in the Superficial Dorsal Horn of the Spinal Cord, held May
22–27, 1988, in El Escorial, Spain"—T.p. verso.
    "Published in cooperation with NATO Scientific Affairs Division."
    Includes bibliographies and indexes.
    ISBN 0-306-43258-7
    1. Spinal cord—Congresses. 2. Afferent pathways—Congresses. I. Cervero,
Fernando. II. Bennett, G. J.(Gary J.) III. Headley, P. M. IV. North Atlantic Treaty
Organization. Scientific Affairs Division. V. Title. VI. Series.
QP371.N37   1989
599′.0188—dc20
DNLM/DLC   89-16161
for Library of Congress   CIP

© 1989 Plenum Press, New York
A Division of Plenum Publishing Corporation
233 Spring Street, New York, N.Y. 10013

All rights reserved

No part of this book may be reproduced, stored in a retrieval system, or transmitted
in any form or by any means, electronic, mechanical, photocopying, microfilming,
recording, or otherwise, without written permission from the Publisher

Printed in the United States of America

PREFACE

This book constitutes the proceedings of a NATO Advanced Research Workshop held in El Escorial (Spain) from 22 - 27 May 1988 with the title *Processing of sensory information in the superficial dorsal horn of the spinal cord*. Included in the book are reports of most of the main lectures given at the meeting, section introductions written by each session Chairman, section reports compiled by session rapporteurs and some short papers invited from authors of communications given in poster form. The latter were selected on the basis of being immediately relevant to the topic of the workshop and of originating from a laboratory not represented by the main speakers. All in all we believe that the reader can get a fair idea of the structure and general character of this Workshop.

The overall aim of the meeting was to review the current state of knowledge on the role of the superficial dorsal horn of the mammalian spinal cord as a nucleus of relay and modulation of the somatic and visceral sensory input to the central nervous system. In this context, the contribution of this spinal cord region to the appreciation of pain was a central topic of discussion.

Over the last decade there has been a considerable increase in anatomical, physiological and neurochemical studies of the superficial dorsal horn. This surge of interest has had the beneficial effect of exposing the limitations of the old concepts and of forcing a change of direction of research in this field. However, such major revision has also produced a plethora of publications and a number of different views and contradictory opinions. With this Workshop and through the vehicle of its proceedings we hope to provide a review of the new data so as to test the strength of the ideas emerging from recent work and to identify directions for future research.

Unfortunately, not every scientist working in the field has contributed to our book. Some could not come to the meeting, a few speakers did not submit a paper and, inevitably, limitations of time, space and funds meant a restricted programme of invited speakers and talks. We regret the gaps but believe that the reader will nevertheless find that most of the new data and ideas and virtually all the active research groups are represented in this volume.

Contrary to common practice with this type of publication, we have had all the submitted papers refereed. Reviewers were selected mainly from the participants to the meeting so that they could provide an informed view on the papers from their direct knowledge of the presentation and of the subsequent discussion. Although refereeing has inevitably lengthened publication time we firmly believe that it has been worth it since many papers have been improved and clarified following the reviewers comments.

The meeting was sponsored by the Scientific Affairs Division of NATO and we wish to express our appreciation to NATO for their help and financial support, and particularly to Dr Craig Sinclair who shared with us a few days of the Workshop and provided helpful comments and advice. Two UK organizations, the Wellcome Trust and The Physiological Society helped to fund the attendance of young British scientists and we are most grateful for their help. Finally two members of the pharmaceutical industry - Merck Sharp and Dohme and Parke Davis - also provided funds to help with the running of the meeting.

A number of individuals have helped beyond the call of duty with the organization of the meeting and with the editing of this book. We have been particularly fortunate to have the secretarial help of Mrs Ruth Alexander throughout the running of the Workshop and the preparation of this book. To her, to the referees of the contributions and to everyone else who has helped us with this project we offer our thanks.

F. Cervero
G.J. Bennett
P.M. Headley

CONTENTS

SECTION VI: SUPERFICIAL DORSAL HORN CHANGES FOLLOWING
PERIPHERAL INJURY

THE SUPERFICIAL DORSAL HORN

Fernando Cervero

Department of Physiology, University of Bristol, Medical School, University Walk
Bristol BS8 1TD, U.K.

The superficial dorsal horn is a morphologically distinct region of the grey matter of the spinal cord that has been recognized as a separate anatomical entity for over 150 years. It contains the first synaptic relay of fine afferent fibres from skin, muscle and viscera and for this reason has been regarded as an important site for the initial processing of signals directly related to the transmission and modulation of pain. Every neurobiological technique (light microscopy, immunohistochemistry, single unit electrophysiology, electron microscopy) has shown more and more distinct features of this region of the dorsal horn which make it clearly different from the rest of the spinal grey matter. Moreover, some of these peculiarities point to fundamental differences - functional as well as anatomical - in the processing of the sensory information mediated by fine afferent fibres as opposed to the processing of the signals carried by large myelinated afferents.

HISTORICAL BACKGROUND

The superficial dorsal horn was the first region of the spinal cord to be described as a separate anatomical entity. This was done in 1824 by the anatomist L. Rolando who was impressed by the gelatinous appearance of the dorsalmost region of the grey matter. His description led to the naming of this zone as the *Substantia Gelatinosa* and by the end of the nineteenth century the superficial dorsal horn had been subdivided into a more dorsal Marginal Zone and a larger and more ventral Substantia Gelatinosa proper (see Cervero and Iggo, 1980 for references). Our current nomenclature originates from the work of Rexed (1952) who divided the entire grey matter of the spinal cord into ten laminae of which the superficial dorsal horn took the first two: lamina I for the Marginal Zone and lamina II for the Substantia Gelatinosa.

The light microscopic anatomy of the superficial dorsal horn was examined in great detail in the second half of the nineteenth century. In 1859, J.L. Clarke (of Clarke's column fame) published a thorough study of the grey matter of the spinal cord using, for the first time, fixed specimens of cords (largely from cattle) rendered transparent with the help of clearing agents. He described all the neuronal elements of the superficial dorsal horn and illustrated his descriptions with drawings of outstanding artistic quality (Fig. 1). Included in his illustrations are the fusiform cells of the Marginal Zone whose dendritic trees extend in a medio-lateral orientation. These cells were rediscovered 30 years later by Waldeyer in a study of the spinal cord of the gorilla and have been known

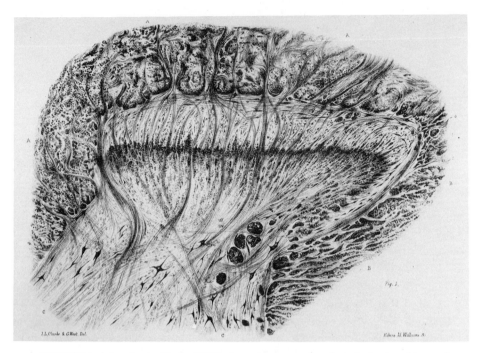

FIGURE 1: A drawing by Clarke (1859) of a transverse section through the dorsal horn of a calf. Note the clear border between the superficial and deep dorsal horns and the different cell types including marginal and substantia gelatinosa cells.

ever since as *Waldeyer cells*. Clarke also described and illustrated the boundary between the superficial and deep dorsal horn as well as the small cells of the Substantia Gelatinosa whose dendritic trees show a dorso-ventral orientation.

All these cellular elements were described in considerable detail, and in the light of the neuron theory, by Ramón y Cajal (1890, see Fig. 2). Cajal's descriptions of fibres and nerve cells and, to some extent, his nomenclature - Marginal Cells, Central Cells, Limiting Cells - have survived almost untouched until this day (see Beal *et al*, this volume). He also highlighted the close relationship between fine primary afferents and superficial dorsal horn neurones, a concept that was further developed at the beginning of this century by Ranson (1914) and Ranson and von Hess (1915). Using combined anatomical and physiological techniques they demonstrated that the gelatinous appearance of the superficial dorsal horn was due to the presence of large numbers of unmyelinated fibres and axons; they proposed that this region of the cord was the relay of fine afferent fibres concerned with the transmission of pain.

In the mid 1960's and as a result of the first single unit recordings of neuronal activity in the dorsal horn, the small neurones of the Substantia Gelatinosa were given a protagonist's role in the *Gate Control theory* of pain mechanisms (Melzack and Wall, 1965). This hypothesis, an elaboration of the older *Pattern theory* of pain, denied the existence of specific nociceptors and of neurones specifically concerned with the transmission of nociceptive signals and hypothesized that the small neurones of the Substantia Gelatinosa controlled the flow of convergent inputs onto non-specific dorsal horn neurones.

Experimental evidence was already available at the time of the *Gate Theory* on the existence of specific cutaneous nociceptors, and more recent work has produced evidence for the presence of specific nociceptor-driven cells in the superficial dorsal

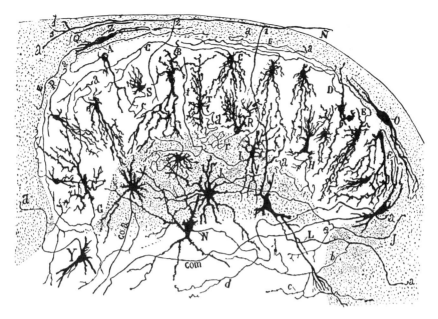

FIGURE 2: A drawing by Ramón y Cajal (1890) of the different cells and fibres seen in a transverse section of the dorsal horn of a newborn dog (Golgi stain). Note the illustration of Marginal (O, Z), Limiting (A, F) and Central (S, T, H) cells of the superficial dorsal horn.

horn (Christensen and Perl, 1970). These observations and the numerous electrophysiological studies on the properties of superficial and deep dorsal horn neurones have fuelled a controversy on the roles in pain perception of the two main types of nociceptive dorsal horn neurone: specific and convergent. The reader will be able to appreciate the intensity of the arguments in some of the following chapters.

A very recent development in the history of the superficial dorsal horn has been the discovery of numerous neuropeptides in the fibres and nerve cells of this region of the cord. The functional significance of most of these compounds is far from clear, but this is a very active area of research and several of the contributions to this symposium deal with the presence, biochemistry and putative functions of many of these biologically active peptides.

CURRENT OPINIONS

It is hard to summarise in a few paragraphs the considerable amount of information about the superficial dorsal horn that has emerged from recent studies; much of this information is, indeed, reviewed in detail in the following chapters. At the risk of gross oversimplification, it is, nevertheless, possible to highlight a few main conclusions which represent points of general agreement on the anatomical and functional organization of the superficial dorsal horn.

1. The superficial dorsal horn (laminae I and II) is the main region of termination of small myelinated and unmyelinated afferent fibres from skin, muscle and viscera. However, lamina II does not receive a major projection of fine afferent fibres from muscle and viscera whereas many of these fibres and some small myelinated afferents from skin nociceptors project directly to the deep dorsal horn (mainly lamina V). Because of the nociceptive nature of many of the fine afferent fibres that terminate in

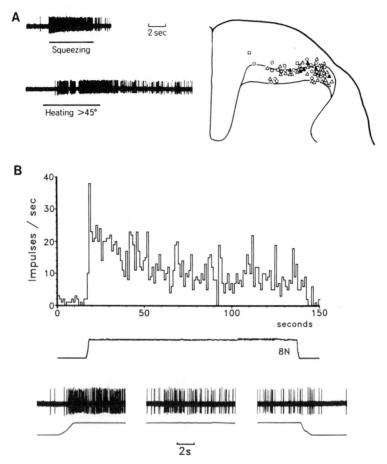

FIGURE 3: Nocireceptive neurones of the superficial dorsal horn. A: Neurones recorded in cat's lumbar cord. Note the absence of background activity and the strong responses to noxious stimuli applied to the cutaneous receptive field. The recording sites of 61 such cells are also illustrated. Closed symbols indicate intracellular recordings. Circles: neurones with only an Aδ input; Triangles: neurones with Aδ and C fibre inputs; Squares: fibre input not established. Data from Cervero *et al* (1979). B: Neurone recorded in the sacral spinal cord of the rat. The histogram shows the response of the cell to a 2 minute noxious pinch of the tail of 8N intensity. Selected portions of the original record are also shown. Data from Laird and Cervero (unpublished).

the superficial dorsal horn it is believed that this region of the spinal grey matter is concerned with the relay and modulation of pain-related signals.

2. There are essentially two main categories of nociceptive dorsal horn neurone: those with an exclusive input from skin nociceptors (Nocireceptive, Class 3 or Nociceptor-specific) and those with convergent inputs from peripheral nociceptors and sensitive mechanoreceptors (Multireceptive, Class 2 or Wide-dynamic-range). Both categories of cell are represented in the superficial dorsal horn with a concentration of Nocireceptive cells in the Marginal Zone or lamina I. Both categories of cell include interneurones and projection neurones, the latter being able to transmit their specific or convergent information to supraspinal centres via a number of ascending pathways.

3. The synaptic terminals of the fine primary afferents that project to the superficial dorsal horn, and many of the neurones of this region, contain a variety of putative

neurotransmitter compounds including several neuropeptides. These substances are produced, released and taken up as a result of functional activity in the primary afferents that terminate in the superficial dorsal horn. However, their specific functional roles are not fully understood.

4. Most superficial and deep dorsal horn neurones are under some form of descending control from supraspinal centres. This control can take the form of excitation as well as inhibition of transmission through the spinal relay. It is assumed that this descending control represents some form of central modulation of the sensory message as it is first processed in the spinal cord.

5. The input properties of certain classes of superficial and deep dorsal horn neurones can be altered by repetitive noxious stimulation of the periphery or by injury or lesion of peripheral nerves and of central pathways. Thus, the responses of some dorsal horn neurones and the sensory consequences of their activation can vary depending on the past experience of the subject and on the presence of a lesion in the sensory pathway.

THE SUPERFICIAL DORSAL HORN AND PAIN

As it has been pointed out in previous paragraphs, the superficial dorsal horn is regarded as an important area of relay and modulation of nociceptive signals. The existence of two classes of nociceptive neurone in the dorsal horn - Nocireceptive and Multireceptive - and the concentration of Nocireceptive cells in the most dorsal layer of the superficial dorsal horn have produced substantial differences of opinion as to the roles of the two classes of cells in nociception and pain.

Nocireceptive cells were first described by Christensen and Perl (1970) and have been the object of numerous further investigations (for reviews see Cervero and Iggo, 1980 and, in this volume, Hylden et al, Kniffki, McMahon and Wall, Dubner et al). They constitute a well defined population of neurons located mainly in lamina I, having small cutaneous receptive fields, little or no spontaneous activity, an input from Aδ and C afferent fibres and being exclusively activated by noxious stimulation of the skin (see examples in Fig. 3). Nocireceptive cells include some with axons projecting to supraspinal regions. In addition some of them can also be driven by non-cutaneous inputs such as those originating in muscle or viscera (Cervero 1983, Craig and Kniffki, 1985).

Nocireceptive cells are concentrated in lamina I which also contains Multireceptive neurones. Cervero and Tattersall (1987) have recently shown that when consideration is given to additional inputs from viscera some important properties of lamina I neurones appear. Thus, most lamina I neurones with an exclusive somatic input were found to be Nocireceptive whereas lamina I neurones responding to both somatic and visceral inputs included many Multireceptive cells. In another study Cervero and Lumb (1988) have also shown that lamina I neurones with a restricted ipsilateral visceral input are all Nocireceptive whereas those with bilateral visceral inputs are largely Multireceptive cells. These results suggest that the more restricted the input to lamina I cells - somatic only rather than viscero-somatic, ipsilateral visceral rather than bilateral visceral - the higher the chances of the cell being Nocireceptive. On the other hand the greater the convergence of inputs from different peripheral sources the higher the chances of the cell being Multireceptive. These observations show further differences between Nocireceptive and Multireceptive cells in the superficial dorsal horn and highlight the Nocireceptive system of neurones as a distinct group of cells with restricted inputs and little afferent convergence.

There is, of course, the possibility that Nocireceptive cells normally have low threshold inputs that are weakened or inhibited by the other inputs to the cell or by the anaesthetics given to the experimental animal. This is the thinking behind interpretations of dorsal horn function contrary to any idea of a modality labelled line of sensory transmission in the dorsal horn (see for instance McMahon and Wall, this volume). However, there is enough experimental evidence to support the view that Nocireceptive cells constitute a separate category of dorsal horn neurons whose peripheral inputs are dominated in the normal animal by inputs from nociceptors. Nocireceptive cells have been recorded in the superficial dorsal horn of several species of higher mammals and at all spinal cord levels. They have been described in animals under a variety of anaesthetic regimes as well as in decerebrate and spinal animals. They show a number of fundamental differences from Multireceptive cells in receptive field size, level of spontaneous activity and fibre input threshold and latency.

In a recent examination of the responses of dorsal horn neurones to prolonged noxious mechanical stimuli (Cervero et al, 1988) it was found that Nocireceptive cells were better suited to encode these stimuli than were Multireceptive cells. This conclusion was reached by analysing the phasic and tonic components of the responses of dorsal horn neurones of both kinds to a noxious pinch stimulus applied to the receptive fields of the cells for 2 minutes (see Fig. 3B). Little evidence of encoding was found in the phasic component of the responses; however, the stimulus response curves for the tonic components showed that the slopes of Nocireceptive cells were considerably steeper than those of Multireceptive neurones (Cervero et al, 1988). Moreover, the cutaneous receptive fields of Nocireceptive cells are more stable than those of Multireceptive neurons and are less likely to be influenced by a previous noxious stimulus (Laird and Cervero, this volume). Although we have observed small increases in the receptive fields of Nocireceptive cells after a noxious pinch, these could easily be explained by changes in the responses of the peripheral receptor rather than by central alterations of responsiveness. These observations have led us to the suggestion that Nocireceptive cells are a more hard-wired system of sensory neurones than are Multireceptive cells.

The existence of two nociceptor-driven systems of cells in the dorsal horn - a convergent and plastic system of Multireceptive cells and a specific and relatively hard-wired system of Nocireceptive cells - does not necessarily give immediate clues as to the role of these two systems in pain and nociception. Hylden et al and Dubner et al (this volume) argue that Multireceptive cells are concerned with the sensory-discriminative aspects of pain whereas Nocireceptive neurones are part of the pathway that deals with the autonomic and emotional reactions evoked by injury. Because of their ability to relay nociceptive signals in a consistent and stable way, it could also be argued that Nocireceptive neurones carry the sensory signal and Multireceptive neurones play a part in its modulation and discrimination. These questions cannot be definitively answered on the basis of current experimental evidence. To a large extent the opinions on this matter are heavily tinted with individual views about the neurophysiological mechanisms of pain. However, the existence of the two separate populations of nociceptive dorsal horn neurone must be taken into account by all pain models.

Recent reports have shown that the input properties and receptive fields of Nocireceptive cells of the superficial dorsal horn can change after damage to peripheral nerves or after cutaneous inflammation (see Hylden et al and Dubner et al, this volume). These are interesting results, for they clearly show a reactive capacity of the Nocireceptive system to nerve damage or to persistent noxious stimuli applied to its peripheral receptive field. Such properties can also help to explain the mechanisms of the abnormal sensations that sometimes follow either damage to nerve pathways or persistent noxious states. However, these abnormal sensations are not part of the normal set of responses of the Nocireceptive system to acute injury, nor of the reactions of its cells to brief noxious events.

It is extremely important to separate what is part of the physiological repertoire of responses of dorsal horn cells from what is the consequence of continuing damage to the periphery or of lesion of the nerve pathways that mediate nociceptive transmission. The responses of a cell to a brief noxious stimulus express the capacity of the nociceptive system to signal the onset of a pain-evoking event. Changes induced by noxious states are due to a continuous noxious input or to a lesion somewhere along the nerve pathway. It is indeed possible that a hard-wired system involved in the signalling of noxious events could become hyperexcitable as a reaction to a noxious state and thus lead to pathological sensations including persistent, abnormal or intractable pains.

NON-CUTANEOUS INPUTS TO THE SUBSTANTIA GELATINOSA

Over the last few years a number of anatomical studies using transport of horseradish peroxidase (HRP) along a variety of visceral and muscle nerves have shown that afferent fibres from non-cutaneous structures do not terminate in significant numbers in lamina II (the Substantia Gelatinosa) of the dorsal horn, for reviews see deGroat (1986) and Mense (1986). The more recent results of Sugiura (this volume), based on injections of individual visceral afferents with tracer substances show that lamina II receives not more than 10% of the total number of terminals generated by visceral afferent fibres in the dorsal horn. In addition, electrophysiological recordings in the dorsal horn have failed to detect significant numbers of neurones in lamina II driven by visceral afferents (Cervero and Tattersall, 1987).

Since the majority of muscle and visceral afferent fibres are small myelinated or unmyelinated, these findings have called into question traditional interpretations of the Substantia Gelatinosa as the region of termination of all unmyelinated afferent fibres. Moreover, these results have also raised the question of whether or not lamina II neurons are only concerned with the processing of sensory information from the skin.

It is now very clear that unmyelinated afferent fibres from deep and visceral organs terminate outside lamina II, particularly in laminae I and V (see Sharkey et al, this volume). It is also well established that lamina II receives little input from non-cutaneous structures and that the balance of its inputs is definitely tilted towards a substantial cutaneous projection of fine afferent fibres. These observations suggest that the Substantia Gelatinosa is mainly (or exclusively) concerned with the processing of sensory information from the skin. Also, they indicate that the spinal processing of nociceptive inputs from muscle and viscera differs substantially from the processing of nociceptive signals of cutaneous origin.

FUTURE TRENDS

Much progress has been made in the understanding of the functions of the superficial dorsal horn but much more remains to be done. A good deal of the scientific interest in this region of the spinal cord stems from its relation to pain processing and it is obvious that a detailed knowledge of dorsal horn function will provide new leads for the treatment of certain pain conditions. However, we should not lose sight of the fact that other sensory modalities are also well represented in the superficial dorsal horn and that a nociceptive input to the spinal cord could be involved in functions other than the appreciation of pain.

Many of the recent results from superficial dorsal horn studies point to the inadequacies of our current techniques. For instance, the observation that brief periods of noxious stimulation can alter the responses of some spinal neurones argues against the use of extensive surgery in acute preparations. Moreover, acute electrophysiological experiments require the use of anaesthetics or decerebration, procedures that are known to alter the responsiveness of spinal neurones to their peripheral inputs.

Some of these problems can be bypassed by the use of awake animal models (e.g. Collins, this volume). This is a relatively new field in dorsal horn studies and more of this kind of work is therefore expected in the future. An alternative approach is to conduct minimally invasive experiments in humans where the subjects can report their sensory experiences in parallel with the recording of neural activity. Microneurography of peripheral nerves has already helped to settle many questions about the specificity of cutaneous receptors and the elementary sensations evoked by the stimulation of single afferent fibres. Studies of the response properties of thalamic neurones to peripheral stimuli in patients undergoing neurosurgery have also been reported (Lenz et al, 1987). More of these kinds of studies could perhaps help us to understand better the spinal processing of afferent information.

An interesting development that has taken place over the last few years has been the introduction of many new neurochemical techniques for the labelling and identification of neuronal elements and of their chemical contents. Some of the more recent developments permit the identification of neurones and pathways activated by specific stimuli and of the sites of release of biologically active neuropeptides. In combination with traditional physiological techniques, or applied to some of the recent models of neuropathic pain, they may prove a valuable new tool for the analysis of the spinal afferent relay.

Most of the new techniques currently used in studies of the superficial dorsal horn are represented in the following chapters and are described in some detail by the scientists that have developed them. It is hoped that the review of the advances made in this field over the last decade, and the description of the new directions of study, will help and stimulate further research in this important area.

REFERENCES

CERVERO, F. (1983). Somatic and visceral inputs to the thoracic spinal cord of the cat: effects of noxious stimulation of the biliary system. *Journal of Physiology* **337**, 51-67.

CERVERO, F., HANDWERKER, H.O. AND LAIRD, J.M.A. (1988). Prolonged noxious stimulation of the rat's tail: responses and encoding properties of dorsal horn neurones. *Journal of Physiology* **404**, 419-436.

CERVERO, F. AND IGGO, A. (1980). The substantia gelatinosa of the spinal cord. A critical review. *Brain* **103**, 717-772.

CERVERO, F., IGGO, A. AND MOLONY, V. (1979). Ascending projections of nociceptor-driven lamina I neurones in the cat. *Experimental Brain Research* **35**, 135-149

CERVERO, F. AND LUMB, B.M. (1988). Bilateral inputs and supraspinal control of viscero-somatic neurones in the lower thoracic spinal cord of the cat. *Journal of Physiology* **403**, 221-237.

CERVERO, F. AND TATTERSALL, J.E.H. (1986). Somatic and visceral sensory integration in the thoracic spinal cord. In **Visceral Sensation**; *Progress in Brain*

Research vol. **67**, eds. F. Cervero and J.F.B. Morrison, pp 189-205. Amsterdam: Elsevier.

CERVERO, F. AND TATTERSALL, J.E.H. (1987). Somatic and visceral inputs to the thoracic spinal cord of the cat: marginal zone (lamina I) of the dorsal horn. *Journal of Physiology* **388**, 383-395.

CHRISTENSEN, B.N. AND PERL, E.R. (1970). Spinal neurones specifically excited by noxious or thermal stimuli: marginal zone of the dorsal horn. *Journal of Neurophysiology* **33**, 293-307.

CLARKE, J.L. (1859). Further researches on the grey substance of the spinal cord. *Philosophical Transactions of the Royal Society. Series B*, **149**, 437-468.

CRAIG, A.D. AND KNIFFKI, K-D. (1985). Spinothalamic lumbosacral lamina I cells responsive to skin and muscle stimulation in the cat. *Journal of Physiology* **365**, 197-221.

DE GROAT, W.C. (1986). Spinal cord projections and neuropeptides in visceral afferent neurones. In **Visceral Sensation**; *Progress in Brain Research* vol. **67**, eds. F. Cervero and J.F.B. Morrison, pp 165-187. Amsterdam: Elsevier.

LENZ, F.A., TASKER, R.R., DOSTROVSKY, J.P., KWAN, H.C., GORECKI, J., HIRAYAMA, T. AND MURPHY, J.T. (1987). Abnormal single unit activity recorded in the somatosensory thalamus of a quadriplegic patient with central pain. *Pain* **31**, 225-236.

MELZACK, R. AND WALL, P.D. (1965). Pain mechanisms: a new theory. *Science* **150**, 971-979.

MENSE, S. (1986). Slowly conducting afferent fibres from deep tissues: neurobiological properties and central nervous actions. *Progress in Sensory Physiology* **6**, 139-219.

RAMÓN Y CAJAL, S. (1890). Nuevas observaciones sobre la estructura de la médula espinal de los mamíferos. *Laboratorio Anatomico de la Facultad de Medicina.* Barcelona: Casa Provincial de Caridad.

RANSON, S.W. (1914). An experimental study of Lissauer's tract and the dorsal roots. *Journal of Comparative Neurology* **24**, 531-545.

RANSON, S.W. AND VON HESS, C.L. (1915). The conduction within the spinal cord of the afferent impulses producing pain and the vasomotor reflexes. *American Journal of Physiology* **38**, 128-152.

REXED, B. (1952). The cytoarchitectonic organization of the spinal cord in the cat. *Journal of Comparative Neurology* **96**, 415-495.

SECTION I

AFFERENT INPUTS TO THE SUPERFICIAL
DORSAL HORN

INTRODUCTION TO SECTION I

The Editors

   It has been known for almost a century that fine afferent fibres from the skin, muscle and viscera terminate in the superficial dorsal horn of the spinal cord. The close relationship between these afferent fibres and the transmission of nociceptive information gave support to the notion that the superficial dorsal horn plays an important role in the initial modulation and integration of pain-related signals. Recent anatomical and functional studies have, indeed, confirmed that many fine afferent fibres terminate in the superficial layers of the dorsal horn but have also increased our knowledge about the detailed mode of termination of individual afferent fibres and of groups of fibres from skin, muscle and viscera. The papers presented in this section discuss these recent studies and attempt to answer three basic questions: i) do all fine afferent fibres terminate in the superficial dorsal horn? ii) do fine afferent fibres from skin, muscle and viscera show different patterns of termination in the spinal cord? and iii) what are the structure and ultrastructure of the terminals of individual fine afferent fibres in the superficial dorsal horn?

DISTRIBUTION OF UNMYELINATED PRIMARY AFFERENT FIBERS IN THE DORSAL HORN

Y. Sugiura*, N. Terui, Y. Hosoya and K. Kohno

Institute of Basic Medical Sciences, University of Tsukuba, Tsukuba, Ibaraki 305, Japan

Primary afferent neurons with fibers in peripheral nerve encode sensory information from many tissues and organs. They represent the first step in processing information about peripheral events. Peripheral afferent fibers can be divided into two major groups on the basis of size and structure, myelinated or unmyelinated. These two categories account for the principal conduction velocity subsets, A (myelinated) and C (unmyelinated) of both somatic and visceral afferent fibers.

During the past decade, direct evidence on the central projections of myelinated primary afferent fibers has been obtained by the use of neuronal tracing techniques based upon axoplasmic transport of marker substances, e.g. horseradish peroxidase (HRP), wheatgerm-agglutinin conjugated HRP and fluorescent dyes. Intracellular deposition of markers has permitted demonstration of the terminal patterns of single fibers (Snow et al, 1976; Light and Perl, 1979, Brown 1981a; for reviews see Fitzgerald, 1984; Fyffe, 1984). The central terminations of a primary afferent neuron closely relates to its functional properties (Light and Perl, 1979; Brown 1981a; Sugiura et al, 1986). This kind of evidence on the terminations of myelinated afferent fibers with known physiological characteristics has partially clarified the functional organization of the lamination of the dorsal horn as described by Rexed (1952). In particular, the terminations of myelinated (A) and unmyelinated (C) afferent fibers from skin exhibit different arrangements in the superficial dorsal horn (Réthelyi 1977; Gobel et al, 1981; Sugiura et al, 1986). So far only certain kinds of myelinated fibers from skin or muscle have been found to project to lamina I (marginal zone) and to parts of lamina II (substantia gelatinosa), and they lack the dense concentration of terminations in that lamina noted for C-fiber units of the skin (Sugiura et al, 1986). In contrast, visceral afferent fibers of all diameters studied by HRP application to abdominal organs are reported to end in laminae I, IV and V with little or no projection to lamina II (DeGroat 1978; Morgan et al, 1981; Nadelhaft et al, 1983; Cervero and Connell, 1984a, b; Nadelhaft and Booth, 1984; Morgan et al, 1986; Nunez 1986). It should be noted that up to now there has been no information about the central projections of individual visceral afferent fibers.

* Present address: Department of Anatomy, Fukushima Medical College, 1-Hikarigaoka, Fukushima City, Fukushima 960-12, Japan

TERMINATIONS OF MYELINATED PRIMARY AFFERENT COLLATERALS

Central projections of myelinated fibers have been comprehensively reviewed elsewhere (Brown, 1981 a,b; Fyffe, 1984). The following briefly summarizes this literature. Large diameter afferent fibers from muscle (Ia and Ib) terminate in laminae IV, V, VI and in the interneuron and motoneuron pools of laminae VII and IX (Brown and Fyffe, 1977, 1979, Ishizuka *et al*, 1979). Afferent fibers associated with skin but not with muscle, e.g. from hair follicle, RA and SA of glabrous skin and D-hair receptors project to laminae III and IV with some endings in inner II (IIi) (Brown, 1981 a,b; Light and Perl, 1979). The central termination of cutaneous high threshold mechanoreceptors, that is mechanical nociceptors, however, is unlike that of other myelinated cutaneous or muscle sensory units. High threshold mechanoreceptors with thin myelinated fibers terminate in laminae I, outer II (IIo) as well as having scattered endings dorsal to the central canal and, on occasion, collaterals crossing to contralateral lamina V (Light and Perl, 1979). In summary, many myelinated fibers end in the N. proprius, i.e. laminae III-IV and others terminate in the marginal layer of the dorsal horn and in the intermediate part of the spinal cord. Thus, myelinated fibers terminate in most regions of the dorsal horn but do not form a concentrated pattern of projection in lamina II (substantia gelatinosa). These observations represent the basis for proposing an organization of myelinated afferent fibers in respect to their region of termination which is related to fiber diameters and the types of sensory units with which they are associated (Fyffe, 1984).

TECHNICAL CONSIDERATIONS

Labelling and identifying central terminals from unmyelinated primary afferent fibers has difficulties not encountered with the myelinated fiber population. Several procedures can be used to mark a population of primary afferent fibers of a given segment or a fascicle of dorsal root fibers, including unmyelinated elements, using techniques based upon degeneration or the transport of foreign substances such as HRP and HRP-lectin combinations (Sprague and Ha, 1964; Brown, 1981 a,b; Light and Perl, 1979; Abrahams *et al*, 1984; Arvidsson and Thomander, 1984). Approaches for tracing the central projections of primary afferent fibers using marker substances depend upon anterograde transport and require application of the indicator molecule close to the termination zone in the spinal cord. Intracellular application of HRP in single primary afferent fibers whose receptive characteristics had been determined by electrophysiological recording is a powerful variation of this technique. However, this latter approach has been successful only for myelinated fibers (Snow *et al*, 1976; Light and Perl, 1979). The major difficulty with its use for unmyelinated fibers is their small cross-sectional diameter which makes stable intracellular recording essentially impossible even with the finest of pipette microelectrodes. Attempts to overcome this problem by electrophysiologically recording in the dorsal root ganglia and application of HRP intracellularly at this location have been largely unsuccessful because the peroxidase reaction product became undetectable at points of bifurcation of these thin fibers or when the fibers decreased in diameter as they approached terminal zones (Sugiura *et al*, 1985).

Neuronal labelling techniques based upon HRP take advantage of a relatively rapid axoplasmic transport system that in primary afferent fibers carries the molecules at rates of 1mm per hour or faster. Our approach to projection of the unmyelinated fibers evolved from the use of another marker molecule, a plant lectin. The lectin derived from phaseolus vulgaris, which aggutinates white blood cells, has been proposed as a means of studying the configuration and connections of central nervous system neurons (Gerfen and Sawachenko, 1984; Sawachenko and Gerfen, 1985; Ter Horst *et al*, 1985). As in the case of HRP, phaseolus vulgaris leuko-agglutinin (PhA-L) can be delivered iontophoretically. The PHA-L marker can be detected at very low concentrations by immunocytochemistry utilizing antibodies directed against it. The antibody, in turn, is indicated by a sequence of procedures utilizing avidin-biotin and peroxidase-antiperoxidase (Hsu *et al*, 1981 a,b). The PHA-L molecule is carried by a relatively slow transport system (1-2 mm per day); however, it is transported to the very finest terminals of neurons including those of unmyelinated primary afferent fibers without the blockage at junctions or apparent loss of detectability noted for HRP. Thus, labelling dorsal root ganglion cells established to have unmyelinated primary afferent fibers by electrophysiological recording proved practical (although difficult). This approach was used to successfully stain and describe the central terminations of several different kinds of cutaneous primary afferent units with C-afferent fibers (Sugiura *et al*, 1986). The following reviews these earlier results and presents new data on differences in the termination patterns between C-afferent fibers originating from somatic structure and those whose receptive terminals are in the viscera.

CENTRAL TERMINATION OF CUTANEOUS C-FIBER SENSORY UNITS

At least six functionally different kinds of primary afferent units with unmyelinated (C) fibers from the skin of mammalian species have been identified. These include three kinds of nociceptors (polymodal, high threshold mechanical and mechanical-cold), two thermoreceptors (cooling and warming) and a low threshold mechanoreceptor (Bessou and Perl, 1969; Kumazawa and Perl, 1977; Shea and Perl 1985). The central projections of three kinds of nociceptors and of low threshold mechanoreceptors with C-afferent fibers were determined using the PHA-L marker in the second cervical (C-2) and/or the sixth lumbar spinal segment (L-6) of the guinea pig (Sugiura *et al*, 1986). The three types of nociceptors did not differ in any obvious way from those reported for the rabbit ear (Shea and Perl, 1985). They responded selectively, the mechanical nociceptors only to intense, usually tissue-damaging, mechanical stimuli and two types only to thermal stimuli. They did not exhibit ongoing activity at room temperature. The noxious stimuli used for evaluation of receptive characteristics consisted of radiant heat sufficient to damage the skin, contact or evaporative cooling sufficient to cause temperatures to drop below 20° C and pinch with tissue forceps.

Low threshold mechanoreceptors also exhibited the characteristics described in other species in being very vigorously excited by gentle brushing or sudden cooling of the skin with no greater response evoked by noxious mechanical stimulation (Bessou and Perl, 1969). Table I gives the results of the analyses of the central terminal domains for seven cutaneous C-fiber units and Fig. 1 shows schematically their terminal arborization. Comments on the individual types follow.

One high threshold mechanoreceptor was studied at the C-2 level. Its receptive field was on the ear. The axon of this dorsal root neuron was found to run in Lissauer's tract for a short distance rostrally from the point of entry into the spinal cord and then it passed through lamina I to lamina II. Second or third order branches diverged from the root fiber and ran caudally. Terminal branches, enlargements of these branches and boutons were located in the lateral part of the substantia gelatinosa in the deep part of lamina IIo and the adjacent part of lamina IIi (Fig. 1A). The terminal domain extended 280 μm in the rostral-caudal direction and 100 μm dorsal-ventrally.

TABLE I

Sensory modality of receptive field	Segmental level (ganglion)	Conduction velocity (m/sec)	Terminal Area			
			Rostro-caudal (μm)	Dorso-ventral (μm)	Medio-lateral (μm)	Laminae
High-threshold mechanoreceptor	C2	0.5	280	100	150	IIo part of IIi
Polymodal nociceptor	C2	0.5	300	50	200	IIi
	L6	0.5	600	150	200	I,IIo III,IV
Mechanical cold nociceptor	C2	0.5	400	300	150	I part of IIo
Low-threshold mechanoreceptor	C2	0.5	380	50	120	IIo part of IIi
	C2	0.6	300	50	100	IIi,IIo

A summary of the locations and dimensions for terminal regions of identified C-afferent fibers from the skin. Neurons stained in the C-2 ganglion were processed immunohistologically after two days of survival. Cells stained in L-6 ganglion were processed histologically after 5-6 days of survival. The indicated extension of each of the terminal areas represents the dense area of terminal enlargements. These were measured from histological sections with an ocular micrometer or calculated by a digital computer-based three-dimensional graphics program. The overall extent of the central branches of a given fiber were greater than those listed for the major terminal domains. The laminae of termination were based upon a classification following Rexed (1952). (Data from Sugiura et al., 1986).

Two C-fiber polymodal nociceptors (CPM) were analyzed. One from the C-2 ganglion had a fiber that ran caudally in Lissauer's tract for almost 2000 μm and terminated in the lateral part of lamina II. Lamina II curves at this point, and is distorted relative to lamination more caudally because of the trigeminal nucleus caudalis. The terminal region was clearly within lamina II. Secondary branches from the main fiber passed for another several hundred μm before forming a concentrated distinctly circumscribed terminal plexus (Fig. 1). The terminal plexus extended some 300 μm rostrocaudally and 150 μm in the medial-lateral direction. A polymodal nociceptor of the sixth lumbar ganglion had some different termination features. At the junction of the dorsal root with the spinal cord, the fiber bifurcated into a rostral and a caudal branch. These ascended and descended from this point sending collaterals at approximately 200-400 μm intervals. A large terminal plexus with closely packed end branch enlargement and boutons was located in lamina I and IIo at the level of the dorsal root entrance. The ascending and descending branches of this fiber ran close to the surface of the dorsal funiculus laterally and then sent branches back to join the main terminal plexus in the very large terminal array. The only collateral not joining this array passed into deeper layers (lamina III-IV). This was the sole deep collateral observed from any of the cutaneous unmyelinated fibers. Reconstruction of this CPM of the lumbar cord indicated that the terminal fiber and branches totalled over 40,000 μm on which 2,805 distinct enlargements were counted.

Two mechanical-cold nociceptors were analyzed. One, from the C-2 ganglion had a fiber that ran caudally in Lissauer's tract for almost one full segment. Secondary branches left the stem fiber with further branching to form a compact terminal plexus in lamina I and IIo at the lateral margin of the superficial dorsal horn. The terminal region of this fiber extended some 400 μm rostrocaudally and 150 μm in the medial-lateral direction. The total length of the fiber and all of its branches was 16,300 μm. As in the case of the CPM, the mechanical-cold nociceptor of the 6th lumbar ganglion had a stem that divided into branches running rostrally and caudally. This mechanical-cold nociceptor also formed a dense terminal arborization with many terminal swellings at the segmental level of the fiber's entry into the spinal cord. The major terminal branches came together to form the dense plexus extending 450 μm in the rostral caudal direction and 150 μm in the medial-lateral dimension in lamina I and IIo.

In the guinea pig among cells excited by electrical stimulation of the auricular nerve, low threshold mechanoreceptors or C-mechanoreceptors appeared relatively commonly in recordings from the C-2 ganglion; however, they were very rare in L-6 ganglion. Detailed labelling of two such units at the C-2 level were successful. Both elements showed a similar geometry in their termination pattern. Such C-mechanoreceptor units had a fiber that passed caudally in Lissauer's tract after joining the spinal cord. The stem fiber sent collaterals following the curve of the lateral surface of lamina II. At the

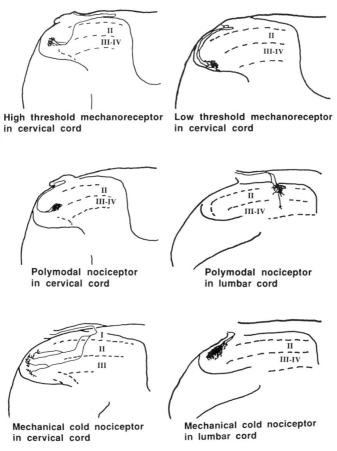

High threshold mechanoreceptor in cervical cord

Low threshold mechanoreceptor in cervical cord

Polymodal nociceptor in cervical cord

Polymodal nociceptor in lumbar cord

Mechanical cold nociceptor in cervical cord

Mechanical cold nociceptor in lumbar cord

FIGURE 1: Schematic diagrams illustrating the locations of arborizations of physiologically-identified unmyelinated afferent fibers from the skin. The transverse plane drawings were reconstructed from distributions observed in parasaggital histological sections of the cervical or the lumbar spinal cord. Functional properties of each type of sensory unit were based upon criteria given in Shea and Perl (1985). See text for additional details. (Data from Sugiura *et al*, 1986.)

transition of lamina IIi and IIo a terminal plexus was formed that took the form of a slender rod. The total fiber length and branch length stained in the example shown in Fig. 1 was 13,200 μm. The swellings and boutons of the fibers from C-mechanoreceptors were unusually large and in the example shown in Fig. 1 a total of 1,149 were counted.

SINGLE UNMYELINATED FIBER DISTRIBUTIONS AT THORACIC LEVEL

The following are new data from C-cells of the 13th thoracic dorsal root ganglion (DRG) obtained using similar procedures as in the study of cutaneous afferent fibers (Sugiura et al, 1986). Primary afferent fibers with a somatic distribution were identified by electrical stimulation of the subcostal nerve distributed to muscle and skin. Unfortunately under the circumstances of these experiments, it was not possible to utilize natural stimulation of tissue to identify further the characteristics of the receptive units. Visceral afferent fibers of the same segment were identified by electrical stimulation of the coeliac ganglion and its associated nerves. The onset latency of neuronal action potentials recorded from the 13th thoracic dorsal root ganglion separated into several distinct groups to electrical stimulation of these somatic and visceral afferent nerves. One group responded with a latency of less than 2 msec. Given the conduction distances of 7 to 13 mm, this short latency group was judged to be DRG neurons with myelinated fibers. (It should be noted that conduction velocities in the guinea pigs used (150-250 grams) were considerably slower than those observed in larger mammalian species.) A second set of responses appeared at latencies of 12-35 msec. These were presumed to be conducting at C (unmyelinated) conduction velocities. Responses over 20 msec typically came from the visceral nerve stimulation where the conduction distances were uncertain because of the network formed by the sympathetic fibers and nerves contributing to the paravertebral plexi.

The somatic C-afferent fibers labelled in the 13th thoracic DRG typically had major ascending and descending branches that passed either along the dorsal surface of the dorsal funiculus and/or through Lissauer's tract. Such splitting of a primary fiber upon entry into the spinal cord into a rostrally and caudally directed branch, therefore, appears to be typical for the lumbosacral spinal cord for both myelinated and unmyelinated elements (Réthelyi, 1977; Light and Perl, 1979; Sugiura et al, 1986). Each C-fiber stem had several collateral branches that in turn had multiple branches and terminal enlargements concentrated in a circumscribed, distinctive distribution within lamina II. As was noted for the functionally-identified cutaneous C-afferent fibers, several collateral branches of a parent often came together to form the concentrated terminal plexus. The terminal regions typically extended approximately 400 μm in the rostral-caudal direction and 100 μm or less in the medial-lateral direction. It is noteworthy that in these experiments four out of eight examples of well-stained somatic C-afferent fibers from the T-13 DRG had a branch passing through Lissauer's tract while the other fibers passed in the rostral-caudal direction on the surface of the dorsal funiculus or within the dorsal horn itself. From this it is obvious that not all unmyelinated fibers pass through Lissauer's tract as has been implied by some classical anatomists (Earle, 1952; Szentagothai, 1964). This would be in keeping with modern concepts suggesting that Lissauer's tract represents a mixture of primary afferent fibers and fibers of intraspinal origin (Light and Perl, 1979).

CENTRAL TERMINALS OF VISCERAL C-AFFERENT FIBERS

Units whose latency of action potential from stimulation at the ceoliac ganglion exceeded 15 msec were classified as having C-fibers. The central distribution of the visceral C-afferent fibers at the T-13 level differed distinctively from the C-fiber somatic units excited by the subcostal nerve of the same segment. Typically, the visceral C-units had terminal enlargements at many sites along their rostral-caudal extension. A single C-visceral fiber typically bifurcated into ascending and descending branches. Each of these branches then travelled to some 2-3 thoracic segments superficially in the dorsal funiculus. Each major branch had several collaterals that then terminated in lamina I and lamina II along this considerable rostral-caudal extension. These collaterals appeared periodically at intervals ranging from 2-300 to 1000 μm. The result was that each of the visceral afferent fibers had terminals in the superficial dorsal horn from the 10th thoracic to the 2nd lumbar segments. There were also terminals in lamina V and lamina X. The terminal branches showed *en passant* and large bouton endings but at each terminal region only one or two terminal branches were present. The concentrated, distinct terminal plexus seen for the somatic C-fibers was never found for any of the visceral C-afferent fibers.

Termination in lamina II showed enlargements of an unusual shape with a single string of separated enlargements extending over 1000 μm in the rostrocaudal direction within lamina II. The diagram in Fig. 2 schematically shows the termination of a typical T-13 visceral C-unit. Some terminal branches were found in the white matter of the dorsal and lateral funiculi. A few branches of the visceral afferent units penetrated medially to reach lamina X (the dorsal, commissural nucleus) and then crossed over to lamina V on the contralateral side. In the sense of reaching the midline region above the central canal and then passing contra-laterally to lamina V, these visceral afferent units mimicked the behavior of the cutaneous myelinated high-threshold mechanoreceptors described by Light and Perl (1979). The terminal enlargements in the lateral funiculus, the lateral part of lamina V and in lamina X clearly had a spatial relationship to locations of dendrites and somata of preganglionic sympathetic neurons.

SOMA SIZE OF SOMATIC AND VISCERAL C-AFFERENT NEURONS

While the total number of C-fiber units recorded at the T-13 level was relatively small, a distinct difference in the cell body size of the two populations was noted. Somatic C-afferent units in the T-13 ganglion in our sample averaged 22.5 μm in diameter, a size that appears similar to that described for the rat and found in other experiments in the guinea pig (Harper and Lawson, 1985; Sugiura *et al*, 1988). On the other hand, the C-fiber units of visceral distribution averaged an almost 50% greater diameter, 32.5 μm. Perhaps this difference in size is correlated with the far more extensive central distributions at the same segmental level shown by the visceral afferent units compared with the somatic units.

COMMENTS AND SUMMARY

Combining the previous observations on cutaneous primary afferent units with C-fibers (Sugiura *et al*, 1986) with our present data on somatic and visceral afferent fibers leads us to the following general conclusions. Somatic C-afferent fibers terminate largely in the superficial dorsal horn, particularly in lamina II (the substantia gelatinosa). The area of termination of somatic C-afferent fibers typically is a highly concentrated region of terminal enlargements and boutons which is well circumscribed. The terminal region typically extends approximately 4-500 μm in the rostro-caudal direction and less than 200 μm in the medio-lateral dimension. There is a clear relationship between the central projection zone of somatic C-afferent units and the

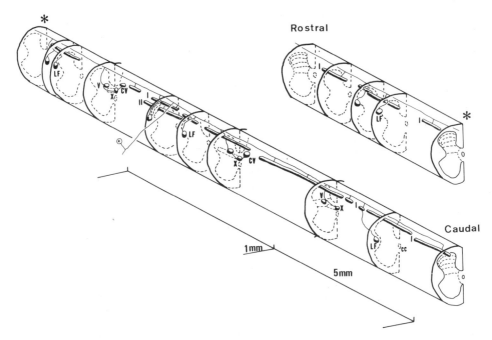

FIGURE 2: A schematic three-dimensional drawing of the central collateral distribution from a single unmyelinated visceral afferent fiber from the T-13 dorsal root ganglion of guinea pig. The visceral afferent unit in the T-13 ganglion was identified as having a C-fiber by the 75 msec latency of its response to electrical stimulation of the ceoliac ganglion. Terminals in lamina I were distributed over the entire extension of the primary afferent fiber. Terminals in lamina II extended over 1mm in the rostrocaudal dimension. The circular areas marked as I,II,V,X indicate the location of terminals in laminae of the same designation. The asterisk indicates the point at which the spinal cord drawing was interrupted. CV and CX indicate lamina V and X contra-laterally. LF - lateral funiculus; CC - central canal.

type of sensory unit. Nociceptors tend to terminate most superficially, in lamina I and lamina IIo, while the low-threshold mechanoreceptors have their circumscribed terminal plexus more deeply in lamina IIi. In contrast, visceral C-afferent fibers have a distributed sparse set of enlargements and terminal boutons in lamina I, lamina II and bilaterally in laminae V and X.

These conclusions show some distinct differences in the terminal regions for myelinated and unmyelinated afferent fibers. Myelinated afferent fibers of all functional types have relatively few terminals in lamina II, the substantia gelatinosa. The exceptions are the thinly myelinated fibers from nociceptors that invade the interface between lamina I and lamina IIo and also the thinly myelinated low-threshold mechanoreceptors (D-hair) that have terminals at the interface between lamina III and lamina IIi. Visceral afferent fibers on the other hand, appear to avoid laminae III and IV, the nucleus proprius. (Light and Perl, 1979; Brown, 1981b; Abrahams *et al*, 1984; Cervero and Connell, 1984; Craig and Mense, 1983; Craig and Kniffki, 1985; Mense and Probhakar, 1986; Molander and Grant, 1987). The information currently missing on these distinctions is that on the central projections of myelinated afferent fibers from visceral regions.

In spite of the evidence that there is some segregation in the primary afferent distributions of somatic and visceral afferent units, we have in fact added to the data showing that there is a substantial convergence of projection to given laminae from somatic and visceral tissues. Thus, somatic and visceral afferent fibers related to several kinds of functionally definable receptive elements distribute terminals to laminae I, II and V. Furthermore, at least some fibers of somatic origin and also visceral afferent fibers terminate in lamina X and in lamina V bilaterally. These converging patterns offer multiple opportunities for integration of visceral and somatic sensory inputs, a point made by a number of previous commentators (Pomeranz et al, 1968; Selzer and Spencer, 1969; Fields et al, 1970; Cervero, 1983; Cervero and Tattersall, 1984; Ness and Gebhart, 1987). Furthermore, the extensive longitudinal distribution of the visceral C-afferent fibers in the superficial dorsal horn, over 5 lumbar-thoracic segments, also offers the opportunity for extensive interplay between visceral and somatic afferent inputs. One is tempted to think in terms of nociceptive and pain mechanisms for certain of these interactions since a substantial proportion of the identified somatic terminal distributions in the superficial dorsal horn are from nocireceptive types of primary afferent units. The poorly localized nature of visceral sensation and of referred pain from the viscera fits with the anatomical multi-segmental distribution of visceral input (Seltzer and Spencer, 1969a). Our observations on single C-afferent units of visceral origin agree with the results of labelling of entire visceral nerves or organs that also suggested extensive rostro-caudal distribution (Kuo et al, 1983; Sharkey et al, 1983; Ciriello and Calaresu, 1984). As was suggested by Seltzer and Spencer some years ago (1969b), visceral and afferent distribution over a number of segments could play an important part in facilitating action by somatic afferent input.

The significance of the observed projection to common regions by visceral and somatic afferent nerves will depend upon the nature of the afferent information coming in from each source as well as the mechanisms that may be put into play by such inputs. At least one view suggests that visceral afferent neurons are a homogeneous group or at least have a continuum of receptive characteristics with no specific or distinctive separation of the selectivity of one element from that of another (Jänig and Morrison, 1986); however, there is strong evidence suggesting a substantial selectivity in the activation of certain visceral afferent units (e.g., Bessou and Perl, 1966; Beacham and Kunze, 1969, Moss, 1987). An obvious next step for such considerations would be to combine analyses of the behavior of functionally-studied units from visceral regions with their particular central distribution patterns.

ACKNOWLEDGEMENTS

We wish to thank Dr E.R. Perl for his critical and helpful suggestions and Mrs. Junko Sakamoto for technical assistance. We are also grateful to Ms Sherry Derr and Ms Nancy Freeman for preparing the manuscript. This study was supported by grants from the Ministry of Education, Science and Culture of Japan, Japan Society of The Promotion of Science and The Ichiro Kanehara Foundation.

REFERENCES

ABRAHAMS, V.C., RICHMOND, F.J., AND KEANE, J. (1984). Projections from C2 and C3 nerves supplying muscles and skin of the cat neck: A study using transganglionic transport of horseradish peroxidase. *Journal of Comparative Neurology* 230, 142-154.

ARVIDSSON, J. AND THOMANDER, L. (1984). An HRP study of the central course of sensory intermediate and vagal fibers in peripheral facial nerve branches in the cat. *Journal of Comparative Neurology* 223, 35-45.

BEACHAM, W.S. AND KUNZE, D.L. (1969). Renal receptors evoking a spinal vasometer reflex. *Journal of Physiology* **201**, 73-85.

BESSOU, P. AND PERL, E.R. (1966). A movement receptor of the small intestine. *Journal of Physiology* **182**, 404-426.

BESSOU, P. AND PERL, E.R. (1969). Response of cutaneous sensory units with unmyelinated fibers to noxious stimuli. *Journal of Neurophysiology* **32**, 1025-1043.

BROWN, A.G. (1981a). The terminations of cutaneous nerve fibers in the spinal cord. *Trends in Neuroscience* **4**, 64-67.

BROWN, A.G. (1981b). *Organization in the spinal cord.* Springer-Verlag. New York.

BROWN, A.G. AND FYFFE, R.E.W. (1977). The morphology of group Ia afferent fibre collaterals in the spinal cord of the cat. *Journal of Physiology* **274**, 111-127.

BROWN, A.G. AND FYFFE, R.E.W. (1979). The morphology of group Ib afferent fibre collaterals in the spinal cord of the cat. *Journal of Physiology* **296**, 215-228.

CERVERO, F. (1983). Somatic and visceral inputs to the thoracic spinal cord of the cat: effects of noxious stimulation of the biliary system. *Journal of Physiology* **337**, 51-67.

CERVERO, F. AND CONNELL, L.A. (1984a). Fine afferent fibers from viscera do not terminate in the substantia gelatinosa of the thoracic spinal cord. *Brain Research* **294**, 370-374.

CERVERO, F. AND CONNELL, L.A. (1984b). Distribution of somatic and visceral primary afferent fibres within the thoracic spinal cord of the cat. *Journal of Comparative Neurology* **230**, 88-98.

CERVERO, F. AND TATTERSALL, J.E.H. (1987). Somatic and visceral inputs to the thoracic spinal cord of the cat: Marginal zone (lamina I) of the dorsal horn. *Journal of Physiology* **383**, 383-395.

CIRIELLO, J. AND CALARESU, F.R. (1983). Central projections of afferent renal fibers in the rat: An anterograde transport study of horseradish peroxidase. *Journal of the Autonomic Nervous System* **8**, 273-285.

CRAIG, A.D. AND KNIFFKI, K.D. (1985). Spinothalamic lumbosacral lamina I cells responsive to skin and muscle stimulation in the cat. *Journal of Physiology* **365**, 197-221.

CRAIG, A.D. AND MENSE, S. (1983). The distribution of afferent fibers from the gastrocnemius-soleus in the dorsal horn of the cat, as revealed by the transport of horseradish peroxidase. *Neuroscience Letters* **41**, 233-238.

DEGROAT, W.C., NADELHAFT, I., MORGAN, C. AND SCHAUBLE, T. (1978). Horseradish peroxidase tracing of visceral efferent and primary afferent pathways in the cats sacral spinal cord using benzidine processing. *Neuroscience Letters* **10**, 103-108.

EARLE, K.M. (1952). The tract of Lissauer and its possible relation to the pain pathway. *Journal of Comparative Neurology* **96**, 93-111.

FIELDS, H.L., MEYER, G.A. AND PARTRIDGE, Jr., L.D. (1970). Convergence of visceral and somatic input onto spinal neurons. *Experimental Neurology* **26**, 36-52.

FITZGERALD, M. (1984). The course and termination of primary afferent fibres. In *Textbook of Pain*, eds. Wall, P.D. and Melzack, R., Churchill, Livingstone.

FYFFE, R.E.W. (1984). Afferent fibres. In *Handbook of the Spinal Cord.* Vol. **2** and **3.**, ed. Davidoff, R.A. pp. 79-136. New York: Marcel Dekker.

GERFEN, C.R. AND SAWACHENKO, P.E. (1984). An anterograde neuroanatomical tracing method that shows the detailed morphology of neurons, their axons and terminals: Immunohistochemical localization of an axonally transported plant lectin, phaseolus vulgaris leucoagglutinin (PHA-L). *Brain Research* **290**, 219-238.

GOBEL, S., FALL, W.M. AND HUMPHREY, E. (1981). Morphology and synaptic connections of ultrafine primary axons in lamina I of the spinal dorsal horn: Candidates for the terminal axonal arbors of primary neurons with unmyelinated (C) axon. *Journal of Neuroscience* **1**, 1163-1179.

HARPER, A.A. AND LAWSON, S.N. (1985). Conduction velocity is related to morphological cell type in rat dorsal root ganglion neurones. *Journal of Physiology* **359**, 31-46.

HSU, S.-H., RAINE, L. AND FANGER, H. (1981a). The use of avidin-bioitinperoxidase complex (ABC) in immunoperoxidase techniques: A comparison between ABC and unlabelled antibody (PAP) procedures. *Journal of Histochemistry and Cytochemistry* **29**, 577-580.

HSU, S.-H., RAINE, L. AND FANGER, H. (1981b). A comparative study of the peroxidase-antiperoxidase method and an avidine-biotin complex method for studying polypeptide hormones with radioimmunoassay antibodies. *American Journal of Clinical Pathology* **75**, 734-738.

ISHIZUKA, N., MANNEN, H., HONGO, T. AND SASAKI, S. (1979). Trajectory of group Ia afferent fibers stained with horseradish peroxidase in the lumbosacral spinal cord of the cat: Three dimensional reconstructions from serial sections. *Journal of Comparative Neurology* **186**, 189-212.

JANIG, W. AND MORRISON, J.F.B. (1986). Functional properties of spinal visceral afferent supplying abdominal and pelvic organs, with special emphasis on visceral nociception. *Progress in Brain Research* 67, 87-114 eds. Cervero, F. and Morrison, J.F.B. Elsevier, Amsterdam.

KUMAZAWA, T. AND PERL, E.R. (1977). Primate cutaneous sensory units with unmyelinated (C) afferent fibers. *Journal of Neurophysiology* **40**, 1325-1338

KUO, D.C., NADELHAFT, I., HISAMITSU, T. AND DEGROAT, W.C. (1983). Segmental distribution and central projections of renal afferent fibers in the cat studied by transganglionic transport of horseradish peroxidase. *Journal of Comparative Neurology*, **216**, 162-174.

LIGHT, A.R. AND PERL, E.R. (1979). Spinal termination of functionally identified primary afferent neurons with slowly conducting myelinated fibers. *Journal of Comparative Neurology* **186**, 133-150.

MENSE, S. AND PROBHAKAR, N.R. (1986). Spinal termination of nociceptive afferent fibers from deep tissues in the cat. *Neuroscience Letters* **66**, 169-174.

MOLANDER, C. AND GRANT, G. (1987). Spinal cord projections form hindlimb muscle nerves in the rat studied by transganglionic transport of horseradish peroxidase, wheat germ agglutinin conjugated horseradish peroxidase, or horseradish peroxidase with dimethylsulfoxide. *Journal of Comparative Neurology* **260**, 246-255.

MORGAN, C., DEGROAT, W.C. AND NADELHAFT, I. (1986). The spinal distribution of sympathetic preganglionic and visceral primary afferent neurons that send axons into the hypogastric nerves of the cat. *Journal of Comparative Neurology* **243**, 23-40.

MORGAN, C., NADELHAFT, I. AND DEGROAT, W.C. (1981). The distribution of visceral primary afferents from the pelvic nerve to Lissauer's tract and the spinal gray matter and its relationship to the sacral parasympathetic nucleus. *Journal of Comparative Neurology* **201**, 415-440.

MOSS, N.G. (1987). Electrophysiological characteristics of sensory mechanisms in the kidney. In *Clinical and Experimental Hypertension* Part A: Theory and Practice, ed. Slater, I.H., pp. 1-13. New York: Marcel Dekker, Inc.

NADELHAFT, I. AND BOOTH, A.M. (1984). The location and morphology of preganglionic neurons and the distribution of visceral afferents from the rat pelvic nerve: A horseradish peroxidase study. *Journal of Comparative Neurology* **226**, 238-245.

NADELHAFT, I., ROPPOLO, J., MORGAN, C. AND DEGROAT, W.C. (1983). Parasympathetic preganglionic neurons and visceral primary afferents in monkey sacral spinal cord revealed following application of horseradish peroxidase to pelvic nerve. *Journal of Comparative Neurology* **216**, 36-52.

NESS, T.J. AND GEBHART, G.H. (1987). Characterization of neuronal responses to noxious visceral and somatic stimuli in the medial lumbosacral spinal cord of rat. *Journal of Neurophysiology* **57**, 1867-1892.

NUNEZ, R., GROSS, G.H. AND SACHS, B.D. (1986). Origin and central projections of rat dorsal penile nerve: Possible direct projection to autonomic and somatic neurons by primary afferents of nonmuscle origin. *Journal of Comparative Neurology* **247**, 417-429.

POMERANZ, B., WALL, P.D. AND WEBER, W.V. (1968). Cord cells responding to fine myelinated afferents from viscera, muscle and skin. *Journal of Physiology* **199**, 511-532.

RÉTHELYI, M. (1977). Preterminal and terminal axon arborizations in the substantia gelatinosa of cat's spinal cord. *Journal of Comparative Neurology* **172**, 511-527.

REXED, B. (1952). The cytoarchitectonic organization of the spinal cord in the cat. *Journal of Comparative Neurology* **96**, 415-495.

PIERAU, F.-K., FELLMER, G. AND TAYLOR, D.C.M. (1984). Somato-visceral convergence in cat dorsal root ganglion neurones demonstrated by double-labelling with fluorescent tracers. *Brain Research* **321**, 63-70.

SAWACHENKO, P.E. AND GERFEN, C.R. (1985). Plant lectins and bacterial toxins as tools for tracing neuronal connections. *Trends in Neuroscience* **8**, 378384.

SELZER, M. AND SPENCER, W.A. (1969a). Convergence of visceral and cutaneous afferent pathways in the lumbar spinal cord. *Brain Research* **14**, 331-348.

SELZER, M. AND SPENCER, W.A. (1969b). Interactions between visceral and cutaneous afferent in the spinal cord: Reciprocal primary afferent fiber depolarization. *Brain Research* **14**, 349-366.

SHARKEY, K.A., WILLIAMS, P.G., SHULTZBERG, M. AND DOCKRAY, G.J. (1983). Sensory substance P-innervation of the urinary bladder: Possible site of action of capsaicin in causing urine retention in rats. *Neuroscience* **10**, 861-868.

SHEA, V.K. AND PERL, E.R. (1985). Sensory receptors with unmyelinated (C) fibers innervating the skin of the rabbit's ear. *Journal of Neurophysiology* **54**, 491-501.

SNOW, P.J., ROSE, P.K. AND BROWN, A.G. (1976). Tracing axon and axon collaterals of spinal neurons using intracellular injection of horseradish peroxidase. *Science* **191**, 312-313.

SPRAGUE, J.M. AND HA, H. (1964). The terminal fields of dorsal root fibers in the lumbosacral spinal cord of the cat, and the dendritic organization of the motor nuclei. In *Organization of the Spinal Cord*, eds. Eccles, J.C. and Schade, J.P., pp. 120-154. Amsterdam: Elsevier.

SUGIURA, Y., HOSOYO, Y., ITO, R. AND KOHNO, K. (1988). Ultrastructural features of functionally identified primary afferent neurons with C (unmyelinated) fibers of the guinea pig. Classification of dorsal root ganglion cell type with reference to sensory modality. *Journal of Comparative Neurology*, (in press).

SUGIURA, Y., LEE, C.L. AND PERL, E.R. (1986). Central projections of identified, unmyelinated (C) afferent fibers innervating mammalian skin. *Science* **234**, 358-361.

SUGIURA, Y., SCHRANK, E. AND PERL, E.R. (1985). Central terminal distribution of unmyelinated afferent fibers. *Society of Neuroscience Abstract* **11**, 118.

SZENTAGOTHAI, J. (1964). Neuronal and synaptic arrangement in the substantia gelatinosa Rolandi. *Journal of Comparative Neurology* **122**, 219-239.

TER HORST, G.J., GROENWEGEN, H.J., KARUST, H. AND LUITEN, P.G.M. (1985). Phaseolus vulgaris leukoagglutinin immunocytochemistry. A comparison between autoradiographic and lectin tracing neuronal efferents. *Brain Research* **307**, 379-383.

SPINAL PROJECTIONS OF THIN MYELINATED DEEP AFFERENTS AND THEIR TOPICAL RELATION TO DORSAL HORN NEURONES PROCESSING DEEP INPUT

U. Hoheisel and S. Mense*

Anatomisches Institut III, Im Neuenheimer Feld 307,D-6900 Heidelberg, FRG

INTRODUCTION

Afferent input from the skin, from deep tissues (e.g. muscle, fascia, joint) and from viscera elicits distinct sensations which differ subjectively in that cutaneous sensations are usually better localizable and - in the case of pain - better tolerable than are sensations of deep or visceral origin. This raises the question as to whether these differences are due to the fact that the afferent information is transmitted via different neuronal systems or is processed differently by the same neuronal population. For addressing this question, both morphological and neurophysiological techniques have been used, but most of the available data concern the organization of afferent neurones possessing receptive fields (RFs) in the skin (Brown, 1981). The present report deals with primary and second order afferent neurones that supply deep tissues and aims at describing the main features of these cells in comparison to cutaneous and visceral neurones.

MATERIALS AND METHODS

The results were obtained from chloralose-anaesthetized adult cats. For studying the spinal terminals of identified primary afferent fibres, single axons supplying the deep tissues of the hindlimb were impaled with glass microelectrodes at the dorsal root entry zone and their electrical activity recorded. Only myelinated units having a maximal conduction velocity of 40 m/s were included in the sample, i.e. fast conducting fibres from muscle spindles and tendon organs were discarded. With the use of graded mechanical stimuli (local pressure, joint movement) the receptive endings in muscles and other deep structures of the hindlimb were characterized as low-threshold mechanosensitive (LTM) if they responded to weak, innocuous pressure, high-threshold mechanosensitive (HTM) if they required noxious stimuli for activation, and muscle spindle secondary if they were activated in the typical manner by muscle stretch. All stimuli were applied by hand using forceps with broadened tips. The intensity of a stimulus was considered to be noxious if it elicited deep pain in humans and aversive reactions in awake animals. In cases where the deep tissues had not been surgically

---

* Author for correspondence

exposed, the deep location of the receptive field was taken for granted if strong stimulation of the overlying skin was ineffective. After physiological identification horseradish peroxidase (HRP) was injected ionophoretically into the axon and was visualized later using diaminobenzidine as a chromogen (cf. Light and Perl, 1979).

Second order (dorsal horn) neurones were examined with the same technique either intracellularly in order to obtain both physiological and morphological data or extracellularly in functional studies. In the latter case the recording site was marked with HRP. In some experiments the spinal cord rostral to the recording level (S1 - L5) was blocked with a cooling thermode (0° C)in contact with the dorsal columns.

RESULTS AND CONCLUSIONS

Spinal trajectory of thin myelinated afferent fibres from deep tissues of the hind-limb

The afferent units were of three functional types: HTM, LTM and muscle spindle secondary endings. The pattern of spinal termination was so typical for the different types that in most cases the function of a given unit could be inferred from its histological appearance (course of collaterals, location of terminal arborizations).

HTM units. Half of the fibres with HTM properties terminated exclusively in lamina I. The parent fibers ascended in Lissauer's tract or the lateral dorsal columns and issued collaterals that entered lamina I laterally. The collaterals were oriented in the medio-lateral direction and often extended over great portions of the lamina (Fig. 1). The other half of the HTM units terminated in both lamina I and deeper laminae of the dorsal horn, namely laminae IV-VI (Fig. 2). At least two of the latter HTM units could be identified as having their origin in the gastrocnemius-soleus (GS) muscle (Fig. 2 D, E); in other cases a muscle origin was probable but could not be proven, since the deep tissues had not been surgically exposed (e.g. Fig. 2 C). These results demonstrate that there is a projection of muscle afferent fibres (of the HTM type) to lamina I.

The data support previous results obtained in experiments employing whole nerve staining techniques: application of HRP to the GS muscle nerves in cats resulted in distinct labelling in lamina I (in addition to other projection areas) the labelling often extending around the lateral edge of the dorsal horn (Craig and Mense, 1983; Mense and Craig; 1988). The present data show that at least some of these fibres have HTM properties. The question as to whether muscle afferent fibres terminate in lamina I has been addressed by several groups of workers, with varying results. In the cat, some fore-limb muscles have been reported to project to this layer (Abrahams and Swett, 1986) while others do not (Nyberg and Blomqvist, 1984). Neck muscles appear to have only faint projections, if any, to the superficial dorsal horn (Abrahams et al, 1984; Bakker et al, 1984).

In the rat, the results are even more controversial. In an early investigation Brushart and Mesulam (1980) reported that afferent fibres from hind-limb muscles terminate in lamina II, but these results have to be questioned, since the HRP had been injected intramuscularly. The same is true for a study by Kalia et al (1981) who reported a diffuse projection of muscle afferent units to laminae I-V. The method of intramuscular injection of HRP is likely to result in leakage of the tracer out of the muscle and consequently to artifactual labelling (cf. Craig and Mense, 1983). Other authors have emphasized that rat hind-limb muscles (particularly the GS) do not project to the superficial dorsal horn (Molander and Grant, 1987). In the rat - as in the cat - there is some evidence that the spinal pattern of termination might differ between individual muscles. Thus, at the cervical level, some neck muscles of the rat have been reported to

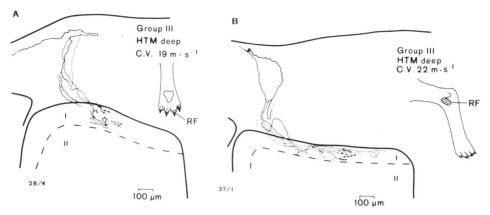

FIGURE 1: Spinal terminal arborizations of deep HTM units projecting exclusively to lamina I. In A and B, the afferent fibre enters the spinal cord via the dorsal root to the left, approaches the dorsal horn laterally and issues collaterals which terminate with boutons in lamina I. The receptive fields (RFs) were located in the deep tissues of the third toe (A) and of the lateral aspect of the ankle joint (B), respectively. The conduction velocity (C.V.) of the afferent fibres was in the upper group III range. The figures are reconstructions from serial sections. Thick lines mark the dorsal border of the spinal cord and of the dorsal horn. The approximate border between laminae I and II is indicated by the dashed line.

project to the superficial dorsal horn whereas others do not (Mysicka and Zenker, 1981; Ammann *et al*, 1983). At the time being it is hard to decide whether there are real differences between rat and cat and between individual muscles, or whether differences in the techniques employed are responsible for the conflicting results.

LTM units. The LTM units differed from the HTM ones in that they did not terminate in lamina I. The main projection areas were laminae IV-VI with some additional collaterals terminating in lamina II. In general, the LTM units were more heterogeneous in appearance than the other types, i.e. the differences in the pattern of termination were greater.

Fibres from muscle spindle secondary endings. These units exhibited a termination pattern identical to that described for spindle secondaries of faster conduction velocity (about 50-60 m/s; cf. Fyffe, 1979). The fibres had no terminal arborizations in laminae dorsal to lamina IV, the main projection areas being laminae VI/VII and the ventral horn.

Thus, the main histological difference between the three functional types concerned the laminae in which they terminated, whereas the appearance of the collaterals and boutons was very similar.

A consistent finding in all these experiments was that lamina III was free of terminals. The only exception to this rule was a HTM unit that possessed a few large boutons in lamina III (Fig. 2 E). Thus it appears that lamina III is not an important relay for primary afferent information from deep tissues. Of course it is theoretically possible that non-myelinated muscle afferent fibres, which have not yet been stained as single units, terminate in lamina III. However, the available evidence from experiments employing whole nerve staining techniques speaks against a strong projection of these fibres to lamina III in the cat (Craig and Mense, 1983; Abrahams and Swett, 1986). Since visceral afferent fibres likewise do not project to this layer (Morgan *et al*, 1981; Cervero and Connell, 1984), lamina III can be considered to be a dorsal horn region which is reserved for the processing of primary afferent information from the skin.

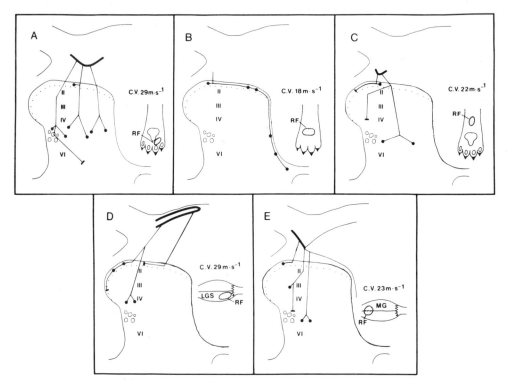

FIGURE 2: Schematic reconstructions of HTM units terminating in both lamina I and deeper layers of the dorsal horn. The parent fibre is marked by a thick line, the collaterals by thin lines. Terminal arborizations with boutons are indicated by filled circles, fibres terminating without visible boutons by a short bar. The size and location of the receptive fields in the deep tissues of the left hind-limb is given by the hatched areas in the inserts. The border between laminae I and II is indicated by a dotted line, the reticulated lateral portion of lamina V by open circles. MG, medial gastrocnemius muscle; LGS, lateral gastrocnemius-soleus muscle.

In the arrangement of the spinal terminations no clear somatotopy could be detected. This is particularly true for the endings in lamina I which did not show a systematic shift when the location of the RF changed. However, the units projecting to the deep dorsal horn tended to terminate laterally in laminae IV/V if the RF was located in the GS muscle, i.e. rather proximal and post-axial in the hind-limb.

A comparison with afferent units from the deep tissues of the cat tail (Mense *et al*, 1981) shows that the results obtained from the lumbo-sacral level cannot be transferred to all segmental levels. The caudal deep afferent units differed from the lumbo-sacral ones by showing frequent contralateral projections - which were totally missing in the lumbo-sacral fibres - and by having additional terminations in lamina X. In comparison with thin myelinated afferent fibres from the cat caudal skin (Light and Perl, 1979), the deep afferent units from the same region looked similar if they were HTM, but differed by not projecting to lamina III if they had LTM properties.

Properties of dorsal horn cells processing deep input

Physiology. Only neurones that received input from deep tissues and that were not dominated by muscle spindles or tendon organs were selected for this study. Most of the neurones (about 70%) had RFs in both skin and deep tissues (convergent neurones), while the rest responded only to stimulation of deep tissues. In both input categories, cells with LTM and HTM properties were found (cf. Fig. 3 A). Neurones having HTM RFs in both skin and deep tissues might be responsible for the cutaneous hyperalgesia that often accompanies deep pain (Hockaday and Whitty, 1967). In the present study, cooling of the spinal cord rostral to the recording site was found to increase the chance of finding cells with deep input. Therefore, some of the experiments were carried out in cats with a cold block of the spinal cord. Even so, only a few cells responded to stimulation of deep tissues while the great majority had either a pure cutaneous input or no detectable RFs. As can be seen from Fig. 3 B, the cold block did not change the proportions of neurones with convergent or deep input. Among the cells with deep input only, there was a trend to have lower mechanical thresholds under this condition, but the main effect of the cold block was an increase in cells having double RFs in either skin or deep tissues. Surprisingly, the overall proportion of LTM RFs was not increased but was decreased by the cold block. Thus it is possible that under the influence of the cold block new HTM RFs appeared, particularly in the convergent cells.

In contrast to the cells of the present study, some of which had a purely deep input, all dorsal horn neurones with input from the thoracic viscera have been described to be convergent (viscerosomatic), i.e. there were no cells having a purely visceral input (Cervero and Tattersall, 1985; Foreman *et al*, 1981). At the sacral level, however, a few cells in lamina X have been reported to have an exclusively visceral input (Honda, 1985). Some of the viscerosomatic cells could be driven from RFs in deep tissues. Therefore, an unknown proportion of these cells in the present study that were classified as having deep input only, might possess additional visceral input. On the other hand, other authors studying dorsal horn cells with muscle input have found (a

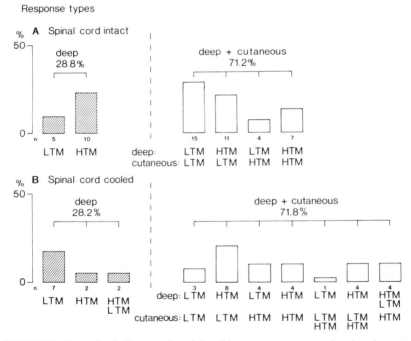

FIGURE 3: Receptive field properties of dorsal horn neurones processing deep input. A, data from anaesthetized animals with intact spinal cord. Hatched columns, neurones having exclusively deep input; stippled columns, cells having convergent input from both deep tissues and skin. B, data from animals with a cold block of the spinal cord. The number of cells making up each column is given by n.

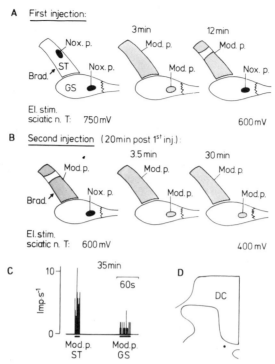

FIGURE 4: Changes in the response properties of a dorsal horn neurone following injection of bradykinin into one of its receptive fields (RFs). A, left panel: situation before injection of bradykinin. The neurone had two RFs, one in the semitendinosus (ST), the other one in the gastrocnemius-soleus (GS) muscle. Both had high mechanical thresholds and required noxious pressure (Nox. p.) for activation. Middle panel: 3 min after infiltration of the ST muscle with bradykinin. The RF is greatly enlarged and now has a low mechanical threshold. The RF in the GS muscle likewise shows a decrease in mechanical threshold; in the ST muscle an insensitive strip has appeared. B, left panel: 20 min after injection of bradykinin; time of second injection of the algesic agent in to the ST muscle. After the second chemical stimulation the mechanical threshold of the RF in the GS muscle was lowered for more than 30 min. The electrical threshold of the neurone dropped from 750 mV at the beginning of A to 400 mV at the end of B. C, neuronal responses to stimulation of the RFs with Mod. p. 35 min after the second injection of bradykinin. The Mod. p. stimulus was totally ineffective before injection of bradykinin. D, location of recording site. RFs marked in black have a high, shaded RFs a low mechanical threshold.

few) neurones that responded exclusively to stimulation of deep tissues (Craig and Kniffki, 1985). Dorsal horn cells processing input from articular nerves appear to be of the convergent type (with additional input from the skin, cf. Schaible *et al*, 1986), so that a pure input from deep tissues or viscera may be the exception rather than the rule.

When comparing descriptions of dorsal horn neurones of different laboratories it has to be kept in mind that the response properties of the cells are not constant but can be modulated by descending influences and by primary afferent input. Therefore, the classification of dorsal horn neurones into different response types also depends on the history of the neurones. Previous noxious stimulations and of course surgical operations may alter the response properties for prolonged periods. Slowly conducting afferent fibres from skeletal muscle have been found to be particularly effective in this respect (Wall and Woolf, 1984). In our experiments an injection of a painful dose of bradykinin into a muscle RF of a neurone that had two HTM RFs was followed by a decrease in mechanical stimulation threshold of both the injected RF and the other (remote) RF, the effect lasting for about one hour (Fig. 4). Extensive operations at the beginning of an experiment and repeated noxious stimulations during the experiment are likely to produce a higher proportion of convergent cells and of cells responding to weak stimuli (Hoheisel and Mense, 1988). The "real" threshold and degree of convergence are therefore difficult to determine in an animal experiment.

Morphology. The available data on the morphology of dorsal horn neurones processing input from the skin indicates that there is no close correlation between morphological and functional properties (Light *et al,* 1979; Bennett *et al,* 1980; Brown and Fyffe, 1981; Woolf and King, 1987). The same is true for the neurones with deep RFs studied in the authors' laboratory. Among these cells all known morphological types were found to be present: Waldeyer cells in lamina I, islet cells and stalked (limit-roph) cells in lamina II, and mostly multipolar cells in deeper laminae. Thus, cells being driven from deep tissues appear to belong to the same gross histological types as neurones having cutaneous input.

The only morphological difference between cells having deep and those having cutaneous input seems to be that the former have either no or only a few dendritic spines (Hoheisel and Mense, unpublished). However, this comparison is based on indirect evidence derived from the literature and cannot be quantified. In our study, two neurones with purely cutaneous input were stained for reasons of comparison; both of them had large numbers of dendritic spines.

Morphological differences between neurones with LTM and HTM properties could not be detected. The cell shown in Fig. 5 was driven by HTM receptors in the deep tissues of the sole of the left hind-paw; it had the appearance of a Waldeyer cell. Another neurone in lamina I had similar morphological features but totally different

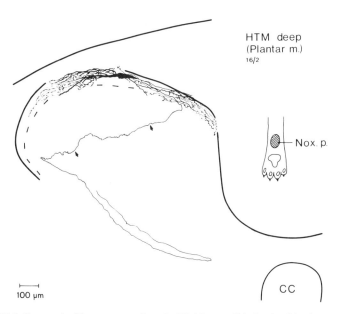

FIGURE 5: Camera lucida reconstruction of a Waldeyer cell in lamina I having exclusively deep input with a high mechanical threshold. The axon (arrows) ascended in the grey matter of the deep dorsal horn.

response properties in that it responded to light touch applied to the fascia of the GS muscle. This was a consistent finding: cells of the same morphological type could have different physiological properties and, conversely, cells with identical response properties could exhibit different morphology. Of course it can be argued that such a result was to be expected, since all cells with deep input had been accepted for study, irrespective of their being interneurones or projecting neurones. As it is well known that cells of a given ascending tract may show great differences in response properties, it might be more appropriate to look for correlations between function and morphology among cells belonging to the same tract, thus eliminating gross differences in basic morphology. In some neurones of our sample the axon was stained for a sufficiently long distance to allow a statement to be made concerning the tract the cell projected into. Two neurones with somata in laminae III/IV had axons that issued a network of collaterals with many boutons ventral to the soma. The axon could be followed for several mm in the dorsal columns; it moved away from the dorsal horn on its way rostrally. These cells probably belonged to the postsynaptic dorsal column (PSDC) system. Although their morphology was similar, their functional properties differed clearly. One neurone had a pure deep LTM input, whereas the other one had two RFs, one with HTM properties in the deep tissues and another (LTM) in the skin. At the time being it appears to be impossible to infer the function of a dorsal horn neurone from its morphology.

Topical relationship between primary afferent fibres and dorsal horn cells processing information from deep tissues

Lamina I. The well developed and medio-laterally oriented collaterals of nociceptive afferent fibres in lamina I (cf. Fig. 1) are suitable for making monosynaptic contacts with second order neurones in this layer (cf. Fig. 5). Results of other groups have shown that many neurones in lamina I of the cat project to the thalamus (Craig and Burton, 1981). This could mean that at the spinal level a direct connection with higher centres exists for deep pain. On the other hand, the deep LTM input to other cells in lamina I cannot be monosynaptic, since no LTM fibres from deep tissues terminated in lamina I.

Lamina II. The only input from deep primary afferent fibres to lamina II was derived from LTM units. Their terminals could make monosynaptic connections with LTM cells in this lamina. Again, the deep input to HTM neurones in lamina II has to be polysynaptic, since no HTM primary afferent units terminated in this lamina. The contribution of non-myelinated deep afferent fibres as an input source to the superficial dorsal horn (cf. Sugiura *et al*, 1986) is hard to assess, since the great majority of the neurones having deep input did not respond to electrical activation of group IV fibres.

Lamina III. This layer was virtually free of deep afferent terminals. Therefore, any input from deep tissues to neurones in this lamina has to be polysynaptic.

Laminae IV/V. These laminae contained numerous terminal fields of both LTM and HTM primary afferent fibres. Surprisingly, the number of second order cells encountered in these laminae was small. In fact, if the locations of the stained neurones with deep input are plotted on a scheme of the dorsal horn, a gap appears in laminae IV/V (Fig. 6). The reasons for the lack of cells driven by deep input in these layers are obscure. Possibly, the primary afferent terminals located in this area elicit subthreshold effects only, form inhibitory synapses, or are postsynaptic to dendrites or axons (Maxwell and Rethelyi, 1987). (Postsynaptic potentials were not evaluated in this study, since the aim was to quickly characterize the cells with suprathreshold stimuli and then

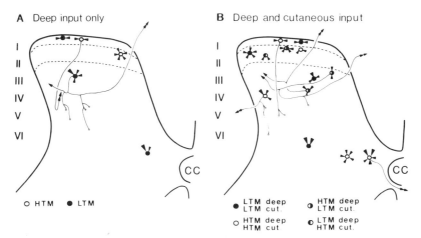

A Deep input only

B Deep and cutaneous input

○ HTM ● LTM

● LTM deep / LTM cut.
○ HTM deep / HTM cut.
◑ HTM deep / LTM cut.
◐ LTM deep / HTM cut.

FIGURE 6: Locations of intracellularly stained dorsal horn cells plotted on a schematic cross section of the dorsal horn. A, neurones having input from deep tissues only. B, convergent neurones with input from both skin and deep tissues. The soma is marked by an open or closed circle according to the code at the bottom of the figure. The main orientation of the dendrites is indicated by the arrowheads surrounding the soma. Thin lines represent axons, open circles areas of local terminal fields with boutons. Single arrowheads indicate caudally directed axonal projections, double ones rostral projections.

to inject HRP). Another possibility would be that the terminal arborizations do not form synapses but release a modulator substance into the interstitial space (cf. Honda *et al*, 1983; Hunt and Rossi, 1985). Such a mechanism could explain the changes in response behaviour of dorsal horn cells described above (cf. Fig. 4). The two cells encountered in laminae IV/V were recorded in cats in which the spinal cord was blocked with cold. In animals with an intact spinal cord not a single neurone with deep input was found in these layers. This finding confirms the results of an early investigation by Pomeranz *et al* (1968) who were unable to activate cells in lamina V with electrical stimulation of muscle nerves. Thus, laminae IV/V receive a strong primary afferent projection from deep tissues, but there is little change in discharge frequency of second order cells in response to this input. Interestingly, many viscero-somatic cells have been reported to be located in lamina V (Cervero and Tattersall, 1985), so that the neck of the dorsal horn may constitute an integrative centre for visceral and cutaneous information.

Laminae VI/VII. Both LTM and HTM afferent fibres projected to these laminae. Second order neurones in laminae VI/VII likewise had LTM or HTM properties. The cells usually possessed long dorsal dendrites, which could also pick up activity from terminals in laminae V. This arrangement again offers the possibility of monosynaptic connections between deep primary afferent fibres and dorsal horn neurones (e.g. those belonging to the ventral spinocerebellar tract).

Ventral horn. Some collaterals of afferent fibres from muscle spindle secondary endings reached the lateral ventral horn (lamina IX) and thus supported the data of other authors showing that muscle spindle secondary endings can be monosynaptically connected to motoneurones (Kirkwood and Sears, 1974). Apparently, this statement is also true for secondary endings with a slow conduction velocity in the group III range.

Generally speaking, the input from deep tissues to dorsal horn neurones appears to be much less effective than input from the skin. Consequently, during the experiments many neurones driven by cutaneous receptors had to be discarded before a neurone responding to deep input was encountered. This may be one of the reasons for the scarcity of reports dealing with neurones having deep input. Descending inhibitory influences appear to be of great importance, since a cold block of the spinal cord largely increased the efficacy of the deep input. The topical arrangement of deep primary afferent fibres and dorsal horn neurones is far from being understood. Particular hard to answer is the question as to why laminae IV/V receive strong projections from deep afferent fibres but contain only few cells responding to this input.

REFERENCES

ABRAHAMS, V.C., RICHMOND, F.J.R. AND KEANE, J. (1984). Projections from C2 and C3 nerves supplying muscles and skin of the cat neck: a study using transganglionic transport of horseradish peroxidase. *Journal of Comparative Neurology* **230**, 142-154.

ABRAHAMS, V.C. AND SWETT, J.E. (1986). The pattern of spinal and medullary projections from a cutaneous nerve and a muscle nerve of the forelimb of the cat: A study using the transganglionic transport of HRP. *Journal of Comparative Neurology* **246**, 70-84.

AMMANN, B., GOTTSCHALL, J. AND ZENKER, W. (1983). Afferent projections from the rat longus capitis muscle studied by transganglionic transport of HRP. *Anatomy and Embryology* **166**, 275-289.

BAKKER, D.A., RICHMOND, F.J.R. AND ABRAHAMS, V.C. (1984). Central projections from cat suboccipital muscle: a study using transganglionic transport of horseradish peroxidase. *Journal of Comparative Neurology* **228**, 409-421.

BENNETT, G.J., ABDELMOUMENE, M., HAYASHI, H. AND DUBNER,R. (1980). Physiology and morphology of substantia gelatinosa neurons intracellularly stained with horseradish peroxidase. *Journal of Comparative Neurology* **194**, 809-827.

BROWN, A.G. (1981). Organization in the spinal cord. The anatomy and physiology of identified neurones. *Springer, Berlin, Heidelberg, New York* 238 pp.

BROWN, A.G. AND FYFFE, R.E.W. (1981). Form and function of dorsal horn neurones with axons ascending the dorsal columns in cat. *Journal of Physiology* **321**, 31-47.

BRUSHART, T.M. AND MESULAM, M.-M. (1980). Transganglionic demonstration of central sensory projections from skin and muscle with HRP-lectin conjugates. *Neuroscience Letters* **17**, 1-6.

CERVERO, F. AND CONNELL, L.A. (1984). Fine afferent fibers from viscera do not terminate in the substantia gelatinosa of the thoracic spinal cord. *Brain Research* **294**, 370-374.

CERVERO, F. AND TATTERSALL, J.E.H. (1985). Cutaneous receptive fields of somatic and viscerosomatic neurones in the thoracic spinal cord of the cat. *Journal of Comparative Neurology* **237**, 325-332.

CRAIG, A.D. AND BURTON, H. (1981) Spinal and medullary lamina I projection to nucleus submedius in medial thalamus: a possible pain center. *Journal of Neurophysiology* **45**, 443-466.

CRAIG, A.D. AND KNIFFKI, K.-D. (1985). Spinothalamic lumbosacral lamina I cells responsive to skin and muscle stimulation in the cat. *Journal of Physiology* **365**, 197-221.

CRAIG, A.D. AND MENSE, S. (1983). The distribution of afferent fibers from the gastrocnemius-soleus muscle in the dorsal horn of the cat, as revealed by the transport of horseradish peroxidase. *Neuroscience Letters* **41**, 233-238.

FOREMAN, R.D., HANCOCK, M.B. AND WILLIS, W.D. (1981) Responses of spinothalamic tract cells in the thoracic spinal cord of the monkey to cutaneous and visceral inputs. *Pain* **11**, 149-162.

FYFFE, R.E.W (1979). The morphology of group II muscle afferent fibre collaterals. *Journal of Physiology* **296**, 39P-40P.

HOCKADAY, J.M. AND WHITTY, C.W.M. (1967). Patterns of referred pain in the normal subject. *Brain* **90**, 481-496.

HOHEISEL, U. AND MENSE, S. (1988). Long-term changes in discharge behaviour of cat dorsal horn neurones following noxious stimulation of deep tissue. *Pflügers Archiv* 411, Suppl. 1, R 128.

HONDA, C.N. (1985). Visceral and somatic afferent convergence onto neurons near the central canal in the sacral spinal cord of the cat. *Journal of Neurophysiology* **53**, 1059-1078.

HONDA, C.N., RETHELYI, M. AND PETRUSZ, P. (1983). Preferential immunohistochemical localization of vasoactive intestinal polypeptide (VIP) in the sacral spinal cord of the cat: light and electron microscopic observations. *Journal of Neuroscience* **3**, 2183-2196.

HUNT, S.P. AND ROSSI, J. (1985). Peptide and non-peptide-containing unmyelinated primary afferents: the parallel processing of nociceptive information. *Philosophical Transactions of the Royal Society London, Series B* **308**, 283-289.

KALIA, M., MEI, S.S. AND KAO, F.F. (1981). Central projections from ergoreceptors (C fibers) in muscle involved in cardiopulmonary responses to static exercise. *Circulation Research* **48**, Suppl. I, 48-62.

KIRKWOOD, P.A. AND SEARS, T.A. (1974). Monosynaptic excitation of motoneurons from secondary endings of muscle spindles. *Nature* **252**, 243-244.

LIGHT, A.R. AND PERL, E.R. (1979). Spinal termination of functionally identified primary afferent neurons with slowly conducting myelinated fibers. *Journal of Comparative Neurology* **186**, 133-150.

LIGHT, A.R., TREVINO, D.L. and PERL, E.R. (1979). Morphological features of functionally defined neurons in the marginal zone and substantia gelatinosa of the spinal dorsal horn. *Journal of Comparative Neurology* **186**, 151-171.

MAXWELL, D.J. AND RETHELYI, M. (1987). Ultrastructure and synaptic connections of cutaneous afferent fibres in the spinal cord. *Trends in Neuroscience* **10**, 117-122.

MENSE, S. AND CRAIG, A.D. (1988). Spinal and supraspinal terminations of primary afferent fibers from the gastro-cnemius-soleus muscle in the cat. *Neuroscience*, in press.

MENSE, S., LIGHT, A.R. AND PERL, E.R. (1981). Spinal terminations of subcutaneous high-threshold mechanoreceptors.In A.G. Brown and M. Rethelyi (Eds.), *Spinal Cord Sensation*, pp. 79-86. Scottish Academic Press, Edinburgh .

MOLANDER, C. AND GRANT, G. (1987). Spinal cord projections from hindlimb muscle nerves in the rat studied by transganglionic transport of horseradish peroxidase, wheat germ agglutinin conjugated horseradish peroxidase, or horseradish peroxidase with dimethylsulfoxide. *Journal of Comparative Neurology* **260**, 246-255.

MORGAN, C., NADELHAFT, I. AND DE GROAT, W.C. (1981). The distribution of visceral primary afferents from the pelvic nerve to Lissauer's tract and the spinal gray matter and its relationship to the sacral parasympathetic nucleus. *Journal of Comparative Neurology* **201**, 415-440.

MYSICKA, A. AND ZENKER, W. (1981). Central projections of muscle afferents from the sternomastoid nerve in the rat. *Brain Research* **211**, 257-265.

NYBERG, G. AND BLOMQVIST, A. (1984). The central projection of muscle afferent fibres to the lower medulla and upper spinal cord: An anatomical study in the cat with the transganglionic transport method. *Journal of Comparative Neurology* **230**, 99-109.

POMERANZ, B., WALL, P.D. AND WEBER, W.V. (1968). Cord cells responding to fine myelinated afferents from viscera, muscle and skin. *Journal of Physiology* **199**, 511-532.

SCHAIBLE, H.-G., SCHMIDT, R.F. AND WILLIS, W.D. (1986). Responses of spinal cord neurones to stimulation of articular afferent fibres in the cat. *Journal of Physiology* **372**, 575-593.

SUGIURA, Y., LEE, C.L. AND PERL, E.R. (1986). Central projections of identified, unmyelinated (C) afferent fibers innervating mammalian skin. *Science* **234**, 358-361.

WALL, P.D. AND WOOLF, C.J. (1984). Muscle but not cutaneous C-afferent input produces prolonged increases in the excitability of the flexion reflex in the rat. *Journal of Physiology* **356**, 443-458.

WOOLF, C.J. AND KING, A.E. (1987). Physiology and morphology of multireceptive neurons with C-afferent fiber inputs in the deep dorsal horn of the rat lumbar spinal cord. *Journal of Neurophysiology* **58**, 460-479.

THE DISTRIBUTION OF MUSCLE AND CUTANEOUS PROJECTIONS TO THE DORSAL HORN OF THE UPPER CERVICAL CORD OF THE CAT

Vivian C. Abrahams

Department of Physiology, Queen's University Kingston, Ontario, Canada K7L 3N6

INTRODUCTION

In 1952 Rexed published his seminal paper entitled *The Cytoarchitectonic Organisation of the Spinal Cord in the Cat*. Rexed pointed out that the cytoarchitectonics of the cord were relatively consistent and organised in laminae along the length of the cord. Two years later, in 1954, Rexed published his complete cytoarchitectonic atlas of the cat spinal cord detailing the laminar organisation of the cord, segment by segment. Rexed's (1954) description of spinal cord architecture has become the effective road map for spinal cord research since that time.

The recognition that the cytoarchitecture of the spinal cord is relatively consistent in all segments of the spinal cord was an important advance in the understanding of the anatomy of the cord. It has also been an important advance in modern spinal cord physiology and it is now common to talk of neurons as having the characteristics of a particular lamina. The emphasis on a longitudinally organised plan within segments has sometimes obscured the disparate segmental functions within the spinal cord. For example, the lumbosacral cord in almost all mammals gives rise to the nerves that control the major muscles of locomotion. The same spinal segments innervate those pelvic viscera concerned with reproduction and elimination. The thoracic cord has a very different intrinsic functional role and is important in the control of the muscles of respiration and of posture and also plays a major role in sympathetic function. The lower cervical cord is of unique importance in the specialised motor and sensory processes that characterise function in the forepaws and digits. The spinal segments of the upper cervical cord contain the motoneurons that directly control head movement. Thus, this part of the spinal cord is critical for the execution of movements of the head that bring the special senses to bear on a target. This part of the spinal cord also participates in major sensory functions, for it receives a major input from a wealth of neck proprioceptors important in segmental reflexes such as the cervico-collic reflex (Ezure *et al*, 1983) and also in reflexes of posture and locomotion (Abrahams and Falchetto, 1969; Biemond and DeJong, 1969; Richmond *et al*, 1976; DeJong *et al*, 1977; Manzoni *et al*, 1979). It is at the upper cervical level that the functional continuum of brain and spinal cord is most obvious and one key question from both a functional and an anatomical standpoint, is where does the spinal cord end and the medulla begin?

41

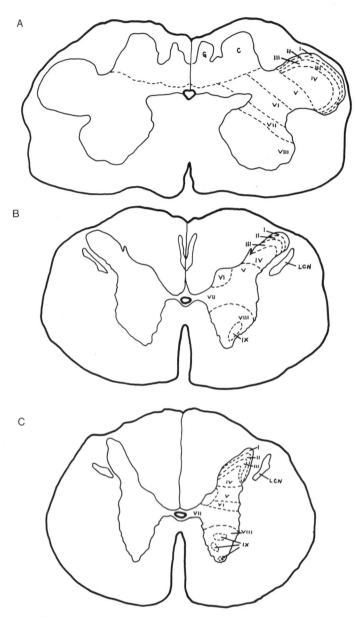

FIGURE 1: Diagram to illustrate the laminar organisation of the dorsal horn of the lower medulla and the dorsal horn of the upper spinal cord. A). Transverse section of medulla caudal to obex and rostral to the C1 roots. B). Transverse section at C1. C). Transverse section at C2. After Rexed (1954) and Gobel *et al* (1977).

THE SPINO-MEDULLARY JUNCTION

The upper cervical cord is not only functionally specialised, but has some anatomically distinct characteristics which reflect the merging of the medulla and the spinal cord. Figure 1 diagrams segments of the upper cervical cord and lower medulla.

The C1 segment in particular can be seen to be a transitional segment between spinal cord and medulla so that the region is sometimes called the spino-medullary junction. The spinal cord in C1 becomes enlarged and flattened and begins to assume the characteristic morphology of the medulla. The gray matter of the dorsal horn at this level is also enlarged and broadened and becomes rectangular in outline. The bulk of the gray matter of the ventral horn is greatly reduced compared with C2 and C3, and is only vestigial in rostral C1. The dorsal surface of the dorsal horn comes close to the surface of the spinal cord and the separation, which is about 500 μm in C2 and C3, is reduced to about 50 μm in rostral C1 (Abrahams, Richmond and Keane, 1984b).

Although it is convenient to talk of the medulla and the spinal cord as though they are separate entities, both anatomically and functionally there is no clear point in C1 at which it can be said that the spinal cord ends and the medulla begins. The anatomic contiguity between the morphology of the medulla and spinal cord is most evident in the dorsal horn. The dorsal medullary region of gray matter contiguous with the spinal dorsal horn has for many years been called the subnucleus caudalis of the spinal nucleus of the trigeminal system. This gray matter represents the most caudal penetration of the trigeminal system. Yet, the anatomical contiguity between subnucleus caudalis and the spinal dorsal horn has been commented on many times since it was first noted by Ramón y Cajal (1909). In their meticulously prepared atlas of the human brainstem, Olszewski and Baxter (1954) pointed out that subnucleus caudalis is an *oral prolongation of the apical gray substance of the dorsal horn of the cervical spinal cord* and also noted that *the cytoarchitecture of the nucleus tractus spinalis trigemini caudalis is essentially the same as that of the apex of the dorsal horn of the spinal cord.* Rexed (1952) in his cytoarchitectonic analysis identified the typical first 4 laminae of the dorsal horn in subnucleus caudalis. A more detailed cytoarchitectural study of the spino-medullary region of the cat CNS by Gobel, Falls and Hockfield (1977) and Gobel, Hockfield and Ruda (1981) led to the recognition that eight layers with laminar boundaries and the cytological characteristics defined by Rexed for the spinal cord could be identified in subnucleus caudalis of V (Fig. 1). The work of Gobel *et al* (1977, 1981) may be regarded as definitive in establishing the notion that there is an anatomical continuum between the dorsal horn of the spinal cord and the lower medulla. To emphasise the anatomical continuum the term *dorsal horn of the medulla* is currently in use to describe what used to be called subnucleus caudalis (Gobel *et al*, 1981; Hoffman, Dubner, Hayes and Medline, 1981; Hu, Dostrovsky and Sessle, 1981).

The anatomical continuum between spinal cord and medulla also reflects a functional continuum. The dorsal horn of the medulla and the dorsal horn of upper cervical segments share extensive connections from both cervical and trigeminal primary afferent fibres. It has been known for some time that many primary afferent fibres of the trigeminal system penetrate caudally several segments into the cervical spinal cord and many cervical primary afferent fibres track rostrally to terminate high in the medulla (Kerr, 1961, 1963, 1972). These findings, which were based on degeneration experiments, have been confirmed and extended in more recent experiments in which the transganglionic transport of horseradish peroxidase (HRP) was used to trace the pathways and destinations of trigeminal (Arvidsson and Gobel, 1981; Marfurt, 1981; Hayashi, 1982) and upper cervical primary afferent fibres (Abrahams *et al*, 1984b).

The earlier anatomical experiments suggested that there was a non-overlapping somatotopic organisation of trigeminal and cervical primary afferent fibre input within both the dorsal horn of the upper cervical and lower medullary dorsal horn (Kerr, 1961, 1963, 1972). Early electrophysiological experiments confirmed the anatomical findings and it was found that the neurons in these regions receiving cervical and trigeminal input were largely segregated. Some convergence was reported, but it was uncommon (Kerr and Olafson, 1961). More recent electrophysiological experiments have shown that convergence in the dorsal horn of both the medulla and the upper cervical cord is common with about 40% of neurons receiving input from both trigeminal and cervical systems (Abrahams et al, 1979).

The dorsal horn of the medulla has long been implicated in the perception of facial pain (for review see Sessle, 1987). The presumption was that the descending tract was a small fibre pathway containing fibres subserving nociception. More recent work shows that a much wider range of facial cutaneous receptors project to this region and trigeminal input to the dorsal horn of the medulla and the upper cervical cord includes a mixture of both non-noxious and noxious inputs. Nociceptive afferents from facial skin were found in lamina I, II, V and VI, low threshold afferents in lamina III - VI (Sessle et al, 1986; Sessle, 1987), a situation analogous to that in lower segmental levels of the spinal cord. Most of the available evidence thus emphasises that the dorsal horn of the medulla is not only an anatomical homologue of the spinal dorsal horn but a functional homologue.

One aspect of spinal cord function in the upper cervical region which is rarely considered is that this part of the cord is subjected to considerable bending because of the mobility of the head and neck (Richmond and Vidal, 1988). In species such as the lamprey, with particularly mobile spinal cords, it has been found that the cord contains peripherally located mechanoreceptors which monitor movements of the spinal cord (Grillner, Williams and Lagerbäck, 1984), something which might also be true in higher mammals.

Although the functional homology between the upper cervical dorsal horn and the dorsal horn of the medulla has been stressed, there are some unique cell groups in other regions of the upper cervical cord. The lateral cervical nucleus which lies in white matter lateral to the dorsal horn (Rexed, 1954) has no obvious homologue at other spinal levels. The lateral cervical nucleus does not receive any significant input from the upper cervical cord and is a target for axons from spino-cervical tract neurons located in lumbosacral cord (Brown, 1973). The anatomical location of the lateral cervical nucleus seems to have little to do with functional relationships with the upper cervical cord. There is also a central cervical nucleus located medially in the intermediate gray of the upper cervical segments (Wiksten, 1979a). In the cat this nucleus appears to be entirely a precerebellar nucleus (Matsushita and Ikeda, 1975; Wiksten, 1979b) and is very much concerned with proprioceptive function in the upper cervical cord, for it is a major target of muscle primary afferent fibres entering the upper cervical cord (Hirai et al, 1984).

TRIGEMINAL INPUT TO THE UPPER CERVICAL CORD AND TRIGEMINO-NECK REFLEXES

Most studies of the dorsal horn of the medulla have been concerned with the sensory characteristics of the trigeminal input and the relationship between trigeminal and cervical inputs. However, the trigeminal input to the lower medulla and upper cervical cord also subserves a motor function. The trigeminal projection to the cervical dorsal horn activates many neurons in the upper cervical cord at short latencies. One third of cervical neurons activated by trigeminal nerve stimulation have latencies of 5 msec or less and virtually all have latencies less than 20 msec (Abrahams et al, 1979). This short latency trigeminal input to the upper cervical cord is of significance in head movement, for many of the cervical neurons that are activated are motoneurons. Thus, stimulation of branches of the trigeminal nerve in anaesthetised cats is very effective in initiating short latency upper cervical motoneuron activity (Abrahams and Richmond, 1977; Sumino and Nozaki, 1977; Abrahams *et al*, 1979). The cervical motoneuron response to trigeminal nerve stimulation has been named the trigemino-neck reflex (Sumino and Nozaki, 1977). It has been suggested that this electrically recorded reflex is the analogue of the aversion movements of the head following stimulation of facial skin (Abrahams and Richmond, 1977; Sumino and Nozaki, 1977). The notion that the trigeminal projections to the upper cervical cord are the anatomical substrate for this reflex is not a new idea. Kerr and Olafson (1961) in their discussion of trigeminal projections to the upper cervical cord cite a 1924 publication of Van Valkenburg which suggested that the spinal trigeminal tract was a pathway for reflex turning of the head in response to tactile and noxious stimuli applied to the face.

PHYSIOLOGICAL STUDIES OF SENSORY RECEPTORS ENTERING THE UPPER CERVICAL CORD

In order to understand the physiology and anatomy of the dorsal horn of the upper cervical cord, it is first necessary to understand the source of sensory input to those spinal segments. The cutaneous input to the upper cervical cord has not been systematically explored, but the experiments done to date suggest that input includes all the usual well-recognised classes of cutaneous receptors including nociceptors. The skin regions served by these nerves include the pinna, the neck and the occiput (Abrahams *et*

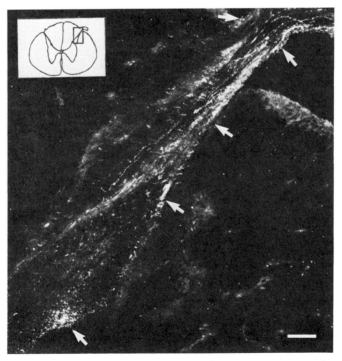

FIGURE 2: Dark field photograph of transverse section at root entry zone of caudal C2 after transport of HRP by C2 cutaneous nerve. Arrows show lateral distribution of HRP deposit in lateral dorsal root and in lateral regions of dorsal horn. Note narrow shape of C2 dorsal horn. Inset diagram shows region photographed. (From Abrahams *et al*, 1984b, with permission.)

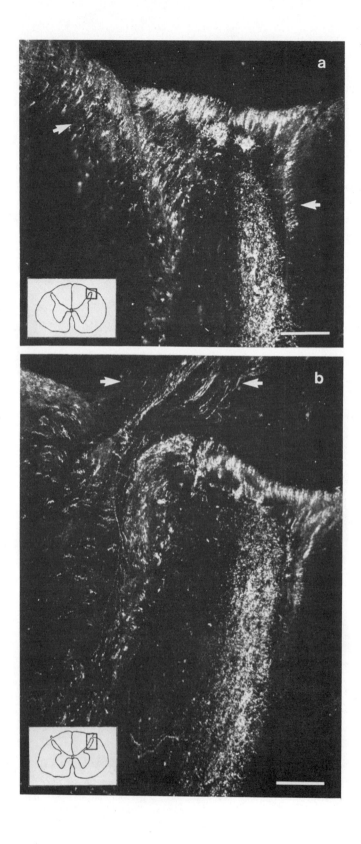

al, 1984a; Abrahams et al, 1988). The C1 dorsal root, however, is unique since it appears to be entirely free of cutaneous input (Hekmatpanah, 1961). Perhaps the most unusual aspect of the sensory input to the upper cervical cord is the dense input from muscle receptors. The system of deep neck receptors is one of great abundance and remarkable order: unusually high concentrations of receptors including muscle spindles, Golgi tendon organs, Pacinian and paciniform corpuscles and free nerve endings are found in deep and superficial muscles (Richmond et al, 1988). There is compelling evidence that this remarkable system of muscle receptors is the heart of the neck proprioceptive system, a system of great importance in the maintenance of posture and in normal locomotion (Peterson and Richmond, 1988).

What is of particular importance to those concerned with the organisation of the superficial dorsal horn is that there is a significant muscle input to the upper cervical cord from group III and group IV fibres (Richmond et al, 1976; Abrahams et al, 1984a). The usual classification of muscle receptors assigns spindle afferent fibres to group I and II. In neck muscles this categorisation does not hold and a significant number of muscle spindles and other encapsulated receptors are served by small myelinated group III fibres (Richmond and Abrahams, 1979). In the limited studies that have been performed, it was found that group III fibres from neck muscles that do not serve spindles serve high threshold mechanoreceptors, with no evidence for group III nociceptors (Abrahams et al, 1984a). These group III mechanoreceptors do not seem to be randomly distributed and are located in tissue close to the tendinous intersections that separate the compartments of the large dorsal neck muscles (Richmond and Abrahams, 1975; Richmond et al, 1985). Despite the absence of evidence for the presence of group III nociceptors, the few group IV receptors that were recorded from had properties consistent with nociceptive function (Abrahams et al, 1984a). It is a reasonable assumption that the group III fibres of neck muscle are almost entirely from mechanoreceptors including muscle spindles and that some or all group IV fibres have functions that include nociception. However, it is quite likely that small sensory fibres from muscle that enter the upper cervical cord contain an unusually high proportion of non-nociceptors.

ORGANISATION OF CUTANEOUS PROJECTIONS TO THE DORSAL HORN OF THE UPPER CERVICAL CORD

The introduction of the technique of pathway tracing based on the anterograde transport of horseradish peroxidase (HRP) (Grant et al, 1979; Mesulam and Brushart, 1979) has provided a powerful anatomical tool for the analysis of the pathways and targets of primary afferent fibres. By dipping the central cut end of appropriate nerves in HRP solution, we have been able to use this technique extensively to follow the

FIGURE 3: Dark field photograph through mid (top) and rostral C2 (bottom) dorsal horn to show pattern of HRP reaction product after transport by C2 cutaneous nerve. Note the large number of transected axons and the deposition of HRP within the lateral dorsal horn, and the change in shape of the dorsal horn between rostral and caudal C2. Arrow on left in (a) shows obliquely cut axons entering dorsal columns. Arrow on right in (a) shows obliquely cut axons which terminate in the substantia gelatinosa. Arrows in (b) show extent of the dorsal root. Calibration bar = 100 μm. Inset diagrams show area photographed. (Reprinted from Abrahams et al, 1984b, with permission.)

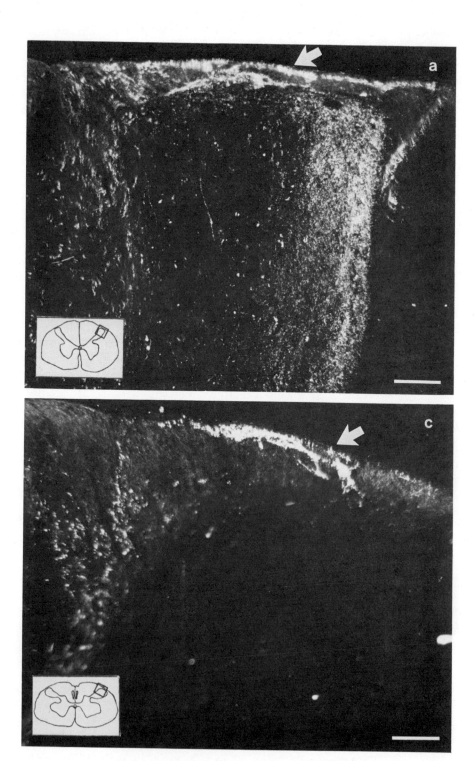

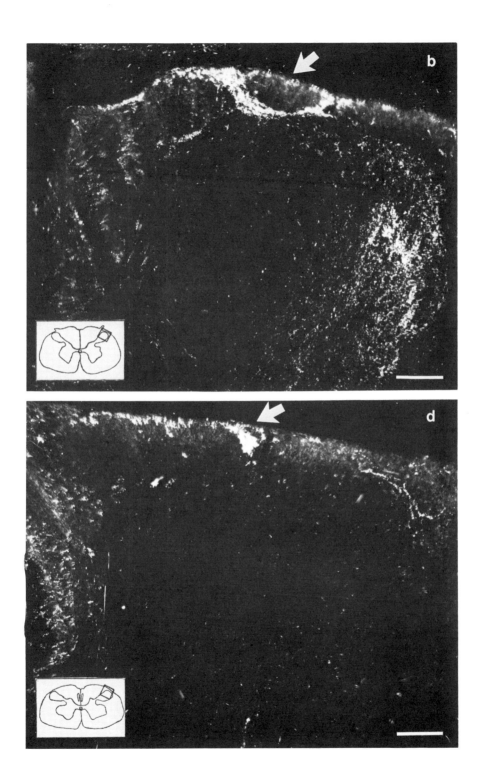

course of primary afferents entering the upper cervical cord. Figures 2 and 3 show cutaneous projections to the upper cervical cord of the cat demonstrated by this technique. As at other levels of the cord (Brown and Fuchs, 1975) primary afferents terminate in the dorsal horn somatotopically so that the projections from neck and pinna skin occupy only the lateral half of the dorsal horn. There is a strong deposit of HRP reaction product in all layers of the lateral half of the dorsal horn with HRP reaction product at its most dense in the segment of dorsal root entry. Projections are seen caudal to the root of entry, but are weak and do not penetrate more than 1 or 2 segments below the segment of entry. In contrast, rostral projections are extensive and prominent, and HRP reaction product is present throughout the cervical segments and extends rostrally into the dorsal horn of the medulla (Abrahams et al, 1984b). Here too somatotopy is preserved and in the dorsal horn of the medulla fibres from neck skin terminate only in the more lateral regions of the gray matter (Fig. 3).

In both upper cervical and lower medullary regions, HRP reaction product transported by cutaneous nerves is particularly prominent in the superficial dorsal horn and many axons entering dorsal roots can be seen to project to and enter Lissauer's tract. These fibres can be seen entering dense accumulations of granular reaction product in lamina II (the substantia gelatinosa) suggesting that many of the Lissauer tract axons terminate there. As in other layers of the dorsal horn, the projections in the superficial layers of the upper cervical cord extends only one or two segments caudally. However, the rostral projections to the superficial dorsal horn of the medulla are prominent and extensive and are found even more rostrally than the deeper projections. As in lower regions of the cord, the patterns of axonal HRP in the ascending fibres of the tract of Lissauer indicate a complex fibre organisation. Fibres in this region can be seen tracking in many directions in the fashion first illustrated by Ranson (1913, 1914) in his degeneration experiments. As in the deeper layers of the dorsal horn, the superficial dorsal horn projections are not evenly distributed but are somatotopically organised with the reaction product occupying only the lateral regions of the superficial dorsal horn in both cord and medulla.

An unusual and prominent feature in the superficial layers of the medullary dorsal horn was the presence of small intense accumulations of HRP reaction product in laminae I and II continuous with deposits around clumps of neurons just dorsal to lamina I (Fig. 4c and d). Cells in this region were described by Ramón y Cajal (1909) and were called by him interstitial cells. Kerr (1970) and Gobel et al (1977) extended those anatomical observations, Gobel et al (1977) preferring the term *islet cells* for the neuron groups which they believed to be extensions of lamina I. These same neurons were studied electrophysiologically by Hubbard and Hellon (1980) and by Dawson et al, (1980). They found the neurons to have the characteristics of lamina I cells, except for the presence of spontaneous discharge. However, it is worth remembering that the dorsal surface of the lower medulla in most vertebrates is a region subject to flexion and extension movements with the movements of the head. It would be of interest to know if

FIGURE 4 (Previous 2 pages): Dark field photograph of a series of transverse sections through rostral C1 (a and b) and caudal medulla (c and d) to show extent of HRP distribution seen after exposure of C2 cutaneous nerve. The arrows indicate the more superficial accumulation of HRP which lies on the surface of the medulla in c and d. Inset diagrams show area photographed. Calibration bar 100 μM. (Reprinted, with permission from Abrahams et al, 1984b.)

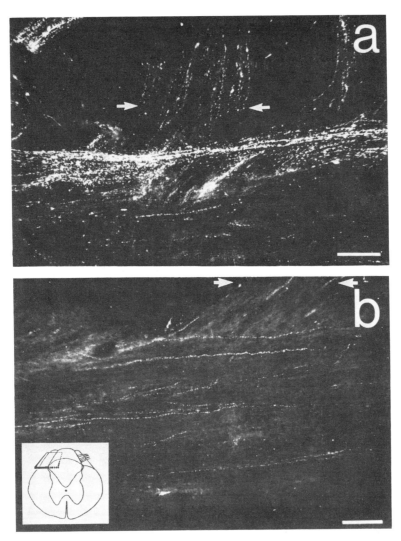

FIGURE 5: Dark field photograph of root entry zone in C2 after exposure of a cutaneous (a) and a muscle (b) nerve to HRP. Inset diagram shows area photographed. Calibration bar 100 μM. (Reprinted from Abrahams *et al*, 1984b, with permission.)

the islet cells of the cat share with the similar cells in the lamprey the intrinsic mechanosensitive properties referred to earlier (Grillner *et al*, 1984).

MUSCLE AFFERENT PROJECTIONS TO THE SUPERFICIAL DORSAL HORN

The property of the HRP transganglionic transport technique that permits the selective demonstration of input from specific nerves supplying specific organs has made it possible to examine the organisation of primary afferent fibres to the dorsal horn of the upper cervical cord from muscle nerves separately to that from cutaneous input (Brushart and Mesulam, 1980; Mysicka and Zenker, 1981; Ammann *et al*, 1983; Craig and Mense, 1983; Bakker *et al*, 1984; Abrahams *et al*, 1984b; Abrahams and Swett, 1986). This work has shown, in virtually all species and at all levels of the cord that, in contrast to cutaneous input, muscle input to the superficial dorsal horn is minimal. Projections to the upper cervical cord from large dorsal neck muscles proved to be no exception (Abrahams *et al* 1984b). In experiments in which neck muscle nerves were

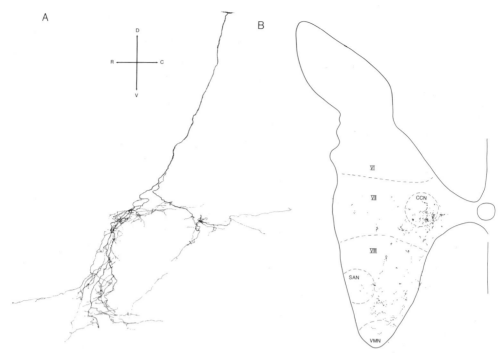

FIGURE 6: A). Reconstruction in the sagittal plane of a C2 collateral from a presumed group 1A axon from a large dorsal neck muscle. Note the absence of boutons in the dorsal horn. B). Transverse section to show distribution of boutons from the single collateral in the intermediate and ventral gray matter. (From Rose and Keirstead, *Canadian Journal of Physiology and Pharmacology* (1986), **64**, 505-586, with permission.)

exposed to HRP, the dorsal horn was almost devoid of HRP reaction product. When nerves supplying superficial muscles were exposed (Abrahams *et al*, 1984b) a few fibres were found tracking through the tract of Lissauer and some HRP deposits were present in lamina I (Fig. 5). In experiments in which deep neck muscles were exposed to HRP, no reaction product could be found in the superficial dorsal horn (Bakker *et al*, 1984).

The HRP reaction product that was present in the cervical cord after muscle nerve exposure was mainly found in fibres which travelled alongside the lateral and medial margins of the dorsal horn and which terminated in lamina V and in the central cervical nucleus. Consistent with these observations, Rose and Keirstead (1986) have visualised large axons from neck muscle group Ia fibres by filling them with HRP intra-axonally. These axons give rise to large numbers of boutons in the regions of the central cervical nucleus and the ventral horn, but provide no boutons, and presumably no synaptic connections to the dorsal horn (Fig. 6). Thus the tract of Lissauer and the substantia gelatinosa receive no primary afferent input from muscle and deep receptors either at upper cervical levels or at the level of the dorsal horn of the medulla. In the upper cervical cord and medulla, the functional importance of the tract of Lissauer and the substantia gelatinosa seems uniquely related to aspects of cutaneous sensation.

Despite all the differences in morphological and physiological detail, it seems that the spectrum of sensory information entering the upper cervical cord and lower medulla and the targets of that information are not significantly different from those found at other levels of the spinal cord. Only time will tell if this is due to the relatively small amount of physiological study of this area, or whether we should assume that function as well as structure in the dorsal horn (and particularly the superficial dorsal horn) is consistent throughout the length of the spinal cord.

Supported by the Medical Research Council of Canada.

REFERENCES

ABRAHAMS, V.C., ANSTEE, G., RICHMOND, F.J.R. AND ROSE, P.K. (1979). Neck muscle and trigeminal input to the upper cervical cord and lower medulla of the cat. *Canadian Journal of Physiology and Pharmacology* **57**, 642-651.

ABRAHAMS, V.C., CLINTON, R.J. AND DOWNEY, D. (1988). Somatosensory projections to the superior colliculus of the anaesthetised cat. *Journal of Physiology* **396**, 563-580.

ABRAHAMS, V.C. AND FALCHETTO, S. (1969). Hind leg ataxia of cervical origin and cervico-lumbar spinal interactions with a supratentorial pathway. *Journal of Physiology* **203**, 435-447

ABRAHAMS, V.C., LYNN, B. AND RICHMOND, F.J.R. (1984a). Organisation and sensory properties of small myelinated fibres in the dorsal cervical rami of the cat. *Journal of Physiology* **347**, 177-187.

ABRAHAMS, V.C. AND RICHMOND, F.J.R. (1977). Motor role of the spinal projections of the trigeminal system. In *Pain in the Trigeminal Region*, eds. Anderson, D.J. and Matthews, B., pp. 405-413. Amsterdam: Elsevier.

ABRAHAMS, V.C., RICHMOND, F.J.R. AND KEANE, J. (1984b). Projections from C2 and C3 nerves supplying muscles and skin of the cat neck: a study using transganglionic transport of horseradish peroxidase. *Journal of Comparative Neurology* **230**, 142-154.

ABRAHAMS, V.C. AND SWETT, J.E. (1986). The pattern of spinal and medullary projections from a cutaneous nerve and a muscle nerve of the forelimb of the cat: a study using the transganglionic transport of HRP. *Journal of Comparative Neurology* **246**, 70-84.

AMMANN, B., GOTTSCHALL, J. AND ZENKER, W. (1983). Afferent projections from the rat longus capitis muscle studied by transganglionic transport of HRP. *Anatomy and Embryology* **166**, 275-289.

ARVIDSSON, J. AND GOBEL, S. (1981). An HRP study of the central projections of primary trigeminal neurons which innervate tooth pulps in the cat. *Brain Research* **210**, 1-16.

BAKKER, D.A., RICHMOND, F.J.R. AND ABRAHAMS, V.C. (1984). Central projections from cat suboccipital muscles: a study using transganglionic transport of horseradish peroxidase. *Journal of Comparative Neurology* **228**, 409-421.

BIEMOND, A. AND DEJONG, J. (1969). On cervical nystagmus and related disorders. *Brain* **92**, 437-458.

BROWN, A.G. (1973). Ascending and long spinal pathways: dorsal columns, spinocervical tract and spinothalamic tract. In Handbook of Sensory Physiology, section, *Somatosensory system*, vol. II, pp. 315-338, Berlin: Springer Verlag.

BROWN, P.B. AND FUCHS, J.L. (1975). Somatotopic representation of hindlimb skin in cat dorsal horn. *Journal of Neurophysiology* **38**, 1-19.

BRUSHART, T.M. AND MESULAM, M.-M. (1980). Transganglionic demonstration of central sensory projections from skin and muscle with HRP-lectin conjugates. *Neuroscience Letters* **17**, 1-6.

CRAIG, A.D. AND MENSE, S. (1983). The distribution of afferent fibers from the gastrocnemius-soleus muscle in the dorsal horn of the cat, as revealed by the transport of horseradish peroxidase. *Neuroscience Letters* **41**, 233-238.

DAWSON, N.J., HELLON, R.F. AND HUBBARD, J.I. (1980). Cell responses evoked by tooth pulp stimulation above the marginal layer of the cat's trigeminal nucleus caudalis. *Journal of Comparative Neurology* **193**, 983-994.

DEJONG, P., DEJONG, J., COHEN, B. AND JONGKEES, L. (1977). Ataxia and nystagmus induced by injection of local anaesthetics in the neck. *Annals of Neurology* **1**, 240-246.

EZURE, K., FUKUSHIMA, K., SCHOR, R.H. AND WILSON, V.J. (1983). Compartmentalisation of the cervicocollic reflex in cat splenius muscle. *Experimental Brain Research* **51**, 397-404.

GOBEL, S., FALLS, W.M. AND HOCKFIELD, S. (1977). The division of the dorsal and ventral horns of the mammalian caudal medulla into eight layers using anatomical criteria. In *Pain in the Trigeminal Region*, eds. Anderson, D.J. and Matthews, B., pp. 443-453. Amsterdam: Elsevier.

GOBEL, S., HOCKFIELD, S. AND RUDA, M.A. (1981). Anatomical similarities between medullary and spinal dorsal horns. In *Oral-facial Sensory and Motor Functions*, eds. Kawamura, Y. and Dubner, R., pp. 211-223. Tokyo: Quintessence.

GRANT, G., ARVIDSSON, J., ROBERTSON, B. AND YGGE, J. (1979). Transganglionic transport of horseradish peroxidase in primary sensory neurons. *Neuroscience Letters* **12**, 23-28.

GRILLNER, S., WILLIAMS, T. AND LAGERBACK, P.-A. (1984). The edge cell, a possible intraspinal mechanoreceptor. *Science* **223**, 500-503.

HAYASHI, H. (1982). Differential terminal distribution of single large cutaneous afferent fibres in the spinal trigeminal nucleus and in the cervical spinal dorsal horn. *Brain Research* **244**, 173-177.

HEKMATPANAH, J. (1961). Organisation of tactile dermatomes C1 through L4, in cat. *Journal of Neurophysiology* **24**, 129-140.

HIRAI, N., HONGO, T., SASAKI, S., YAMASHITA, M. AND YOSHIDA, K. (1984). Neck muscle afferent input to spinocerebellar tract cells of the central cervical nucleus in the cat. *Experimental Brain Research* **55**, 286-300.

HOFFMAN, D.S., DUBNER, R., HAYES, R.L. AND MEDLINE, T.P. (1981). Neuronal activity in a thermal discrimination task. 1. Responses to innocuous and noxious thermal stimuli. *Journal of Neurophysiology* **46**, 409-427.

HU, J.W., DOSTROVSKY, J.O. AND SESSLE, B.J. (1981). Functional properties of neurons in cat trigeminal subnucleus caudalis (medullary dorsal horn). 1. Responses to oral-facial noxious and non-noxious stimuli and projections to thalamus and subnucleus oralis. *Journal of Neurophysiology* **45**, 173-192.

HUBBARD, J.I. AND HELLON, R.F. (1980). Excitation and inhibition of marginal layer and interstitial interneurons in cat nucleus caudalis by mechanical stimuli. *Journal of Comparative Neurology* **193**, 995-1007.

KERR, F.W.L. (1961). Structural relation of the trigeminal spinal tract to upper cervical roots and the solitary nucleus in the cat. *Experimental Neurology* **4**, 134-148.

KERR, F.W.L. (1963). The divisional organization of afferent fibres of the trigeminal nerve. *Brain* **86**, 721-732.

KERR, F.W.L. (1970). The fine structure of subnucleus caudalis of the trigeminal nerve. *Brain Research* **23**, 129-145.

KERR, F.W.L. (1972). Central relationships of trigeminal and cervical primary afferents in the spinal cord and medulla. *Brain Research* **43**, 561-572.

KERR, F.W.L. AND OLAFSON, R. (1961). Trigeminal and cervical volleys: convergence on single units in the spinal gray at C1 and C2. *Archives of Neurology* **5**, 171-178.

MANZONI, D., POMPEIANO, O. AND STAMPACCIA, G. (1979). Tonic cervical influences on posture and reflex movements. *Archives Italiennes de Biologie* **117**, 81-110.

MARFURT, C.F. (1981). The central projections of trigeminal primary afferent neurons in the cat as determined by the transganglionic transport of horseradish peroxidase. *Journal of Comparative Neurology* **203**, 785-798.

MATSUSHITA, M. AND IKEDA, M. (1975). The central cervical nucleus as cell origin of a spinocerebellar tract arising from the cervical cord: a study in the cat using horseradish peroxidase. *Brain Research* **100**, 412-417.

MESULAM, M.-M. AND BRUSHART, T.M. (1979). Transganglionic and anterograde transport of horseradish peroxidase across dorsal root ganglia: a tetramethylbenzidine method for tracing sensory connections of muscles and peripheral nerves. *Neuroscience* **4**, 1107-1117.

MYSICKA, A. AND ZENKER, W. (1981). Central projections of muscle afferents from the sternomastoid muscle in the rat. *Brain Research* **211**, 257-265.

OLSZEWSKI, J. AND BAXTER, D. (1954). Cytoarchitecture of the human brain stem. Karger, Basel

PETERSON, B. AND RICHMOND, F.J.R. (1988). Control of Head Movement, eds. Peterson, B. and Richmond, F.J.R., Oxford University Press.

RAMÓN Y CAJAL (1909). Histologie du système nerveux de l'homme et des vertébrés. Consejo de Investigaciones Cientificas, Madrid.

RANSON, S.W. (1913). The course within the spinal cord of the non- medullated fibers of the dorsal roots: a study of Lissauer's tract in the cat. *Journal of Comparative Neurology* **23**, 259-281.

RANSON, S.W. (1914). The Tract of Lissauer and the Substantia Gelatinosa Rolandi. *American Journal of Anatomy* **16**, 97-126.

REXED, B. (1952). The cytoarchitectonic organisation of the spinal cord of the cat. *Journal of Cell and Comparative Neurology* **96**, 415-496.

REXED, B. (1954). A cytoarchitectonic atlas of the spinal cord in the cat. *Journal of Comparative Neurology* **100**, 297-380.

RICHMOND, F.J.R. AND ABRAHAMS, V.C. (1975). Morphology and enzyme histochemistry of dorsal muscles of the cat neck. *Journal of Neurophysiology* **38**, 1312-1321.

RICHMOND, F.J.R. AND ABRAHAMS, V.C. (1979). Physiological properties of muscle spindles in dorsal neck muscles of the cat. *Journal of Neurophysiology* **42**, 604-617.

RICHMOND, F.J.R., ANSTEE, G.C.B., SHERWIN, E.A. AND ABRAHAMS, V.C. (1976). Motor and sensory fibres of neck muscle nerves in the cat. *Canadian Journal of Physiology and Pharmacology* **54**, 294-304.

RICHMOND, F.J.R., BAKKER, D.A. AND STACEY, M.S. (1988). The sensorium: receptors of neck muscles and joints. In *Control of Head Movement*, eds. Peterson, B.W. and Richmond, F.J.R., pp. 49-62. New York: Oxford.

RICHMOND, F.J.R., MacGILLIS, D.R.R. AND SCOTT, D.A. (1985). Muscle-fiber compartmentalization in cat splenius muscles. *Journal of Neurophysiology* **53**, 868-885.

RICHMOND, F.J.R. AND VIDAL, P.P. (1988). The motor system: joints and muscles of the neck. In *Control of Head Movement*, eds. Peterson, B.W. and Richmond,

F.J.R., pp. 1-21. New York, Oxford.

ROSE, P.K. AND KEIRSTEAD, S.A. (1986). Segmental projection from muscle spindles: a perspective from the upper cervical cord. *Canadian Journal of Physiology and Pharmacology* **64**, 505-508.

SESSLE, B.J. (1987). The neurobiology of facial and dental pain: present knowledge, future directions. *Journal of Dental Research* **66**, 962-981,

SESSLE, B.J., HU, J.W., AMANO, N. AND ZHONG, G. (1986). Convergence of cutaneous, tooth pulp, visceral neck and muscle afferents onto nociceptive and non-nociceptive neurons in trigeminal subnucleus caudalis (medullary dorsal horn) and its implications for referred pain. *Pain* **27**, 219-235.

SUMINO, R. AND NOZAKI, S. (1977). Trigemino-neck reflex: its peripheral and central organisation. In *Pain in the Trigeminal Region*, eds. Anderson, D.J. and Matthews, B., pp. 365-375. Amsterdam: Elsevier.

WIKSTEN, B. (1979a). The central cervical nucleus in the cat. I. A Golgi study. *Experimental Brain Research* **36**, 143-154.

WIKSTEN, B. (1979b). The central cervical nucleus in the cat. II. The cerebellar connections studied with retrograde transport of horseradish peroxidase. *Experimental Brain Research* **36**, 155-173.

ELECTRON MICROSCOPIC LOCALIZATION OF PEPTIDE-LIKE IMMUNOREACTIVITY IN LABELLED DORSAL ROOT TERMINALS IN THE SPINAL SUBSTANTIA GELATINOSA OF THE MONKEY

Alan R. Light and Anahid M. Kavookjian

Department Physiology, UNC-Chapel Hill, Chapel Hill, NC 27599-7545, USA

INTRODUCTION

During the past 15 years, there has been an explosion of information about the localization of peptide substances in the peripheral and central nervous system. This information has been derived largely from immunocytochemical studies which use antibodies that are specific for certain peptides to label the peptides *in situ* in fixed brain tissue.

The substantia gelatinosa of the spinal cord dorsal horn is a region which contains many of these newly discovered neuropeptides; see for example (Hunt, 1983; Lynn and Hunt, 1984; Dodd *et al*, 1983; Ruda *et al*, 1986; DiFiglia *et al*, 1982; Honda *et al*, 1983; Hökfelt *et al*, 1982; Hökfelt *et al*, 1980). Many of these peptides have been localized to nerve terminals in the substantia gelatinosa which have been shown to stem from dorsal root ganglion cells because of their disappearance following dorsal root section (Dodd *et al*, 1983; Jessell *et al*, 1979; Ju *et al*, 1987; Carlton *et al*, 1987; DiFiglia *et al*, 1982; Hökfelt *et al*, 1982). Several of these peptides seem to be contained in specific subsets of small diameter dorsal root ganglion cells (Hökfelt *et al*, 1976; Ju *et al*, 1987; Hökfelt *et al*, 1982). Because nociceptors terminate heavily in the substantia gelatinosa (Rethelyi *et al*, 1982; Light and Perl, 1979a; Mense and Prabhakar, 1986; Sugiura *et al*, 1986) investigators have suggested that several of the neuropeptides may be localized in specific subsets of nociceptive primary afferents . Further, some have speculated that these neuropeptides may be involved in synaptic transmission or modulation of transmission between primary afferent nociceptors and second-order spinal cord neurons (Yaksh, 1986; Carlton *et al*, 1987; Hökfelt *et al*, 1982; Iversen, 1984). However, the substantia gelatinosa and marginal zone are not concerned only with nociception. Instead, in addition to nociceptive afferents, thermoreceptive afferents end here, as well as low threshold, mechanoreceptive C-fibers and a variety of, as yet, uncharacterized visceral primary afferents (Sugiura *et al*, 1986; Morgan *et al*, 1986). Thus, the identification of a particular neuropeptide with a specific primary afferent modality requires a combination of physiological recording and peptide localization techniques. While the anatomical localization of neuropeptides has progressed rapidly, the determination of the physiological properties of the neurons which contain specific peptides has been more difficult. Most of the attempts to double label physiologically identified primary afferents have concentrated on the dorsal root ganglion cell, which, because of its large size, can be easily recorded from and labelled with a variety of intracellular dyes. Unfortunately, the concentration of neuropeptides in the dorsal root ganglion cells is very low in cats and monkeys, often being at undetectable levels. Therefore, in order to increase the number of dorsal root ganglion cells labelled with antibodies to neuropeptides, many investigators have used transport blockers such as colchicine, so as to increase the concentration of neuropeptide in the cell bodies, e.g. (Ju *et al*, 1987; Hökfelt *et al*, 1977; Hökfelt *et al*, 1975).

The results obtained from studies in which intracellular recording and labelling of physiologically identified dorsal root ganglion cells was combined with colchicine treatment to increase peptide content have been somewhat puzzling (Leah *et al*, 1985). Substance P, for example, was rarely found to be localized in nociceptor dorsal root ganglion cells. Perhaps more puzzling was the identification of VIP in D-Hair dorsal root ganglion cells. This is puzzling because D-Hair primary afferents terminate in the inner substantia gelatinosa and lamina III while VIP-like immunoreactivity is found mostly in the sacral spinal cord marginal zone (Honda *et al*, 1983).

These paradoxical results may be explained by the recent suggestion that administration of colchicine induces the transduction of messenger RNA which are normally not present, or only present in very low concentrations (Rethelyi, Metz, Petrusz and Lund, submitted to Brain Res.)

A more direct approach in attempts to associate the physiological properties of neurons with neuropeptides is to label the nerve terminals of a physiologically identified primary afferent , and then visualize the neuropeptide within the synaptic bouton. Since the concentration of neuropeptide within the synaptic boutons is very high, they are easily demonstrable with immunocytochemical methods. Unfortunately, the primary afferent nerve terminals are difficult to label with intra-axonal recording techniques and are also very small. The small size makes unequivocal demonstration at the light microscopic level very difficult. Electron microscopic demonstration has also been problematic because reasonable ultrastructure is difficult to obtain in the presence of agents which enhance the penetration of the antibodies used for labelling the peptides.

Recently, Dr. Silvia De Biasi, working in Dr. Rustioni's laboratory, has improved the technique for immunocytochemical labelling of peptides on ultrathin sections, which are suitable for electron microscopy (De Biasi and Rustioni, submitted). We report here on the use of this technique on primary afferent fibers and their terminations which have been either bulk labelled by crushing HRP into the dorsal root or individually labelled following physiological identification via intra axonal recording and labelling with HRP.

METHODS

The spinal cord tissue was obtained in previous experiments reported by Light and Perl (1979b), and as part of a control series of experiments in a program project grant on neuroplasticity in the spinal dorsal horn. Briefly, monkeys were anesthetized with sodium pentobarbital (I.V.) and were maintained under anesthesia during all surgical and experimental procedures. A laminectomy was performed exposing the lumbosacral spinal cord and dorsal roots. For anatomical experiments, several dorsal rootlets were freed at the dorsal root entry zone, placed on a plastic platform, and HRP pledgets were crushed into the roots. For physiological labelling experiments, the dorsal roots were placed on stimulating and recording electrodes for electrical activation and observation of the compound action potential, respectively. Fine micropipettes filled with 5% HRP in buffered 0.5 M KCl were lowered into the dorsal root entry zone while stimulating the dorsal roots as a search stimulus for primary afferent axons. When an axon was impaled, the receptive field was located, and the type of stimulus which best excited the receptor was determined. The receptor was classified according to Burgess and Perl (1973) and the axon was labelled with HRP by making the electrode positive with 10-30 nA square wave pulses at 100 Hz for 1-10 minutes. The two fibers selected for double labelling had conduction velocities in the C fiber range. One fiber (PP-20) had a conduction velocity of 0.75 m/sec and had a mechanical nociceptive receptive field localized to a small spot on the distal one third of the tail. The response of this unit to noxious thermal stimuli or noxious chemicals was not tested. The other fiber (HDM-37) had a conduction velocity of 0.9 M/sec, but the receptive field could not be found in the short time available while recording from the single fiber.

In both experiments, the animals were allowed to survive for 6-8 hours under anesthesia following which they were perfused with buffered 2% paraformaldehyde and 2.5% glutaraldehyde. The spinal cord was removed and postfixed overnight in the perfusion fixative. Transverse or parasagittal sections were cut at 50 microns on a Vibratome, reacted with DAB + H_2O_2, and scanned for the presence of labelled axons and terminals. Sections containing labelled structures were post fixed in osmium tetroxide, dehydrated, infiltrated with Epon-Araldite, and embedded between teflon coated coverslips. (Details can be found in Metz et al, 1982). Selected sections were reconstructed with a drawing tube, photographed, and recut into serial, ultrathin sections. These ultrathin sections were collected on formvar coated, one slot, nickel grids. Appropriate grids were located by scanning sections with the electron microscope. Subsequently, these grids were labelled for peptide immunoreactivity with the following protocol which is essentially the same as that demonstrated to us by Dr. De Biasi. (see De Biasi and Rustioni, submitted).

Briefly, grids were etched with $NaIO_4$ and $NaBH_4$, then placed in a blocking solution of normal goat serum. Grids were incubated with primary antisera for 1 hour. The primary antisera were 1) anti-Substance P , obtained from Dr Peter Petrusz of the UNC Department of Cell Biology and Anatomy (this antiserum has been well characterized; submitted). 2) anti-Calcitonin Gene Related Peptide (CGRP) obtained from three different sources (Peninsula Labs, Cambridge Biochemical, and Dr Catia Sternini, UCLA, see characterization in Sternini and Brecha, 1986; Sternini et al, 1987), 3) anti-somatostatin obtained from Dr Robert Elde, Dept. of Anatomy, University of Minnesota. Following washes, the grids were incubated with 5 or 10 nanometer gold particles which had been coated with goat anti-rabbit immunoglobulin. After more washes, the grids were either viewed not post stained so that HRP labelled profiles were easily visible or post stained with uranyl acetate and lead citrate for well contrasted ultrastructure. Grids were then viewed on a Zeiss 10C electron microscope. Quantitative measurements of the percentages of labelled boutons with each antiserum were not made in this study. For some quantitative measures see De Biasi and Rustioni, submitted. Controls were performed on adjacent ultrathin sections. These included substituting buffer for the primary antisera, and preabsorbing primary antisera with excess antigen. In all cases, controls were nearly blank, i.e. almost no gold particles were present in control sections.

RESULTS

The HRP labelled fibers and synaptic boutons were readily visible in ultrathin sections before post staining. After the immunostaining, the HRP reaction product

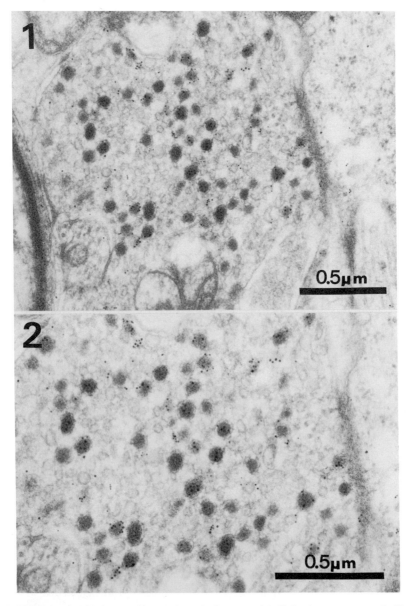

FIGURE 1: Electron micrograph of bouton labelled for somatostatin-like immunoreactivity with 5 nanometer gold particles. Note gold particles over large granular and large dense-core vesicles. From substantia gelatinosa of monkey spinal cord.

FIGURE 2: Higher power electron micrograph of portion of same bouton as in figure 1.

remained intact. Immunolabelling with the 5 and 10 nanometer gold particles was also easily discerned. These particles were usually found overlying large, granular or dense-core vesicles in both the fibers and boutons. Immunolabelling was also found overlying large granular and dense-core vesicle within HRP labelled fibers and boutons, unequivocally demonstrating that they were of dorsal root origin. The labelling results of each primary antiserum are described below. For each of these antisera, tissue from two monkeys was examined. The sections were cut from the caudal lumbar and first sacral segments. The ultrathin sections were cut from transverse blocks which contained laminae I-III.

Anti-somatostatin

Boutons labelled with the somatostatin antibody were found in various parts of the substantia gelatinosa and marginal zone. Labelled boutons contained a mixture of small, round, clear vesicles and large, dense-core vesicles. The boutons were of both large and medium size and established asymmetric contacts with dendritic profiles. Immunolabelling was almost entirely restricted to the large dense-core population (Figures 1 and 2). Profiles which were labelled both with HRP (confirming their dorsal root origin) and gold particles (confirming somatostatin-like immunoreactivity) were difficult to find. Boutons labelled only with gold particles were, however, easy to find. Whether this represents a true negative finding, or whether HRP fails to label this sub-population of primary afferent boutons well, or the immunostaining with anti-somatostatin fails to label HRP profiles could not be discerned. Because the majority of the antiserum labelling was in the inner substantia gelatinosa (lamina IIi) and because the inner substantia gelatinosa primary afferent labelling tends to be patchy, we suspect that our ultrathin sections did not include many HRP labelled profiles in this lamina, making the chances for double label poor.

Anti-substance P

Boutons labelled with the substance P antibody were mostly confined to the outermost portion of the substantia gelatinosa and were found throughout the marginal zone. The deeper portions of the dorsal horn were not examined in this study. As with the anti-somatostatin labelling, the gold particles were found mostly over large dense-core and granular vesicles. Immunolabelling varied from bouton to bouton. In some boutons, nearly every large dense-core vesicle was heavily labelled. This was found both in boutons which contained numerous dense-core vesicles, and other boutons in which only one or two dense-core vesicles were present. In others boutons, only a few dense-core vesicles were labelled even when many were present in a single ultrathin section. In still other boutons, even when many dense-core vesicles were present, immunolabelling was absent. This was especially apparent in the deeper substantia gelatinosa where many boutons contained large dense-core vesicles, but almost none exhibited immunolabelling. Boutons which were labelled with HRP via the root crush method were also found to contain labelled dense-core vesicles (Figure 3 and 4). As with the non-HRP labelled profiles, the number of dense-core vesicles labelled varied from bouton to bouton. Labelled boutons also usually contained many small, clear, round vesicles. Synaptic articulations were usually of the asymmetric type with prominent post-synaptic specializations.

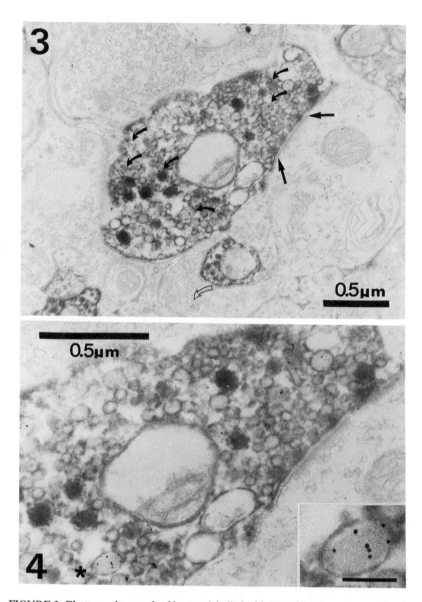

FIGURE 3: Electron micrograph of bouton labelled with HRP/DAB reaction product by crushing HRP into a dorsal rootlet. Large granular and dense-core vesicles (curved arrows) are labelled with substance P-like immunoreactivity by 5 nanometer gold particles. Straight arrow indicates limits of asymmetric synaptic specialization. Open curved arrow points to large dense-core vesicle labelled with gold particles (substance P-like immunoreactivity) in bouton unlabelled with HRP.

FIGURE 4: Higher power electron micrograph showing details from figure 3. Asterisk indicates gold particle-labelled vesicle shown at even higher power in insert at lower right. Scale bar in insert is 0.1 microns. Figures 3 and 4 are from superficial, spinal substantia gelatinosa of monkey.

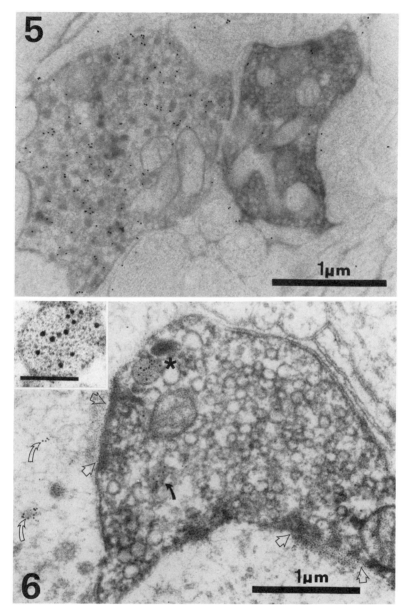

FIGURE 5: Electron micrograph of boutons labelled with HRP/DAB reaction product and labelled for CGRP-like immunoreactivity with 10 nanometer gold particles. Note labelling mostly over large dense-core vesicles. Ultrathin section not post stained with lead citrate and uranyl acetate so that HRP reaction product is easily visible.

FIGURE 6: Electron micrograph of another labelled primary afferent bouton demonstrating 5 nanometer gold particles which indicate CGRP-like immunoreactivity. Asterisk indicates labelled vesicle shown at higher power in insert at upper left. Calibration in insert is 0.1 micron. Dark curved arrow indicates another gold labelled vesicle. Open curved arrows indicate labelled vesicles in adjacent, non-HRP labelled bouton. Open arrows indicate possible synaptic specializations.

63

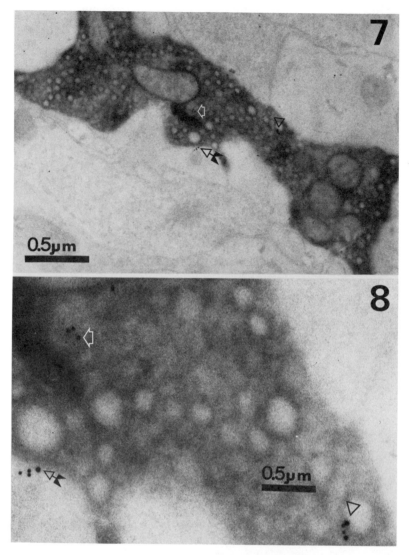

FIGURE 7: Electron micrograph of bouton from physiologically identified, single C-nociceptor axon (PP-20). Overall electron density is HRP reaction product. Section was reacted for substance P-like immunoreactivity with 5 nanometer gold particles. A few gold particles can be seen overlying a large dense-core vesicle (open, white arrow) and adjacent to another vesicle (triangle). Open arrow with flights points to gold particles over a dense-core vesicle in an adjacent, non-HRP labelled bouton. This light, gold labelling may not indicate specific immunoreactivity. Fiber from monkey spinal substantia gelatinosa. Section not post stained with lead citrate or uranyl acetate.

FIGURE 8: Higher power electron micrograph showing details of figure 7. All markings as in figure 7.

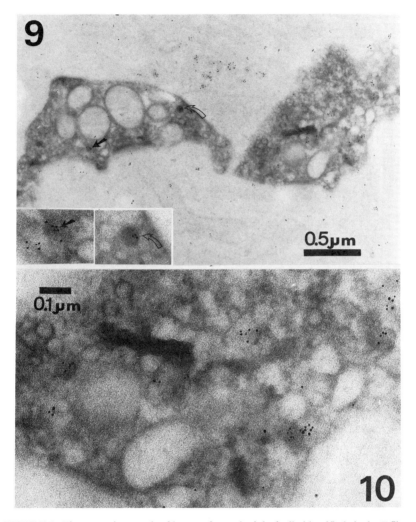

FIGURE 9: Electron micrograph of bouton from physiologically identified single C-fiber (HDM-37). Section was reacted for CGRP-like immunoreactivity with 5 nanometer gold particles. Arrows point to labelled, large dense-core vesicles shown at higher power in inserts at lower left. Note also gold labelling of dense-core vesicles in profile above HRP labelled bouton.

FIGURE 10: Higher power electron micrograph of right side of bouton in figure 9. Calibration in this figure is also calibration for inserts in figure 9. Figures 9 and 10 from monkey spinal substantia gelatinosa. Section not post stained with lead citrate or uranyl acetate.

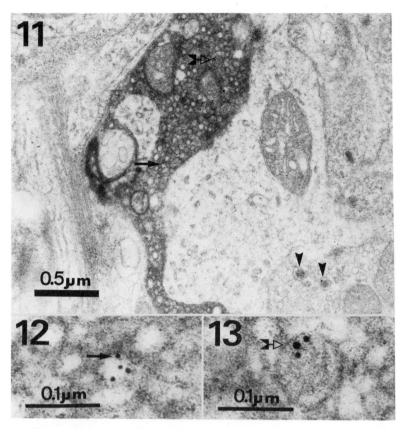

FIGURE 11: Electron micrograph of bouton from physiologically identified single C-nociceptor (PP-20). Section reacted for CGRP-like immunoreactivity with 5 nanometer gold particles. Arrows point to gold labelled vesicles. Arrow heads point to gold labelled vesicles in adjacent, non-HRP labelled profile.

FIGURE 12: Higher power electron micrograph showing gold labelled vesicle indicated by same type of arrow in figure 11.

FIGURE 13: Higher power electron micrograph showing gold labelled vesicle indicated with same type of arrow in figure 11. Figures 11-13 from monkey spinal substantia gelatinosa. Section post stained with lead citrate and uranyl acetate.

Anti-CGRP

Anti-CGRP labelled profiles were also found in superficial dorsal horn. The appearance of these boutons was nearly identical to those with anti substance P labelling. They were, however, more numerous than the anti substance P profiles. Again, most of the labelling was confined to large granular and dense-core vesicles. However, labelling was also occasionally found over small, clear vesicles (see figures 5 and 6). As with anti-substance P labelling, not all boutons containing dense-core vesicles were labelled. Instead, only those in the superficial substantia gelatinosa were found heavily labelled. Also, as with the substance P antibody, not every dense-core vesicle in a profile was labelled.

Immunolabelling in single C fibers

The positive immunolabelling of substance P- and CGRP-like substances in synaptic boutons identified as primary afferents by the presence of HRP served as positive controls which demonstrated that such labelling could be obtained in the spinal dorsal horn. We then attempted to immunolabel with anti-substance P and anti-CGRP C-fibers which were physiologically identified by staining with intraaxonal HRP. Anti-somatostatin was not attempted because of the poor labelling of HRP profiles obtained with this antibody as described above.

Anti-substance P labelling was very sparse in both of the single labelled fibers. Only the examples shown in figures 7 and 8 from PP-20 demonstrated much labelling. However, this labelling was not considered dense enough to rule out possible false labelling due to background.

Anti-CGRP labelling was much more dense. Several examples of labelled dense-core vesicles were found in both the identified nociceptor (PP-20) and the unidentified C fiber (HDM-37) (figures 9-13). As in the whole dorsal root labelled population, the labelling was largely confined to the large, dense-core population. In addition, not every large, dense-core vesicle within the HRP labelled profiles was labelled.

DISCUSSION

This study confirms the suitability of the post-embedding, immunostaining procedure for labelling putative peptides with immunogold in HRP labelled profiles in the spinal cord dorsal horn.

The results of this study confirm the presence of substance P- and CGRPlike immunoreactivity within primary afferent boutons in the superficial dorsal horn of the spinal cord. The detectable immunoreactivity for each antibody was largely confined to the large dense-core population. Whether this represents the entire intra-axonal store of these peptides or whether the peptide content in the cytoplasm or clear vesicle store has been lost or become inaccessible due to tissue processing could not be determined in the present study. The distribution of these peptides in the dorsal horn is consistent with light-level immunostaining studies in the primate dorsal horn. The presence of CGRP-like-immunoreactivity in the single stained C fiber and C nociceptor also directly demonstrates an association which has been postulated by others (Colin and Kruger, 1986; Carlton *et al*, 1987). Surprisingly little evidence for substance P immunolabelling was found in these single, physiologically identified fibers. This evidence is consistent with the results of Leah *et al*, (1985) who found it difficult to label the dorsal root ganglion cells of C nociceptors with substance P immunoreactivity. However, the present sample is extremely limited and, thus, the generality of these results is questionable. Further analysis is needed to determine the suitability of this technique, and to answer fundamental questions about the localization of peptides in primary afferent nerve terminals.

ACKNOWLEDGEMENTS

The authors would like to thank Mr Scott Donaghy for service beyond the call of duty in helping to prepare the figures for this manuscript as well as for his usual technical expertise during and after the experiments. Supported by NINCDS grant #RO1-NS16433 and #P01-NS14899 and NIDA grant #R01-DA04420.

REFERENCES

BURGESS, P.R. AND PERL, E.R. (1973). Cutaneous mechanoreceptors and nociceptors. In *Handbook of Sensory Physiology. Somatosensory System*, ed. IGGO, A., pp. 2978. Berlin: Springer-Verlag.

CARLTON, S.M., MCNEILL, D.L., CHUNG, K. AND COGGESHALL, R.E. (1987). A light and electron microscopic level analysis of calcitonin gene-related peptide (CGRP) in the spinal cord of the primate: an immunohistochemical study. *Neurosci.Lett.* **82**, 145-150.

COLIN, S. AND KRUGER, L. (1986). Peptidergic nociceptive axon visualization in whole-mount preparations of cornea and tympanic membrane in rat. *Brain Res.* **398**, 199-203.

DIFIGLIA, M., ARONIN, N. AND LEEMAN, S.E. (1982). Light microscopic and ultrastructural localization of immunoreactive substance P in the dorsal horn of monkey spinal cord. *Neuroscience* **7**, 1127-1139.

DODD, J., JAHR, C.E., HAMILTON, P.N., HEATH, M.J., MATTHEW, W.D. AND JESSELL, T.M. (1983). Cytochemical and physiological properties of sensory and dorsal horn neurons that transmit cutaneous sensation. *Cold Spring Harbor Symp.Quant.Biol.* **48**, 685-695.

HÖKFELT, T., KELLERTH, J.O., NILSSON, G. AND PERNOW, B. (1975). Experimental immunohistochemical studies on the localization and distribution of substance P in cat primary sensory neurons. *Brain Res.* **100**, 235-252.

HÖKFELT, T., ELDE, R., JOHANSSON, O., LUFT, R., NILSSON, G. AND ARIMURA, A. (1976). Immunohistochemical evidence for separate populations of somatostatin-containing and substance P-containing primary afferent neurons in the rat. *Neuroscience* **1**, 131-136.

HÖKFELT, T., LJUNGDAHL, A., TERENIUS, L., ELDE, R. AND NILSSON, G. (1977). Immunohistochemical analysis of peptide pathways possibly related to pain and analgesia: enkephalin and substance P. *Proc.Natl.Acad.Sci.USA* **74**, 3081-3085.

HÖKFELT, T., LUNDBERG, J.M., SCHULTZBERG, M., JOHANSSON, O., SKIRBOLL, L., ANGGARD, A., FREDHOLM, B., HAMBERGER, B., PERNOW, B., REHFELD, J. AND GOLDSTEIN, M. (1980). Cellular localization of peptides in neural structures. *Proc.R.Soc.Lond.[Biol]* **210**, 63-77.

HÖKFELT, T., VINCENT, S., DALSGAARD, C.J., SKIRBOLL, L., JOHANSSON, O., SCHULTZBERG, M., LUNDBERG, J.M., ROSELL, S., PERNOW, B. AND JANCSO, G. (1982). Distribution of substance P in brain and periphery and its possible role as a co-transmitter. *Ciba.Found.Symp.* 84-106.

HONDA, C.N., RETHELYI, M. AND PETRUSZ, P. (1983). Preferential immunohistochemical localization of vasoactive intestinal polypeptide (VIP) in the sacral spinal cord of the cat: light and electron microscopic observations. *J.Neurosci.* **3**, 2183-2196.

HUNT, S.P. (1983). Cytochemistry of the Spinal Cord. In *Chem. Neuroanatomy*, ed. EMSON, P.C., pp. 53-84. Raven Press.

IVERSEN, L.L. (1984). Amino acids and peptides: fast and slow chemical signals in the nervous system?. *Proc.R.Soc.Lond.[Biol]* **221**, 245-260.

JESSELL, T.M., TSUNOO, A., KANAZAWA, I. AND OTSUKA, M. (1979). Substance P: depletion in the dorsal horn of rat spinal cord after section of the peripheral processes of primary sensory neurons. *Brain Res.* **168**, 247-259.

JU, G., HÖKFELT, T., BRODIN, E., FAHRENKRUG, J., FISCHER, J.A., FREY, P., ELDE, R.P. AND BROWN, J.C. (1987). Primary sensory neurons of the rat showing calcitonin gene-related peptide immunoreactivity and their relation to substance P-, somatostatin-, galanin-, vasoactive intestinal polypeptide- and cholecystokinin-immunoreactive ganglion cells. *Cell Tissue Res.* **247**, 417-431.

LEAH, J.D., CAMERON, A.A. AND SNOW, P.J. (1985). Neuropeptides in physiologically identified mammalian sensory neurones. *Neurosci.Lett.* **56**, 257263.

LIGHT, A.R. AND PERL, E.R. (1979a). Spinal termination of functionally identified primary afferent neurons with slowly conducting myelinated fibers. *J.Comp.Neurol.* **186**, 133-150.

LIGHT, A.R. AND PERL, E.R. (1979b). Reexamination of the dorsal root projection to the spinal dorsal horn including observations on the differential termination of coarse and fine fibers. *J.Comp.Neurol.* **186**, 117-131.

LYNN, B. AND HUNT, S.P. (1984). Afferent C-fibres: physiological and biochemical correlations. *Trends in Neurosci.* **7**, 186-188.

MENSE, S. AND PRABHAKAR, N.R. (1986). Spinal termination of nociceptive afferent fibres from deep tissues in the cat. *Neurosci.Lett.* **66**, 169-174.

METZ, C.B., KAVOOKJIAN, A.M. AND LIGHT, A.R. (1982). Techniques for HRP intracellular staining of neural elements for light and electron microscopic analyses. *Journal of Electrophysiological Techniques* **9**, 151-163.

MORGAN, C., NADELHAFT, I. AND DEGROAT, W.C. (1986). The distribution within the spinal cord of visceral primary afferent axons carried by the lumbar colonic nerve of the cat. *Brain Res.* **398**, 11-17.

RETHELYI, M., LIGHT, A.R. AND PERL, E.R. (1982). Synaptic complexes formed by functionally defined primary afferent units with fine myelinated fibers. *J.Comp.Neurol.* **207**, 381-393.

RUDA, M.A., BENNETT, G.J. AND DUBNER, R. (1986). Neurochemistry and neural circuitry in the dorsal horn. *Prog.Brain Res.* **66**, 219-268.

STERNINI, C. AND BRECHA, N. (1986). Immunocytochemical identification of islet cells and nerve fibers containing calcitonin gene-related peptide-like immunoreactivity in the rat pancreas. *Gastroenterology* **90**, 1155-1563.

STERNINI, C., REEVE, J.R. Jr. AND BRECHA, N. (1987). Distribution and characterization of calcitonin gene-related peptide immunoreactivity in the digestive system of normal and capsaicin-treated rats. *Gastroenterology.* **93**, 852-862.

SUGIURA, Y., LEE, C.L. AND PERL, E.R. (1986). Central projections of identified, unmyelinated (C) afferent fibers innervating mammalian skin. *Science* **234**, 358-361.

YAKSH, T.L. (1986). The central pharmacology of primary afferents with emphasis on the disposition and role of primary afferent substance P. *In Spinal Afferent Processing*, ed. YAKSH, T.L., pp. 165-195. New York: Plenum.

IMMUNOREACTIVITY OF RAT PRIMARY AFFERENT NEURONES WITH C- AND A-FIBRES

Sally Lawson, Peter McCarthy and Pamela Waddell

Department of Physiology, The Medical School, University Walk, Bristol BS8 1TD, U.K.

Sensory neurones are commonly classified into conduction velocity (CV) groups, the C-, Aδ- and Aα/β- fibre groups. If the functional significance of these groups is to become clear, the borderlines between the groups need to be clearly defined. However, fibres are sometimes classified as C on the basis of their CV in the periphery, although, as we show below, some of these may conduct in the Aδ range nearer the ganglion. Furthermore, an assumption is sometimes made that small dorsal root ganglion (DRG) neurones have C-fibres and thus that some peptides found predominantly in small neurones are only in C-fibre cells. However it has been shown in the rat that, although C-fibres arise from small neurones, A-fibres can arise from all sizes of neurones including the very small ones (Harper and Lawson 1985). Therefore, we have correlated the fibre CV of neurones directly with their immunoreactivity. The antibodies we have used are anti-substance P, anti-calcitonin gene related peptide, 2C5 and RT97.

Substance P may be a neuromodulator or neurotransmitter for some primary afferent nerves (eg Pernow, 1983) and may have a role in neurogenic inflammation (Lembeck and Holzer, 1979). Substance P-like immunoreactivity (SP-LI) is found in about 20% of neurones in rat DRGs (Hökfelt *et al*, 1976, Lawson *et al*, 1985), and these are mostly small. In the cat SP-LI was found in 12/26 C-fibre neurones and in 0/4 Aδ neurones (Leah *et al*, 1985). There is no direct information on CV of SP-LI cells in the rat.

Calcitonin gene-related peptide (CGRP) released from sensory neurones may be involved directly in neurogenic vasodilation (Brain *et al*, 1985) as well as in potentiating the action of the tachykinins in neurogenic inflammation (Gamse and Saria, 1985). Its relationship to sensory function is not clear, although it is present in some nociceptive neurones (Silverman and Kruger, 1988). CGRP-LI is found in 40-50% of neurones in rat lumbar DRGs, mostly small, but also in some medium and large neurones (Lee *et al*, 1985).

2C5, an antibody against a lactoseries carbohydrate chain labels 30-50% of all DRG neurones. These are mainly small plus a few medium and large neurones (Lawson *et al*, 1985). The 2C5 positive neurones are particularly sensitive to the neurotoxic effects of neonatal capsaicin, being more greatly reduced in number than SP-LI or CGRP-LI neurones (Lawson, 1987).

RT97 is a monoclonal antineurofilament antibody which labels only the *light* subpopulation of DRG neurones of the rat leaving the *small dark* neurones unlabelled (Lawson *et al*, 1984).

Electrophysiological experiments were performed on L4, L5 and L6 DRGs of 6-8 week old female Wistar rats. The ganglia with attached peripheral nerves and dorsal roots were removed under pentobarbitone anaesthesia (40-60 mg/kg Sagatal intraperitoneally), placed in a perspex recording chamber (McCarthy and Lawson, 1988) and superfused with oxygenated balanced salt solution at 36.5°C, which contained: NaCl 140 mM; KCl 5 mM; CaCl 2 mM; MgCl 2 mM; glucose 5 mM; Hepes buffer 5 mM; pH 7.4. The nerves were led into adjacent paraffin-filled troughs also at 36.5°C, and were laid over stimulating electrodes. Intracellular voltage recordings were made from the somata of the DRG neurones. Stimuli to the nerve were 0.1-1 ms duration square wave pulses of 1-50 V at 1 Hz. An estimate of peripheral nerve and/or dorsal root CV was made from the latency from nerve stimulation to the start of the intracellular action potential. The distribution of peripheral nerve CVs in cells recorded from L4, L5 and L6 ganglia is shown in Figure 1.

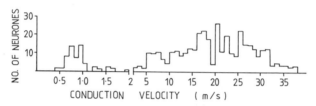

FIGURE 1: For explanation see text

Conduction Velocity: Neurones with CVs of <1.3 m/s were classified as having C-fibres on the basis of the clear peak below 1.3 m/s (see histogram). A-fibre neurones were divided into Aδ (1.3 m/s) and Aα/β (12 m/s). The 12 m/s boundary between Aδ- and Aα/β- fibres was chosen from this data (histogram) and from the more prominent Aδ peak in L6 neurones, which had an upper limit of 12 m/s. Dorsal root CVs are on average slightly slower than peripheral nerve CVs in the rat, but for a particular neurone usually fall into the same CV group.

Changes in CV along the peripheral nerve: This possibility was examined by measuring *accurate* CV from several points along the nerve. *Accurate* measurements were calculated from the difference in conduction time and distance from two stimulation points to the DRG. There was no consistent change in CV in Aα/β- fibres (n=11) along the length of the nerve, up to about 30 mm from the DRG. Over this distance, however, 2/3 slow Aδ-fibres slowed to conduct in the C-fibre range more peripherally, and 5/6 C-fibres slowed by 30-50% (average 43%) between 14-28 mm from the ganglion. It has also been shown that more than half the fibres conducting in the Aδ range between the sciatic notch and the DRG conducted in the C-fibre range, from the tibial nerve to the sciatic notch (Harper and Lawson 1985). Thus there is clear slowing towards the periphery in a high proportion of C- and Aδ-fibres.

Immunocytochemistry: In neurones to be studied immunocytochemically, intracellular dye injections were made following electrophysiological characterisation of the neurones. Dyes used were Lucifer yellow or ethidium bromide (see McCarthy and Lawson 1988). DRGs were fixed in Zamboni's fixative and were incubated overnight at 4°C in 30% sucrose in 0.1M phosphate buffered saline, pH 7.4. Serial cryostat sections

(7 μm) were cut and the sections with profiles of dye injected neurones were incubated at 4°C for 48 hours with primary antibodies. The antibodies were: polyclonal anti-SP antibody donated by P.Keen, a polyclonal anti-CGRP antibody donated by J. Polak, monoclonal antibody RT97 donated by J. Wood or monoclonal antibody 2C5 donated by B. Randle. Sections were later incubated with fluorescence (FITC or TRITC) conjugated second layer antibodies for 30 minutes at room temperature. The second layer antibodies were goat anti-rabbit IgG for SP and CGRP, goat anti-mouse IgG for RT97 or goat anti-mouse IgM for 2C5. The cells were visualised under epifluorescence. Colchicine was not used in any of these studies.

For each antibody used, the range of cross sectional areas of these immunoreactive dye-injected cells was similar to the range for immunoreactive cells in histological studies of lumbar ganglia in rats of the same age. This indicates that dye injection *per se* did not affect cell size or cause false positives for these antibodies.

TABLE 1: POSITIVE CELLS IN EACH CONDUCTION VELOCITY RANGE

	RANGE	C	A δ	A α/β
SP-LI	0.5- 9.5	53% (15)	21% (29)	0% (36)
CGRP-LI	0.5-28.5	42% (12)	40% (23)	14% (36)
2C5	0.4-14.6	73% (11)	12% (25)	8% (34)
RT97	0.8-39.0	23% (17)	100% (31)	100% (39)

Legend to Table 1: Summary of the range (in m/s) of conduction velocities of neurones that were positive for the antibodies shown. The percentages of the injected neurones which were subsequently found to be positive are given with the number of injected cells tested for each antibody in brackets. CV measurements were made from a point 10-25mm from the DRG. It is possible that some of the peripheral nerve Aδ fibres may have conducted in the C-fibre range more peripherally.

In conclusion: We understand the term C-fibre to imply that the fibre conducts in the C-fibre range along its entire length. Fibres conducting the Aδ range near the DRG are therefore properly classified as Aδ even if, as our results indicate, a number of them may conduct in the C-fibre range more peripherally. We have shown that some neurones with C-fibres as well as some with Aδ fibres have SP-LI. CGRP-LI was found in neurones with C-fibres, as well as some with Aδ and some with Aα/β-fibres. It would be extremely interesting to know if the functions of the peptide containing Aδ neurones differ from functions of peptide containing C-fibre neurones. Neurones labelled with 2C5 mostly had C-fibres but a few had Aδ- or Aα/β-fibres. These data also show that all small dark (RT97 negative) neurones have C-fibres although some C-fibre neurones,as well as all A-fibre neurones, belong to the light (RT97 positive) population. Therefore RT97 staining of the soma is a good, but not a perfect, indication of whether the fibre is myelinated, although lack of RT97 staining reliably indicates that the fibre is unmyelinated. These results demonstrate the importance of direct correlation of immunocytochemical and electrophysiological data within the same neurone. Furthermore, assumptions about CV on the basis of cell size or peripheral CV measurements may be misleading.

This research was supported by the MRC, UK.

REFERENCES

BRAIN, S.D., WILLIAMS, T.J., TIPPINS, J.R., MORRIS, H.R. AND MACINTYRE, I. (1985) Calcitonin gene-related peptide is a potent vasodilator. *Nature*, **313**, 54-56.

GAMSE, R. AND SARIA, A. (1985) Potentiation of tachykinin-induced plasma extravasation by calcitonin gene-related peptide. *Eur. J.Pharm.*, **114**, 61-66

HARPER, A.A, AND LAWSON, S.N. (1985) Conduction velocity is related to morphological cell type in rat dorsal root ganglion neurones. *J.Physiol.*, **359**, 31-46

HÖKFELT, T., ELDE, R., JOHANSSON, O., LUFT, R., NILSSON, G. AND ARIMURA, A. (1976) Immunohistochemical evidence for separate populations of somatostatin-containing and substance P containing primary afferent neurons in the rat. *Neurosci.*, 1, 131-136

LAWSON, S.N. (1987) Immunocytochemically defined populations of dorsal root ganglion neurones remaining in the rat after neonatal capsaicin. *Neurol. and Neurobiol.*, **30**, 125-132

LAWSON, S.N., HARPER, A.A., HARPER, E.I., GARSON, J.A. AND ANDERTON, B.H. (1984) A monoclonal antibody against neurofilament specifically labels a subpopulation of rat sensory neurones. *J. Comp. Neurol.*, **228**, 263-272

LAWSON, S.N., HARPER, A.A., HARPER, E.I., GARSON, J.A., COAKHAM, H.B. AND RANDLE, B.J. (1985) Monoclonal antibody 2C5: a marker for a subpopulation of small neurones in rat dorsal root ganglia. *J. Neurosci.*, **16**, 365-374

LEAH, J.D., CAMERON, A.A. AND SNOW, P.J. (1985) Neuropeptides in physiologically identified mammalian sensory neurones. *Neuroscience Letters*, **56**, 257-263

LEE, Y., TAKAMI, Y., KAWAI, Y., GIRGIS, S., EMSON, P.C. AND TOHYAMA, M. (1985) Distribution of calcitonin gene-related peptide in the rat peripheral nervous system with reference to its coexistence with substance P. *Neurosci.*, **15**, 1227-1237

LEMBECK, F. AND HOLZER, P. (1979) Substance P as neurogenic mediator of antidromic vasodilation and neurogenic plasma extravasation. *Naunyn Schmiedebergs Arch. Pharm.*, **310**, 175-183

MCCARTHY, P.W. AND LAWSON, S.N. (1988) Differential intracellular labelling of identified neurones with two fluorescent dyes. *Brain Res. Bull.*, **20**, 261-265

PERNOW, B. (1983) Substance P. *Pharmacol. Rev.*, **35**, 85-141

SILVERMAN, J.D. AND KRUGER, L. (1988) Lectin and neuropeptide labelling of separate populations of dorsal root ganglion neurones and associated *nociceptor* thin axons in rat testis and cornea whole-mount preparations. *Somatosens. Res.*, **5**, 259-267

COEXISTENCE OF PEPTIDES IN PRIMARY AFFERENT NEURONS

Virginia S. Seybold, *Mary M. Tuchscherer and Mary G. Garry

Department of Cell Biology and Neuroanatomy, University of Minnesota, Minneapolis
and *Northwestern College of Chiropractic, Minneapolis, MN, USA

Primary afferent neurons have been shown with immunohistochemistry to contain a variety of peptide-like substances. In fact, some neurons contain more than one peptide (Dalsgaard *et al*, 1982; Wiesenfeld-Hallin *et al*, 1984; Leah *et al*, 1985; Lee *et al*, 1985; Skofitsch and Jacobowitz, 1985; Tuchscherer and Seybold, 1985; Gibbins *et al*, 1987). We are interested in the possibility that particular peptides, alone or in combination, may be markers for functional categories of sensory neurons or targets of these neurons. Toward this end, we have studied the expression of peptide-immunoreactivity in dorsal root ganglion cells of cat and rat. Post-translational modification of amino acid sequences contained in the peptide precursor molecules, however, may alter the antigenic determinants expressed in a perikaryon. An antigenic determinant visualized in a neuronal perikaryon by immunohistochemistry may be cleaved or modified to an unrecognizable sequence, or the epitope recognized by an antibody may be created. For this reason we have also investigated the coexistence of peptide-immunoreactivities in axonal varicosities of primary afferent neurons in the spinal cord.

Since the cat is a common model for studies of the spinal cord, and there are relatively few studies of cat dorsal root ganglia, we were interested in neurochemical studies of primary afferent neurons in this species. Data on cat can add to our appreciation of similarities and differences among species in the expression of coexistence of peptides by primary afferent neurons. Immunofluorescence was used to determine the extent to which several peptides coexist with substance P (SP) or with somatostatin (SOM) in neurons within selected lumbar dorsal root ganglia of cat. Two antigens were visualized simultaneously in each tissue section using the approach outlined by Wessendorf and Elde (1985). Complete details concerning the antisera and methods of analysis are presented in Garry *et al*, (1989). We focused on dorsal root ganglia (DRG) L5 and L6 of cat because their somatotopy approximates that of rat ganglion L4, which has been the focus of previous studies (Tuchscherer and Seybold, 1985, 1988). Furthermore, these ganglia contain sensory neurons whose axons traverse the sciatic nerve in cat and rat, respectively, and these ganglia are minimally associated with visceral afferent neurons (Brown and Fuchs, 1975; Morgan *et al*, 1981; Kuo *et al*, 1984; Nadelhaft and Booth, 1984; Swett and Wolf, 1985; Molander and Grant, 1986; Schmalbruch, 1986).

When cat DRG L5 and L6 were treated with colchicine (500 μg total dose), intrathecally, 48 hours prior to perfusion, neuronal perikarya were immunoreactive for

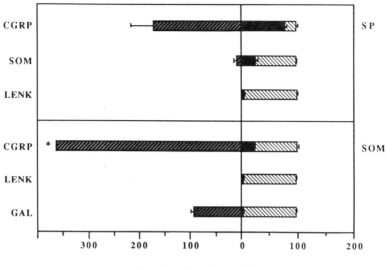

Relative Number of Cells

FIGURE 1: Histograms illustrating coexistence of peptides with substance P or somatostatin in perikarya of cat lumbar dorsal root ganglia. Each line of bars represents observations for combinations of one substance (listed to the left of the histograms) with substance P (upper group) or somatostatin (lower group). The bars to the left of zero represent the relative numbers of cells which were immunoreactive for each substance alone. The bars to the right of zero are stacked. Inside bars represent the relative number of cells which were immunoreactive for the substance+SP or SOM. The outside bars represent the relative numbers of cells which were immunoreactive for SP or SOM alone. Data were normalized to 100 cells immunoreactive for SP or SOM with each combination of antibodies used. Values represent the mean±S.E.M.; n=4 for the SP group; n=3 for the SOM group. (*) Actual value was 460±224.

calcitonin gene-related peptide (CGRP), galanin (GAL), leu-enkephalin (LE), SOM and SP. Our negative results were also noteworthy: we did not observe immunoreactivity for bombesin, dynorphin A1-8 (DYN), met-enkephalin, serotonin, vasopressin, or vasoactive intestinal polypeptide (VIP) in these ganglia. Since bombesin and VIP immunoreactivities have been visualized in perikarya of more caudal DRG of cat (Basbaum and Glazer, 1983; Leah *et al*, 1985; Cameron *et al*, 1988), it is likely that these peptides are associated with sensory neurons that innervate pelvic viscera.

Among the antisera that were immunoreactive with cat DRG, we obtained data indicating that three peptides coexist with SP (CGRP/SP, LE/SP and SOM/SP), and an additional two peptides coexist with SOM (CGRP/SOM and LE/SOM). Data on combinations of peptides which coexisted in lumbar DRG of cat are summarized in Figure 1. Coexistence was not complete for any combinations studied, with the exception of LE-immunoreactive perikarya. This population of cells, however, was sparse. Similarly, a few cells were immunoreactive for GAL/SOM, but these were less than 2% of the total populations of GAL or SOM immunoreactive perikarya. Cells that were immunoreactive for only one of the peptides examined in a combination were frequently observed. The proportions of coexistence of SOM/SP and CGRP/SP determined for populations of perikarya analyzed in our study were comparable to those reported by Snow and co-workers (Leah *et al*, 1985; Cameron *et al*, 1988). Since these earlier reports focused on more caudal ganglia, the similarities in data suggest that CGRP, SOM and SP may be preferentially associated with cutaneous, vascular or skeletal muscle afferent neurons as compared with visceral afferents.

Immunofluorescence was also the optimal method for addressing the coexistence of peptides in neuronal varicosities visualized with the light microscope. There is no direct marker for primary afferent neuron varicosities that would be compatible with the two fluorophores used in immunohistochemistry. We therefore used the disappearance of peptide immunoreactivity after dorsal rhizotomy to infer which populations of immunoreactive varicosities within the superficial laminae of the dorsal horn are associated with primary afferent neurons. Computerized image processing was used to quantify changes in the densities of immunoreactive varicosities and the coexistence of two peptides within varicosities. The image processing system and approach are described in a previous publication (Tuchscherer *et al*, 1987). Densities of immunoreactive varicosities in laminae I and II were selected for analysis because peptides have been localized to predominantly small diameter perikarya in dorsal root ganglia (Hökfelt *et al*, 1976; Tuchscherer and Seybold, 1985), and small diameter primary afferent neurons are known to terminate within these laminae (Kumazawa and Perl, 1978; Sugiura *et al*, 1986). A computer program was used to count the number of singly- and doubly-labelled varicosities within the superficial laminae. Details concerning antisera and analysis of data are reported in Tuchscherer and Seybold (1988).

Figure 2 summarizes data concerning coexistence of substances with SP in varicosities of primary afferent neurons of rat. These data are based on material obtained from spinal segment L4 after multiple unilateral dorsal rhizotomies (L2-L6)

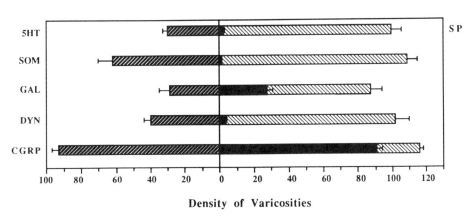

Density of Varicosities

FIGURE 2: Histogram illustrating coexistence of peptides and serotonin with substance P in varicosities associated with primary afferent axons within laminae I and II outer of rat spinal cord. Densities of varicosities were calculated by subtracting values obtained from the dorsal horn ipsilateral to the lesion from values obtained contralateral to the lesion. Each line of bars represents observations for combinations of one substance (listed to the left of the histogram) with SP. The bars to the left of zero represent the density of varicosities which were immunoreactive for each substance alone. The bars to the right of zero are stacked. Inside bars represent the density of varicosities that were immunoreactive for each substance + SP; the outside bars represent the density of varicosities which were immunoreactive for SP alone. Thus, the difference between 0 and the outer limit of the outside bars represents the total density of SP immunoreactive varicosities. Values represent a mean±S.E.M. (n=6). The actual area quantified for laminae I + II(outer) averaged $8000 \pm 170 \, \mu m^2$ in control animals. Data were normalized to $6600 \, \mu m^2$.

and a 10-day survival period.   Densities of varicosities were calculated by subtracting values obtained from the dorsal horn ipsilateral to the lesion from values obtained contralateral to the lesion. Data were corrected for changes in volume of laminae I and II as a result of primary afferent axon degeneration. Consistent with observations of dorsal root ganglia of rat, SP did not coexist to an appreciable extent with SOM, however, coexistence of CGRP/SP and GAL/SP were observed.   Coexistence of CGRP/SP in perikarya within rat DRG has been described (Lee *et al*, 1985). Interestingly, the values for GAL/SP and CGRP/SP were equal to values observed in control animals (Tuchscherer and Seybold, 1988).   This suggests that the total populations of varicosities which are immunoreactive for these combinations of peptides in the superficial laminae of the dorsal horn of normal animals may be associated with primary afferent neurons. Also noteworthy was that a portion of the DYN-immunoreactive varicosities was depleted by dorsal rhizotomy suggesting that DYN is contained in primary afferent neurons of rat. Although SP and DYN coexisted in varicosities within control animals, there was no significant change in the density of DYN/SP immunoreactive varicosities in laminae I and II with dorsal rhizotomy. Therefore, varicosities in the dorsal horn which contain DYN/SP most likely arise from intrinsic   or   descending   sources.   Importantly,   the   density   of   neurotensin-immunoreactive varicosities was not changed by dorsal rhizotomy indicating that none of the changes observed on the side ipsilateral to the lesion were nonspecific due to ischemia.

The comparative studies briefly described above are relevant to two issues regarding the neurochemistry of primary afferent neurons. Firstly, there are species differences in the expression of peptides by primary afferent neurons. At one level, this issue concerns the expression of a peptide by dorsal root ganglion cells in general. For example, some guinea pig sensory neurons express CCK-8 (Buck *et al*, 1983; Gibbins *et al*, 1987), but there is evidence that rat primary afferent neurons do not express the message for CCK-8 (Rethelyi *et al*, 1987). On another level, our data indicate that there is variability among species in the patterns of coexistence of peptides among primary afferent neurons. Substance P and SOM coexist in cat but do not coexist in rat primary afferent neurons (Hökfelt *et al*, 1976; Tuchscherer and Seybold, 1985). Whether these differences have functional significance remains to be determined.

It is also important to note that there are several similarities between rat and cat in the expression of peptides by primary afferent neurons. These include the lack of coexistence of SOM and GAL (see Ju *et al*, 1987 for data on rat) as well as the pattern of coexistence of CGRP/SP. It is especially noteworthy that we have observed similar proportional coexistence of CGRP/SP between rat and cat primary afferent neurons when using the same antibodies and comparable spinal levels. The conservation of both pattern and proportion underscores the potential for function of these substances.

The second issue concerns apparent discrepancies in the visualization of peptides in the perikarya and the varicosities of primary afferent neurons at the site of termination of their axons in the spinal cord. The decrease in DYN immunoreactivity after dorsal rhizotomy suggests DYN is present in primary afferent neurons, but this result is not confirmed by our observations of dorsal root ganglia from rats treated with colchicine. Similarly, we are not able to visualize bombesin immunoreactivity in DRG of cats treated with colchicine, but bombesin immunoreactive varicosities are significantly depleted from the spinal cord following dorsal rhizotomy (Garry *et al*, 1988). These data emphasize the importance of having multiple markers for the synthesis of peptides in neurons.   We cannot exclude the possibility that the decreases in peptide immunoreactivity we observed after dorsal rhizotomy are secondary to the loss of afferent input. *In situ* hybridization studies that use probes for the mRNA that codes the peptide sequence are important for confirming that an epitope (*eg.*, DYN or bombesin) is being created during axonal transport in primary afferent neurons. Alternately, it would be desirable to have a marker that is positive for axons of primary afferent neurons and that can be used in conjunction with immunohistochemistry to determine occurrence of peptides within axonal terminals. Lectin binding visualized with fluorescent labels (Plenderleith *et al*, 1988) may be useful in this regard.

REFERENCES

BASBAUM, A.I. AND GLAZER, E.J. (1983). Immunoreactive vasoactive intestinal polypeptide is concentrated in the sacral spinal cord: A possible marker for pelvic visceral afferent fibers. *Somatosensory Research* **1**, 69-82.

BROWN, P.B. AND FUCHS, J.L. (1975). Somatotopic representation of hindlimb skin in cat dorsal horn. *Journal of Neurophysiology* **38**, 1-9.

BUCK, S.H., WALLSH, J.H., DAVIS, T.P., BROWN, M.R., YAMAMURA, H.I. AND BURKS, T.F. (1983). Characterization of the peptide and sensory neurotoxic effects of capsaicin in the guinea pig. *Journal of Neuroscience* **3**, 2064-2074.

CAMERON, A.A., LEAH, J.D. AND SNOW, P.J. (198X). The coexistence of neuropeptides in feline sensory neurons. *Neuroscience*, in press.

DALSGAARD, C.-J., VINCENT, S.R., HÖKFELT, T., LUNDBERG, J.M., DAHLSTRÖM, A., SCHULTZBERG, M., DOCKRAY, G.J. AND CUELLO, A.C. (1982). Coexistence of cholecystokinin- and substance P-like peptides in neurons of the dorsal root ganglia of the rat. *Neuroscience Letters* **33**, 159-163.

GARRY, M.G., AIMONE, L. D., YAKSH, T.L. AND SEYBOLD, V.S. (1988). Coexistence of peptides in primary afferent neurons in cat spinal cord. *Society for Neuroscience Abstracts* **14**, 354.

GARRY, M.G., MILLER, K.E. AND SEYBOLD, V.S. (1989). Lumbar dorsal root ganglia of cat: A quantitative study of peptide immunoreactivity and cell size. *Journal of Comparative Neurology* (in press).

GIBBINS, I.L., FURNESS, J.B. AND COSTA, M. (1987). Pathway-specific patterns of the co-existence of substance P, calcitonin gene-related peptide, cholecystokinin and dynorphin in neurons of the dorsal root ganglia of the guinea pig. *Cell and Tissue Research* **248**, 417-437.

HÖKFELT, T., ELDE, R., JOHANSSON, O., LUFT, R., NILSSON, G. AND ARIMURA, A. (1976). Immunohistochemical evidence for separate populations of somatostatin-containing and substance P-containing primary afferent neurons in the rat. *Neuroscience* **1**, 131-136.

JU, G., HÖKFELT, T., BRODIN, E., FAHRENKRUG, J., FISCHER, J.A., FREY, P., ELDE, R. P. AND BROWN, J. C. (1987). Primary sensory neurons of the rat showing calcitonin gene-related peptide immunoreactivity and their relation to substance P-, somatostatin-, galanin-, vasoactive intestinal polypeptide- and cholecystokinin-immunoreactive ganglion cells. *Cell and Tissue Research* **247**, 417-431.

KUMAZAWA, T. AND PERL, E.R. (1978). Excitation of marginal and substantia gelatinosa neurons in the primate spinal cord: Indications of their place in dorsal horn functional organization. *Journal of Comparative Neurology* **177**, 417-434.

KUO, D.C., ORAVITZ, J.J., ESKAY, R. AND DEGROAT, W.C. (1984). Substance P in renal afferent perikarya identified by retrograde transport of fluorescent dye.

Brain Research **323**, 168-171.

LEAH, J.D., CAMERON, A.A., KELLY, W.L. AND SNOW, P.J. (1985). Coexistence of peptide immunoreactivity in sensory neurons of the cat. *Neuroscience* **16**, 683-690.

LEE, Y., KAWAI, Y., SHIOSAKA, S., TAKAMI, K., KIJAMA, H., HILLYARD, C.J., GIRGIS, S., MacINTYRE, I., EMSON, P.C. AND TOHYAMA, M. (1985). Coexistence of calcitonin gene-related peptide and substance P-like peptides in single cells of the trigeminal ganglion of the rat: Immunohistochemical analysis. *Brain Research* **330**, 194-196.

MOLANDER, C. AND GRANT, G. (1985). Cutaneous projections from the rat hindlimb foot to the substantia gelatinosa of the spinal cord studied by transganglionic transport of WGA-HRP conjugate. *Journal of Comparative Neurology* **237**, 476-484.

MORGAN, C., NADELHAFT, I. AND DEGROAT, W.C. (1981). The distribution of visceral primary afferents from the pelvic nerve to Lissauer's tract and the spinal gray matter and its relationship to the sacral parasympathetic nucleus. *Journal of Comparative Neurology* **201**, 415-440.

NADELHAFT, I. AND BOOTH, A. (1984). The location and morphology of preganglionic neurons and the distribution of visceral afferents from the rat pelvic nerve: A horseradish peroxidase study. *Journal of Comparative Neurology* **226**, 238-245.

PLENDERLEITH, M.B., CAMERON, A.A., KEY, B. AND SNOW, P.J. (1988). Soybean-agglutinin binds to a subpopulation of primary afferent neurons in the cat. *Neuroscience Letters* **86**, 257-262.

RETHELYI, M., McGEHEE, D. AND LUND, P.K. (1986). Neuronal localization of cholecystokinin mRNAs in rat and guinea pig brain. *Society for Neuroscience Abstracts* **12**, 1041.

SCHMALBRUCH, H. (1986). Fiber composition of the rat sciatic nerve. *Anatomical Record* **251**, 71-81.

SKOFITSCH, G. AND JACOBOWITZ, D.M. (1985). Calcitonin gene-related peptide coexists with substance P in capsaicin sensitive neurons and sensory ganglia of the rat. *Peptides* **6**, 747-754.

SUGIURA, Y., LEE, C.L. AND PERL, E.R. (1986). Central projections of identified, unmyelinated (C) afferent fibers innervating mammalian skin. *Science* **234**, 358-361.

SWETT, J.E. AND WOOLF, C.J. (1985). The somatotopic organization of primary afferent terminals in the superficial laminae of the dorsal horn of the rat spinal cord. *Journal of Comparative Neurology*, **231**, 66-77

TUCHSCHERER, M. M., KNOX, C. AND SEYBOLD, V.S. (1987). Substance P and cholecystokinin-like immunoreactive varicosities in somatosensory and autonomic regions of the rat spinal cord: A quantitative study of coexistence. *Journal of Neuroscience* **7**, 3984-3995.

TUCHSCHERER, M.M. AND SEYBOLD, V.S. (1985). Immunohistochemical studies of substance P, cholecystokinin-octapeptide and somatostatin in dorsal root ganglia of the rat. *Neuroscience* **14**, 593-605.

TUCHSCHERER, M.M. AND SEYBOLD, V.S. (1988). A quantitative study of the coexistence of peptides in varicosities within the superficial laminae of the dorsal horn of the rat spinal cord. *Journal of Neuroscience* , in press.

WESSENDORF, M.W. AND ELDE, R.P. (1985). Characterization of an immunofluorescence technique for the demonstration of coexisting neurotransmitters within nerve fibers and terminals. *Journal of Histochemistry and Cytochemistry* **33**, 984-994.

WIESENFELD-HALLIN, Z., HÖKFELT, T., LUNDBERG, J.M., FORSSMANN, W.G., REINECKE, M., TSCHOPP, F.A. AND FISCHER, J.A. (1984). Immunoreactive calcitonin gene-related peptide and substance P coexist in sensory neurons to the spinal cord and interact in spinal behavioral responses of the rat. *Neuroscience Letters* **52**, 199-204.

LAMINAR AND SEGMENTAL TERMINATION IN THE DORSAL HORN OF THE SPINAL CORD OF AN ARTICULAR NERVE OF THE FOREPAW IN THE CAT

E. Rausell and C. Avendaño

Department of Morphology, Faculty of Medicine, Autonoma University, 28029 Madrid, Spain

The primary afferent fibers conveying information from skin, muscles and tendons have been studied thoroughly in recent years, and the picture of their terminations in the spinal cord is beginning to be unravelled (Brown, 1981; Nyberg and Blomqvist, 1985; Abrahams and Swett, 1986; Molander and Grant, 1987). Less well understood, however, is the spinal distribution of the afferents arising from joints.

Electrophysiological experiments carried out on the cat's knee joint, both *in vivo* and *in vitro* (Grigg, 1975; Grigg *et al*, 1982; Grigg and Hoffman, 1982) suggest that Ruffini and Golgi-Mazzoni capsular mechanoreceptors relay information concerning stress of the joint capsule (indicating the limit of joint rotation) and perpendicular compression onto the joint capsule (signaling deep pressure) respectively. The distribution of afferents from this joint within the spinal dorsal horn was unknown until very recently (Schaible, this volume). Comparable anatomical data are lacking altogether for afferents from other joints. One reason for this apparent neglect of joint afferents is to be found in the relative difficulty in producing specific physiological stimulation of the joints, without unwanted stimulation of neighboring structures. Another - and perhaps more important reason - is that afferent fibers from articular structures often mix, very close to their origin, with those that mediate muscle and tendon inputs. Both groups of fibers are usually ensheathed in the same nerve, so that the former cannot easily be dissected from the latter.

In the present study, we isolated what appears to be a *pure* articular nerve of the wrist joint. We found that the cranial interosseus branch of the median nerve (Crouch, 1969), after innervating the pronator quadratus muscle, perforates the interosseus membrane and crosses the distal radio-ulnaris joint, and then ramifies reaching the articular spaces between the proximal carpal bones. This nerve had been also described in the human wrist joint (Cunningham, 1964). We named these terminal fibers the Carpal Branch of the Interosseus Nerve (CBIN), and we investigated their terminal distribution in the spinal dorsal horn, by means of the method of transganglionic transport of HRP.

The nerve was transected just when it leaves the distal radio-ulnaris joint, and the cut end was introduced into a plastic tube filled with a solution of 50% HRP and 2% WGA-HRP, and the tube was sealed either with paraffin or HystoacrilR, to prevent leakage of the tracer into the surrounding tissue. The same procedure was applied

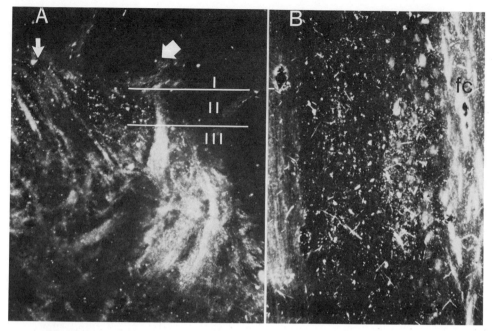

FIGURE 1: A: Photomicrograph under dark field and polarized illumination showing the dorso-medial corner and the medial edge of the dorsal horn, in a coronal section at segmental level C8. In this case, terminal labelling after CBIN impregnation is concentrated in the medial most portion of laminae I, II, and outer part of lamina III (large white arrow). Small white arrow indicates the location of other lateral patch of labelling occupying mainly lamina II. B: Photomicrograph of a horizontal section through laminae II-III in another experiment. Notice the concentration of terminal labelling after CBIN impregnation with HRP plus WGA-HRP in a medial region (right side of the photomicrograph), which corresponds to laminae II-III, and a lateral, less dense patch of labelling located in lamina II . fc, fasciculus cuneatus.

either to the median nerve or to the superficial branch of the radial nerve in the contralateral forepaw. After 72 h survival, the animals were perfused transcardially with a 1% paraformaldehyde, 1.25% glutaraldehyde solution in 0.1M phosphate buffer, pH7.4, followed by a sucrosed cryoprotective solution. The spinal cord and the dorsal root ganglia (DRG) were dissected out between segmental levels C4-T1. Horizontal or coronal 50 μm thick frozen sections from both structures were processed histochemically according to Mesulam's TMB protocol (1978). The retrograde and the transganglionic transport of the tracer into the spinal cord and into DRG were examined microscopically under dark-field and polarized illumination.

After CBIN impregnation, a small but consistent number of labelled neurons was found solely in DRG C8. This number ranged between 29 and 35 neurons, in a sample of 13 experiments in which every ganglion was studied from C4 to T1. These neurons were large or medium-sized, and they formed a loose, crescent-shaped group in the medial face of the ganglion (Fig. 2A). Transganglionic transport of HRP was observed only at the C8 segment of the spinal cord (Fig. 2 A,B). The reaction product was concentrated in the medial-most portion of laminae I, II, and outer part of III (Figs. 1A,B and 2A,B). Additionally, the inner region of lamina II contained a continuous band of labelling throughout its medio-lateral extent (Fig. 1B). No retrogradely labelled motoneurons were found in the ventral horn at any segmental level.

To our knowledge, this is the first report on the distribution in the spinal cord of afferents from the wrist joint. Physiological data on this joint are lacking altogether. Studies on the knee joint have revealed that the articular nerves are composed mainly of afferent fibres arising from Ruffini and Golgi-Mazzoni mechanoreceptors (Clark and Burgess, 1975; Clark, 1975), as well as of small diameter fibers with free endings, probably related to nociception (Clark, 1975). On the other hand, afferents of similar diameter and arising from similar skin mechanoreceptors, have been demonstrated to be distributed in specific laminae of the dorsal horn. Thus, using intraaxonal injections of HRP (see Brown, 1981, for data and references), it has been shown that thin fibers supposedly arising from cutaneous Golgi-Mazzoni receptors terminate mainly in lamina I, whereas thicker fibers arising from Ruffini receptors arborize preferentially in lamina III and in the outer part of lamina IV. Small diameter cutaneous myelinated fibers distribute in laminae I, II and V (Light and Perl, 1979b).

With respect to deep tissues, it is known that large diameter muscle afferents reach lamina V and deeper strata of the dorsal horn. In turn, it has been shown by Mense and Hoheisel (this volume) that thin myelinated fibers arising from muscles are distributed not only within deep laminae of the dorsal horn, but also in lamina I (afferents from high threshold mechanoreceptors) and in lamina II (from low threshold

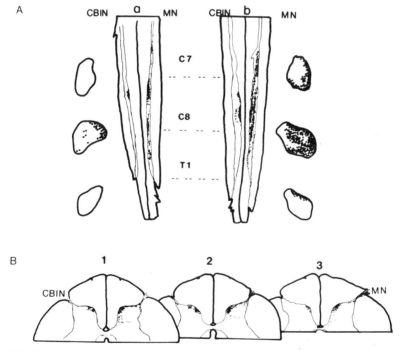

FIGURE 2: Diagrams showing the distribution of anterogradely transported HRP after impregnation of CBIN (left hand side) and median nerve (MN; right hand side). A: Projection-drawings from horizontal sections of the spinal cord (levels C6-T1) and dorsal root ganglia (C7-T1) Section (a) cuts through laminae I and II. Section (b) is more ventrally placed, passing trough laminae II and III. Diagrams of the dorsal root ganglia show the ganglion cells labelled from a number of sections. B: Coronal sections of the dorsal part of the spinal cord at segmental level C8 in other experiment. The reaction product is located in laminae I, II and outer part of III on the CBIN-side, and in laminae I-V on the median nerve (MN) side. For the latter, neither terminal labelling located deeper than lamina V, nor motoneurons are shown in these diagrams.

mechanoreceptors), among others. Besides, these authors report laminae I to III to contain more second order cells receiving deep input than do laminae IV to VI. On the other hand, the spinal distribution of the afferent fibers arising from the subcutaneous tissue of the cat's tail (muscles, tendons, fascia, and joint capsules) had been investigated by means of intra-axonal electrophysiological recording and neuroanatomical tracing methods (Mense *et al*, 1981). The authors reported that thin myelinated fibers (from high threshold mechanoreceptors) were distributed in laminae I and V, while fibers arising from low threshold mechanoreceptors terminated mainly in lamina IV. Lamina V has also been reported to contain terminations of both thin myelinated fibers arising from muscles (Mense and Hoheisel, this volume), and of fibers carried in the medial and posterior articular nerves of the cat's knee joint (Schaible *et al*, this volume). We have not seen such terminations of afferents from the wrist joint, although we cannot discard the possibility; CBIN is a very thin nerve (the number of CBIN ganglion cells ranges between 29 and 35), and HRP labelling resulting from transganglionar transport is usually very limited (as shown in Fig. 1A) so that a sparser terminal labelling than the one contained in laminae I, II, and III (Fig. 1A) is likely to be indistinguishable from background.

The present results suggest that CBIN is a *pure* articular nerve, which probably arises from more than one type of receptor of the wrist joint. This nerve can provide a good anatomical model for carrying out physiological experiments on joint afferents from the wrist.

ACKNOWLEDGEMENTS

We would like to thank to Dr. Reinoso-Suarez and Dr. C. Honda for their critical reading of this manuscript. Supported by CAICyT grant 512/84.

REFERENCES

ABRAHAMS, V.C. AND SWEET J.E. The Pattern of Spinal and Medullary Projections From a Cutaneous Nerve and a Muscle Nerve of the Forelimb of the Cat: A Study using the Transganglionic Transport of HRP. *Journal of Comparative Neurology* 246: 70-84, 1986.

BROWN, A.G. *Organization in the Spinal Cord: The Anatomy and Physiology of Identified Neurones.* Springer Verlag, Berlin Heidelberg, 1981.

CLARK, F.J. Information Signaled by Sensory Fibers in Medial Articular Nerve. *Journal of Neurophysiology*, 38: 1464-1472, 1975.

CLARK, F.J. AND BURGESS P.R. Slowly Adapting Receptors in Cat Knee Joint: Can They Signal Joint Angle?. *Journal of Physiology*, 38: 1448-1463, 1975.

CROUCH, J.E. *Text Atlas of Cat Anatomy.* Lea and Febiger. Philadelphia, 1969.

CUNNINGHAM, E. *Cunningham's Textbook of Anatomy.* Ed G. J. Romanes, Oxf. Univ. Press, London, 10th Edit., 1964.

GRIGG, P. Mechanical Factors Influencing Response of Joint Afferent Neurons From Cat Knee. *Journal of Physiology*, 38: 1473-1484, 1975.

GRIGG, P., HOFFMAN A.H. AND FOGARTY K.E. Properties of Golgi-Mazzoni Afferents in Cat Knee Joint Capsule, as Revealed by Mechanical Studies of Isolated Joint Capsule. *Journal of Physiology*, 47: 31-40,1982.

GRIGG, P. AND A.H. HOFFMAN. Properties of Ruffini afferents Revealed by Stress Analysis of Isolated Sections of Cat Knee Joint Capsule. *Journal of Physiology*, 47: 41-54, 1982.

LIGHT, A. R. AND PERL E. R. Spinal Termination of Functionally Identified Primary

Afferent Neurons With Slowly Conduction Myelinated Fibers. *Journal of Comparative Neurology*, **186**: 133-150, 1979.

MENSE, S., LIGHT A. R., AND PERL E. R. Spinal Terminations of Subcutaneous high threshold Mechanoreceptors. In: *Spinal Cord Sensation*, Ed. A. G. Brown and M. Rethelyi, Scottish Academic Press, pp: 79-83, 1981.

MESULAM, M.M. Tetramethyl Bencidine For Horseradish Peroxidase Neurohystochemistry: A non Carcinogenic Blue Reaction Product With Superior Sensitivity for Visualizing Neural Afferents and Efferents. *Journal of Histochemistry and Cytochemistry*, **26**: 106-117,1978.

MOLANDER, C. AND GRANT G. Spinal Cord Projections From Hindlimb Muscle Nerves in the Rat Studied by Transganglionic Transport of Horseradish Peroxidase, Wheat Germ Agglutinin Conjugated Horseradish Peroxidase, or Horseradish Peroxidase With Dimethylsulfoxide. *Journal of Comparative Neurology*, **260**: 246-255, 1987.

NYBERG, G. AND BLOMQVIST A. The Somatotopic Organization of Forelimb Cutaneous Nerves in the Braquial Dorsal Horn: An Anatomical Study in the Cat. *Journal of Comparative Neurology*, **242**: 28- 39, 1985.

SPINAL TERMINATION OF PRIMARY AFFERENTS OF THE CAT'S KNEE JOINT

Hans-Georg Schaible, Bernd Heppelmann, Arthur D. Craig* and Robert F. Schmidt

Physiologisches Institut der Universität Würzburg, Röntgenring 9, D-8700 Würzburg F.R.G.

INTRODUCTION

Afferent inflow via the articular nerves of the cat's knee trans-synaptically excites neurons in superficial and deep layers of the spinal cord (cf. Schaible *et al*, 1986, 1987a,b). In order to map histologically the afferent input from the knee to the spinal cord we have now investigated the spinal projection of afferent fibres of the medial and posterior articular nerves (MAN and PAN) using transganglionic transport of horseradish peroxidase.

METHODS AND RESULTS

In barbiturate-anaesthetized cats either the MAN or PAN were dissected and were incubated with horseradish peroxidase (HRP, 40%, w/v, Sigma Type VI) in a trough both ends of which were sealed with wax. The nerves were cut whilst submerged in the solution. After 1-4 hours the horseradish peroxidase was removed, the trough was rinsed with a 10% serum albumin solution and was covered with a small sheath of plastic and a drop of agarose. Three to 5 days later the animals were perfused using a 0.5% paraformaldehyde and 2.5% glutaraldehyde solution. The dorsal root ganglia and the caudal spinal cord were removed and cut into $75\mu m$ and $50\mu m$ sections, respectively. The tissue was processed with tetramethylbenzidine (TMB) and was counterstained with thionin.

1) Labelling of dorsal root ganglia. After exposure of MAN to HRP, labelled fibres and perikarya were found in dorsal root ganglia L5/L6 and after treatment of PAN in dorsal root ganglia L6/L7. The labelled neurons were scattered throughout the ganglia without exhibiting any preferential localization. Determination of the diameters of the labelled cell bodies showed that for both nerves most labelled somata were medium to small, reflecting the distribution of the afferents in the joint nerves (Heppelmann *et al*, 1988).

2) Labelling in the spinal cord. The central endings of the primary joint afferents of

---

* Present address: Divisions of Neurobiology and Neurosurgery, Barrow Neurological Institute, Phoenix, Arizona 85013, USA

both nerves showed their most dense distribution in the spinal segments that corresponded to their roots of entry, but from both nerves less dense projections were found up to
L1 and down to S2. This is displayed in Fig. 1 for the PAN (the data were superimposed
from 4-5 adjacent sections of two experiments). Within the segments the laminar
distribution of the projections was similar except for the most rostral segments (see
below). Labelled fibres were found in Lissauer's tract, along the lateral side of the
dorsal horn and within the gray matter. After entering the gray matter the afferents
formed termination fields characterized by branching into a fine network. In all
segments these were located in two areas, in the superficial dorsal horn and in deep
laminae of the dorsal horn.

Projection into the superficial dorsal horn. Figure 2 illustrates in a sagittal section the
dense projection of MAN afferents into the superficial dorsal horn of segment L4.
Labelled fibres were observed in Lissauer's tract and in the gray matter of the
superficial dorsal horn. Within the superficial gray matter labelled afferents were found

POSTERIOR ARTICULAR NERVE

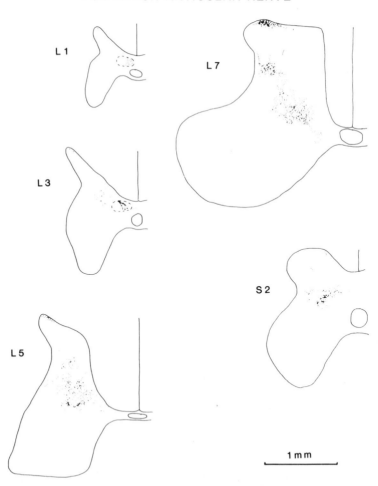

FIGURE 1: Rostrocaudal extent of the projection of PAN afferents into segments of the
lumbosacral spinal cord of the cat. The dots show location and density of the labelled
fibres in the gray matter (from Craig *et al*, 1988).

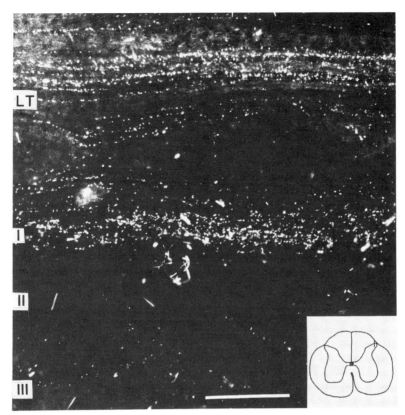

FIGURE 2: Sagittal section of the spinal cord (segment L4) with labelled afferents of MAN. The fibres were distributed in Lissauer's tract (LT) and in lamina I (I) forming a network. No termination of labelled fibres were seen in laminae II or III (II, III). Calibration = 100 μm (from Craig *et al*, 1988).

exclusively in the lateral part of lamina I (the lateral cap). There they formed a network of labelled branches. Similarly, the PAN projected only to the lateral part of lamina I of the same segments. There was no consistent evidence for termination of afferents in laminae II, III and IV. Figure 1 shows the large rostro-caudal extent of this superficial spinal projection: labelled articular fibres of both nerves were observed in lamina I of several segments.

Projections into the deep dorsal horn. The second projection field of both nerves was located in the deep dorsal horn extending from the lateral half of lamina V to the medial part of lamina VII (Figure 1). Fibres traversed the superficial dorsal horn and formed termination fields in laminae VI and VII. Other afferents ran along the lateral side of the dorsal horn entering the gray matter from there. In general the projection to the deep dorsal horn was more dense for PAN than for MAN. In the most rostral segments fibers terminated in Clarke's Column. The projection into this area was much more pronounced for PAN than for MAN.

DISCUSSION AND CONCLUSIONS

The present results show that the spinal projection of joint afferents of the knee of the cat exhibits strong similarities to the spinal projection of afferents from other deep tissues. Afferent fibres from skeletal muscles as well as from visceral organs project mainly to two areas of the spinal cord, namely into lamina I and into deeply located laminae, with an apparent gap of terminations in laminae II, III and IV (Cervero and Connell, 1984; Craig and Mense, 1983; Molander and Grant, 1987; Morgan *et al*, 1986). In contrast, cutaneous afferents project to laminae I to V including the substantia gelatinosa (Réthelyi *et al*, 1982). Whether these anatomical differences are related to the characteristic parameters of cutaneous and deep tissue sensations remains to be shown.

Both joint nerves contain non-nociceptive, nociceptive and mechano-insensitive afferent fibres (Schaible and Schmidt, 1983). The present HRP-study does not allow a definition of the spinal projections of these various fibre types. However, electrophysiological data show that neurons in lamina I require a noxious intensity of stimulation of the joint to be activated (Schaible *et al*, 1986). Thus, lamina I may be the target of nociceptive joint afferents which possibly converge with afferents of other peripheral nerves onto lamina I neurons (Schaible *et al*, 1986). Spinal neurons that are activated exclusively by noxious stimuli to the joints and muscles (and not by stimulation of the skin) are also found in laminae VII and VIII of the cat spinal cord (Schaible *et al*, 1987a). They are dramatically influenced by acute inflammation in the knee (Schaible *et al*, 1987b) so that it is possible that some of the nociceptive afferents project to the deep laminae where both joint nerves form termination fields.

REFERENCES

CERVERO, F. AND CONNELL, L.A. (1984). Distribution of somatic and visceral primary afferents within the thoracic spinal cord of the cat. *Journal of Comparative Neurology* **23**, 88-98.

CRAIG, A.D., HEPPELMANN, B. AND SCHAIBLE, H.-G. (1988). The projection of the medial and posterior articular nerves of the cat's knee to the spinal cord. *Journal of Comparative Neurology*, in press.

CRAIG, A.D. AND MENSE, S. (1983). The distribution of afferent fibers from the gastrocnemius-soleus muscle in the dorsal horn of the cat, as revealed by transport of horseradish peroxidase. *Neuroscience Letters* **41**, 233-238.

HEPPELMANN, B., HEUSS, C. AND SCHMIDT, R.F. (1988). Fiber Size Distribution of Myelinated and Unmyelinated Axons in the Medial and Posterior Articular Nerves of the Cat's Knee Joint. *Somatosensory Research* **5**, 273-281.

MOLANDER, C. AND GRANT, G. (1987). Spinal cord projections from hindlimb muscle neurons in the rat studied by transganglionic transport of horseradish peroxidase, wheat germ agglutinin conjugated horseradish peroxidase, or horse radish peroxidase with dimethylsulfoxide. *Journal of Comparative Neurology* **259**, 246-255.

MORGAN, C., DEGROAT, W.C. AND NADELHAFT, I. (1986). The spinal distribution of sympathetic preganglionic and visceral primary afferent neurons that send axons into the hypogastric nerves of the cat. *Journal of Comparative Neurology* **243**, 23-40.

RÉTHELYI, M., LIGHT, A.R. AND PERL, E.R. (1982). Synaptic Complexes Formed by Functionally Defined Primary Afferent Units With Fine Myelinated Fibers. *Journal of Comparative Neurology* **207**, 381-393.

SCHAIBLE, H.-G. AND SCHMIDT, R.F. (1983). Responses of fine medial articular nerve afferents to passive movements of knee joint. *Journal of Neurophysiology* **49**, 1118-1126.

SCHAIBLE, H.-G., SCHMIDT, R.F. AND WILLIS, W.D. (1986). Responses of spinal cord neurons to stimulation of articular afferent fibres in the cat. *Journal of Physiology* **372**, 575-593.

SCHAIBLE, H.-G., SCHMIDT, R.F. AND WILLIS, W.D. (1987a). Convergent inputs from articular, cutaneous and muscle receptors onto ascending tract cells in the cat spinal cord. *Experimental Brain Research* **66**, 479-488.

SCHAIBLE, H.-G., SCHMIDT, R.F. AND WILLIS, W.D. (1987b). Enhancement of the responses of ascending tract cells in the cat spinal cord by acute inflammation of the knee joint. *Experimental Brain Research* **66**, 489-499.

CELL SIZE AND NISSL PATTERN ANALYSES OF PRIMARY AFFERENT NEURONS INNERVATING THE MOLAR TOOTH PULP AND CORNEA OF THE RAT

Tomosada Sugimoto, Satoshi Wakisaka*, Motohide Takemura and Masaharu Aoki

Second and *First Departments of Oral Anatomy, Osaka University Faculty of Dentistry, 1-8 Yamadaoka, Suita, Osaka 565, Japan

The tooth pulp and the cornea are peculiar in that their major sensibility is pain. It is thus assumed that the primary afferent neurones innervating these trigeminal receptive fields are mostly nociceptors. In the present study, the primary afferent neurones innervating the tooth pulp of three mandibular molars (MTP) and the cornea (COR) were labelled by retrograde transport of horseradish peroxidase (HRP) in young (b.w. = 200g) male rats of the Sprague-Dawley strain. Labelled cell bodies were studied with reference to their size and Nissl pattern. The numerical data from the cell size analysis were compared with those obtained from a similar analysis on the primary afferent neurones comprising a trigeminal cutaneous nerve, the cutaneous branch of the mylohyoid nerve (MhN).

HRP application was performed under anesthesia with ethyl carbamate (urethane 1.3 g/kg, i.p.). HRP was applied as a 50% solution in 2% DMSO and 0.9% NaCl either unilaterally to the pulp chamber from which the coronal pulp had been removed, or to the corneal surface which had been scratched several times with the tip of a sharp instrument, or to the proximal stump of the transected MhN. In preliminary experiments, it was ascertained that uptake of HRP from the periodontal space was minimal after the above HRP application procedure for tooth pulp; i.e., no neuron was labelled in the mesencephalic nucleus after tooth pulp application unless HRP solution was injected through a needle firmly attached to the orifice of the root canal. HRP uptake through the uninjured surface of conjunctivum was also negligible since very few cell bodies in the ganglion (less than one on average) were labelled after corneal application. In contrast, after scratching the cornea about 200 cells per ganglion were labelled after HRP application. Between 24 and 30 hours after HRP application, the animals were re-anesthetized with ether and were fixed by vascular perfusion with 1.25% glutaraldehyde and 1% formaldehyde in 0.1M phosphate buffer (pH 7.3).

For cell size measurement, 60 μm-thick horizontal frozen sections were incubated with tetramethylbenzidine (Mesulam and Brushart, 1979), dehydrated, mounted on glass slides, and cover-slipped with Permount. The photomicroscopic image was projected onto a digitizer and the cross-sectional area of all labelled cell bodies in all sections through the ganglion were measured for the MTP (4 rats) and COR (3 rats), while only two sections which contained the most numerous labelled neurones were

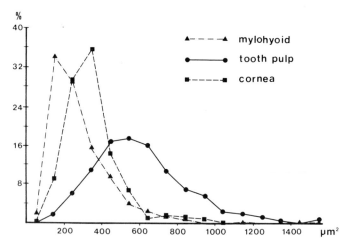

FIGURE 1: Percentage distribution diagrams of the MTP, COR and MhN cells. Cell bodies larger than 1500 μm^2 are put together. Reproduced from Sugimoto *et al*, (1988) by courtesy of Elsevier Biomedical Press.

counted for each animal with HRP applied to the MhN (3 rats). The commonly accepted norm for measurement (to measure only those neuronal profiles which contained a nucleolus) was not acceptable because heavy cytoplasmic label often obscured the nuclear profile.

Each population showed a skewed unimodal percentage distribution with more than 90% falling in the range 100-1000 μm^2 (sample sizes were 661, 834 and 608 cells for MTP, COR and MhN, respectively). The modes of the MTP, COR and MhN cells were 400-700 μm^2 (50%), 300-400 μm^2 (35%) and 100-200 μm^2 (34%), respectively (see Fig. 1). Comparison of cell size spectra of MTP and MhN cells indicated that the trigeminal primary afferent neurons are composed of at least two distinct populations in terms of cell body size. If there were only two types of primary afferent neurons, namely small and large cell groups, the percentage distributions PMhN, j and PMTP, J for a class j (e.g., 200-300 μm^2,...) for MhN and MTP samples can be expressed as:

$$PMhN, j = a1 \cdot PS, j + (1-a1) \cdot PL, j \quad \text{and} \quad PMTP, j = a2 \cdot PS, j + (1-a2) \cdot PL, j$$

where PS, j and PL,j are the percentage distributions for the class j of pure populations of small (S) and large (L) cells; and a1 and a2 are the proportions of small cells in MhN and MTP populations, respectively.

If a given sample i was composed of the same two types, its percentage distribution for the class j would be:

$$Pi, j = a \cdot PS, j + (1-a) \cdot PL, j \quad \text{where a is the proportion of small cells or}$$

$$Pi, j = b \cdot PMhN, j + (1-b) \cdot PMTP, j \quad \text{where } b = (a-a2)/(a1-a2).$$

Because the mode of COR cells was larger than that of MhN and smaller than that of MTP, coefficient b for COR cells should be: $0 < b < 1$. Using the above formula, the theoretical maximum of percentage distribution of COR cells for the range 300-400 μm^2 is calculated to be about 16%, which is only about 1/2 of the actual measurement

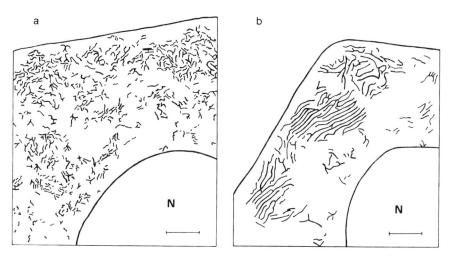

FIGURE 2: Tracings of ER cisternae in electron micrographs of typical MTP (a) and COR (b) cells. In MTP cells, many small aggregations of short, bifurcated ER cisternae are scattered all over the cytoplasm. In COR cells, large parallel arrays of long ER cisternae are restricted to the periphery of the cytoplasm. N: nucleus. Scale bar = 2 μm.

(35.1%). Therefore, a third population, the medium-sized cell group, is considered to contribute to the large percentage distribution of COR cells for the range 300-400 μm^2.

For Nissl pattern analysis, 30 μm-thick vibrating microtome sections were incubated with diaminobenzidine with a modification by Adams (1977), and osmicated in 2% OsO_4. The sections were then dehydrated in alcohols and flat embedded in epoxy resin. Thin sections were cut with a diamond knife on an LKB ultratome and were examined with or without increasing contrast with uranyl acetate and lead citrate.

The MTP and COR cells showed entirely different Nissl patterns. The MTP cells were characterized by ubiquitous small aggregations of rough endoplasmic reticulum (ER). The ER aggregations were separated by strands of neurofilaments, and the ER cisternae were short and often bifurcated (Fig. 2a). This Nissl pattern is a characteristic of large light cells of the A type (Duce and Keen, 1977). In contrast, the ER cisternae of COR cells were much longer than those of MTP cells and formed large parallel arrays which were located in the periphery of the cytoplasm. The perinuclear zone was mainly occupied by the mitochondrion, Golgi complex and lysosome, and was relatively free from ER cisternae (Fig. 2b). The COR cells were thus judged to be small dark cells of the B type (Duce and Keen, 1977).

Ultrastructural and histochemical studies strongly suggest that large light cells of the A type emit thick myelinated fibres, and that small dark cells of the B type emit either finely myelinated or unmyelinated fibres (Rambourg, Clermont and Beaudet, 1973; Duce and Keen, 1977; Sommer, Kazimierczak and Droz, 1985). This implies that the large cells, which constituted a large proportion of MTP cell sample, had thick myelinated fibres probably conducting in Aβ range. It is also probable that the medium-sized COR cells do not have Aβ-fibres but either Aδ- or C-fibres. In the past, however, no ultrastructural or histochemical feature of the cell body has provided a criterion for distinguishing primary afferent neurons with C-fibres from those with Aδ-fibres.

A combined electrophysiological and morphological study in young rats revealed a clear linear correlation between peripheral conduction velocity and cell body size of primary afferent neurons, especially for C- and Aδ-primary afferent neurons (Harper and Lawson, 1985). If this correlation applies to the trigeminal primary afferent neurons, the small cells, which were abundant in the MhN sample, should have smaller peripheral conduction velocities than the medium-sized COR cells. Therefore, the separation of the small and medium-sized cell groups in this study may represent the separation of C- and Aδ-fibres.

In summary, cell size analysis of primary afferent neurons innervating the molar tooth pulp, cornea and cutaneous branch of the mylohyoid nerve distinguished 3 distinct groups of trigeminal primary afferent neurons. Small cells were most frequent in the cutaneous branch of mylohyoid nerve and are assumed to have C-fibres. Most of corneal primary afferents were medium-sized and probably correspond to cells with Aδ-fibres. Many of the tooth pulp primary afferents had large cell bodies corresponding to cells with Aβ-fibres, and small-cell or C-fibre afferents were uncommon. Recent electrophysiological studies support the present conclusions; e.g., Cadden *et al*, (1983) for the tooth pulp and Tanelian and Beuerman (1974) for the cornea.

REFERENCES

ADAMS, J.C. (1977). Technical considerations on the use of horseradish peroxidase as a neuronal marker. *Neuroscience* **2**, 141-145.

CADDEN, S.W., LISNEY, S.J.W. AND MATTHEWS, B. (1983). Thresholds to electrical stimulation of nerves in cat canine tooth-pulp with Aβ-, Aδ- and C-fibre conduction velocities. *Brain Research* **261**, 31-41.

DUCE, I.R. AND KEEN, P. (1977). An ultrastructural classification of the neuronal cell bodies of the rat dorsal root ganglion using zinc iodide-osmium impregnation. *Cell and Tissue Research* **185**, 263-677.

HARPER, A.A. AND LAWSON, S.N. (1985). Conduction velocity is related to morphological cell type in rat dorsal root ganglion neurones. *Journal of Physiology* **359**, 31-46.

MESULAM, M.-M. AND BRUSHART, T.M. (1979). Transganglionic and anterograde transport of horseradish peroxidase across dorsal root ganglia: a tetramethylbenzidine method for tracing central sensory connections of muscles and peripheral nerves. *Neuroscience* **4**, 1107-1117.

RAMBOURG, A., CLERMONT, Y. AND BEAUDET, A. (1983). Ultrastructural features of six types of neurons in rat dorsal root ganglia. *Journal of Neurocytology* **12**, 47-66.

SOMMER, E.W., KAZIMIERCZAK, J. AND DROZ, B. (1985). Neuronal subpopulations in the dorsal root ganglion of the mouse as characterized by combination of ultrastructural and cytochemical features. *Brain Research* **346**, 310-326.

SUGIMOTO, T., TAKEMURA, M. AND WAKISAKA, S. (1988). Cell size analysis of primary neurons innervating the cornea and tooth pulp of the rat. *Pain* **32**, 375-381.

TANELIAN, D.L. AND BEUERMAN, R.W. (1984). Responses of rabbit corneal nociceptors to mechanical and thermal stimulation. *Experimental Neurology* **84**, 165-178.

VISCERAL AND SOMATIC AFFERENT ORIGIN OF CALCITONIN GENE-RELATED PEPTIDE-IMMUNOREACTIVITY IN THE SUPERFICIAL AND DEEP LAMINAE OF THE THORACIC DORSAL HORN OF THE RAT

K. A. Sharkey*, J. A. Sobrino** and F. Cervero

Department of Physiology, Medical School, University of Bristol, University Walk
Bristol BS8 1TD, U.K.

INTRODUCTION

Calcitonin gene-related peptide-immunoreactivity (CGRP-IR) is found in cell bodies of dorsal root ganglia and in the gray matter of the dorsal horn of the spinal cord, in regions associated with the terminals of primary afferent fibres (Carlton *et al*, 1987; Franco-Cereceda *et al*, 1987; McNeil *et al*, 1988; Skofitsch and Jacobowitz, 1985a). The majority of CGRP-IR in the dorsal horn is depleted by dorsal rhizothomy (Gibson *et al*, 1984) and in adult rats treated at birth with capsaicin, suggesting it is of primary afferent origin (Skofitsch and Jacobowitz, 1985b; Franco-Cereceda *et al*, 1987). However, it is not known whether CGRP-IR is of somatic or visceral afferent origin (Dockray and Sharkey, 1986). We have examined the origin of CGRP-IR in the lower thoracic spinal cord of the rat.

EXPERIMENTAL PROCEDURES

Experiments were conducted on 14 adult male Wistar rats (300-500 g). Three groups of rats were used as follows:
a) 5 normal stock rats.
b) 4 rats in which the left splanchnic nerve was sectioned 16-19 days before perfusion.
c) 4 rats in which the left thoracic spinal nerves (intercostal and dorsal ramus) from T8-T12 were sectioned 16-19 days before perfusion.

Animals were anaesthetized with sodium pentobarbitone and were fixed by perfusion through the ascending aorta with Tyrode's solution immediately followed by 4% paraformaldehyde at 4°C (pH 7.4). A laminectomy was performed and the T10-T11 spinal segments were removed and processed for immunohistochemistry with an anti-CGRP antiserum at a dilution 1:1000 (antiserum L-271 donated by G. J. Dockray), as

---

* Present address: Department of Medical Physiology, University of Calgary, Canada
** Present address: Departamento de Fisiologia, Facultad de Medicina, Universidad Complutense, Madrid, Spain

previously described (Sharkey *et al*, 1987), on transverse and parasagittal frozen sections.

RESULTS

a) Normal animals

In normal rats there was dense staining in laminae I and II of the dorsal horn (Fig. 1 A and C). This was seen as rostro-caudally orientated fibres in parasagittal sections and as punctuate immunoreactivity in transverse sections. Dorso-ventrally orientated fibres running from the superficial laminae to lamina V could also be seen. In lamina V, in parasagittal sections, CGRP-IR was seen as an almost continuous rostro-caudally orientated bundle of fibres connected at intervals by a denser plexus of immunoreactivity (clusters); in transverse sections moderately dense punctate immunoreactivity was seen in all sections. In most transverse sections two bundles of CGRP-IR were seen along the lateral and medial borders of the dorsal horn; the medial bundle often appeared to cross the midline. In lamina X two bundles of CGRP-IR could also be seen, one ventral and one dorsal to the central canal; in parasagittal sections they were orientated rostro-caudally.

b) Animals with unilateral thoracic spinal nerve section

After section of the intercostal nerves and dorsal rami there was a small reduction in CGRP-IR in lamina I and a virtual absence of CGRP-IR in lamina II (Fig. 1B). In lamina V clusters of CGRP-IR were still present, though probably reduced in density, but, as can be observed in parasagittal sections, the CGRP-IR *connecting* the clusters was reduced or even absent. There were no obvious changes in lamina X immunoreactivity.

c) Animals with unilateral splanchnic section

After section of the splanchnic nerve there was also a small reduction of CGRP-IR in lamina I, but lamina II was largely unaffected (Fig. 1D). In lamina V there was a reduction or absence of CGRP-IR clusters but no apparent loss of the continuous rostro-caudally orientated bundles *connecting* them. Again, no changes were seen in lamina X immunoreactivity.

CONCLUSIONS

1. CGRP-IR in the superficial and deep dorsal horn is of visceral and somatic afferent origin.
2. Virtually all the CGRP-IR in laminae I and II as well as the continuous bundle of CGRP-IR in lamina V is of somatic origin.
3. CGRP-IR found in clusters in lamina V is mostly of visceral afferent origin.

ACKNOWLEDGEMENTS

This work was supported by the Wellcome Trust and the British MRC.

BIBLIOGRAPHY

CARLTON, S. M., MCNEILL, D. L. AND COGGESHALL, R. E. (1987). A light and electron microscopic level analysis of CGRP in the spinal cord of the primate. *Soc. Neurosci.*, **13**:225.

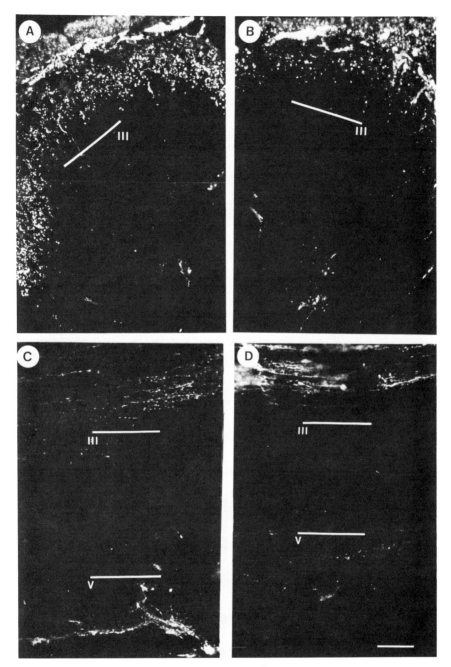

FIGURE 1: CGRP-like immunoreactivity both in transverse sections of the thoracic spinal cord from a rat after thoracic spinal nerve section and in parasagittal sections from a rat after splanchnic nerve section. Note that after thoracic spinal nerve section there was a marked reduction in immunoreactivity in lamina II (B) and that after splanchnic nerve section the CGRP-immunoreactive plexus in lamina V is virtually abolished leaving only immunoreactive fibres (D). Solid white lines indicate the approximate boundaries between laminae II and III (III) and laminae IV and V (V). Bar = 50 μm.

DOCKRAY, G. J. AND SHARKEY, K. A. (1986). Neurochemistry of visceral afferent neurones. In *Visceral sensation*, ed. F. Cervero and J. F. B. Morrison, *Progr. Brain Res.*, **67**, pp. 133-148, Amsterdam Elsevier.

FRANCO-CERECEDA, A., HENKE, H., LUNDBERG, J. M., PETERMANN, J. B., HÖKFELT, T. AND FISCHER, J. A. (1987). Calcitonin Gene-Related Peptide (CGRP) in capsaicin-sensitive Substance P-immunoreactive sensory neurons in animals and man: Distribution and release by capsaicin. *Peptides*, **8**, 399-410.

GIBSON, S. J., POLAK, J. M., BLOOM, S. R., SABATE, I. M., MULDERRY, P. M., CHATEI, M. A., MCGREGOR, G. P., MORRISON, J. F. B., KELLY, J. S., EVANS, R. M. AND ROSENFELD, M. G. (1984). Calcitonin gene-related peptide immunoreactivity in the spinal cord of man and of eight other species. *J. Neurosci.*, **4**, 3101-3111.

MCNEILL, D. L., COGGESHALL, R. E. AND CARLTON, S. M. (1988). A light and electron microscopic study of calcitonin gene-related peptide in the spinal cord of the rat. *Exp. Neurol.*, **99**, 699-708.

SHARKEY, K. A., SOBRINO, J. A. AND CERVERO, F. (1987). Evidence for a visceral afferent origin of substance P-like immunoreactivity in lamina V of the rat thoracic spinal cord. *Neuroscience*, **22**, 1077-1083.

SKOFITSCH, G. AND JACOBOWITZ, D. M. (1985a). Calcitonin gene-related peptide. Detailed immunohistochemical distribution in the central nervous system. *Peptides* **6**, 721-745.

SKOFITSCH, G. AND JACOBOWITZ, D. M. (1985b). Calcitonin gene-related peptide coexists with substance P in capsaicin sensitive neurons and sensory ganglia of the rat. *Peptides* **6**, 747-754.

DISCUSSION ON SECTION I

Rapporteur: Gunnar Grant

Karolinska Institute, Department of Anatomy, Solnavagen 1, Stockholm, Sweden

DIFFERENTIAL CENTRAL PROJECTIONS OF AFFERENTS FROM DIFFERENT PERIPHERAL TARGETS

Results presented during this session gave further support to the view that somatic and visceral afferent fibers differ with regard to their projections to the superficial layers of the dorsal horn. Y. Sugiura, who is the first, together with his collaborators, to have been able to label physiologically-identified C-fiber units, gave examples of such units both of somatic and of visceral types. Differences were demonstrated between the two types, with regard to both their patterns of ramification and to their laminar sites of termination. Both types gave rise to terminals in lamina I, but whereas lamina II is the main site of termination in the superficial two laminae for cutaneous afferents, only occasional ramifications and terminals were demonstrated in this lamina for visceral C-fiber units. This sparse representation of terminals from visceral C-fiber afferents in lamina II was stressed by F. Cervero, who also pointed out that not all of the 7 visceral C-fiber units that had been analyzed by Sugiura really had labelled terminals in lamina II, and that only very occasional termination would be expected, given what is known from earlier physiological studies.

The demonstration by S. Mense of the central projections of thin myelinated deep afferents was another contribution which supports the view of differential central projections of afferents from different peripheral targets. This principle seems to apply not only to mammalian species. Interestingly, differential spinal projections of cutaneous and visceral afferent fibers have also been demonstrated in birds (Ohmori et al, 1987), and of cutaneous and muscle afferent fibers also in the bullfrog (Jhaveri and Frank, 1983). Although a common general principle of organization of the primary afferent projections therefore seems to exist, certain differences may still occur. These may be not only between species but also regionally within a particular species. An example of an inter-species difference may be the gastrocnemius nerve projection to lamina I. In the cat such a projection clearly exists, as was described by Mense, but it has not been possible to demonstrate it in the rat (Molander and Grant, 1987). Regional differences were found by Sugiura and collaborators for the projections of cutaneous polymodal nociceptor afferents to the superficial dorsal horn in the guinea pig. The pattern of termination in the cervical spinal cord was different from that at the lumbar level. Another example of regional differences may be the projections of neck muscle afferents to lamina I in the cat, as was described by V.C. Abrahams. Thus, the superficial neck muscle nerves were found to have some projections to lamina I, whereas no such projections could be demonstrated for deep neck muscle afferents. In addition to inter-species and regional differences in the patterns of primary afferent projections, sex differences might also occur. Such differences should be expected primarily for afferents supplying the genital organs.

LIMITATIONS OF THE LABELLING METHODS PRESENTLY USED FOR STUDYING AFFERENT INPUTS TO THE SUPERFICIAL DORSAL HORN

An important issue which was raised by P.D. Wall concerned the reliability of the labelling techniques. As was pointed out by E.R. Perl, most investigators agree that with no technique can a complete filling of all terminals be claimed to have occurred. This will thus be true not only for the transganglionic labelling methods but will also apply to the refined methods of intra-axonal or intracellular labelling of physiologically identified units. If these two main approaches are compared, it is clear that there is a sampling problem with the intra-axonal/intracellular methods, at least in the short-term perspective. The transganglionic methods are, however, faced with other problems. Especially when free horseradish peroxidase (HRP) is used, spread of tracer creates a problem. This is particularly true if the tracer is applied by injections, for instance into muscle or skin. The use of conjugates, such as wheat germ agglutinin (WGA)-HRP will restrict this problem: the uptake of the conjugates is by way of specific binding sites on the neuronal membrane, and this results in less spread of the tracer and also allows the use of much lower concentrations than when free HRP is used. It is important, however, to be aware of the fact that not all neuronal populations have binding sites for, and transport all, of these conjugates. An example of this is offered by B-HRP (chloragenoid-HRP), which has been found not to label fine calibre afferent projections to the superficial dorsal horn (Robertson and Grant, 1985). A lack of uptake of tracer has also been found to occur from encapsulated endings (muscle spindle and Golgi tendon organ afferents) following tracer injections directly into muscle. Nonetheless such afferents from muscle nerves have been labelled (e.g. Molander and Grant, 1987). Another factor to take into account when HRP-conjugates are used, is that transneuronal transfer may take place. This may occur even after short survival periods, as has been shown for WGA-HRP in the trigeminal system of the rat (Marfurt and Adams, 1984).

Although it is of crucial importance to be aware of the limitations of the different methods, it is still quite obvious what important tools they represent for the further detailed analysis of the primary afferent projections to the spinal cord. The results presented by A.R. Light illustrate how these methods can be used in combination with other methods, so as to provide valuable additional information on the organization of primary afferent projections to the superficial dorsal horn.

REFERENCES

JHAVERI, S. AND FRANK, E. (1983) Central projections of the brachial nerve in bullfrogs: Muscle and cutaneous afferents project to different regions of the spinal cord. *The Journal of Comparative Neurology* **221**, 304-312.

MARFURT, C. AND ADAMS, C.E. (1984) Transneuronal and transcellular transport of horseradish peroxidase-wheat germ agglutinin (HRP-WGA) in rat trigeminal sensory neurons. *Society of Neuroscience Abstracts* **10**,483.

MOLANDER, C AND GRANT, G (1987) Spinal cord projections from hindlimb muscle nerves in the rat studied by transganglionic transport of horseradish peroxidase, wheat germ agglutinin conjugated horseradish peroxidase, or horseradish peroxidase with dimethylsulfoxide. *The Journal of Comparative Neurology* **260**, 246-255.

OHMORI, Y., WATANABE, T. AND FUJIOKA, T. (1987) Projections of visceral and somatic afferents to the sacral spinal cord of the domestic fowl revealed by transganglionic transport of horseradish peroxidase. *Neuroscience Letters* **74**, 175-179.

ROBERTSON, B. AND GRANT, G. (1985) A comparison between wheat germ agglutinin- and choleragenoid-horseradish peroxidase as anterogradely transported markers in central branches of primary sensory neurones in the rat with some observations in the cat. *Neuroscience* **14**, 895-905.

SECTION II

RECEPTIVE FIELD PROPERTIES OF LAMINA I NEURONES

INTRODUCTION TO SECTION II

Ainsley Iggo

Department of Preclinical Veterinary Sciences, University of Edinburgh, U.K.

INTRODUCTION

The anatomical basis of the dorsal root afferent input to the superficial dorsal horn has been laid in the previous chapters of this book. Essentially the majority of the axons are small myelinated ($A\delta$) or unmyelinated (C). The larger myelinated axons or their collaterals pass through lamina I on their way to terminate in deeper laminae. It is, therefore, reasonable to consider the receptive characteristics of the finer afferent fibres since these will determine the kind of stimuli able to affect lamina I neurones most directly. In the cat, the common laboratory animal used in neurophysiological experiments, and especially when the lumbo-sacral spinal cord is considered, most of the fine afferent fibres come from the skin, with a much smaller proportion from the subcutaneous and deep tissues and the pelvic viscera. The $A\delta$ cutaneous afferent units in the cat include a) type D hair follicle afferents; b) mechano-nociceptors, including those effectively excited by needle-like punctiform stimuli and c) some slowly-conducting $A\delta$ axons with receptors responding to intense pressure and to high temperatures. The C afferent units include a) sensitive C-mechanoreceptors, excited by brushing hairs; b) C-nociceptors (some primarily responding to noxious temperatures, others also excited by firm pressure); c) sensitive thermoreceptors, either cold units or warm units.

This diversity of afferent unit types with axons in the $A\delta$ and C groups raises difficulties in the analysis of receptive field characteristics, especially if electrical stimulation of peripheral nerve trunks is used as the major search stimulus. It is for this reason that the use of natural stimuli is mandatory if the functional significance of sensory receptive fields is to be assessed. Fortunately, it is possible, with some degree of precision, to use quantitatively controlled thermal or mechanical stimuli to excite specified groups of sensory receptors (Cervero *et al*, 1976). A further complication arises if either before or during an experiment a condition of inflammation is generated in the peripheral tissues. Inflammation can greatly modify the receptive properties of peripheral receptors, for example, in adjuvant-induced polyarthritis, nociceptors in the ankle joint capsule may have thresholds similar to sensitive cutaneous C-mechanoreceptors (Guilbaud *et al*, l985). The application of a mild mechanical stimulus to such an inflamed joint could induce a massive afferent inflow in nociceptors and lead to confusing results and conclusions, unless the changes in afferent properties are taken into account.

Finally, the receptive field of a lamina I neurone may be excitatory, inhibitory or mixed in relation to dorsal root afferent input. The nature and extent of the field may also be influenced by both segmental and supra-segmental inputs that affect the excitability of the neurone by selectively or non-selectively altering its ability to respond to sensory afferent inflow.

When we turn to consider actual results, as we will in the ensuing presentations, it is also imperative that the conditions of the experiments are clearly borne in mind. Factors such as anaesthesia and anaesthetic, extent of preparative surgery, degree of excision of parts of the CNS or interruption (reversible or otherwise) of the spinal cord and the physiological state of the animal can all dramatically affect the properties of lamina I neurones. I sometimes feel that much of the published information suffers the disadvantage of emerging from moribund rather than physiologically normal preparations, but perhaps that is an insufficiently sanguine view!

My last general point concerns the method of recording. Knowledge of receptive field properties of lamina I neurones must perforce come from electrophysiological recordings of the neurones. An immediate point of contention, and one with a long if undistinguished history, is the actual location of the neurones from which records of activity are being made or considered. The use of extracellular recording, particularly from the relatively small neurones of lamina I, provides information only about the discharge of individual neurones, or using larger electrodes, of a pool of neurones. It also lacks precision when the location of the cell body is to be established. Intracellular recording, on the other hand, can provide information about afferent inputs that are sub-threshold for discharge of the neurone, about post-synaptic inhibitory activity and, by the use of cell labelling markers released from the electrode, the actual location of the cell body. For these reasons it is clearly preferable, even if very tedious, to build-up knowledge of receptive fields using the latter approach. Such knowledge may then provide a secure data-base to assist in the interpretation of data obtained using extracellular recording methods.

NOCICEPTOR-SPECIFIC NEURONES IN LAMINA I

The majority of the neurones reported for lamina I share the characteristic of being excited only by noxious sensory stimuli, as first reported by Christensen and Perl (1970). Two broad categories were recognised by Cervero et al (1976):- class 3a, excited only by noxious mechanical stimuli, such as squeezing the skin with serrated-tip forceps or pin-prick (stimuli known to excite Aδ mechano-nociceptors), and a second group, class 3b, excited in addition by noxious radiant thermal stimuli (thresholds for neuronal excitation were 40°C and for sustained discharges were >45°C). The use of radiant heat as a stimulus had the advantage that the afferent input was caused in C-fibres from C-thermal nociceptors. The use of controlled mechanical stimulation made it possible to exclude an excitatory input in Aδ axons from D-hair follicle mechanoreceptors for both these groups of nociceptor-driven lamina I neurones and also of C-mechanoreceptor input for the 3(b) group of nociceptor-driven lamina I neurones.

ORGANISATION OF RECEPTIVE FIELDS

There is a well-established somatotopy in the representation of the skin in the dorsal horn (Brown, 1981) evident at several laminar levels, including lamina I (Cervero et al, 1976). The more peripheral on a limb the receptive field of a nociceptive lamina I dorsal horn neurone, the smaller the extent of the excitatory receptive field; on the foot the excitatory receptive field could be restricted to part of one toe pad. The limited sizes of receptive fields was mirrored in the limited number of peripheral nerves that on electrical stimulation can excite a neurone. The effective nerve-evoked input showed a difference when the two sub-classes of nociceptor-specific lamina I neurones were compared. The A -driven group (class 3a) could only be excited by cutaneous nerves, whereas the A and C-driven group (class 3b) could also be excited by nerves innervating deeper tissues, including muscle. Although there is no direct evidence, this latter result could be due to the C-fibre input being indirect, i.e. polysynaptic.

The receptive field includes, of course, inhibitory fields. The nociceptor-driven lamina I neurones, can be inhibited by an input from sensitive mechanoreceptors. This segmental inhibition can completely suppress the vigorous response of a lamina I neurone to a noxious input (Cervero *et al*, 1976). The inhibitory action is presumably mediated via interneurones, since the large myelinated afferent fibres terminate principally below lamina II, and the inhibitory neuronal soma were in the deeper laminae. Less attention has been paid to the inhibitory receptive fields, and often they were evoked by electrical stimulation of peripheral nerves.

MULTI-RECEPTIVE NEURONES IN LAMINA I

These have received less detailed attention than the nociceptor-specific neurones. Their receptive fields include both sensitive mechanoreceptors and nociceptors. As with multi-receptive neurones in the deeper laminae they can be excited by movement of hairs on the body surface, and can also be inhibited by similar stimuli in the same general area, an example, perhaps, of monosynaptic excitation and di-synaptic inhibition. Problems of neuronal location and afferent pathway remain to be resolved.

CONCLUSION

In the presentations to follow in this session we will be hearing more about the nociceptor-specific neurones that project directly to the thalamus and midbrain parabrachial area (Hylden *et al*, 1988), and thus carry forward precise information about the location and characteristics of nociceptive receptive fields. As Kniffki (1988) will be telling us, the central projections from lamina I preserve, by their trajectory and destination, the characteristics of the original receptive fields. Thus we see emerging a highly differentiated system, involving lamina I, that is capable of preserving the original encoding of noxious stimuli delivered to the peripheral tissues. Its role vis-à-vis the multi-receptive system continues to provoke us, and to call for a resolution.

REFERENCES

BROWN, A.G. (1981). *Organization in the Spinal Cord*. Berlin: Springer.

CHRISTENSEN, B.N. AND PERL, E.R. (1970). Spinal neurones specifically excited by noxious or thermal stimuli: marginal zone of dorsal horn. *Journal of Neurophysiology*, **33**, 293-307.

CERVERO, F., IGGO, A. AND OGAWA, H. (1976). Nociceptor-driven dorsal horn neurones in the lumbar spinal cord of the cat. *Pain*, **2**, 5-24.

GUILBAUD, G., IGGO, A. AND TEGNER, R. (1985). Sensory receptors in the ankle joint capsules of normal and arthritic rats. *Experimental Brain Research*, **58**. 29-40.

HYLDEN, J.L.K., NAHIN, R.L., ANTON, F. AND DUBNER, R. (1988). Characterization of lamina I projection neurones: Physiology and Anatomy. *This volume*.

KNIFFKI, K.D. (1988). Input to and output from lamina I neurones in the cat spinal cord. *This volume*.

CHARACTERIZATION OF LAMINA I PROJECTION NEURONS: PHYSIOLOGY AND ANATOMY

Janice L. K. Hylden, Richard L. Nahin, Fernand Anton and Ronald Dubner

Neurobiology and Anesthesiology Branch, National Institute of Dental Research
National Institutes of Health, Bethesda, Maryland 20892, USA

The primary afferent input to the most superficial part of the dorsal horn has been shown to originate from slowly conducting (Aδ and C) fibers. Recordings from individual slowly conducting myelinated (Burgess and Perl, 1967; Perl, 1968) and unmyelinated (Bessou and Perl, 1969; Beitel and Dubner, 1976; Kumazawa and Perl, 1977) fibers demonstrated that a large proportion of these small fibers required high threshold cutaneous stimulation for their activation and could be classified as various types of nociceptors. Thus, it follows that regions in which small diameter afferents terminate play a role in pain mechanisms. Christensen and Perl (1970), in a study designed specifically to discover cells responding to high-threshold mechanoreceptors, found a concentration of such cells in the marginal zone (lamina I) of the cat. Their report concluded that *lamina I represents a specialized sensory nucleus containing neurons important for nociception and for detection of thermal changes in the skin* (Christensen and Perl, 1970). Although some lamina I neurons appear to receive primary afferent input exclusively from nociceptors, others receive convergent input from a variety of peripheral receptors (Willis *et al*, 1974; Price and Browe, 1975; Cervero *et al*, 1976 Price *et al* 1976).

Early evidence from human material suggested that some lamina I cells projected rostrally in the spinothalamic tract (Kuru, 1949). Dilly *et al* (1968) gave the first description of the physiology of a lamina I thalamic projection cell in the cat. This early observation was later replicated by other investigators in rat (Giesler *et al*, 1976), cat (Hu *et al*, 1981; Craig and Kniffiki, 1985) and monkey (Willis *et al*, 1974; Price *et al*, 1976). In all cases, the lamina I component of the spinothalamic and trigeminothalamic tracts was made up primarily of high threshold neurons with slower central conduction velocities as compared to deeper cells.

With the introduction of horseradish peroxidase (HRP) retrograde labelling techniques, the cells of origin of the spinothalamic tract were again shown to include lamina I cells (Trevino, 1976; Carstens and Trevino, 1978; Giesler *et al*, 1979). In addition, a number of reports suggested that a second site of termination for lamina I cells was the midbrain (Trevino, 1976; Willis *et al*, 1979; Menétrey *et al*, 1982; Wiberg and Blomqvist, 1984).

We were particularly impressed by the magnitude of the lamina I spinomesencephalic projection as shown in the cat by Wiberg and Blomqvist (1984).

These investigators demonstrated a dense projection from the lumbar spinal cord to the parabrachial nuclei, the adjacent cuneiform nuclei and the ventrolateral periaqueductal gray (PAG). The majority of the cells of origin of this tract were located in lamina I. Therefore, subsequent experiments in our laboratory were directed toward the physiological and anatomical characterization of those lamina I neurons with projections to the mesencephalic parabrachial area (PBA); the PBA was described as a region of the caudal midbrain surrounding the brachium conjunctivum that included portions of the parabrachial nuclei, nucleus cuneiformis and PAG (Hylden et al, 1985, 1986a) and extended into the dorsolateral pons (Cechetto et al, 1985; Panneton and Burton, 1985).

PHYSIOLOGY OF LAMINA I PROJECTION NEURONS

Lamina I Neurons Projecting to the Parabrachial Area of the Cat

All lumbar lamina I neurons that were antidromically activated from the midbrain PBA in the cat responded to high threshold stimuli. The vast majority of these (92%) were classified as nociceptive-specific; these cells responded exclusively to noxious mechanical stimuli or to noxious mechanical and noxious heat stimuli. The remaining cells were of the wide-dynamic-range type (Hylden et al, 1985, 1986b); these cells responded maximally to high threshold stimuli, but could also be activated by low threshold stimuli. The primary afferent input to recorded lamina I projection neurons was from myelinated and/or unmyelinated fibers in the sciatic nerve. Receptive fields were generally small, and often consisted of the surface of one or more toes or toe pads. Central conduction velocities were slow, ranging from 1.0 to 18 m/s; this is in the range of previously reported central conduction velocities of lamina I neurons projecting two or more segments rostrally (Kumazawa et al, 1975; Cervero et al, 1979) and corresponds to a population of cells with small myelinated, and perhaps some unmyelinated, axons.

Figure 1 depicts data obtained from one representative nociceptive-specific lamina I projection neuron including the extent of the receptive field and the site of antidromic activation in the PBA. This particular neuron was also stained by intracellular iontophoresis of HRP. Of 19 PBA projection neurons stained with HRP, all had cell bodies located in lamina I and all were oriented rostrocaudally, but various cell body shapes, cell sizes and densities of dendritic spines were represented (Hylden et al, 1985, 1986b).

Light et al (1987) have also examined the projection from the superficial lumbar dorsal horn to the PBA in the cat. In agreement with our observations, these authors found that most of the PBA projection neurons were nociceptive-specific and fewer had wide-dynamic-range properties. Central conduction velocities were quite low (0.7-23.2 m/s). The antidromic stimulating electrode placement in the study by Light et al (1987) was slightly caudal to what we have used, but would be included in the area that we have defined as the PBA and certainly is a region of termination for numerous lamina I neurons (Cechetto et al, 1985; Panneton and Burton, 1985). Yezierski and Schwartz (1986) have also examined the spinomesencephalic projection in cats and, although they did not restrict their investigation to the superficial dorsal horn, reported on the properties of a few lamina I neurons that were antidromically activated from the caudal midbrain; 2 high-threshold and 2 wide-dynamic-range cells were observed.

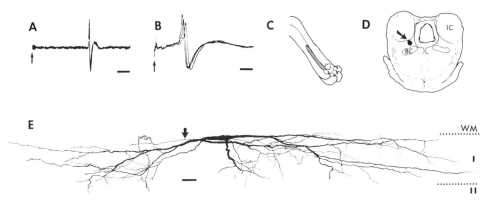

FIGURE 1: Example of a nociceptive-specific PBA projection neuron recorded in the cat. A: antidromic response to stimulation of the ipsilateral PBA at a latency of 45 ms-4 traces are superimposed; scale bar, 10 ms. B: orthodromic spikes occurred at 4.5 ms after electrical stimulation of the sciatic nerve-3 traces are superimposed; scale bar, 2 ms. Arrows in A and B indicate time of stimulation. C: nociceptive excitatory receptive field (shaded area). D: site of lesion (arrow) made with the stimulating electrode following completion of the experiment. BC: brachium conjunctivum; IC: inferior colliculus. E: camera lucida drawing of the neuron in the parasagittal plane. Only a portion of the axon (arrow) is shown. The axon was followed down through the dorsal horn to lamina VI, where it issued a collateral that coursed toward the central canal, then the axon moved dorsal and lateral toward the DLF. Scale bar, 50 μm. Dotted lines at the right indicate the borders of the white matter (WM), lamina I and lamina II. (From Hylden *et al*, 1985)

Lamina I Projection Neurons in the Rat

In the rat, the physiology of lamina I projection neurons follows that observed in the cat. In a recent study, we recorded from lamina I neurons that were antidromically activated from the upper cervical spinal cord of rats (Hylden *et al*, 1988b). All neurons received primary afferent drive from Aδ and/or C-fibers in the sciatic nerve and were classified as nociceptive-specific (93%) or wide-dynamic-range (7%). The majority of cells responded to thermal as well as mechanical stimuli; thresholds for activation by heat were in the noxious range (43-50°C). Central conduction velocities ranged from 0.8 to 16.2 m/s. The receptive fields of lamina I projection neurons with sciatic input were usually located either on one or more toes, occasionally including an adjacent foot pad, or on a small patch of skin on the dorsal, ventral or lateral surface of the paw (Fig. 2). More proximally located receptive fields were generally larger than distal fields. The cells examined in this study were identified as lamina I projection neurons, but we did not determine their site of termination. They are likely to be spinomesencephalic (Ménétrey *et al*, 1980; McMahon and Wall, 1985) or spinothalamic (Giesler *et al*, 1976; Ménétrey and Besson, 1981) projection neurons.

The arrangement of receptive fields of lumbar dorsal horn cells forms a somatotopic map of the hindlimbs and caudal body parts. This has been described in detail by several authors for dorsal horn cells in general (Brown and Fuchs, 1975; Pubols and Goldberger, 1980; Light and Durkovic, 1984) and by Cervero *et al* (1976) and Hylden *et al* (1987) for nociceptive lamina I neurons. Cells with toe receptive fields, which have comprised the majority of sciatic nerve-innervated cells in our studies, primarily occupy the medial two-thirds of lamina I. Cells with receptive fields on the foot and/or ankle

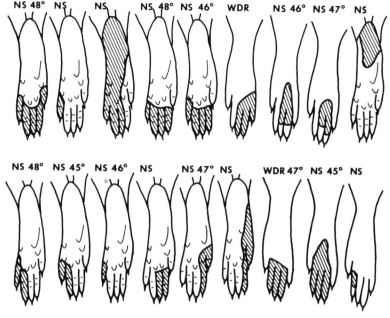

FIGURE 2: Examples of receptive fields for lumbar lamina I projection neurons recorded in the rat. Shaded regions indicate the area from which a response could be elicited by mechanical stimulation. The majority of cells (16 of the 18 shown here) were nociceptive-specific (NS). Two of the 18 cells were of the wide-dynamic-range type (WDR). These 2 cells responded to light touch, but had a more vigorous response to pressure and pinch. Mechanical (von Frey) thresholds for these WDR neurons were less than 10 mN and for the NS neurons were greater than 50 mN. Eleven of the 18 cells shown here responded to noxious heat applied to the receptive field with a contact thermode: thresholds ranged from 45 to 48°C as indicated.

are concentrated more laterally. Cells with receptive fields on the leg and thigh are normally recorded in the most lateral part of the dorsal horn. This arrangement correlates closely with the distribution of hindlimb nerve small diameter primary afferent terminals labelled by transganglionic transport of HRP as demonstrated by Swett and Woolf (1985) in the rat.

RETROGRADE LABELLING OF LAMINA I PROJECTION NEURONS

Lamina I Neurons Project their Axons via the Dorsolateral Funiculi

An interesting aspect of the lamina I projection system was brought to our attention by McMahon and Wall (1983) in a report on lamina I cells projecting through the dorsolateral funiculi (DLF). In this report, a majority of lamina I neurons in rats were antidromically activated from the contralateral DLF and not from the ventrolateral quadrant where the spinothalamic tract is known to travel. In a subsequent paper, these authors reported that these lamina I neurons terminated in the midbrain and in fact some cells appeared to have multiple collaterals terminating in the ventrolateral PAG and adjacent nucleus cuneiformis (McMahon and Wall, 1985). The question arises as to the functional role of a DLF pathway for nociceptive projection neurons. Lesions of the DLF in rat leave nociceptive responses apparently intact (Basbaum *et al*, 1977). Therefore, what does a nociceptive projection pathway have to do with pain if, when the axons of such a system are cut the response of the animal to painful stimuli remains?

We performed retrograde labelling experiments in cats (Hylden *et al*, 1986a) and rats (Hylden *et al*, 1988a) to examine the extent of the lamina I PBA projection via the DLF. Injection of WGA-HRP (wheat germ agglutinin conjugated to HRP) into the PBA resulted in labelling of cells bilaterally (contralateral predominance) throughout the length of the spinal cord in animals with intact spinal cords. A particularly high concentration of cells was noted in lamina I. In rats, more than one-third of the labelled cells in the cervical and lumbar enlargements were located in lamina I; in cats, 40-60% were located in lamina I. In animals with bilateral lesions of the DLF at lower thoracic levels there was a significant decrease in the percentage of labelled cells located in lamina I caudal to the lesions. Figure 3 presents examples of data obtained from two rats with injections of WGA-HRP into the PBA, one control rat and one rat with bilateral DLF lesions. The decrease in labelling of lamina I neurons ranged from 71 to 94%, depending on the extent of the DLF lesions. Lesions including the dorsal-most two-thirds of the DLF resulted in a smaller, but significant decrease in the number of lamina I cells labelled. DLF lesions did not reduce the labelling of cells located in deeper laminae.

Our observation of a DLF projection for lamina I spinomesencephalic neurons in the cat and rat agrees with the electrophysiological evidence for such a projection in the rat (McMahon and Wall, 1983). The earliest descriptions of a DLF projection for lamina I neurons were made by Molenaar and Kuypers (1978) in the cat and monkey and by Zemlan *et al* (1978) in the rat. Both sets of authors used spinal cord white matter applications of HRP to demonstrate labelling in more caudal segments.

Spinothalamic/Spinomesencephalic Collateralization of Lamina I Neurons

Recent reports have demonstrated that, in addition to the spinomesencephalic lamina I neurons discussed so far, spinothalamic lamina I neurons also project via the DLF. In both cats (Jones *et al*, 1985, 1987) and monkeys (Apkarian *et al*, 1987) retrograde labelling of lamina I spinothalamic neurons was blocked caudal to DLF lesions but was not altered by lesions of the ventrolateral quadrant. Lamina I spinomesencephalic and lamina I spinothalamic tract neurons also have similar response properties to natural and electrical stimuli. Recent reports that have concentrated on characterizing the lamina I component of the spinothalamic tract have given us some detailed information on this projection system. Craig and Kniffki (1985) have reported on a population of lamina I spinothalamic tract neurons in the cat that were primarily nociceptive-specific with small receptive fields and slow central conduction velocities (mean 3.7 m/s). Lamina I spinothalamic tract neurons in the monkey appear to have somewhat faster central conduction velocities (mean 17 m/s), but as in the cat, receptive fields are small and the majority of cells respond exclusively or maximally to noxious cutaneous stimuli (Ferrington *et al*, 1987).

In light of these similarities it is not surprising that we (Hylden *et al*, 1986b) and others (Price *et al*, 1978; Girardot *et al*, 1987; Yezierski *et al*, 1987) have seen neurons that were antidromically activated from both the midbrain and the thalamus. We have examined the collateral projection of lamina I cells to the midbrain and thalamus by retrograde labelling and have attempted to estimate the magnitude of collateralization (Hylden *et al*, 1988a). For these experiments, relatively large injections of Fluoro-gold were made into the lateral thalamus of rats and rhodamine-labelled latex microspheres were injected into the PBA ipsilateral to the thalamic injection. Sagittal sections of the contralateral cervical and lumbar enlargements were examined for the presence of cells containing one or both fluorescent retrograde tracers.

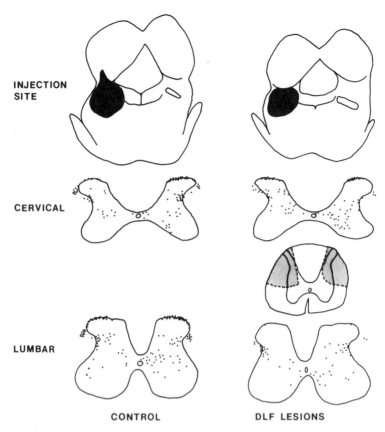

INJECTION SITE

CERVICAL

LUMBAR

CONTROL   DLF LESIONS

FIGURE 3: Camera lucida drawings depicting the data obtained from two rats with injections of WGA-HRP into the PBA: one control rat and one rat that had bilateral DLF lesions. The distribution of retrogradely labelled cells in the cervical and lumbar enlargements is indicated. Note that in the rat with DLF lesions few lamina I neurons are labelled caudal to the lesion. (Adapted from Hylden *et al*, 1988a).

All rats that had reasonable retrograde labelling from both injection sites (n = 10 rats) demonstrated some degree of collateral labelling. The observed distribution of single and double labelled neurons in the lumbar enlargement is presented diagrammatically in Fig. 4. Double labelled neurons were especially abundant in lamina I. In seven rats, the percentage of lamina I spinothalamic tract cells double-labelled from the PBA ranged from 50% to 98%. Thus, the majority of lamina I spinothalamic tract neurons in the cervical and lumbar enlargements had collateral branches terminating in the PBA. The converse relationship was not true-the majority of lamina I PBA projection neurons (50-96%) were only single labelled (Hylden *et al*, 1988a).

The high proportion of lamina I spinothalamic neurons double labelled from the midbrain has been seen following more discrete injections into the PAG. Pechura (1987a, 1987b) demonstrated significant collateralization to the PAG in the rat of both laterally projecting and medially projecting spinothalamic tract cells. This was especially striking for lamina I cells projecting to the lateral thalamus; approximately one-third of such cells were double labelled from the PAG. Since the mesencephalic terminal field of lamina I PBA projection neurons extends into the PAG, double

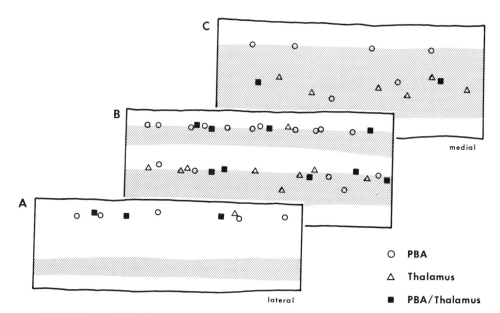

FIGURE 4: The locations of PBA projection neurons (open circles), thalamic projection neurons (open triangles) and neurons having collateral projections to both PBA and thalamus (filled squares) are indicated in schematic drawings of 3 representative parasagittal sections trough the lateral spinal nucleus (A), lateral dorsal horn (B) and medial dorsal horn (C) of the lumbar enlargement of one rat that was injected with Fluoro-gold in the lateral thalamus and rhodamine-labelled microspheres in the PBA.

labelled cells described by Liu (1983), Pechura (1987a, 1987b) and Harmann *et al* (1987) in the rat and by Zhang *et al* (1987) in the monkey can be considered to be a subset of the larger population of PBA/thalamic projection neurons. Our study using more general PBA injections has served to emphasize the magnitude of this collateral projection.

Neurochemistry of Lamina I Projection Neurons

One further point concerning lamina I projection neurons that has received some attention in the current literature is the neurochemistry of these cells. Recent studies have identified some neuropeptide-containing cells in the rat spinal cord with projections to the medullary reticular formation (Nahin, 1987) or the thalamus (Coffield and Miletic, 1987; Ju *et al*, 1987; Nahin, 1988). Neurons in the marginal zone of the spinal cord have been observed to stain immunohistochemically for opioid peptides using antibodies directed toward either enkephalin (Aronin *et al*, 1981; Glazer and Basbaum, 1981) or dynorphin (Khachaturian *et al*, 1982; Cruz and Basbaum, 1985; Cho and Basbaum, 1988; Ruda *et al*, 1988). Therefore, opioid peptides are potential transmitter substances for lamina I projection neurons. Standaert *et al*, (1986) have combined retrograde labelling of lamina I cells from the dorsolateral pons with immunocytochemical staining for opioid peptides and have observed that as many as 50% of retrogradely labelled cells also stained with one or more antisera directed toward either dynorphin, enkephalin, pro-enkephalin or peptide E. Our own investigations of PBA projection neurons have indicated that only a small percentage of retrogradely labelled lamina I neurons contain enkephalin or dynorphin (between 1 and 10%; Nahin and Hylden, 1986; Nahin *et al*, 1988).

119

SUMMARY AND CONCLUSIONS

The studies described above, from both our and other laboratories, have demonstrated the presence of a direct projection system from lamina I through the DLF to the PBA with major collateralization to the thalamus. The cells making up this system are largely nociceptive-specific, have small receptive fields and slow central conduction velocities. It is apparent from these studies that the lamina I projection system is involved in distributing information to various brainstem sites. We have discussed terminations in the midbrain and lateral thalamus, but lamina I projection neurons are also known to terminate in the medial thalamus, especially in nucleus submedius (Craig and Burton, 1981), in the hypothalamus (Burstein *et al*, 1987) and the nucleus of the solitary tract (Menétrey and Basbaum, 1987). A significant number, and perhaps the vast majority, of lamina I neurons have multiple termination sites, including cells that terminate in both midbrain and thalamus (see above) and cells that terminate at multiple midbrain sites (McMahon and Wall 1985; Hylden el al., 1986b; Yezierski and Schwartz, 1987).

The small receptive fields and nociceptive properties of these cells suggest that they may be important in the localization of noxious stimuli. Although this may make up one component of their function, we believe that the role of lamina I projection neurons is much more complex.

The fact that lamina I neurons project their axons through the DLF argues against a simple sensory role for these neurons. Classically, pain and temperature sensations have been considered to be transmitted by the crossed spinothalamic tract in the anterolateral quadrant of the spinal cord. This viewpoint has been supported by the clinical success of anterolateral cordotomy for pain relief (see references in Vierck *et al*, 1985) and by the apparent analgesia produced by such lesions in monkeys (Vierck *et al*, 1983). Lesions of the DLF do not produce analgesia in rats (Basbaum *et al*, 1977) or monkeys (Vierck *et al*, 1971), but may in fact result in hyperalgesia. However, in cats dorsal hemisection has been reported to attenuate pain reactivity and thermosensitivity (Kennard, 1954; Casey *et al*, 1981). We have observed that lamina I PBA projection neurons in both the cat and the rat send their axons through the DLF. Due to the high degree of collateralization, a DLF projection for the majority of rat lamina I spinothalamic projection neurons can also be inferred. Thus, a dorsolateral spinothalamic pathway has now been demonstrated in monkey, cat and rat. These observations of a DLF projection for lamina I neurons, together with a demonstrated lack of involvement of DLF pathways in the detection of noxious stimuli (Vierck *et al*, 1971), suggest that lamina I projection neurons are not necessary for the rostral conduction of pain sensations.

A second characteristic of lamina I projection neurons, their primarily nociceptive-specific nature, also argues against an important role for these neurons in the sensory-discriminative aspects of pain. Recent evidence has indicated that nociceptive-specific neurons are not involved in the encoding process by which monkeys perceive the intensity of noxious stimuli (Maixner *et al*, 1986). In these experiments, the neuronal discharge of wide-dynamic-range type neurons in the medullary dorsal horn correlated closely with behavioral detection latency in a thermal detection task conducted in the noxious range (temperatures at which monkeys and humans normally choose to escape the stimulus); the neuronal discharge of nociceptive-specific neurons did not correlate with the ability of the animal to detect a noxious heat stimulus in this temperature range.

It appears likely from the above discussion that nociceptive-specific lamina I spinomesencephalic/spinothalamic projection neurons do not play an important role in pain sensation *per se*, but may be involved in other aspects of the pain response. The potential importance and functional complexity of the lamina I projection system may become more evident upon consideration of the data available on the physiology, pharmacology and anatomy of the termination sites of these neurons.

Electrical stimulation of the midbrain PAG produces analgesia in rats and cats (Reynolds, 1969; Liebeskind *et al*, 1973; Oliveras *et al*, 1974), and this same area has been shown to be important for the analgesic action of morphine (Yaksh *et al*, 1976; Abbott and Melzack, 1982). A direct projection from the PAG to the serotonin-rich nucleus raphe magnus of the medulla (Ruda, 1975) is believed to be the connection through which electrical or pharmacological manipulations in the midbrain activate an antinociceptive medullospinal pathway (Basbaum *et al*, 1976, 1978). Injections of retrograde tracer into the rostral ventral medulla result in the labelling of cells in the PAG and adjacent nucleus cuneiformis of the caudal midbrain (Gallager and Pert, 1978; Abols and Basbaum, 1981). This cell group overlaps with the terminal fields of spinal lamina I projection neurons. Thus, the terminals of nociceptive lamina I spinomesencephalic projection neurons are ideally situated to provide input onto cells in the ventral medulla and thereby activate a descending pain inhibitory system. We have also observed that lamina I projection neurons receive serotonergic afferents (Hylden *et al*, 1986c) and are often inhibited by stimulation of descending fibers. It is therefore probable that nociceptive lamina I projection neurons represent an initial link in an ascending-descending pain modulation system that functions as a negative feedback control loop. Basbaum and Fields (1978) originally proposed that noxious stimuli were critical for the activation of the medullospinal pain modulatory system.

Stimulation in various midbrain areas has also been shown to elicit complex emotional reactions and painful sensations in humans (Nashold *et al*, 1969) as well as fear-motivated behavior in animals (Spiegel *et al*, 1954; Delgado *et al*, 1956; Liebman *et al*, 1970; Kiser *et al*, 1978). Midbrain areas also are important in the control of locomotion (Skultety, 1963; Sinnamon, 1984). The midbrain PAG and cuneiform nuclei receive input from multiple sources including gustatory afferents (Norgren and Leonard, 1973), and general visceral afferents (Loewy and Burton, 1978; Norgren, 1978) as well as the spinal nociceptive input already discussed. This area of the midbrain has multiple efferent connections including those to hypothalamic, diencephalic and limbic structures (Chi, 1970; Edwards, 1975; Edwards and DeOlmos, 1976; Hopkins and Holstege, 1978; Saper *et al*, 1978; Fulwiler and Saper, 1984). Thus, it follows that nociceptive input to the midbrain PBA may be important in the motivational-affective aspects of pain (Spiegel *et al*, 1954; Melzack and Casey, 1968; Bowsher, 1976). In addition, lamina I projection neurons are possibly involved in the activation of visceral reflexes via input to the dorsolateral pons/caudal mesencephalon (Saper and Loewy, 1980) and to the nucleus of the solitary tract (Menétrey and Basbaum, 1987).

REFERENCES

ABBOTT, F.V. AND MELZACK, R. (1982). Brain stem lesions dissociate neural mechanisms of morphine analgesia in different kinds of pain. *Brain Research* **251**, 149-155.

ABOLS, I.A. AND BASBAUM, A.I. (1981). Afferent connections of the rostral medulla of the cat: a neural substrate for midbrain-medullary interactions in the modulation of pain. *Journal of Comparative Neurology* **201**, 285-297.

APKARIAN, A.V., STEVENS, R.T. AND HODGE, C.J. (1987). The primate dorsolateral spinothalamic pathway. *Society for Neuroscience Abstracts* **13**, 580.

ARONIN, N., DIFIGLIA, M., LIOTTA, A.S. AND MARTIN, J.B. (1981). Ultrastructural localization and biochemical features of immunoreactive leu-enkephalin in monkey dorsal horn. *Journal of Neuroscience* **1**, 561-577.

BASBAUM, A.I., CLANTON, C.H. AND FIELDS, H.L. (1976). Opiate and stimulus-produced analgesia: functional anatomy of a medullospinal pathway. *Proceedings of the National Academy of Science USA* **73**, 4685-4688.

BASBAUM, A.I., CLANTON, C.H. AND FIELDS, H.L. (1978). Three bulbospinal pathways from the rostral medulla of the cat. An autoradiographic study of pain modulating systems. *Journal of Comparative Neurology* **178**, 209-224.

BASBAUM, A.I. AND FIELDS, H.L. (1978). Endogenous pain control mechanisms: review and hypothesis. *Annals of Neurology* **4**, 451-462.

BASBAUM, A.I., MARLEY, N.J.E., O'KEEFE, J. AND CLANTON, C.H. (1977). Reversal of morphine and stimulus-produced analgesia by subtotal spinal cord lesions. *Pain* **3**, 43-56.

BEITEL, R.E. AND DUBNER, R. (1976). Responses of unmyelinated (C) polymodal nociceptors to thermal stimuli applied to monkey's face. *Journal of Neurophysiology* **39**, 1160-1175.

BESSOU, P. AND PERL, E.R. (1969). Response of cutaneous sensory units with unmyelinated fibers to noxious stimuli. *Journal of Neurophysiology* **32**, 1025-1043.

BOWSHER, D. (1976). Role of the reticular formation in responses to noxious stimulation. *Pain* **2**, 361-378.

BROWN, P.B. AND FUCHS, J.L. (1975). Somatotopic representation of hindlimb skin in cat dorsal horn. *Journal of Neurophysiology* **38**, 1-9.

BURGESS, P.R. AND PERL, E.R. (1967). Myelinated afferent fibres responding specifically to noxious stimulation of the skin. *Journal of Physiology* **190**, 541-562.

BURSTEIN, R., CLIFFER, K.D. AND GIESLER, G.J., Jr. (1987). Direct somatosensory projections from the spinal cord to the hypothalamus and telencephalon. *Journal of Neuroscience* **7**, 4159-4164.

CARSTENS, E. AND TREVINO, D.L. (1978). Laminar origins of spinothalamic projections in the cat as determined by the retrograde transport of horseradish peroxidase. *Journal of Comparative Neurology* **182**, 151-166.

CASEY, K.L., HALL, B.R. AND MORROW, T.J. (1981). Effect of spinal cord lesions on responses of cats to thermal pulses. *Pain* (Suppl. **1**), S130.

CECHETTO, D.F., STANDAERT, D.G. AND SAPER, C.B. (1985). Spinal and trigeminal dorsal horn projections to the parabrachial nucleus in the rat. *Journal of Comparative Neurology* **240**, 153-160.

CERVERO, F., IGGO, A. AND OGAWA, H. (1976). Nociceptor-driven dorsal horn neurones in the lumbar spinal cord of the cat. *Pain* **2**, 5-24.

CERVERO, F., IGGO, A. AND MOLONY, V. (1979). Ascending projections of nociceptor-driven lamina I neurones in the cat. *Experimental Brain Research* **35**, 135-149.

CHI, C.C. (1970). An experimental silver study of the ascending projections of the central gray substance and adjacent tegmentum in the rat with observations in the cat. *Journal of Comparative Neurology* **139**, 259-270.

CHO, H.J. AND BASBAUM, A.I. (1988). Increased staining of immunoreactive dynorphin cell bodies in the deafferented spinal cord of the rat. *Neuroscience Letters* **84**, 125-130.

CHRISTENSEN, B.N. AND PERL, E.R. (1970). Spinal neurons specifically excited by noxious or thermal stimuli: marginal zone of the dorsal horn. *Journal of*

Neurophysiology **33**, 293-307.

COFFIELD, J.A. AND MILETIC, V. (1987). Immunoreactive enkephalin is contained within some trigeminal and spinal neurons projecting to the rat medial thalamus. *Brain Research* **425**, 38-383.

CRAIG, A.D. AND BURTON, H. (1981). Spinal and medullary lamina I projection to nucleus submedius in medial thalamus: a possible pain center. *Journal of Neurophysiology* **45**, 443-466.

CRAIG, A.D. AND KNIFFKI, K.-D. (1985). Spinothalamic lumbosacral lamina I cells responsive to skin and muscle stimulation in the cat. *Journal of Physiology* **365**, 197-221.

CRUZ, L. AND BASBAUM, A.I. (1985). Multiple opioid peptides and the modulation of pain: immunohistochemical analysis of dynorphin and enkephalin in the trigeminal nucleus caudalis and spinal cord of the cat. *Journal of Comparative Neurology* **240**, 331-348.

DELGADO, J.M.R., ROSVOLD, H.E. AND LOONEY, E. (1956). Evoking conditional fear by electrical stimulation of subcortical structures in the monkey brain. *Journal of Comparative Physiology and Psychology* **49**, 373-380.

DILLY, P.N., WALL, P.D. AND WEBSTER, K.E. (1968). Cells of origin of the spinothalamic tract in the cat and rat. *Experimental Neurology* **21**, 550-562.

EDWARDS, S.B. (1975). Autoradiographic studies of the projections of the midbrain reticular formation: descending projections of nucleus cuneiformis. *Journal of Comparative Neurology* **161**, 341-358.

EDWARDS, S.B. AND DEOLMOS, J.S. (1976). Autoradiographic studies of the projections of the midbrain reticular formation: ascending projections of nucleus cuneiformis. *Journal of Comparative Neurology* **165**, 417-432.

FERRINGTON, D.G., SORKIN, L.S. AND WILLIS, W.D. (1987). Responses of spinothalamic tract cells in the superficial dorsal horn of the primate lumbar spinal cord. *Journal of Physiology* **388**, 681-703.

FULWILER, C.E. AND SAPER, C.B. (1984). Subnuclear organization of the efferent connections of the parabrachial nucleus in the rat. *Brain Research Reviews* **7**, 229-259.

GALLAGER, D.W. AND PERT, A. (1978). Afferents to brain stem nuclei (brain stem raphe, nucleus reticularis pontis caudalis and nucleus gigantocellularis) in the rat as demonstrated by microiontophoretically applied horseradish peroxidase. *Brain Research* **144**, 257-275.

GIESLER, G.J., Jr., MÉNÉTREY, D., GUILBAUD, G. AND BESSON, J.M. (1976). Lumbar cord neurons at the origin of the spinothalamic tract in the rat. *Brain Research* **118**, 320-324.

GIESLER, G.J., Jr., MÉNÉTREY, D. AND BASBAUM, A.I. (1979). Differential origins of spinothalamic tract projections to medial and lateral thalamus in the rat. *Journal of Comparative Neurology* **184**, 107-125.

GIRARDOT, M.-N., BRENNEN, T.J., MARTINDALE, M.E. AND FOREMAN, R.D. (1987). Effects of stimulating the subcoeruleus-parabrachial region on the non-noxious and noxious responses of T1-T5 spinothalamic tract neurons in the primate. *Brain Research* **409**, 19-30.

GLAZER, E.J. AND BASBAUM, A.I. (1981). Immunohistochemical localization of leucine-enkephalin in the spinal cord of the cat: Enkephalin-containing marginal neurons and pain modulation. *Journal of Comparative Neurology* **196**, 377-389.

HARMANN, P.A., CARLTON, S.M. AND WILLIS, W.D. (1987). Collaterals of spinothalamic tract cells to the periaqueductal gray: a fluorescent double-labelling study in the rat. *Brain Research* **441**, 87-97.

HOPKINS, D.A. AND HOLSTEGE, G. (1978). Amygdaloid projections to the mesencephalon, pons and medulla oblongata in the cat. *Experimental Brain Research* **32**, 529-547.

HU, J.W., DOSTROVSKY, J.O. AND SESSLE, B.J. (1981). Functional properties of neurons in cat trigeminal subnucleus caudalis (medullary dorsal horn). I. Responses to oral-facial noxious and non-noxious stimuli and projections to thalamus and subnucleus oralis. *Journal of Neurophysiology* **45**, 173-192.

HYLDEN, J.L.K., HAYASHI, H., BENNETT, G.J. AND DUBNER, R. (1985). Spinal lamina I neurons projecting to the parabrachial area of the cat midbrain. *Brain Research* **336**, 195-198.

HYLDEN, J.L.K., HAYASHI, H. AND BENNETT, G.J. (1986a). Lamina I spinomesencephalic neurons in the cat ascend via the dorsolateral funiculi. *Somatosensory Research* **4**, 31-41.

HYLDEN, J.L.K., HAYASHI, H., DUBNER, R. AND BENNETT, G.J. (1986b). Physiology and morphology of the lamina I spinomesencephalic projection. *Journal of Comparative Neurology* **247**, 505-515.

HYLDEN, J.L.K., HAYASHI, H. RUDA, M.A. AND DUBNER, R. (1986c). Serotonin innervation of physiologically identified lamina I projection neurons. *Brain Research* **370**, 401-404.

HYLDEN, J.L.K., NAHIN, R.L. AND DUBNER, R. (1987). Altered responses of nociceptive cat lamina I spinal dorsal horn neurons after chronic sciatic neuroma formation. *Brain Research* **411**, 341-350.

HYLDEN, J.L.K., ANTON, F. AND NAHIN, R.L. (1988a). Spinal lamina I projection neurons in the rat: collateral innervation of parabrachial area and thalamus. *Neuroscience* (in press).

HYLDEN, J.L.K., NAHIN, R.L., TRAUB, R.J. AND DUBNER, R. (1988b). Physiological characterization of spinal lamina I projection neurons in rats with unilateral adjuvant-induced inflammation. (in preparation)

JONES, M.W., HODGE, C.J., Jr., APKARIAN, A.V. AND STEVENS, R.T. (1985). A dorsolateral spinothalamic pathway in cat. *Brain Research* **335**, 188-193.

JONES, M.W., APKARIAN, A.V., STEVENS, R.T. AND HODGE, C.J., JR. (1987). The spinothalamic tract: an examination of the cells of origin of the dorsolateral and ventral spinothalamic pathways in cats. *Journal of Comparative Neurology* **260**, 349-361.

JU, G., MELANDER, T., CECCATELLI, S., HOKFELT, T. AND FREY, P. Immunohistochemical evidence for a spinothalamic pathway co-containing cholecystokinin- and galanin-like immunoreactivities in the rat. *Neuroscience* **20**, 439-456.

KENNARD, M.A. (1954). The course of ascending fibers in the spinal cord of the cat essential to the recognition of painful stimuli. *Journal of Comparative Neurology* **100**, 511-524.

KHACHATURIAN, H., WATSON, S.J., LEWIS, M.E., COY, D., GOLDSTEIN, A. AND AKIL, H. (1982). Dynorphin immunocytochemistry in the rat central nervous system. *Peptides* **3**, 941-954.

KISER, R.S., LEBOVITZ, R.M. AND GERMAN, D.C. (1978). Anatomic and pharmacologic differences between two types of aversive midbrain stimulation. *Brain Research* **155**, 331-342.

KUMAZAWA, T., PERL, E.R., BURGESS, P.R. AND WHITEHORN, D. (1975). Ascending projections from marginal zone (lamina I) neurons of the spinal dorsal horn. *Journal of Comparative Neurology* **162**, 1-12.

KUMAZAWA, T. AND PERL, E.R. (1977). Primate cutaneous sensory units with unmyelinated (C) afferent fibers. *Journal of Neurophysiology* **40**, 1325-1338.

KURU, M. (1949). *Sensory Paths in the Spinal Cord and Brain Stem.* Tokyo: Sogensya.

LIEBESKIND, J.C., GUILBAUD, G., BESSON, J.-M. AND OLIVERAS, J.-L. (1973). Analgesia from electrical stimulation of the periaqueductal gray matter in the cat: behavioral observations and inhibitory effects on spinal cord interneurons. *Brain Research* **50**, 441-446.

LIEBMAN, J.M., MAYER, D.J. AND LIEBESKIND, J.C. (1970). Mesencephalic central gray lesions and fear-motivated behavior in rats. *Brain Research* **23**, 353-370.

LIGHT, A.R. AND DURKOVIC, R.G. (1984). Features of laminar and somatotopic organization of lumbar spinal cord units receiving cutaneous inputs from hindlimb receptive fields. *Journal of Neurophysiology* **52**, 449-458.

LIGHT, A.R., CASALE, E.J. AND SEDIVEC, M. (1987). The physiology and anatomy of spinal laminae I and II neurons which project to the parabrachial region of the midbrain and pons. In *Fine Afferent Nerve Fibers and Pain*, eds. Schmidt, R.F *et al.* pp. 347-356. Weinheim: VCH.

LIU, R.P.C. (1983). Laminar origins of spinal projection neurons to the periaqueductal gray of the rat. *Brain Research* **264**, 118-122.

LOEWY, A.D. AND BURTON, H. (1978). Nuclei of the solitary tract: efferent projections to the lower brain stem and spinal cord of the cat. *Journal of Comparative Neurology* **181**, 421-450.

MAIXNER, W., DUBNER, R., BUSHNELL, M.C., KENSHALO, D.R., Jr. and OLIVERAS, J.-L. (1986). Wide-dynamic-range dorsal horn neurons participate in the encoding process by which monkeys perceive the intensity of noxious heat stimuli. *Brain Research* **374**, 385-388.

McMAHON, S.B. AND WALL, P.D. (1983). A system of rat spinal cord lamina I cells projecting through the contralateral dorsolateral funiculus. *Journal of Comparative Neurology* **214**, 217-223.

McMAHON, S.B. AND WALL, P.D. (1985). Electrophysiological mapping of brainstem projections of spinal cord lamina I cells in the rat. *Brain Research* **333**, 19-26.

MELZACK, R. AND CASEY, K.L. (1968). Sensory, motivational and central control determinants of pain. A new conceptual model. In *The Skin Senses*, ed. Kenshalo, D.R., pp. 423-443. Springfield, IL: Thomas.

MENÉTREY, D. AND BASBAUM, A.I. (1987). Spinal and trigeminal projections to the nucleus of the solitary tract: a possible substrate for somatovisceral and viscerovisceral reflex activation. *Journal of Comparative Neurology* **255**, 439-450.

MENÉTREY, D. AND BESSON, J.M. (1981). Electrophysiology and location of dorsal horn neurones in the rat, including cells at the origin of the spinoreticular and spinothalamic tracts. In *Spinal Cord Sensation. Sensory Processing in the Dorsal Horn*, eds. Brown, A.G. and Rethelyi, M., pp. 179-188. Edinburgh: Scottish Academic Press.

MENÉTREY, D., CHAOUCH, A. AND BESSON, J.-M. (1980). Location and properties of dorsal horn neurons at origin of spinoreticular tract in lumbar enlargement of the rat. *Journal of Neurophysiology* **44**, 862-877.

MENÉTREY, D., CHAOUCH, A., BINDER, D. AND BESSON, J.-M. (1982). The origin of the spinomesencephalic tract in the rat: an anatomical study using the retrograde transport of horseradish peroxidase. *Journal of Comparative Neurology* **206**, 193-207.

MOLENAAR, I. AND KUYPERS, H.G.J.M. (1978). Cells of origin of propriospinal fibers and of fibers ascending to supraspinal levels. A HRP study in cat and rhesus monkey. *Brain Research* **152**, 429-450.

NAHIN, R.L. (1987). Immunocytochemical identification of long ascending peptidergic neurons contributing to the spinoreticular tract in the rat. *Neuroscience* **23**, 859-869.

NAHIN, R.L. (1988). Immunocytochemical identification of long ascending, peptidergic lumbar spinal neurons terminating in either the medial or lateral thalamus in the rat. *Brain Research* **443**, 345-349.

NAHIN, R.L. AND HYLDEN, J.L.K. (1986). Immunocytochemical investigations of long ascending somatosensory pathways in the rat and cat. *Society for Neuroscience Abstracts* **12**, 228.

NAHIN, R.L., HYLDEN, J.L.K. AND DUBNER, R. (1988). Adjuvant-induced inflammation is associated with increased dynorphin immunoreactivity in both local circuit and projection neurons in lumbar spinal lamina I of the rat. *Society for Neuroscience Abstracts* **14**, (in press).

NASHOLD, B.S., Jr., WILSON, W.P. AND SLAUGHTER, D.G. (1969). Sensations evoked by stimulation in the midbrain of man. *Journal of Neurosurgery* **30**, 14-24.

NORGREN, R. (1978). Projections from the nucleus of the solitary tract in the rat. *Neuroscience* **3**, 207-218.

NORGREN, R. AND LEONARD, C.M. (1973). Ascending central gustatory pathways. *Journal of Comparative Neurology* **150**, 217-238.

OLIVERAS, J.-L., BESSON, J.-M., GUILBAUD, G. AND LIEBESKIND, J.C. (1974). Behavioral and electrophysiological evidence of pain inhibition from midbrain stimulation in the cat. *Experimental Brain Research* **20**, 32-44.

PANNETON, W.M. AND BURTON, H. (1985). Projections from the paratrigeminal nucleus and the medullary and spinal dorsal horns to the peribrachial area in the cat. *Neuroscience* **15**, 779-797.

PECHURA, C.M. (1987a). Lateral versus medial spinothalamic neurons and their axon collaterals to the periaqueductal gray and medullary reticular formation in the rat. *Society for Neuroscience Abstracts* **13**, 113.

PECHURA, C.M. (1987b). Laterally versus medially projecting spinothalamic neurons and their axon collaterals to the periaqueductal gray and medullary reticular formation in the rat. Uniformed Services University of the Health Sciences: *Ph.D. dissertation*.

PERL, E.R. (1968). Myelinated afferent fibres innervating the primate skin and their response to noxious stimuli. *Journal of Physiology* **197**, 593-615.

PRICE, D.D. AND BROWE, A.C. (1975). Spinal cord coding of graded non-noxious and noxious temperature increases. *Experimental Neurology* **48**, 201-221.

PRICE, D.D., DUBNER, R. AND HU, J.W. (1976). Trigeminothalamic neurons in nucleus caudalis responsive to tactile, thermal, and nociceptive stimulation of monkey's face. *Journal of Neurophysiology* **39**, 936-953.

PRICE, D.D., HAYES, R.L., RUDA, M.A. AND DUBNER, R. (1978). Spatial and temporal transformations of input to spinothalamic tract neurons and their relation to somatic sensation. *Journal of Neurophysiology* **41**, 933-947.

PUBOLS, L.M. AND GOLDBERGER, M.E. (1980). Recovery of function in dorsal horn following partial deafferentation. *Journal of Neurophysiology* **43**, 102-117.

REYNOLDS, D.V. (1969). Surgery in the rat during electrical analgesia induced by focal brain stimulation. *Science* **164**, 444-445.

RUDA, M,A. (1975). Autoradiographic study of the efferent projections of the midbrain central gray of the cat. University of Pennsylvania: *Ph. D. dissertation.*

RUDA, M.A., IADAROLA, M.J., COHEN, L.V. AND YOUNG, S.W., III (1988). In situ hybridization histochemistry and immunocytochemistry reveal an increase in spinal dynorphin biosynthesis in a rat model of peripheral inflammation and hyperalgesia. *Proceedings of the National Academy of Science USA* **85**, 622-626.

SAPER, C.B. AND LOEWY, A.D. (1980). Efferent connections of the parabrachial nucleus in the rat. *Brain Research* **197**, 291-317.

SAPER, C.B., SWANSON, L.W. AND COWAN, W.M. (1978). The efferent connections of the anterior hypothalamic area of the rat, cat and monkey. *Journal of Comparative Neurology* **182**, 575-600.

SINNAMON, H.M. (1984). Forelimb and hindlimb stepping by the anesthetized rat elicited by electrical stimulation of the diencephalon and mesencephalon. *Physiology and Behavior* **33**, 191-199.

SKULTETY, F.M. (1963). Stimulation of periaqueductal gray and hypothalamus. *Archives of Neurology* **8**, 608-620.

SPIEGEL, E.A., KLETZKIN, M. AND SZEKELY, E.G. (1954). Pain reactions upon stimulation of the tectum mesencephali. *Journal of Neuropathology and Experimental Neurology* **13**, 212-220.

STANDAERT, D.G., WATSON, S.J., HOUGHTEN, R.A. AND SAPER, C.B. (1986). Opioid peptide immunoreactivity in spinal and trigeminal dorsal horn neurons projecting to the parabrachial nucleus in the rat. *Journal of Neuroscience* **6**, 1220-1226.

SWETT, J.E. AND WOOLF, C.J. (1985). The somatotopic organization of primary afferent terminals in the superficial laminae of the dorsal horn of the rat spinal cord. *Journal of Comparative Neurology* **231**, 66-77.

TREVINO, D.L. (1976). The origin and projections of a spinal nociceptive and thermoreceptive pathway. In *Sensory Functions of the Skin of Primates with Special Reference to Man*, ed. Zotterman, Y., pp. 367-376. Oxford: Pergamon Press.

VIERCK, C.J., Jr., COOPER, B.Y., FRANZEN, O., RITZ, L.A. AND GREENSPAN, J.D. (1983). Behavioral analysis of CNS pathways and transmitter systems involved in conduction and inhibition of pain sensations and reactions in primates. In *Progress in Psychobiology and Physiological Psychology*, Vol.1, eds. Sprague, J. and Epstein, A., pp. 113-165. New York: Academic Press.

VIERCK, C.J., Jr., GREENSPAN, J.D., RITZ, L.A. AND YEOMANS, D.C. (1985). The spinal pathways contributing to the ascending conduction and the descending modulation of pain sensations and reactions. In *Spinal Systems of Afferent Processing*, ed. Yaksh, T.L., pp. 275-329. New York: Plenum Press.

VIERCK, C.J., Jr., HAMILTON, D.M. AND THORNBY, J.I. (1971). Pain reactivity of monkeys after lesions to the dorsal and lateral columns of the spinal cord. *Experimental Brain Research* **13**, 140-158.

WIBERG, M. AND BLOMQVIST, A. (1984). The spinomesencephalic tract in the cat: its cells of origin and termination pattern as demonstrated by the intraaxonal transport method. *Brain Research* **291**, 1-18.

WILLIS, W.D., KENSHALO, D.R., Jr. AND LEONARD, R.B. (1979). The cells of origin of the primate spinothalamic tract. *Journal of Comparative Neurology* **188**, 543-574.

WILLIS, W.D., TREVINO, D.L., COULTER, J.D. AND MAUNZ, R.A. (1974). Responses of primate spinothalamic tract neurons to natural stimulation of hindlimb. *Journal of Neurophysiology* **37**, 358-372.

YAKSH, T.L., YEUNG, J.C. AND RUDY, T.A. (1976). Systematic examination in the rat of brain sites sensitive to the direct application of morphine: observation of differential effects within the periaqueductal gray. *Brain Research* **114**, 83-103.

YEZIERSKI, R.P. AND SCHWARTZ, R.H. (1986). Response and receptive field properties of spinomesencephalic tract (SMT) cells in the cat. *Journal of Neurophysiology* **55**, 76-96.

YEZIERSKI, R.P., SORKIN, L.S. AND WILLIS, W.D. (1987). Response properties of spinal neurons projecting to midbrain or midbrain-thalamus in the monkey. *Brain Research* **437**, 165-170.

ZEMLAN, F.P., LEONARD, C.M., KOW, L.M. AND PFAFF, D.W. (1978). Ascending tracts of the lateral columns of the rat spinal cord: a study using the silver impregnation and horseradish peroxidase techniques. *Experimental Neurology* **62**, 298-334.

ZHANG, D., CARLTON, S.M., SORKIN, L.S., HARMANN, P.A. AND WILLIS, W.D. (1987). Collaterals of spinothalamic tract (STT) neurons to the PAG: a double labelling study in the monkey. *Society for Neuroscience Abstracts* **13**, 113.

INPUT TO AND OUTPUT FROM LAMINA I NEURONES IN THE CAT SPINAL CORD

K.-D. Kniffki

Physiologisches Institut der Universität Würzburg,Röntgenring 9, D-8700 Würzburg
F.R.G.

INTRODUCTION

Is there a dorsolateral nociceptive lamina I-spino-thalamo-cortical pathway? In recent years evidence has accumulated suggesting that the answer to this question might be yes. Since the functional and anatomical organization of the nociceptive spino-thalamic system differs fundamentally in some aspects in the species so far investigated, this account will limit itself to the situation in the cat.

Lamina I of the dorsal horn receives input from $A\delta$- and C-fibres including those associated with nociceptors, and lamina I is a major source of the spinothalamic tract (STT).

Recent experiments have indicated the existence of two distinct components of the STT, the classical ventral STT (VSTT) and a new dorsolateral STT (DSTT). The DSTT originates almost exclusively in lamina I, whereas the VSTT has its source in deeper laminae (Jones *et al*, 1987).

In the cat the DSTT terminates in a region of the lateral thalamus which is termed the ventral periphery of the ventrobasal complex (VBvp; Apkarian *et al*, 1987; Kniffki and Vahle-Hinz, 1987). There is evidence from several laboratories that VBvp contains nociceptive neurones (Kniffki and Mizumura, 1983; Honda *et al*, 1983; Yokota and Matsumoto, 1983a,b; Yokota *et al*, 1985; Hodge *et al*, 1987).

In the lateral part of VBvp, the ventral periphery of the ventral posterolateral nucleus (VPLvp), nociceptive neurones have been found to project to the cortical postcruciate area, but not to area 3b, the target of neurones of VPL proper (Craig and Kniffki, 1985c). In addition, a projection from VPLvp to the second somatosensory cortex has been revealed.

In Fig. 1 a composite view is shown of the results described. The question marks indicate our current lack of knowledge about the input and output connections between cat peripheral VB and spinal, thalamic and cortical structures.

THE DORSOLATERAL LAMINA I-SPINO-THALAMO-CORTICAL PATHWAY

Spinothalamic Lamina I Neurones

Christensen and Perl (1970) concluded from their demonstration of the response properties of cat lamina I neurones, that lamina I in the spinal dorsal horn represents a specialized sensory nucleus containing neurones important for nociception and for detection of thermal changes in the skin. It was subsequently demonstrated that lamina I receives direct input from small-diameter Aδ- and C-fibres from skin, muscle, viscera and joint (Craig and Mense, 1983; Cervero and Connell, 1984; de Groat, 1986; Craig *et al*, 1988) including those associated with nociceptors (Light and Perl, 1979). Anatomical investigations have established that lamina I is also a major source of the STT in other species than the cat (Willis, 1985), and furthermore, it contains a high concentration of both nociceptive-specific and thermoreceptive neurones (Perl, 1984).

The major response characteristics of those lamina I cells that project into the spinothalamic tract of the cat are reviewed below (Craig and Kniffki, 1985a,b).

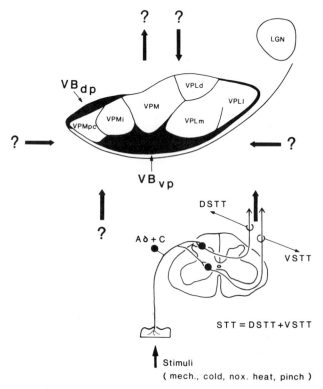

FIGURE 1: Composite view of the pathway from afferent Aδ- and C-fibres to the spinal cord, via the neurones of origin of the spinothalamic tract (STT) by way of its dorsolateral (DSTT) and ventral parts (VSTT), to the lateral part of the ventral periphery of the cat ventrobasal complex (VBvp). The drawing of VB proper was composed from several frontal planes to show the subnuclei and the fibre laminae separating them. VBdp = dorsal periphery of VB. VPL = ventral posterolateral nucleus; m, l, and d indicate the subdivisions of VPL, where forelimb, hindlimb, and trunk are represented by neurones responding to innocuous mechanical stimulation of the skin. VPM = ventral posteromedial nucleus; i represents the subdivision of VPM that contains neurones responding to innocuous mechanical stimulation with ipsi- and contralateral intraoral receptive fields. VPMpc = parvocellular part of VPM, which is assumed to be a relay nucleus for gustation. LGN = lateral geniculate nucleus. The question marks indicate our current lack of knowledge about the input and output connections between cat peripheral VB from and to spinal, thalamic and cortical structures (Kniffki and Vahle-Hinz, unpublished).

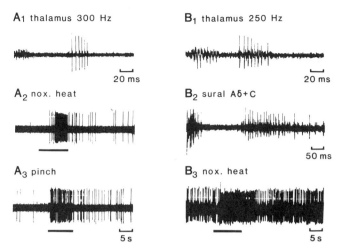

A₁ thalamus 300 Hz

B₁ thalamus 250 Hz

20 ms

20 ms

A₂ nox. heat

B₂ sural Aδ+C

50 ms

A₃ pinch

B₃ nox. heat

5 s

5 s

FIGURE 2: Responses of two nociceptive-specific spinothalamic lamina I neurones. A1, B1: Antidromic response of each cell to a thalamic stimulus train. A2, A3: Responses of cell A to application of noxious heat and pinch within the receptive field. This particular cell had Aδ- and C-fibre input from the tibial nerve; it was initially unresponsive to all forms of innocuous stimulation, and had no background activity in the absence of intentional stimulation. After repeated noxious stimulation of the skin within the receptive field, an ongoing discharge developed and the cell became weakly responsive to application of innocuous pressure and cold stimuli. B2, B3: Cell B responded to Aδ- and C-fibre input from the sural nerve and was only responsive to noxious heat stimulation within a restricted receptive field. After repeated noxious stimulation it also exhibited an ongoing activity (*cf.* beginning of the trace in B3 prior to the noxious heat stimulation indicated by the bar underneath). (From Craig and Kniffki, 1985).

General properties. Based on a total of 218 identified lumbosacral spinothalamic tract lamina I (lamI-STT) cells, their mean central conduction velocity was found to be quite low: 3.7 m/s (range: 1.1 - 16.7 m/s). Of these 218 lamI-STT cells, 47% projected only to medial thalamus, 19% only to lateral thalamus, 26% to both, and 8% to mid-thalamus. About 10% of all cells had an ongoing activity in the absence of intentional stimulation when first isolated.

Response properties. Ninety-three lamI-STT cells responded to electrical stimulation of the sciatic nerve; 47 of these were examined with the complete set of stimuli used.

(1) Nociceptive-specific cells: From the sample of fully characterized lamI-STT cells 47% responded specifically to noxious cutaneous (40%) or deeper tissue stimulation (7%). Cutaneous nociceptive-specific lamI-STT cells responded to pinch or noxious heat, or to both (Fig. 2). In general, the response characteristics of these cells were quite stable over time. In some cells, however, the responses were enhanced following repeated noxious stimulation. None of the cutaneous nociceptive-specific cells displayed ongoing activity upon initial isolation; but about a third developed ongoing activity after noxious stimulation of their receptive fields, which were generally small.

(2) Cold-specific cells: Vigorous responses to innocuous cooling of the skin were observed in 13% of the fully characterized lamI-STT cells (Fig. 3A). Each of these cold-specific cells had a bursting ongoing discharge upon initial isolation, which was inhibited by warming the skin. Their receptive fields were located on the glabrous skin of the paw.

(3) Multireceptive cells: This third class was formed by 28% of the lamI-STT cells and these showed responses to cutaneous noxious stimulation, and, in addition, to innocuous cold stimulation (Fig. 3B), or to deeper tissue stimulation, or to both.

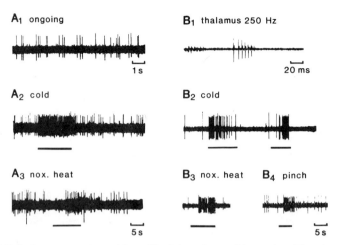

A₁ ongoing

B₁ thalamus 250 Hz

1 s

20 ms

A₂ cold

B₂ cold

A₃ nox. heat

B₃ nox. heat   **B₄** pinch

5 s

5 s

FIGURE 3: Responses of a cold-specific (A) and a multireceptive (B) spinothalamic lamina I neurone. A: Upon initial isolation the cell had a slow bursting ongoing activity (A1); it was activated only by non-noxious cooling of the central pad of the hindpaw (A2). Its ongoing activity was depressed by warming the receptive field; noxious heat evoked a weak response (A3). B: This cell responded immediately and reproducibly to cold applied to the central pad of the hindpaw (B2), to noxious heat (B3) and to pinch (B4); its antidromic response to the thalamic stimulus train is shown in B1. Duration of stimuli marked with bars. (From Craig and Kniffki, 1985).

(4) Unresponsive cells: 13% of the lamI-STT cells did not respond to any of the natural stimuli applied.

Ascending thalamic projections. The neurones of two of the four response categories had distinct thalamic projections. The majority of the cold-specific cells were antidromically activated only from medial thalamus, and almost all multireceptive cold-sensitive cells were activated from both medial and lateral thalamus. The nociceptive-specific cells projected to thalamus in a pattern similar to that of the entire sample of lamI-STT cells.

Subsequently the distribution of STT cells and their thalamic projection sites were studied in the cat with the multiple retrograde fluorescent labelling method (Craig *et al*, 1987). After injecting Diamidino Yellow and Fast Blue at sites in medial and lateral thalamus including the STT projection regions, and after survival times of up to 5 weeks, on average 2088 single- and double-labelled cells were counted contralateral to the injection sites from segments C5-C7 and L5-S2. The distribution of the cells of origin of the STT (Fig. 4) was the following: 46% were located in lamina I, 8% in lamina V, 5% in lamina VI, 20% in lamina VII and 21% in lamina VIII. Of particular note is the large contribution of lamina I cells. The thalamic projections of the entire population was spread with 54% projecting only to the medial thalamus, 30% projecting only to the lateral thalamus, and 16% projecting to both (Fig. 5). As can be seen in Fig. 5 the mean percentage of the labelled lamina I STT population that projected only to medial thalamus was 29%, which is in marked contrast to the average proportion of labelled STT cells that projected only to the lateral thalamus from lamina V, which was just 4%. In particular the same overall projection pattern was found for lamI-STT cells. The projection pattern of lamina I cells observed with the multiple retrograde fluorescent labelling method corroborates the physiological findings.

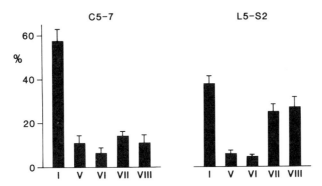

FIGURE 4: Differences in the laminar distribution of fluorescence-labelled STT cells in cervical (C5-7) and lumbosacral segments (L5-S2) of the spinal cord after injecting Diamidino Yellow and Fast Blue at sites in the contralateral medial and lateral thalamus covering the regions of the STT projections. For eight cases the means are shown of the percentages of STT neurones labelled in the individual laminae with respect to the total numbers of cells labelled at each level. Error bars mark standard deviations. (Craig, Linington and Kniffki, unpublished).

The dorsolateral spinothalamic tract (DSTT)

It is remarkable that about half of the entire STT in the cat originates in lamina I and that about half of these cells project only to the medial thalamus. In the anaesthetized animal more than half of the lamI-STT cells generally maintain the functional specificity of small-diameter primary afferent fibres, i.e. 47% were nociceptive-specific cells and 13% were cold-specific cells. This supports the possibility that these neurones are involved in the central representation of nociception and thermoreception as specific sensory modalities. However, about one third of the lamI-STT cells were multireceptive indicating that lamI-STT cells might be involved in other functions as well.

Further evidence that lamI-STT cells form a unique group of projecting cells of the STT comes from the fact that their axons lie outside the funicular confines traditionally assigned to the STT (Jones et al, 1985, 1987). Using retrograde transport of horseradish peroxidase (HRP) combined with lesions in the ventral quadrant (VQ) and in the dorsolateral funiculus (DLF), the authors demonstrated the existence of two distinct components of the STT in the cat: the dorsolateral STT (DSTT) ascending through the DLF, and the ventral STT (VSTT) ascending through the VQ. The cells of origin that contribute to each segmentally crossed pathway are quite distinct from one another. The DSTT originates almost exclusively in lamina I and its axons are spread diffusely throughout the DLF. The VSTT originates from deeper laminae and its axons ascend in the ventrolateral and ventromedial portions of the spinal cord. No axon was found travelling in the dorsal columns.

Thalamic targets of the DSTT

Using anterograde transport of WGA-HRP from the lumbar enlargement combined with thoracic VQ or DLF lesions it was shown by Apkarian et al,(1987) that the terminations of the DSTT and the VSTT overlap along the VPLvp (Fig. 1), whereas the VSTT in addition projects more anteriorly to the caudal ventrolateral nucleus. In the medial thalamus, the DSTT terminates in nucleus submedius, the VSTT terminates in nucleus centralis lateralis, and both tracts have terminations within nucleus reuniens.

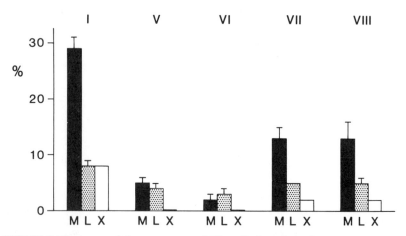

FIGURE 5: The means of the percentages of STT cells in each lamina of the spinal cord fluorescence-labelled either from medial thalamus (M), or from lateral thalamus (L) or from both (X), with respect to the entire labelled STT population in 4 cases. Error bars indicate standard deviations. (Craig, Linington and Kniffki, unpublished).

The ventral periphery of the ventrobasal complex (VBvp)

It should be emphasized that in the cat's lateral thalamus, VBvp is quite a distinct region (Fig. 1). It is this very region in which the STT terminates (Berkley, 1980; Craig and Burton, 1985; but cf. Boivie, 1971), in particular the lamI-DSTT (Apkarian *et al*, 1987), and in which neurones are located responding to activation of somatic nociceptors (Kniffki and Mizumura, 1983; Honda *et al*, 1983; Kniffki *et al*, 1983; Gordon 1983; Yokota and Matsumoto, 1983a,b; Kniffki and Craig, 1985; Craig and Kniffki, 1985c; Yokota *et al*, 1985; Yokota *et al*, 1986; Vahle-Hinz and Kniffki, 1987, 1988; Kniffki and Vahle-Hinz, 1987; Vahle-Hinz *et al*, 1987; Yokota *et al*, 1987; Hodge *et al*, 1987; Brüggemann *et al*, 1988).

Identification of VBvp. Most of the region that lies dorsally adjacent to VB is a portion of the posterior group (PO), here denoted as PO*d*. The dorsal periphery of VB (VB*dp*) is part of PO*d*. With reference to earlier studies in PO (Poggio and Mountcastle, 1960; Berkley, 1973; Guilbaud *et al*, 1977), PO*d* has recently been closely examined (Craig *et al*, 1983). The PO*d*/VB*dp*-VB border is determined by electrophysiological criteria and was subsequently verified histologically (Kniffki and Craig, 1985). Several general observations have begun to emerge from the sample of more than 1200 somatically responsive units recorded within the entire PO*d*. Most of the units (90%) responded to low-threshold cutaneous stimuli. Their receptive fields (RFs) were generally larger than those of VB neurones, and in contrast to those of neurones in the caudal part of PO, were predominantly contralateral; only 5% were found to have an ipsilateral or bilateral RF. Only 8% responded to low-threshold deep stimulation and just 2% responded to noxious cutaneous stimuli and were classified as wide dynamic range (WDR) neurones. There appears to be a coarse topographic ordering of RF locations that parallels medio-laterally the more precise somatotopic organization in VB. An approximate mirror-image reversal in the dorso-ventral progression of the RFs is often observed in comparison to VB proper. It should be noted, however, that the orderly progression of RFs in a vertical electrode penetration can have exceptions in PO*d* (Kniffki and Craig, 1985).

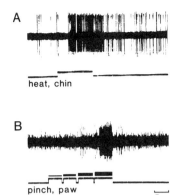

A

heat, chin

B

pinch, paw

5 s

FIGURE 6: Responses of two nociceptive neurones located in the ventral periphery of VPM to noxious stimuli applied within their receptive fields. Beneath the original records a trace of the stimulus duration is shown. In B the increasing stimulus intensity from light pressure to pinch is marked qualitatively by the width of the bars. (From Vahle-Hinz *et al*, 1987; Kniffki and Vahle-Hinz, 1988).

In general, the sensitivity to natural stimulation increased as the POd/VBdp-VB border was approached. The 2% of the neurones that responded in a WDR fashion were intermixed within the sample of low threshold (LT) cells as were 300 other neurones that were unresponsive to somatic stimulation.

Within VB the pattern of somatotopically organized responses was observed to be similar to that described previously (Mountcastle and Henneman, 1949; Gaze and Gordon, 1954; Rose and Mountcastle, 1954; Baker, 1971; Golovchinsky *et al*, 1981; Vahle-Hinz and Gottschaldt, 1983). As the electrode is moved ventrally from the VBdp through VPL the sequence of contralateral RFs progresses distally and the size of the RFs decreases. Using a metal microelectrode near VBvp, large clusters of cells are encountered whose RFs are confined to a small spot at the very distal end of a part of the extremity. The actual border between VB and VBvp is defined by 1) the limit of the progression of RF location and size, 2) the sudden change from cluster responses to unitary responses, and 3) a jump of RF location to more proximal parts and/or an increase in size of the RF associated with the unitary recording. Whenever this transition has been marked, the subsequent histological verification has revealed that the electrode had been in VBvp (Kniffki and Craig, 1985; Vahle-Hinz *et al.*, 1987; Kniffki and Vahle-Hinz, 1987).

Receptive fields of VBvp neurones. VBvp cells have been found with RFs not only in the skin, but also in muscle, viscera, cornea, and teeth (Kniffki and Mizumura, 1983; Honda *et al.*, 1983; Kniffki and Craig, 1985; Vahle-Hinz and Kniffki, 1987, 1988; Vahle-Hinz *et al.*, 1987; Kniffki and Vahle-Hinz, 1987; Yokota *et al.*, 1983, 1985, 1987; Hodge *et al.*, 1987; Brüggemann *et al.*, 1988). However, the greatest effort up to date has been made in delineating the cutaneous receptive field properties.

The excitatory cutaneous receptive fields of VBvp cells vary greatly in size (Kniffki and Mizumura, 1983; Kniffki and Craig, 1985; Vahle-Hinz *et al.*, 1987; Kniffki and Vahle-Hinz, 1987). Only very few of the RFs are very small, covering the surface of a digit or less or for instance, covering a distinct area on the cornea; few are small, covering the area of a foot or less; some are medium covering an area larger than a foot but less than a leg or smaller than the head; a considerable portion of the RFs found so far are large, *i.e.* the area of a foot, leg and part of a thigh or the entire half of the head; and still others are complex occupying areas on more than one limb or being located on the head and part of the forepaw. Some of the VB*vp* cells have cutaneous inhibitory receptive fields (Kniffki and Vahle-Hinz, 1987).

The VPL*vp* cells exhibited a coarse medio-lateral somatotopy: cells with hindlimb RFs were located laterally and those with forelimb RFs were located medially (Kniffki and Craig, 1985). It should be noted, however, that a considerable number of exceptions have been found, particularly for low-threshold VPL*vp* cells (Hebestreit *et al*, in preparation). Corresponding to this overall somatotopic organization, neurones with RFs on the head are located even further medially, i.e. within VPM*vp*. A detailed somatotopy was not obvious within VPM*vp*, although cells with intraoral RFs tend to occur medially and caudally in this region (Vahle-Hinz and Kniffki, 1987; Kniffki and Vahle-Hinz, 1987). Cells with RFs on the cornea were located in the caudo-medial part of VPM*vp* and ventral to VPMi (*cf.* Fig. 1), where the thalamic input from low-threshold mechanoreceptors in intraoral structures is represented (Vahle-Hinz and Kniffki, 1988).

Response categories of VBvp neurones. Based on the activation of the VB*vp* cells by various kinds of stimuli several response types can be recognized in VPL*vp* and VPM*vp*.

(1) VPLvp neurones: In recent studies (Kniffki and Craig, 1985; Brüggemann *et al.*, 1988; Hebestreit *et al*, in preparation), only 5% at most of the VPL*vp* cells were excited exclusively by noxious mechanical and/or thermal stimulation of the skin, 12% at most responded in a WDR fashion and 8% at most had an input from deep structures. The majority, however, required only innocuous tactile stimulation. So far very few cells have been found in VPL*vp* that respond to innocuous cooling of the skin. Some units were unresponsive to any of the stimuli used and these were located predominantly medially in VPL*vp* (Hebestreit *et al.*, in preparation).

(2) VPMvp neurones: In marked contrast to the responses of VPL*vp* cells, only 2% of the VPM*vp* cells responded to innocuous stimulation alone (Vahle-Hinz and Kniffki, unpublished). As defined above (*cf.* Fig. 1), VB*vp* includes the ventroposterior inferior nucleus (VPI; Jones, 1985) and its somewhat extended area as defined by Herron and Dykes (1986), who demonstrated input from Pacinian corpuscles to VPI neurones. This is in contrast to other reports (Yokota *et al.*, 1985; Vahle-Hinz *et al*, 1987; Kniffki and Vahle-Hinz, 1987) and this discrepancy currently remains unexplained.

The high proportion of nociceptive-specific cells (58%) in comparison to multireceptive-nociceptive cells (42%) within VPM*vp* (Kniffki and Vahle-Hinz, 1987) is remarkable in view of the corresponding percentages of cells within VPL*vp*.

Within VPM*vp* recordings were frequently obtained from neurones that were unresponsive to somatosensory stimuli and to stimuli applied to the teeth (Vahle-Hinz and Kniffki, to be published).

Response properties of VBvp neurones. In general, the responses of the nociceptive VB*vp* cells reflect the stimulus parameters, *i.e.* location, duration and intensity of the stimuli applied to an excitatory RF (Figs. 6, 7). But, in contrast to this response type, some of the nociceptive VPM*vp* cells showed quite a different response behaviour, *i.e.* to a noxious stimulus applied to an orofacial RF these cells *switched* to a high frequency discharge which was often maintained for minutes (Vahle-Hinz *et al*, 1987). This stimulus-response relationship does not seem to be appropriate for encoding the stimulus intensity or duration, and thus these neurones may be involved in some sort of a warning system by detecting the location of a potentially damaging stimulus within the receptive periphery of an organism.

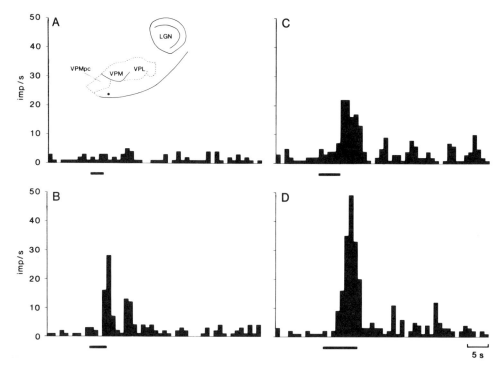

FIGURE 7: Peristimulus time histograms (bin width: 1s) of the graded responses of a nociceptive-specific neurone located within VBvp (see inset) to noxious cutaneous heat stimulation. The bars indicate the duration of the application of radiant heat to the receptive field on the ear. The duration of the heat stimulus is a measure of the actual, but unknown temperature at the receptor sites. The neuronal response latencies correlated rather well with the onset of pain felt by the experimenter who subjected a finger tip to the same stimuli (from Kniffki and Vahle-Hinz, 1987).

Very recently, studies of the reliability of the physiological characterization of VPL*vp* cells revealed that transitions in the response properties of some of the VPL*vp* cells occurred (Fig. 8; Brüggemann *et al.*, 1988). For about half of the VPL*vp* cells the classification into non-nociceptive (nn) and nociceptive (n) response categories was quite reliable. The other half of the VPL*vp* cells did, however, show transitions in their response properties even under a constant level of anaesthesia. The following transitions were observed: nn ⟺ n, n ⟺ 0, nn ⟹ 0, with 0 = no response. It is not clear what mechanisms underlie these transitions of the response properties of VPL*vp* cells.

Morphology of VBvp. Taking into account the available data about VPL*vp*, it is tempting to assume that the regions containing nociceptive neurones have identifiable cytoarchitectural characteristics (Kniffki *et al.*, 1983). In order to determine whether the functional distinction between VB and VBvp neurones is reflected in the neurones' morphology, their soma size, form-factor and excentricity were recently measured in sections stained by Bielschowsky's silver impregnation technique. It turned out that the somata of neurones within VBvp are smaller and more elliptical or spindle-shaped compared to those of neurones within VB proper (Hanesch *et al*, 1987; Brandt *et al*, 1988). A Golgi study is currently in progress to characterize the morphology of VBvp cells more fully.

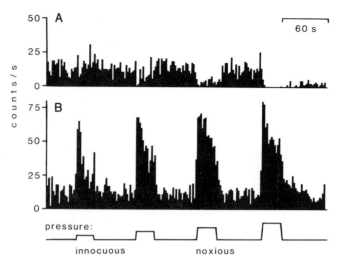

FIGURE 8: Transition in the response properties of a VPLvp neurone under constant pentobarbitone anaesthesia. The interval between the two identical characterizations was 5 minutes; the neuronal activity is displayed as peristimulus time histograms. The trace beneath B represents the graded mechanica; stimuli applied to the skin of the receptive field. (From Brüggemann, Hebestreit and Kniffki, 1988)

Transmitters and neuromodulators within VBvp. Relatively little is known about the thalamic transmitter chemistry (Jones, 1987). Very little is known about the transmitters or neuromodulators involved in the afferent and efferent connections of the cat VB*vp*. Recently, however, substance P immunoreactive terminals were found (Spreafico *et al*, 1986; Battaglia, 1988, personal communication). Whether STT (DSTT, VSTT) neurones contain substance P has not yet been demonstrated.

Cortical projections of VBvp neurones. The recent findings (Craig and Kniffki, 1985c; Craig, Hebestreit and Kniffki, unpublished) regarding the cortical projection of VPL*vp* cells further distinguish VPL*vp* as a distinct region. Antidromic activation was used to locate the cortical projection sites of physiologically characterized cells recorded within VPL*vp*. Ball electrodes that could be moved freely across the cortical surface enabled the identification of foci in the postcruciate cortex, and in some experiments, both the postcruciate and the anterior ectosylvian cortices (AEs).

Almost all (n=28) of a sample of 30 VPL*vp* cells whose projection sites within both regions were determined projected to the postcruciate cortex. Ten of these cells projected also to the AEs, and 2 cells projected only to the AEs.

The projection sites in the postcruciate cortex of 68 VPL*vp* cells were examined. Except for two, the projection sites of VPL*vp* cells were rostral to the first somatosensory cortical area (SI). SI was identified by recording responses to cutaneous stimulation on the cortical surface or intracortically, as well as by determining projection sites of cells within VPL proper. It appears that most projection sites of identified VPL*vp* cells were in cortical area 3a. Whether the adjacent area 4gamma is involved is a matter of debate.

The postcruciate projection sites of VPL*vp* cells with forelimb RFs were in the lateral, forelimb portion of area 3a, whereas those VPL*vp* cells with hindlimb RFs projected to the medial portion of area 3a, just lateral to the hindpaw representation in SI. The projection sites were found to be topographically appropriate, independent of the location of the VPL*vp* cells relative to the somatosensory representation in VPL proper.

Small cortical injections of retrograde tracers at the antidromically identified projection sites of VPL*vp* cells resulted in labelling of one or a few cells at the recording site in VPL*vp*. Larger injections of horseradish peroxidase (HRP) in the forelimb portion of area 3a confirmed that it receives input from VPL*vp* cells ventral to VPLm as well as from the ventrolateral nucleus (VL), the rostral dorsomedial portion of VPLm and other regions. Large injections of HRP in the medial postcruciate cortex resulted in labelling throughout the mediolateral extent of VPL*vp*.

The details of the cortical projections of VPM*vp* cells have yet to be determined.

CONCLUSIONS

The results of the investigations of the functional properties of lamI-STT and VB*vp* neurones, and of their electrophysiologically and neuroanatomically determined projections, support the concept of a dorsolateral nociceptive lamina I-spino-thalamo-cortical pathway. In particular, two of these pathways seem to exist: one ascending from lamina I of the spinal dorsal horn as DSTT via the DLF through nucleus submedius (SM) in the medial thalamus to the middle layer of the ventrolateral orbital (VLO) cortical field (Craig, 1987), and the other one through VB*vp* in the lateral thalamus to the postcruciate somatosensory cortex.

The hypothesis, that SM is the medial thalamic site for interactive information transfer with lateral thalamus and somatosensory cortex (Craig, 1987), might be supported by the findings of 1) the distinct lamI-STT input to the dorsal portion of the nucleus submedius (SMd), which was first revealed by anterograde HRP transport (Craig and Burton, 1981) and 2) the projection of SMd to the VLO cortical field, which is itself reciprocally interconnected with portions of the somatosensory cortices (SI-SIII) excluding area 3b of SI, the projection area of neurones of VB proper, but including the postcruciate area 3a, the target of the VPL*vp* cells.

The pathways from lamina I, the DSTT and the VSTT, via VPL*vp* to the postcruciate area (excluding 3b) with its connection to the VLO cortical field, on the one hand and the projection from VPL*vp* to the AEs on the other hand, with their inherent specific neuronal elements, together with the fact that many STT cells give off collaterals to periaqueductal gray and brainstem reticular formation, may subserve different aspects of sensory discrimination, motor integration and affective or regulatory functions.

As indicated by the question marks in Fig. 1, our current lack of knowledge about the complete input and output connections between cat peripheral VB and spinal, thalamic and cortical structures provides guide-lines for future research as do well designed behavioural studies as for example the recent one of Casey and Morrow (1988).

ACKNOWLEDGEMENTS

I am indebted to my colleagues for the collaborative work. The competent technical assistance of Ms. Heike Brandt and Ms Christa Erhard is deeply appreciated. The projects have been supported by the Deutsche Forschungsgemeinschaft and by the Hermann und Lilly Schilling-Stiftung für Medizinische Forschung im Stifterverband für die Deutsche Wissenschaft.

REFERENCES

APKARIAN, A.V., HODGE, C.J., JONES, M.W. AND STEVENS, R.T. (1987). Thalamic terminations of the dorsolateral and ventrolateral spinothalamic pathways. In: *Effects of injury on trigeminal and spinal somatosensory systems*, eds. Pubols, L.M. and Sessle, B.J., p 513. New York: Alan R. Liss.

BAKER, M.A. (1971). Spontaneous and evoked activity of neurones in the somatosensory thalamus of the waking cat. *Journal of Physiology* **217**, 359-379.

BERKLEY, K.J. (1973). Response properties of cells in ventrobasal and posterior group nuclei of the cat. *Journal of Neurophysiology* **36**, 940-952.

BERKLEY, K.J. (1980). Spatial relationships between the terminations of somatic sensory and motor pathways in the rostral brainstem of cats and monkeys. I. Ascending somatic sensory inputs to lateral diencephalon. *Journal of Comparative Neurology* **193**, 283-317.

BOIVIE, J. (1971). The termination of the spinothalamic tract in the cat. An experimental study with silver impregnation methods. *Experimental Brain Research* **12**, 331-353.

BRANDT, H., BRÜGGEMANN, J., HANESCH, U., KNIFFKI, K.-D. AND VAHLE-HINZ, C. (1988). Morphometrically verified differences between neurones of the thalamic ventral posteromedial nucleus (VPM) and of its ventral periphery (VPMvp). *Pflügers Archiv* **411** Suppl. 1, R131.

BRÜGGEMANN, J., HEBESTREIT, H. AND KNIFFKI, K.-D. (1988). Transitions in the response properties of neurones located in the ventral periphery of the cat ventral posterolateral nucleus (VPLvp). *Pflügers Archiv* **411** Suppl. 1, R132.

CASEY, K.L. AND MORROW, T.J. (1988). Supraspinal nocifensive responses of cats: spinal cord pathways, monoamines, and modulation. *Journal of Comparative Neurology* **270**, 591-605.

CERVERO, F. AND CONNELL, L.A. (1984). Distribution of somatic and visceral primary afferent fibres within the thoracic spinal cord of the cat. *Journal of Comparative Neurology* **230**, 88-98.

CHRISTENSEN, B.N. AND PERL, E.R. (1970). Spinal neurons specifically excited by noxious or thermal stimuli: Marginal zone of the dorsal horn. *Journal of Neurophysiology* **33**, 293-307.

CRAIG, A.D. (1987). Medial thalamus and nociception: The nucleus submedius. In: *Thalamus and pain*, eds. Besson, J.-M., Guilbaud, G. and Peschanski, M., pp. 227-243. Amsterdam: Excerpta Medica.

CRAIG, A.D. AND BURTON, H. (1981). Spinal and medullary lamina I projection to nucleus submedius in medial thalamus: a possible pain center. *Journal of Neurophysiology* **45**, 443-466.

CRAIG, A.D. AND BURTON, H. (1985). The distribution and topographical organization in the thalamus of anterogradely-transported horseradish peroxidase after spinal injections in cat and raccoon. *Experimental Brain Research* **58**, 227-254.

CRAIG, A.D., DUNST, R., KNIFFKI, K.-D. AND SAILER S. (1983). A topographically inverted somatic representation dorsal to VB in the dorsal part of the posterior complex of the cat. *Neuroscience Letters* Suppl. **14**, 78.

CRAIG, A.D., HEPPELMANN, B. AND SCHAIBLE, H.-G. (1988). The projection of the medial and posterior articular nerves of the cat's knee to the spinal cord. *Journal of Comparative Neurology* (in the press)

CRAIG, A.D. AND KNIFFKI, K.-D. (1985a). The multiple representation of nociception in the spinothalamic projection of lamina I cells in the cat. In: *Development, organization and processing in somatosensory pathways*, eds. Rowe, M.J. and Willis, W.D., pp. 347-353, New York: Alan R. Liss.

CRAIG, A.D. AND KNIFFKI, K.-D. (1985b). Spinothalamic lumbosacral lamina I cells responsive to skin and muscle stimulation in the cat. *Journal of Physiology* **365**, 197-221.

CRAIG, A.D. AND KNIFFKI, K.-D. (1985c). Spino-thalamo-cortical mechanisms of nociception. In: *Current trends in pain research and therapy*, Vol. 1, Basic mechanisms and clinical applications, ed. Sharma, K.N. and Usha Nayar, pp. 65-77. New Delhi.

CRAIG, A.D., LININGTON, A.J. AND KNIFFKI, K.-D. (1987). Collateral spinothalamic tract projections to medial and/or lateral thalamus examined with multiple retrograde fluorescent labeling in the cat. *Society for Neuroscience Abstracts* **13**, 581.

CRAIG, A.D. AND MENSE, S. (1983). The distribution of afferent fibres from the gastrocnemius-soleus muscle in the dorsal horn of the cat, as revealed by transport of horseradish peroxidase. *Neuroscience Letters* **41**, 233-238.

DE GROAT, W.C. (1986). Spinal cord projections and neuropeptides in visceral afferent neurones. *Progress in Brain Research* **67**, 165-187.

GAZE, R.M. AND GORDON, G. (1954). The representation of cutaneous sense in the thalamus of cat and monkey. *Quarterly Journal of Experimental Physiology* **39**, 279-304.

GOLOVCHINSKY, V., KRUGER, L., SAPORTA, S.A., STEIN, B.E. AND YOUNG, D.W. (1981). Properties of velocity-mechanosensitive neurons of the cat ventrobasal thalamic nucleus with special reference to the concept of convergence. *Brain Research* **209**, 355-374.

GORDON, G. (1983). Nociceptive cells in ventroposterior thalamus of the cat. *Journal of Neurophysiology* **50**, 1043.

GUILBAUD, G. CAILLE, D. BESSON, J. M. AND BENELLI, G. (1977). Single units activities in ventral posterior and posterior group thalamic nuclei during nociceptive and non nociceptive stimulations in the cat. *Archives of Italian Biology* **115**, 38-56.

HANESCH, U., HAUMANN, P., KNIFFKI, K.-D., MEYERMANN, M. AND VAHLE-HINZ, C. (1987). Differences between neurones in the cat's thalamic ventroposterolateral nucleus (VPL) and its ventral periphery (VPLvp): a morphometric analysis. *Neuroscience* **22**, S805.

HERRON, P. AND DYKES, R. (1986). Connections and function of the thalamic ventroposterior inferior (VPI) nucleus in cats: a relay nucleus in the Pacinian pathway to somatosensory cortex. *Journal of Neurophysiology* **56**, 1475-1497.

HODGE, C.J., APKARIAN, A.V., MARTINI, S. AND MARTIN, R.J. (1987). Lateral thalamic nociception: the effects of interruption of transmission through the ventrolateral and the dorsolateral spinothalamic tracts. In: *Effects of injury on trigeminal and spinal somatosensory systems*, eds. Pubols, L.M. and Sessle, B.J., pp. 313-320. New York: Alan R. Liss.

HONDA, C.N., MENSE, S. AND PERL, E.R. (1983). Neurons in ventrobasal region of cat thalamus selectively responsive to noxious mechanical stimulation. *Journal of Neurophysiology* **49**, 662-673.

JONES, E.G. (1985). *The thalamus*. New York: Plenum Press.

JONES, E.G. (1987). New insights into old concepts of thalamic function. In: *Thalamus and pain*, ed. Besson, J.-M., Guilbaud, G. and Peschanski, M., pp. 1-19. Amsterdam: Excerpta Medica.

JONES, M.W., HODGE, C.J., APKARIAN, A.V. AND STEVENS, R.T. (1985). A dorsolateral spinothalamic pathway in cat. *Brain Research* **335**, 188-193.

JONES, M.W., APKARIAN, A.V., STEVENS, R.T. AND HODGE, C.J. (1987). The spinothalamic tract: an examination of the cells of origin of the dorsolateral and ventrolateral spinothalamic pathways in cats. *Journal of Comparative Neurology* **260**, 349-361.

KNIFFKI, K.-D. AND CRAIG, A.D. (1985). The distribution of nociceptive neurones in the cat's lateral thalamus: the dorsal and ventral periphery of VPL. In: *Development, organization and processing in somatosensory pathways*, eds. Rowe, M.J. and Willis, W.D., pp. 375-382. New York: Alan R. Liss.

KNIFFKI, K.-D. AND MIZUMURA K. (1983). Responses of neurones in VPL and VPL-VL region of the cat to algesic stimulation of muscle and tendon. *Journal of Neurophysiology* **49**, 649-661.

KNIFFKI, K.-D., CRAIG, A.D.AND BERKLEY, K.J. (1983). Nociceptive neurones in cytoarchitecturally identifiable regions in the ventrolateral periphery of the cat's ventroposterolateral nucleus (VPL). *Naunyn-Schmiedeberg's Archiv für Pharmakologie* **322**, R98.

KNIFFKI, K.-D. AND VAHLE-HINZ, C. (1987). The periphery of the cat's ventroposteromedial nucleus (VPMp): nociceptive neurones. In: *Thalamus and pain*, ed. Besson, J.-M., Guilbaud, G. and Peschanski, M., pp. 245-257, Amsterdam: Excerpta Medica.

LIGHT, A.R. AND PERL, E.R. (1979). Spinal termination of functionally identified primary afferent neurons with slowly conducting myelinated fibers. *Journal of Comparative Neurology* **186**, 133-150.

MOUNTCASTLE, V. AND HENNEMAN, E. (1949). Pattern of tactile representation in thalamus of cat. *Journal of Neurophysiology* **12**, 85-100.

PERL, E.R. (1984). Pain and nociception. In Brookhart, J.M. and V.B. Mountcastle (Eds.): *Handbook of Physiology*, Section 1, *The Nervous System*, Vol. III, Darian-Smith, I. (Ed.): Sensory Processes. Bethesda, American Physiological Society, pp. 915-975.

POGGIO, G.F. AND MOUNTCASTLE, V.B. (1960). A study of the functional contributions of the lemniscal and spinothalamic systems to somatic sensibility. Central nervous mechanisms in pain. *Bulletin of the Johns Hopkins Hospital* **106**, 266-316.

ROSE, J.E. AND MOUNTCASTLE, V.B. (1954). Activity of single neurons in the tactile thalamic region of the cat in response to transient peripheral stimulus. *Bulletin of the Johns Hopkins Hospital* **106**, 266-316.

SPREAFICO, R., BATTAGLIA, G. AND RUSTIONI, A. (1986). Is substance P the marker for a population of spinothalamic neurons? *Society for Neuroscience Abstracts* **12**, 956.

VAHLE-HINZ, C., FREUND, I. AND KNIFFKI, K.-D. (1987). Nociceptive neurones in the ventral periphery of the cat's ventro-posteromedial nucleus (VPM). In: *Fine afferent nerve fibres and pain*, ed. Schmidt, R.F., Schaible, H.G. and Vahle-Hinz, C., pp 439-450. Weinheim: VCH Verlagsgesellschaft.

VAHLE-HINZ, C. AND GOTTSCHALDT, K.-M. (1983). Principal differences in the organization of the thalamic face representation in rodents and felids. In: *Somatosensory integration in the thalamus*, ed. Macchi, G., Rustioni, A. and Spreafico, R., pp. 125-145, Amsterdam: Elsevier.

VAHLE-HINZ, C. AND KNIFFKI, K.-D. (1987). Thalamo-cortical system of orofacial nociception. *Pain* Suppl. 4, S265.

WILLIS, W.D. (1985). *The Pain System*. Karger, Basel.

YOKOTA, T., KOYAMA, N. AND MATSUMOTO, N. (1985). Somatotopic distribution of trigeminal nociceptive neurons in ventrobasal complex of the cat thalamus. *Journal of Neurophysiology*, **53**, 1387-1400.

YOKOTA, T. AND MATSUMOTO, N. (1983a). Somatotopic distribution of trigeminal nociceptive specific neurons within the caudal somatosensory thalamus of cat. *Neuroscience Letters* **39**, 125-130.

YOKOTA, T. AND MATSUMOTO, N. (1983b). Location and functional organization of trigeminal wide dynamic range neurons within the nucleus ventralis posteromedialis of the cat. *Neuroscience Letters* **39**, 231-236.

YOKOTA, T., KOYAMA, N. AND NISHIKAWA, Y. (1987). Nociceptive neurons in the shell region of the ventrobasal complex of the thalamus. In: *Effects of injury on trigeminal and spinal somatosensory systems*, ed. Pubols, L.M. and Sessle, B.J., pp. 305-312. New York: Alan R. Liss.

YOKOTA, T., NISHIKAWA, Y. AND KOYAMA, N. (1986). Tooth pulp input to the shell region of nucleus ventralis posteromedialis of the cat thalamus. *Journal of Neurophysiology* **56**, 80-98.

THE INFLUENCE OF CUTANEOUS INPUTS ON THE ACTIVITY OF NEURONES IN THE SUBSTANTIA GELATINOSA

Wilma M. Steedman

Department of Preclinical Veterinary Sciences, Royal (Dick) School of Veterinary Studies, University of Edinburgh, Summerhall, Edinburgh EH9 1QH, U.K.

It is well established that different modalities of sensation are associated with activation of specific types of receptor in the skin. This specificity is preserved in the types of afferent fibre activated and the areas of termination of the central ends of those fibres within the dorsal horn of the spinal cord. Thus in the cat the superficial dorsal horn, and in particular the substantia gelatinosa (lamina II), is the principal area of termination of unmyelinated fibres from cutaneous nociceptors. Intracellular staining of electrophysiologically-characterised C fibres has shown that patterns of terminal arborisation are related to functional attributes (Sugiura *et al*, 1986). In contrast, the majority of neurones recorded within lamina II are multireceptive and may be excited and inhibited from a variety of cutaneous receptors.

Classical Golgi analyses together with degeneration and autoradiographic techniques have demonstrated the hardware basis for such convergence, namely a diversity of possible mono- and poly-synaptic connections between primary afferent fibres and neurones in different regions of the dorsal horn (Ramon y Cajal, 1909; Szentagothai, 1964; Matsushita, 1969; Mannen and Sugiura, 1976). This has been confirmed by intracellular staining of physiologically-characterised neurones (Maxwell and Rethelyi, 1987, for review). Within lamina II many C fibre terminals form the central element of complex glomerular arrangements where they may be presynaptic to dendrites of neurones of lamina II, of interneurones of lamina III and of neurones of the dorsal column postsynaptic system. They can also be postsynaptic to axons immunolabelled for glutamic acid decarboxylase (and therefore assumed to release GABA) and also to dendrites of undetermined origin. Neurones in lamina II have also been demonstrated to be postsynaptic to 5HT-containing axon profiles thought to be of supraspinal origin (Ruda *et al*, 1982; Light *et al*, 1983; Basbaum *et al*, 1982).

Electrophysiological recording has shown that there are neurones in lamina II that receive not only strong, probably monosynaptic, input from nociceptive C afferent fibres but also inhibitory, polysynaptic input from Aβ fibres from innocuous mechanoreceptors (Steedman *et al*, 1985; Steedman and Molony, 1987). In addition, they may be excited and inhibited from a variety of supraspinal sources (e.g. Light *et al*, 1986). Nociceptive afferent input is therefore subject to considerable processing and modulation within lamina II. While some of the output is transmitted directly to higher levels (Giesler *et al*, 1978; Willis *et al*, 1978) the majority of neurones in lamina II appear to have locally projecting axons with *en passant* and terminal swellings. These are in a position to influence cells in adjacent laminae (which give rise to long ascending tracts) as well as making contact with neurones in the ventral horn of the spinal cord.

Three pathways have been described by which sensory input carried by C primary afferent fibres to lamina II could be conveyed to neurones in deeper laminae:

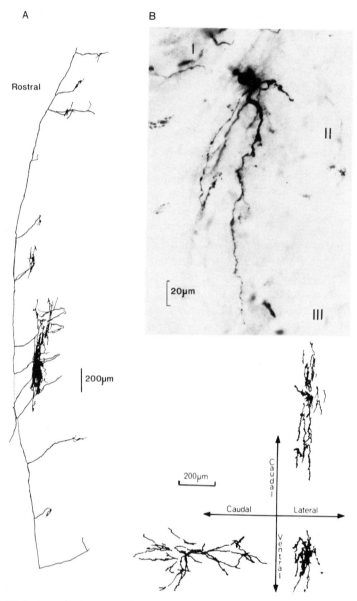

FIGURE 1: A. Sagittal view of the computer-reconstructed termination pattern of a C-polymodal nociceptor within the superficial dorsal horn of the lumbar spinal cord of the guinea-pig (from Sugiura *et al*, 1986; copyright 1986 by the AAAS). B. Photomicrograph of part of a lamina II neurone stained with HRP (in transverse section of the dorsal horn of the lumbar spinal cord of the cat) and computer reconstruction of the dendritic tree represented in three dimensions (from Steedman *et al.*, 1983). The axon projects ventrally into lamina III.

1) direct monosynaptic input from C fibre terminals onto dendrites extending dorsally into lamina II, as has been shown for neurones of the dorsal column postsynaptic system (Bannatyne *et al*, 1987).

2) polysynaptic input through contacts between C-fibre terminals and dendrites of lamina III interneurones (Mannen and Sugiura, 1976; Maxwell *et al*, 1983).

3) polysynaptic input through lamina II neurones with axons projecting ventrally into laminae III-V (Matsushita, 1969; Mannen and Sugiura, 1976; Molony *et al*, 1981; Steedman *et al*, 1983; Light and Kavookjian, 1988).

It is with this last pathway - nociceptive input carried by primary afferent C fibres to the superficial dorsal horn, relayed and processed and then transmitted to the deeper laminae - that this paper is concerned. Recent developments in techniques for intracellular recording and staining have permitted study of the organisation of the pathway and the synaptic relationships involved.

The majority of neurones recorded in the deeper laminae (including cells which project supraspinally through a variety of pathways) demonstrate considerable convergence of input. The functional significance of this apparent loss of specificity has been hotly debated: is modality information encoded within the discharge? do these multireceptive neurones signal merely the general level of activity? is information as to a specific input conveyed along different, dedicated pathways? There is evidence that such multireceptive neurones are involved in the transmission of information which results in the perception of pain (Price and Dubner, 1977; Roberts, 1986) and it has long been recognised that the timing of spikes within trains discharged by neurones at various levels of the somatosensory system can vary with the nature of the activating stimulus (e.g. Brown and Franz, 1970; Angaut-Petit, 1975; Emmers, 1981; Sandner *et al*, 1987). There is also evidence from within the somatosensory system (Salt, 1986; Collingridge *et al*, 1988) that the timing of the presynaptic spikes affects the manner in which synaptic transmission occurs (e.g. the involvement of NMDA receptors). It is possible that multireceptive neurones may encode modality information in the form of specific groupings of action potentials; it is necessary therefore to analyse their responses in terms of the ordering of action potentials rather than simply of the frequency of discharge.

In this paper I shall consider:

1) the synaptic connections between C fibres and neurones in lamina II;

2) modulation of the nociceptive input and the postsynaptic potentials evoked by other inputs;

3) how the ordering of action potentials within the noxious stimulus-evoked discharge of the deeper neurones is determined by the organisation of the pathway and the characteristics of the relay neurone, and how it differs from that within the discharge evoked by non-nociceptive mechanoreceptive input in Aβ fibres.

EXCITATORY PRIMARY AFFERENT INPUTS TO LAMINA II

C fibres have been shown to arborise largely within the superficial dorsal horn; rostrocaudally directed parent fibres send branches which in turn arborise extensively within restricted areas, each branch having numerous *en passant* as well as terminal enlargements (Réthelyi, 1977; Sugiura *et al.*, 1986). The orientations of the terminal arborisations of the C fibres parallel those of the dendritic trees of the neurones in lamina II, *i.e.* extensive rostrocaudally but narrow mediolaterally and restricted dorsoventrally.

This relationship is illustrated in Figure 1 which shows a sagittal view of the

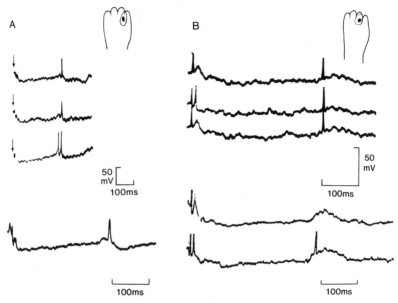

FIGURE 2: Intracellular recordings from two neurones in lamina II. In each case the receptive field (solid) was smaller than and contained within that of a neurone recorded within lamina III (outlined) on the same electrode track. A. Upper traces - intracellular recording of the response to repeated single-shock stimulation of the peroneal nerve (5V 1.2 msec pulse at arrow, once every four seconds). Resting potential was -70 mV. Lower trace - summed responses (n = 10, bin width = 100 μs). B. Upper traces - intracellular recording of the responses to repeated single-shock stimulation of the peroneal nerve (3V, 1.2 msec pulse, once every four seconds). Resting potential was 70 mV but action potentials were attenuated by the recording system. Lower traces - summed responses (n = 15, bin width = 100 μs) to stimuli below and above threshold for an action potential.

termination pattern of a C-polymodal nociceptor in the L-6 segment of guinea-pig spinal cord (Sugiura *et al*, 1986) and the dendritic tree of an HRP-stained neurone of cat spinal cord with its soma in outer lamina II and its axon projecting ventrally into lamina III (Steedman *et al.*, 1983). The concentration of branching within narrow sagittal sheets suggests that one C fibre may make multiple contacts with the dendrites of one neurone, and the variation in extent and density of arborisation of different collaterals suggests a corresponding variation in the density of synaptic contacts made with different neurones.

Our studies of the synaptic potentials evoked in neurones in lamina II by electrical stimulation of peripheral nerves have provided evidence of strong inputs from single C fibres. C fibre-evoked responses arose from a hyperpolarised membrane which in turn resulted from polysynaptic inhibition following activation of low-threshold, fast-conducting inputs in Aβ fibres (Steedman *et al.*, 1985). Two to six discrete e.p.s.p.s lasting up to 25 msec were recorded, one or more of which could reach threshold for an action potential. Averaging showed that there was very little 'jitter' in the responses to stimuli repeated once every 4 seconds (Steedman and Molony, 1987; Iggo *et al*, 1988). In most cases these e.p.s.p.s were superimposed on a longer-lasting, variable e.p.s.p. Examples are shown in Figure 2.

Two components could be distinguished:

1) Short e.p.s.p.s which did not vary in amplitude with stimulus intensity. In the

neurone in Figure 2A each stimulus evoked two e.p.s.p.s, the second of which gave rise to an action potential each time while the first only reached firing threshold in the 18th of 20 repetitions. The averaged trace shows how time-locked and consistent the responses were. No C-evoked response was recorded when stimulus intensity was reduced below the level that elicited an action potential.

2) A long-lasting (60-120 msec) e.p.s.p. which varied in amplitude and duration with stimulus intensity. The neurone in Figure 2B responded with an action potential which arose from the first of four waves of e.p.s.p.s that were superimposed on a long-lasting e.p.s.p. (top traces). When the stimulus intensity was decreased the four short e.p.s.p. waves were still apparent but the first now no longer reached firing threshold because of the decrease in amplitude of the underlying long e.p.s.p. This is shown in the averaged responses (lower traces) which emphasise the regularity of the short e.p.s.p.s.

These recordings can be interpreted in the light of the following observations:

1) the terminal branching of the C fibres is oriented in parallel with the dendritic trees of the lamina II neurones and the density of arborisation of different collaterals varies within that area; this suggests that the different collaterals may provide strongly effective inputs to some neurones and weakly effective inputs to others;

2) the majority of primary afferent input occurs at synapses on dendrites of lamina II neurones;

3) these lamina II neurones are so small that it is likely that prolonged, stable recordings result from impalement of the soma rather than of the dendrites. Attenuation and distortion of synaptic potentials generated at distal loci may therefore be considerable (Iggo et al., 1988);

4) resting membrane potentials recorded in conditions which indicated good sealing of the membrane around the penetrating electrode were considerably more negative than the firing threshold (Iggo et al., 1988);

5) the electrotonic responses to brief rectangular current pulses passed through the recording microelectrode (Iggo et al., 1988) established that the time course of the decay of the response was exponential with a time constant of 0.8 to 2.0 msec, suggesting that axial current flow and temporal summation of short-lived postsynaptic potentials is limited.

These considerations lead to the following suggestions:

1) each all-or-nothing brief e.p.s.p. is the result of spatial summation of a large number of inputs from one C fibre, distorted in shape by the high resistance to axial current flow.

2) the long-lasting, variable e.p.s.p. reflects the activity in a larger number of C fibres each providing a weak input (which may be mono- or poly-synaptic), the greater amplitude in response to stronger stimuli being the result of recruitment of more afferent fibres.

The output of the neurone in response to C fibre stimulation thus consists of action potentials arising singly from discrete e.p.s.p.s. This type of firing is characteristic of both background discharge and that evoked by stimulation of the skin and electrical stimulation of peripheral nerves (Steedman et al., 1985; Iggo et al., 1988). Interspike interval histograms generated from the steady state noxious heat response were accordingly unimodal and symmetric with no very short intervals (Figure 3).

Many of the nocireceptive neurones in lamina II also received an excitatory input from Aβ afferent fibres, although in some cases no non-noxious cutaneous receptive field was found. This input was generally more weakly effective than the C-fibre input. The neurones also received an inhibitory input from sensitive mechanoreceptors in the

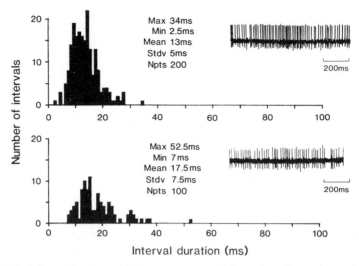

FIGURE 3: Interspike interval histograms generated from the spike trains evoked by noxious heat in two neurones in lamina II of cat lumbar spinal cord.

skin, often from areas overlapping the excitatory receptive fields. Electrical stimulation of peripheral nerves also demonstrated the existence of excitatory and inhibitory inputs from Aβ fibres - e.p.s.p.s which were short-lived and gave rise to single action potentials were almost always immediately followed by long hyperpolarisations (Steedman et al., 1985). While some input from Aβ fibres may be monosynaptic onto distally-located dendrites extending ventrally into lamina III, the majority of Aβ input must be polysynaptic through interneurones in the deeper laminae. Central delays calculated for Aβ inputs to eight nociceptive neurones located within the superficial dorsal horn close to the border between laminae I and II suggested that only one might have received a monosynaptic input (Steedman et al., 1985). Excitatory inputs from Aδ fibres were also recorded, and the central delay times suggested more frequent monosynaptic connections (Steedman et al., 1985).

MODULATION WITHIN LAMINA II

Many investigators have reported that the C fibre input to multireceptive dorsal horn neurones in laminae III-VI is preferentially and profoundly inhibited by activation both of other primary afferent inputs and of inputs of supraspinal origin (e.g. Mendell, 1966; Price et al, 1971; Gregor and Zimmermann, 1972; Brown et al, 1975; Handwerker et al, 1975; Fields and Basbaum, 1978; Willis, 1982). It was originally suggested that this selective inhibition of the nociceptive input was due to presynaptic inhibition of the afferent C fibre terminals in lamina II (Melzack and Wall, 1965). An anatomical basis for presynaptic inhibition exists in the form of axo-axonic and dendro-axonic contacts (Gobel et al, 1980; Maxwell and Rethelyi, 1987) and there is indirect evidence from neurophysiological studies (Calvillo, 1978; Hentall and Fields, 1979; Carstens et al, 1979; Fitzgerald and Woolf, 1981). However, only a very small percentage of synaptic contacts within this cell-packed area of the spinal cord can be presynaptic to an axon terminal, so that postsynaptic mechanisms may be expected to play a major part in inhibition within lamina II. Intracellular recording of nocireceptive neurones in lamina II has in fact provided direct evidence of postsynaptic inhibition, both segmental and suprasegmental in origin. Cutaneous inhibitory receptive fields from which hyperpolarising responses can be elicited were generally more extensive than, and frequently overlapped, the nociceptive excitatory fields (Steedman *et al.*, 1985). We have described i.p.s.p.s (Figure 4A) evoked polysynaptically by electrical activation of Aβ primary afferent fibres; these were voltage-dependent and were reversed at -85mV to -95mV, by the passage of hyperpolarising current(Steedman and Molony, 1987). Similar reversible i.p.s.p.s elicited by stimulation in the nucleus raphe magnus are illustrated in Figure 4B (Light *et al.*, 1986). Thus nocireceptive neurones in lamina II are subject to postsynaptic inhibition both from afferent and from supraspinal sources. Duggan and co-workers have used antibody microprobes to measure immunoreactive substance P released in lamina II in response to noxious stimulation and have found that the release is unaffected by blocking or transecting the spinal cord, suggesting that tonic supraspinal inhibition of noxious input is not due to presynaptic inhibition of nociceptive primary afferent terminals (Duggan *et al*, 1988).

The importance of these inhibitory inputs must not be under-estimated, and intracellular recordings highlight the problems of interpreting experiments using extracellular recording techniques. For example, nocireceptive neurones with the

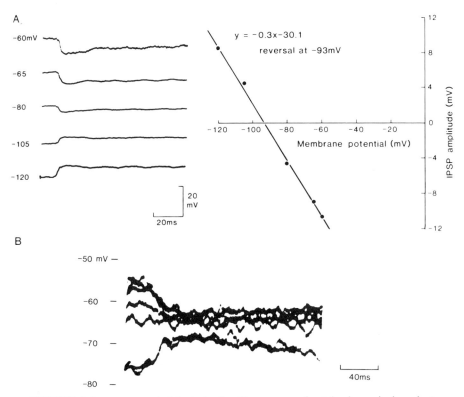

FIGURE 4: I.p.s.p.s recorded from lamina II neurones of cat lumbar spinal cord. A. Responses of a nocireceptive neurone to single-shock electrical stimulation of peroneal nerve (150 mV, 0.2 ms pulses) at different membrane potentials. The amplitude of the i.p.s.p. was plotted as a function of the membrane potential. Resting potential was -60 mV (from Steedman and Molony, 1987). B. Postsynaptic potentials produced by focal stimulation of nucleus raphe magnus at different levels of membrane potential (from Light *et al*, 1986).

following properties, revealed by intracellular recording, are commonly encountered:

1) innocuous mechanical stimulation of the skin elicits e.p.s.p.s but not action potentials - possibly as a result of simultaneous stimulation of an overlapping low threshold inhibitory receptive field;

2) no cutaneous receptive field sensitive to innocuous mechanical stimulation can be identified but electrical stimulation of peripheral nerves reveals excitatory inputs in Aβ fibres. The excitation may arise from receptors in muscles or joints, or may arise from the skin but be concealed by strong inhibitory inputs;

3) trains of action potentials are evoked by noxious stimulation of the skin but electrical stimulation of peripheral nerves at levels which excite C fibres evokes only e.p.s.p.s - presumably due to simultaneous activation of a large number of Aβ fibres which evoked long-lasting polysynaptic i.p.s.p.s that reduce the effectiveness of the C fibre excitatory inputs.

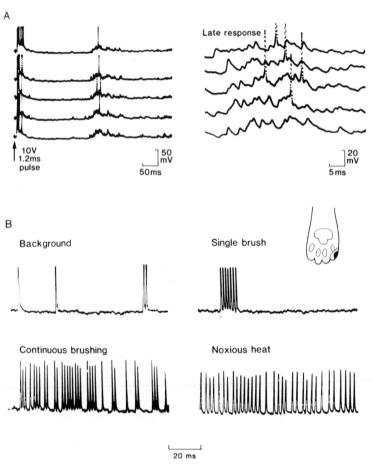

FIGURE 5: Responses of two multireceptive neurones in lamina IV of cat lumbar spinal cord to electrical stimulation of afferent inputs and natural stimulation of the skin. A. Responses to single shocks applied to the peroneal nerve once every four seconds. The late C fibre response is shown on an expanded time base (from Steedman et al., 1985). B. Background activity and responses to natural stimulation of skin. Receptive field (outlined) was larger than that of a neurone recorded within lamina II on the same electrode track (solid).

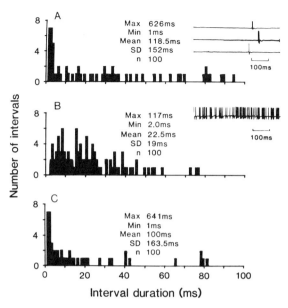

FIGURE 6: Interspike interval histogram generated from spike trains recorded from a multireceptive spinocervical tract neurone in lamina IV of cat lumbar spinal cord. A and C, background activity before and after recovery from stimulus; B, steady state response to noxious heat stimulation of cutaneous receptive field.

In the first two examples extracellular recording would suggest that the neurones were nociceptive-specific rather than multireceptive, and in the third case that the nociceptive input was not conducted by C fibres. These problems are multiplied by the existence of both tonic and phasic inhibitory inputs of supraspinal origin.

OUTPUT FROM LAMINA II TO DEEPER DORSAL HORN

Lamina II neurones with axons which distribute terminal collaterals in the deeper dorsal horn and which make multiple contacts with proximal dendrites and cell somas, have been described (Matsushita, 1969; Mannen and Sugiura, 1976; Light and Kavookjian, 1988). It is probable that some may make multiple contacts with individual deeper neurones, and that the deeper neurones may receive nociceptive input converging from several lamina II neurones. This is confirmed by our observations that:

1) the nociceptive receptive fields of lamina II neurones were smaller than and lay within the boundaries of those of neurones recorded more ventrally in the same recording track (Figures 2 and 5);

2) repeated electrical stimulation of peripheral C fibres which evoked constant latency, consistent responses in neurones in lamina II, elicited, in deeper neurones, more variable, irregular and longer-lasting responses - consisting of a prolonged series of e.p.s.p.s with spikes arising singly and irregularly when the membrane potential reached firing threshold (Figure 5A);

3) the absence of very short intervals and the shape of the interval histogram of noxious heat-evoked activity of deeper neurones (Figure 6B) were consistent with the hypothesis that the discharge was the result of the adding-together of inputs from a number of lamina II neurones which generated interval histograms of the type illustrated in Figure 3.

OUTPUT FROM MULTIRECEPTIVE NEURONES IN THE DEEPER LAMINAE

Many investigators have noted that natural stimulation of the receptive field with different stimuli can evoke quite different patterns of response in a multireceptive neurone. Examples of the types of activity recorded are shown in Figure 5B. This neurone exhibited persistent background activity with occasional irregular bursts of up to five action potentials arising from one complex e.p.s.p. This generated an asymmetric, unimodal interspike interval histogram with rapid rise to mode after a short dead time and a long tail of long intervals, so that mean and modal values were far apart (Figure 6A and C). Brushing hairs in the receptive field increased both the incidence of bursts and the number of action potentials in a burst (Figure 5B). This stimulus activates several receptors so that impulses conducted in several Aβ fibres reach the neurone almost synchronously; in addition individual receptors may activate the neurone along both mono- and polysynaptic pathways and thus elicit a burst of action potentials arising from a complex e.p.s.p. (Hongo and Koike, 1975; Brown et al, 1987). Similar high frequency burst discharges were evoked by the almost synchronous arrival of inputs in a number of Aβ fibres excited by electrical stimulation of peripheral nerves (Figure 5A).

Noxious heat evoked a much more regular discharge which showed no bursts (Figure 5B) and which generated a unimodal, symmetric histogram with no very short intervals and a much reduced tail. Mean and modal values were, therefore, much closer (Figure 6B). The polysynaptic nociceptive drive to the neurone relayed through lamina II thus overrode both the inputs responsible for the bursts occurring in the background discharge (possibly by activation of Aβ afferent fibres as a result of operative procedures) and the influences responsible for the very long intervals (possibly inhibitory inputs).

CIRCUITRY OF THE SYSTEM

The synaptic organisation which we have described is summarised in Figure 7. Neurones in lamina II (cell A) can receive strong input from a small number of C primary afferent fibres, each making multiple contacts. They may also receive inputs from a larger number of C fibres which are effectively weaker, either because they make a smaller number of synaptic contacts or because of the location of the synapses in relation to the recording microelectrode (some of this input may be polysynaptic). Excitatory input from Aβ primary afferent fibres can reach lamina II neurones either monosynaptically (on dendrites which extend ventrally into lamina III) or polysynaptically (probably through lamina III interneurones which send axons dorsally) (cell B). Inhibitory interneurones also relay Aβ input to lamina II - probable candidates would again be interneurones in lamina III (cell C); their axons make synaptic contacts with the dendrites of neurone A and evoke i.p.s.p.s, thus reducing the effectiveness of the nociceptive inputs. Similarly axons descending the spinal cord terminate on neurone A and evoke i.p.s.p.s (descending excitatory inputs have also been defined, Light et al., 1986). The effectiveness of the inhibitory inputs suggests that the synaptic contacts responsible may be on proximal dendrites. The morphology of these neurones - small somas giving rise to a small number of principal dendrites - is such that strategically-located inhibitory synapses could selectively influence inputs to particular areas of the dendritic tree.

In turn the axon of neurone A projects ventrally and can make multiple contacts through collaterals with neurones in laminae III-V (cell D), each of which may also

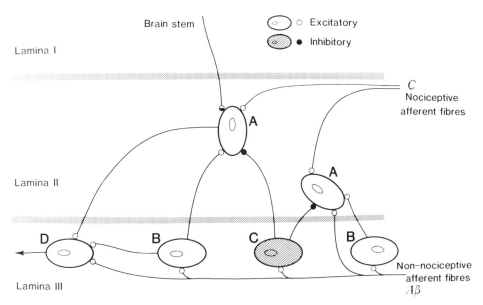

FIGURE 7: Circuitry of the system. Neurones in lamina II (A) may receive: 1) monosynaptic nociceptive inputs from C fibres; 2) non-nociceptive input from Aβ fibres, excitatory - monosynaptically on to ventrally-directed dendrites and/or polysynaptically through lamina III interneurones; (B), and inhibitory - polysynaptically through lamina III inhibitory interneurones (C); 3) excitatory and inhibitory inputs from axons descending from supraspinal sources. In turn these neurones project to cells in deeper laminae (D) which also receive non-nociceptive input from Aβ fibres along mono- and poly-synaptic pathways.

receive inputs from other neurones in lamina II. These deeper neurones also receive input from Aβ primary afferent fibres which may travel along both mono- and poly-synaptic pathways.

CONCLUSIONS

This new knowledge of the organisation and synaptic relationships in the pathway by which nociceptive input in C primary afferent fibres is carried to the substantia gelatinosa (lamina II) and from there transmitted to deeper laminae, has important implications to our understanding of the processing of sensory information. Noxious and innocuous inputs from the skin travel along very different routes before converging on multireceptive neurones in the deeper laminae. The temporal ordering of action potentials in the discharges evoked by different stimuli may therefore be very different, and will depend on the properties of the receptor and afferent fibre on the electrical characteristics of any interneurones as well as on the pattern of synaptic connectivity at each stage. There is now a considerable body of evidence that the timing of action potentials arriving at a synapse affects the manner in which synaptic transmission occurs. Convergence of input may therefore not necessarily mean that specificity of modality is lost - modality information may be encoded in the ordering of intervals within a train of action potentials.

C fibre nociceptive input which is relayed in lamina II is thus subject both to interaction with other excitatory inputs and to modulation by inhibitory inputs, both of which may originate from other primary afferent inputs and from supraspinal sources.

It is not surprising, therefore, that the activity of multireceptive neurones in the deeper laminae is subject to modification in a variety of ways. The nociceptive input through lamina II is subject to modification independently from the non-nociceptive input in $A\beta$ fibres which terminate in the deeper laminae. In addition, non-nociceptive input in a single $A\beta$ fibre may reach the neurone along both mono- and poly-synaptic pathways, so that the polysynaptically conducted input may be affected independently from the monosynaptic input.

The output of neurone D (Fig. 7) should therefore always be examined in terms of the ordering of action potentials within the discharge rather than simply in terms of firing frequency (for example in situations in which one modality of input can be selectively affected).

ACKNOWLEDGEMENTS

This work has been generously supported both by the award of a Kerr-Fry Research Fellowship at the University of Edinburgh and by the Wellcome Trust. I am greatly indebted to V. Molony (without whom the intracellular recordings would never have been made) and S. Zachary for their collaboration. I am also very grateful to D.J. Maxwell for much constructive discussion and to C.R. House and A. Iggo for their continuing and unfailing encouragement and support. I would like to thank H. Anderson, J. Greenhorn, C.M. Warwick and A.M. Stirling-Whyte for all their help

REFERENCES

ANGAUT-PETIT, D. (1975) The dorsal column system: II. Functional properties and bulbar relay of the postsynaptic fibres of the cat's fasciculus gracilis. *Experimental Brain Research* **22**, 471-493.

BANNATYNE, B.A., MAXWELL, D.J. AND BROWN, A.G. (1987). Fine structure of synapses associated with characterized postsynaptic dorsal column neurons in the cat. *Neuroscience* **23**, 597-612.

BASBAUM, A.I., GLAZER, E.J. AND LORD, B.A.P. (1982). Simultaneous ultrastructural localization of tritiated serotonin and immunoreactive peptides. *Journal of Histochemistry and Cytochemistry* **30**, 780-784.

BROWN, A.G. AND FRANZ, D.N. (1970). Patterns of response in spinocervical tract neurones to different stimuli of long duration. *Brain Research* **17**, 156-160.

BROWN, A.G., HAMANN, W.C. AND MARTIN, H.F. (1975). Effects of activity in non-myelinated afferent fibres on the spinocervical tract. *Brain Research* **98**, 243-259.

BROWN, A.G., KOERBER, H.R. AND NOBLE, R. (1987). An intracellular study of spinocervical tract cell responses to natural stimuli and single hair afferent fibres in cats. *Journal of Physiology* **382**, 331-354.

CALVILLO, O. (1978). Primary afferent depolarization of C fibers in the spinal cord of the cat. *Canadian Journal of Physiology and Pharmacology* **56**, 154-157.

CARSTENS, E., TULLOCH, I., ZIEGLGANSBERGER, W. and ZIMMERMANN, M. (1979). Presynaptic excitability changes induced by morphine in single cutaneous afferent C and A fibres. *Pflügers Archiv* **379**, 143-147.

COLLINGRIDGE, G.L., HERRON, C.E. AND LESTER, R.A.J. (1988). Frequency-dependent N-methyl-D-aspartate receptor-mediated synaptic transmission in rat hippocampus. *Journal of Physiology* **399**, 301-312.

DUGGAN, A.W., MORTON, C.R., HUTCHISON, W.D. AND HENDRY, I.A. (1988). Absence of tonic supraspinal control of substance P release in the substantia gelatinosa of the anaesthetized cat. *Experimental Brain Research* (in press).

EMMERS, R. (1981). *Pain, a spike-interval coded message in the brain.* Raven Press, New York.

FIELDS, H.L. AND BASBAUM, A.I. (1978). Brainstem control of spinal pain transmission neurons. *Annual Review of Physiology* **40**, 217-248.

FITZGERALD, M. AND WOOLF, C.J. (1981). Effects of cutaneous nerve and intraspinal conditioning on C-fibre afferent terminal excitability in decerebrate spinal rats. *Journal of Physiology* **318**, 25-39.

GIESLER, G.J., CANNON, J.T., URCA, G. AND LIEBESKIND, J.C. (1978).Long ascending projections from substantia gelatinosa Rolandi and the subjacent dorsal horn in the rat. *Science* **202**, 984-986.

GOBEL, S., FALLS, W.M., BENNETT, G.J., ABDELMOUMENE, M., HAYASHI, H. AND HUMPHREY, E. (1980). An EM analysis of the synaptic connections of horseradish peroxidase-filled stalked cells and islet cells in the substantia gelatinosa of adult cat spinal cord. *Journal of Comparative Neurology* **194**, 781-807.

GREGOR, M. AND ZIMMERMANN, M. (1972). Characteristics of spinal neurones responding to cutaneous myelinated and unmyelinated fibres. *Journal of Physiology* **221**, 555-576.

HANDWERKER, H.O., IGGO, A. AND ZIMMERMAN, M. (1975). Segmental and supraspinal actions on dorsal horn neurones responding to noxious and non-noxious skin stimuli. Pain **1**, 142-165.

HENTALL, I.D. AND FIELDS, H.L. (1979). Segmental and descending influences on intraspinal thresholds of single C-fibres. *Journal of Neurophysiology* **42**, 1527-1537.

HONGO, T. AND KOIKE, H. (1975). Some aspects of synaptic organization in the spinocervical tract cell in the cat. In *The Somatosensory System*, ed. H.H. KORNHUBER. Stuttgart: Georg Thieme.

IGGO, A., MOLONY, V., AND STEEDMAN, W.M. (1988). Membrane properties of nociceptive neurones in lamina II of lumbar spinal cord in the cat. *Journal of Physiology* **400**, 367-380.

LIGHT, A.R., CASALE, E.J. AND MENÉTREY, D.M. (1986). The effects of focal stimulation in nucleus raphe magnus and periaqueductal gray on intracellularly recorded neurons in spinal laminae I and II. *Journal of Neurophysiology* **56**, 555-571.

LIGHT, A.R. AND KAVOOKJIAN, A.M. (1988). Morphology and ultrastructure of physiologically identified substantia gelatinosa (lamina II) neurons with axons that terminate in deeper dorsal horn laminae (III-V). *Journal of Comparative Neurology* **267**, 172189.

LIGHT, A.R., KAVOOKJIAN, A.M. AND PETRUSZ, P. (1983). The ultrastructure and synaptic connections of serotonin-immunoreactive terminals in spinal laminae I and II. *Somatosensory Research* **1**, 33-50.

MANNEN, H. AND SUGIURA, Y. (1976). Reconstruction of neurons of dorsal horn proper using Golgi-stained serial sections. *Journal of Comparative Neurology* **168**, 303-312.

MATSUSHITA, M. (1969). Some aspects of the interneuronal connections in cat's spinal gray matter. *Journal of Comparative Neurology* **136**, 57-80.

MAXWELL, D.J., FYFFE, R.E.W. AND RÉTHELYI, M. (1983). Morphological properties of physiologically characterized lamina III neurones in the cat spinal cord. *Neuroscience* **10**, 1-22.

MAXWELL, D.J. AND RÉTHELYI, M. (1987). Ultrastructure and synaptic connections of cutaneous afferent fibres in the spinal cord. *Trends in Neuroscience* **10**, 117-123.

MELZACK, R. AND WALL, P.D. (1965). Pain mechanisms: a new theory. *Science* **150**, 971-979.

MENDELL, L.M. (1966). Physiological properties of unmyelinated fibre projection to the spinal cord. *Experimental Neurology* **16**, 316-332.

MOLONY, V., STEEDMAN, W.M., CERVERO, F. AND IGGO, A. (1981). Intracellular marking of identified neurones in the superficial dorsal horn of the cat spinal cord. *Quarterly Journal of Experimental Physiology* **66**, 211-223.

PRICE, D.D. AND DUBNER, R. (1977). Neurons that subserve the sensory-discriminative aspects of pain. *Pain* **3**, 307-338.

PRICE, D.D., HULL, C.D. AND BUCHWALD, N.A. (1971). Intracellular responses of dorsal horn cells to cutaneous and sural nerve A and C fibre stimuli. *Experimental Neurology* **33**, 291-309.

RAMÓN Y CAJAL, S. (1909). *Histologie du système nerveux de l'homme et des vertebres.* Vol. **1.**, 1952 reprint. Instituto Ramón y Cajal, Madrid.

RÉTHELYI, M. (1977). Preterminal and terminal axon arborizations in the substantia gelatinosa of cat's spinal cord. *Journal of Comparative Neurology* **172**, 511-528.

ROBERTS, W.J. (1986). A hypothesis on the physiological basis for causalgia and related pains. *Pain* **24**, 297-311.

RUDA, M.A., COFFIELD, AND STEINBUSCH, H.W.M. (1982). Immunocytochemical analysis of serotonergic axons in laminae I and II of the lumbar spinal cord of the cat. *Journal of Neuroscience* **2**, 16601671.

SALT, T.E. (1986). Mediation of thalamic sensory input by both NMDA receptors and non-NMDA receptors. *Nature* **322**, 263-265.

SANDNER, R., HAYASHI, K. AND TSUKADA, M. (1987). Spike trains in rat periaqueductal gray depend on the stochastic properties of interacting electrical stimulation trains. *Brain Research* **421**, 150-160.

STEEDMAN, W.M., IGGO, A., MOLONY, V., KOROGOD, S. AND ZACHARY, S.(1983).Statistical analysis of ongoing activity of neurones in the substantia gelatinosa and in lamina III of cat spinal cord. *Quarterly Journal of Experimental Physiology* **68**, 733746.

STEEDMAN, W.M. AND MOLONY, V. (1987). Intracellularly recorded responses of neurones in lamina II of cat spinal dorsal horn to activation of cutaneous afferent inputs. In *Fine Afferent Nerve Fibres and Pain*, pp. 289-297; ed. SCHMIDT, R.F., SCHAIBLE, H.-G. AND VAHLE-HINZ, C. Weinheim, VCH.

STEEDMAN, W.M., MOLONY, V. AND IGGO, A. (1985). Nociceptive neurones in the superficial dorsal horn of cat lumbar spinal cord and their primary afferent inputs. *Experimental Brain Research* **58**, 171-182.

SUGIURA, Y., LEE, C.L. AND PERL, E.R. (1986). Central projections of functionally identified unmyelinated (C) afferent fibres in mammalian cutaneous nerve. *Science* **234**, 358-361.

SZENTAGOTHAI, J. (1964). Neuronal and synaptic arrangement in the substantia gelatinosa Rolandi. *Journal of Comparative Neurology* **122**, 219-239.

WILLIS, W.D. (1982). Control of nociceptive transmission in the spinal cord. *Progress in Sensory Physiology* **3**. Berlin, Springer-Verlag.

WILLIS, W.D., LEONARD, R.B. AND KENSHALO, D.R. (1978).Spinothalamic tract neurons in the substantia gelatinosa. *Science* **202**, 986-988.

SUPERFICIAL DORSAL HORN NEURONS IN THE RAT RESPONSIVE TO VISCERAL AND CUTANEOUS INPUTS

T.J. Ness and G.F. Gebhart

Department of Pharmacology, College of Medicine, University of Iowa
Iowa City, Iowa 52242, USA

The superficial dorsal horn is widely acknowledged as important to the processing of nociceptive information. As documented in this volume, fine afferent nerve fibers terminate in laminae I and II_O and second order spinal neurons upon which many of these afferents terminate transmit the received message supraspinally. Our current understanding of spinal nociceptive transmission arises primarily from investigations of afferent fibers arising from cutaneous structures. Relatively less is known about afferents arising from deeper structures, particularly viscera. Investigations of visceral afferent projections to the spinal cord describe terminals in the superficial dorsal horn (Cervero and Connell, 1984; DeGroat, 1986) and spinal units in the superficial dorsal horn respond to electrical stimulation of visceral afferents (Blair et al, 1981; Takahashi and Yokota, 1983; Cervero and Tattersall, 1987). In the present study in the rat, colorectal distension was used as a *natural* visceral stimulus to examine the response characteristics and convergent cutaneous receptive fields of neurons in the thoracolumbar spinal cord.

Rats were anesthetized with sodium pentobarbital (45-50 mg/kg) and venous, arterial, and tracheal cannulae inserted. The cervical spinal cord was exposed and rats were irreversibly spinalized at C1 and the brain subsequently pithed. A laminectomy was made to expose the T13-L2 spinal segments and the vertebral column was clamped rostrally and caudally; skin flaps formed a pool for agar and mineral oil. Rats were mechanically ventilated and were paralyzed with pancuronium bromide (0.2 mg/hr) for the duration of the experiment. Single unit recordings were made in the superficial dorsal horn (0.0-0.3 mm from the cord dorsum) using conventional techniques. Colorectal distension (80 mmHg) was used as a search stimulus and was produced by inflating with air a 7-8 cm, flexible latex balloon inserted via the anus. Intracolonic distending pressures were measured with an in-line low volume pressure transducer. Neurons were characterized with respect to responses to graded colorectal distension and of convergent cutaneous inputs (brush, touch, pinch and heat); the sizes of the convergent cutaneous receptive fields were determined and drawn on figurines. To quantify spinal neuronal responses to colorectal distension, the total number of unit discharges were counted beginning with the onset of the distending stimulus. These methods have been described elsewhere in greater detail (Ness and Gebhart, 1987, 1988a).

Neurons (33) in the superficial dorsal horn that were excited by colorectal distension, like neurons in deeper laminae (Ness and Gebhart, 1987, 1988a), were observed to respond at short latency (< 1 sec) following the onset of colorectal distension. The responses of 17 neurons to distension terminated abruptly upon release of the distending stimulus (i.e., short latency-abrupt, SL-A), while 16 neurons exhibited responses which were sustained for an additional 4-30 sec following termination of distension (i.e., short latency-sustained, SL-S; see Fig. 1). All SL-A and SL-S neurons had excitatory convergent cutaneous receptive fields categorized as: very small (<2cm long axis); small (2-4 cm long axis); medium (>4 cm long axis and part of hind limb); large (hindquarter) and very large (> hindquarter with contralateral input). SL-A and SL-S neurons in the superficial dorsal horn exhibited accelerating, monotonic responses to graded distension of the colon (Fig. 1). As with SL-A neurons recorded in deeper laminae (Ness and Gebhart, 1988a), the extrapolated thresholds for response to distension were 0-5 mmHg (Fig. 1) and both noxious and non-noxious stimuli applied in the convergent cutaneous receptive field were excitatory (i.e., SL-A neurons are class 2 or multireceptive in character). Regarding the size of the convergent cutaneous receptive fields, 15 of 17 SL-A neurons had cutaneous receptive fields medium in size or larger. Only two neurons had small receptive fields and none had very small receptive fields (Fig. 2). In contrast, SL-A neurons in the deeper dorsal horn have receptive fields small and very small in size (Ness and Gebhart, 1988a).

SL-S neurons in this study were similar to SL-A neurons in that the mean threshold for response of three SL-S neurons studied was also between 0-5 mm Hg. Like SL-A neurons, SL-S neurons in the superficial dorsal horn were excited by noxious stimuli applied in the convergent cutaneous receptive fields. Most, however, responded only to noxious stimuli (i.e., class 3 or nocireceptive neurons) applied in cutaneous receptive fields small to very large in size (Fig. 2).

This study of neurons in the superficial dorsal horn responsive to noxious colorectal distension further supports an important role for the outer laminae of the spinal dorsal horn in visceral nociceptive transmission. Responses of SL-A and SL-S neurons in the superficial dorsal horn were found to be qualitatively similar to the same classes of neurons previously studied in both thoracolumbar and lumbosacral spinal cord of the

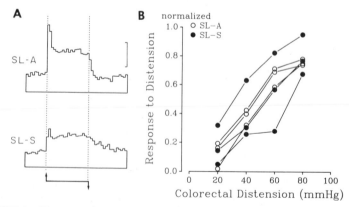

FIGURE 1: Response characteristics of superficial dorsal horn neurons to colorectal distension. A: Mean peristimulus time histograms of 17 SL-A (above) and 16 SL-S (below) neurons to 80 mmHg, 20 s colorectal distension. The period of distension is illustrated below; vertical calibration = 20 Hz. B: Stimulus-response functions of 3 SL-A and 3 SL-S neurons normalized (assigned the value 1) to the response produced by 100 mmHg, 20 s colorectal distension.

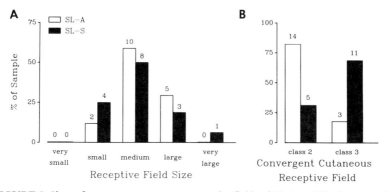

FIGURE 2: Sizes of convergent, cutaneous receptive fields of SL-A and SL-S neurons (A) and proportions considered Class 2 (multireceptive) and Class 3 (nocireceptive) based upon responses to stimuli applied in the convergent, cutaneous receptive field (B). Numbers above the bars indicate the sample size. Definitions of receptive field sizes are given in the text.

rat (Ness and Gebhart, 1987, 1988a). As has been reported for the cat (Blair *et al*, 1981; Cervero and Tattersall, 1987; Takahashi and Yokota, 1983), superficial dorsal horn neurons in the rat are clearly viscerosomatic. All neurons excited by colorectal distension, a stimulus considered to reproduce a natural, noxious visceral stimulus at the intensity and duration applied here (Ness and Gebhart, 1988b), also received convergent cutaneous input. In all cases, noxious stimuli (e.g., heat, pinch) applied in the convergent cutaneous receptive field also excited these neurons. Cervero and Tattersall (1987) reported similar findings; 89% of 36 viscerosomatic units recorded in the superficial dorsal horn in the cat were either multireceptive or nocireceptive. While all units in the present study responded to noxious (nocireceptive) or noxious and non-noxious (multireceptive) inputs from the convergent cutaneous receptive fields, SL-A neurons in the deeper thoracolumbar or lumbosacral spinal cord have been characterized which respond exclusively to non-noxious inputs (Ness and Gebhart, 1987, 1988a).

SL-A and SL-S neurons in the superficial dorsal horn do not differ significantly with respect to the sizes of convergent cutaneous receptive fields. Eighty-two percent of the combined sample of 33 neurons had cutaneous receptive fields medium in size or larger. This result in the rat differs somewhat from that reported by Cervero and Tattersall (1987) who found that 44% of a total 36 viscerosomatic neurons in laminae I in the cat had small cutaneous receptive fields. Based on the finding that a greater percentage of neurons receiving only excitatory cutaneous input in the superficial dorsal horn of the cat have small receptive fields (77%), Cervero and Tattersall (1987) suggest that the cutaneous representation of somatic neurons is more precise than that of viscerosomatic neurons, an interpretation consistent with the general diffuse nature of visceral pains. The results of the present study are not inconsistent with this suggestion.

In previous consideration of other data, we have speculated that, independent of their convergent cutaneous receptive fields, SL-A neurons are visceral analogues of class 2 neurons and SL-S neurons are visceral analogues of class 3 neurons (Ness and Gebhart, 1987, 1988a). Such analogies appear more appropriate to the lumbosacral and deep thoracolumbar spinal cord since neurons which responded to colorectal distension were found which did not have convergent cutaneous receptive fields. However, in the superficial dorsal horn which has clearly been demonstrated to be important to nociceptive transmission, neurons have not been described which are not either somatic or viscerosomatic in character. Perhaps additional examination of neurons in the superficial dorsal horn receiving inputs from other viscera might reveal the presence of *viscerospecific* neurons important to nociceptive transmission.

ACKNOWLEDGMENTS

We would like to thank M. Burcham for technical assistance and T. Fulton for secretarial assistance. Supported by NS 19912 and DA 02879. T.J. Ness was supported by a Life and Health Insurance Medical Research Fellowship.

REFERENCES

BLAIR, R.W., WEBER, R.N. AND FOREMAN, R.D. (1981). Characteristics of primate spinothalamic tract neurons receiving viscerosomatic convergent inputs in T3 T5 segments. *Journal of Neurophysiology* **46**, 797-811.

CERVERO, F. AND CONNELL, L.A. (1984). Distribution of somatic and visceral primary afferent fibers within the thoracic spinal cord of the cat. *Journal of Comparative Neurology* **230**, 88-98.

CERVERO, F. AND TATTERSALL, J.E.H. (1987). Somatic and visceral inputs to the thoracic spinal cord of the cat: marginal zone (laminae I) of the dorsal horn. *Journal of Physiology* **388**, 383-395.

DEGROAT, W.C. (1986). Spinal cord projections and neuropeptides in visceral afferent neurons. In: **Visceral Sensation.** *Progress in Brain Research*, vol. **67**, ed. Cervero, F. and Morrison, J.F.B., pp. 165-187. Amsterdam: Elsevier.

NESS, T.J. AND GEBHART, G.F. (1987). Characterization of neuronal responses to noxious visceral and somatic stimuli in the medial lumbosacral spinal cord of the rat. *Journal of Neurophysiology* **57**: 1867-1892.

NESS, T.J. AND GEBHART, G.F. (1988a). Characterization of neurons responsive to noxious colorectal distension in the T13-L2 spinal cord of the rat. *Journal of Neurophysiology* **60**: in press.

NESS, T.J. AND GEBHART, G.F. (1988b). Colorectal distension as a noxious visceral stimulus: Physiologic and pharmacologic characterization of pseudaffective reflexes in the rat. *Brain Research* **450**: 153-169.

TAKAHASHI, M. AND YOKOTA, T (1983). Convergence of cardiac and cutaneous afferents onto neurons in the dorsal horn of the spinal cord in the cat. *Neuroscience Letters* **38**: 251-256.

IDENTIFICATION OF A SUB-POPULATION OF VISCERO-SOMATIC NEURONES UNIQUE TO THE SUPERFICIAL DORSAL HORN

B. M. Lumb and F. Cervero

Department of Physiology, Medical School, University of Bristol, University Walk
Bristol BS8 1TD, U.K.

The thoracic spinal cord processes somatic and visceral sensory information from the skin and muscles of the thorax and from thoracic and upper abdominal internal organs. The visceral input is mediated by sympathetic nerves and includes afferent fibres that signal visceral pain. Stimulation of visceral afferent fibres activates spinal cord neurones that are also driven by somatic stimulation (viscero-somatic neurones). Viscero-somatic neurones have been shown to contribute axons to ascending sensory pathways and it is generally thought that these cells provide the neurological substrate for the referral of visceral pain (see, Cervero and Tattersall, 1986; Foreman, 1986).

Previous reports from this and other laboratories have shown that viscero-somatic neurones constitute a large proportion (40 - 60%) of all neurones in the lower thoracic spinal cord of the cat. This suggests that visceral afferent information must undergo a considerable degree of central divergence since there are relatively few (10% or less) visceral afferent fibres in thoracic dorsal roots (Cervero *et al*, 1984). We have recently provided evidence to suggest that this divergence may include supraspinal looped pathways and that the spinal transmission of visceral information is under both tonic and phasic descending inhibitory control from the brain stem (Tattersall *et al*, 1986).

In the present study we have extended these investigations by testing whether single thoracic neurones receive bilateral visceral inputs and have determined the extent to which the transfer of this information is modulated by descending control of supraspinal origin.

The experiments were carried out in chloralose-anaesthetised cats. Single-unit recordings were made throughout the grey matter in the lower thoracic spinal cord (T9 - T11). Neurones were classified as viscero-somatic if, in addition to being driven by electrical and/or natural stimulation in their somatic receptive fields, they gave excitatory responses to electrical stimulation of the ipsilateral splanchnic nerve (iSPLN). Excitatory responses of viscero-somatic neurones to electrical stimulation of the contralateral splanchnic nerve (cSPLN) was taken as evidence for bilateral visceral inputs. Phasic descending influences on these cells was tested by electrical stimulation in nucleus raphe magnus (NRM) and the immediately adjacent reticular formation.

Most (89%) of the viscero-somatic neurones recorded could be driven by electrical stimulation of ipsilateral and contralateral splanchnic nerves, i.e. had bilateral visceral inputs. In contrast, a small minority (11%) of viscero-somatic neurones received no

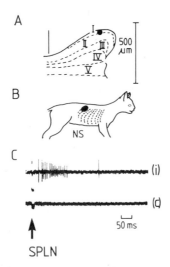

FIGURE 1: Viscero-somatic neurone in the thoracic spinal cord which was excited by stimulation of the ipsilateral splanchnic nerve (iSPLN) but which was not driven by stimulation of the contralateral splanchnic nerve (cSPLN), i.e. had an exclusively ipsilateral visceral input. A: location of the recording site of the neurone in lamina I. B: this cell was excited by noxious stimulation (pinching) of the skin within its somatic receptive field (shaded area). C: single-sweep oscilloscope traces illustrating the response of the cell to single shock stimulation of iSPLN at supramaximal intensity (upper trace) and the failure of cSPLN to evoke activity even when tested with a short train of pulses at supramaximal intensity (lower trace). Arrow indicates the timing of the stimulus.

excitatory drive from the contralateral splanchnic nerve and were therefore considered to have exclusively ipsilateral visceral inputs (Fig.1).

A marked difference between these two populations of viscero-somatic neurones concerns their locations in the spinal grey matter. Cells with bilateral visceral inputs were recorded throughout the spinal grey matter, but predominantly (77%) in laminae VII and VIII, whereas all but one of the neurones with only ipsilateral visceral inputs were recorded in the superficial dorsal horn, predominantly in lamina I, and none in laminae VII and VIII (Fig.2).

These two populations of neurones also differed with respect to the size and characteristics of their somatic receptive fields. Most neurones with bilateral visceral inputs had relatively large somatic receptive fields, were multireceptive and their somatic drives included inputs from deep structures such as muscles and joints. Conversely, neurones with exclusively ipsilateral visceral inputs had small, nocireceptive somatic fields which were confined to cutaneous structures.

When tested for the effects of brain stem stimulation the majority (72%; n=68) of thoracic viscero-somatic neurones gave an initial excitatory response which was followed by a period of reduced responsiveness to stimulation of somatic and visceral afferents. All but one of the cells affected in this way had bilateral visceral inputs and most were located in the deep dorsal horn and in laminae VII and VIII. The remaining neurones exhibited no excitatory drive from the brain stem but their responses to visceral and somatic stimulation were similarly depressed. Cells of this type were recorded throughout the spinal grey matter and included 3 out of 4 cells tested which had exclusively ipsilateral visceral inputs.

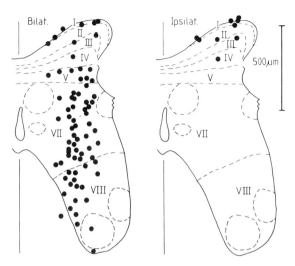

FIGURE 2: Locations of the recording sites of viscero-somatic neurones with bilateral or exclusively ipsilateral visceral inputs. The locations are plotted on a standard transverse section of the T11 grey matter.

The present study has identified two groups of viscero-somatic neurones in the cat thoracic spinal cord; one which has bilateral visceral inputs and a second which cannot be driven by stimulation of cSPLN and is considered to have an ipsilateral visceral input only. Differences in the spinal locations, somatic receptive field properties and descending control of neurones with and without contralateral visceral drives suggests that they represent two distinct populations of neurones which may subserve different roles in the processing of visceral afferent information.

Neurones with bilateral visceral inputs were located predominantly in laminae VII and VIII of the ventral horn. Ventral horn neurones have been implicated in positive feedback loops between the brain stem and spinal cord (see, Lumb, 1986); in the present study, their spinal locations and receptive field properties indicate that neurones with bilateral visceral inputs may contribute to such positive feedback loops. In support of this, in the vast majority of these cells the inhibitory effects of brain stem stimulation were preceded by excitation. Triggering of a positive feedback system by activity in visceral afferent fibres may play a role in maintaining central neuronal activity which could account for the widespread and prolonged increase in sympathetic and motor outflow that accompanies visceral pain.

A small proportion of cells included in this study were found to have exclusively ipsilateral visceral inputs. In contrast to cells with bilateral visceral inputs, they were located mainly in the superficial dorsal horn, had small, nociceptor specific somatic receptive fields and few were excited by stimulation of brain stem sites. Their location in the superficial dorsal horn, an area concerned with the processing and relay of somatic nociceptive information, suggests that cells of this type may be directly involved in the spinal transmission of the sensory aspects of visceral nociceptive information.

ACKNOWLEDGEMENTS

We would like to thank Steve Allen, Rob Wheatley and Simon Lishman for technical assistance. This work was supported by the MRC.

REFERENCES

CERVERO, F., CONNELL, L. A. AND LAWSON, S. N. (1984). Somatic and visceral primary afferents in the lower thoracic dorsal root ganglia of the cat. *Journal of Comparative Neurology* **228** 422-431.

CERVERO, F. AND TATTERSALL, J. E. H. (1986). Somatic and visceral sensory integration in the thoracic spinal cord. In **Visceral Sensation**. *Progress in Brain Research*. vol. **67**. ed. Cervero, F. and Morrison, J. F. B., pp. 189-205. Amsterdam: Elsevier.

FOREMAN, R. D. (1986). Spinal substrates of visceral pain. In *Spinal Afferent Processing*. ed. Yaksh, T. L., pp. 217-242. New York : Plenum Press.

LUMB, B. M. (1986). Brainstem control of visceral afferent pathways in the spinal cord. In **Visceral Sensation**. *Progress in Brain Research*. vol. **67**. ed. Cervero, F. and Morrison, J. F. B., pp. 279-293. Amsterdam : Elsevier.

TATTERSALL, J. E. H., CERVERO, F. AND LUMB, B. M. (1986). Effects of reversible spinalisation on the visceral input to viscero-somatic neurons in the lower thoracic spinal cord of the cat. *Journal of Neurophysiology* **56**, 785-796.

DISCUSSION ON SECTION II

Rapporteur: Daniel Le Bars

Institut National de la Santé et de la Recherche Médicale, Unité de Recherches de Physiopharmacologie du Système Nerveux, INSERM (U.161), 2 rue d'Alésia 75014 Paris, France

THE RECEPTIVE FIELDS OF DORSAL HORN NEURONES; A SIMPLE QUESTION?

The question of what is the receptive field of a single spinal dorsal horn neurone is one which seems very simple at first but which becomes more and more complicated as one's experience increases. Although some of the problems seem at first sight to be of a technical nature, they are in fact derived, directly or indirectly, from the physiological properties of dorsal horn neurones.

During experiments, there is likely to be a bias in the sampling of neurones that will produce an erroneous view of what constitutes the overall population of cells and hence of receptive fields. Such bias is introduced by the types of microelectrode and search stimuli that are used and the way in which the cells are - or are not - backfired from supraspinal structure(s). The search stimuli are of prime importance, not only for trivial reasons such as that the excessive use of non-noxious stimuli can lead to an underestimation of noxious-responding neurones, or that the repeated application of noxious stimuli will damage the stimulated area and produce sensitization phenomena, but also for more fundamental reasons (see Laird and Cervero and Woolf in this volume). For instance, it is well known that the cutaneous receptive fields of spinal neurones are smaller when natural stimuli are used for mapping than when electrical stimulation is used (see Mendell, 1984); synchronisation of inputs by electrical stimuli is likely to be behind such observations.

It is not so easy to perform a careful examination of the receptive field of a neurone. In most experiments, the physiological condition of the animal is monitored by recording heart rate, blood pressure and core temperature. However peripheral temperature and vascular tone could modify the responsiveness of a neurone to a given stimulus; this is particularly relevant in either pharmacological experiments in which the administration of a drug may unintentionally produce such peripheral changes or in physiological experiments in which electrical stimulation of the brain may produce such changes. The use of noxious stimuli can induce sensitization and/or desensitization of peripheral receptors (see Besson and Chaouch, 1987) as well as discrete inflammatory processes. The frequency of application of noxious stimuli to a given area, or to adjacent areas, is therefore critical. In some cases, this frequency has to be very low (see Perl et al, this volume). In this context, previous applications of search stimuli and the testing of previously recorded neurones could both influence later neuronal responses. This is well illustrated by recordings of neurones in the caudal medulla within the subnucleus Reticularis Dorsalis (SRD). These neurones exhibit a convergence of nociceptive information from *whole body* receptive fields but do not show any spontaneous activity at the beginning of experiments; however after long periods of recording or following testing of previous units for their responses to somatic stimuli, the cells progressively build up *spontaneous* activity (Villanueva *et al*, 1988). Interestingly, such activity disappears following systemic morphine (Bing *et al*, 1989). In this case, the convergence of spinal information from the whole body to a single SRD cell probably amplifies the phenomenon. In any case, one has to bear in mind that any part of the body, and in particular the area that is designated the *receptive field* for a given neurone, has its own history before recordings were made from that particular neurone.

Comparison between different experiments can also be difficult for several reasons. Apart from species differences, these relate mainly to the type of preparation and the anaesthetic regime used during the recording sessions. In the spinal preparation, the dorsal horn is free from supraspinal influences while in the decerebrate preparation the descending inhibitory controls are exaggerated. In non-spinal preparations, including the intact preparation, the influence(s) of surgical wounds on the properties of recorded cells must be borne in mind (see below, and Cadden, 1985; Clarke, 1985; Clarke and Matthews, 1985; Matthews, 1985). Finally, in some cases neurones are recorded without anaesthetic (spinal preparations, awake animals) while in others various anaesthetics (chloralose, barbiturates, althesin, nitrous oxide/halothane etc), with different properties, are used by various investigators (see Headley and Parsons, and Molony, in this volume).

The difficulty in determining the receptive field of a dorsal horn neurone is well illustrated by the example of multi-receptive wide-dynamic-range (WDR) neurones whether they are recorded in the superficial or the deep dorsal horn. The first question is to what extent they respond to non-noxious stimuli. It is often believed that these neurones respond under non-pathological conditions, with a higher frequency of firing to any form of noxious stimulation than to any form of innocuous stimulation. Indeed this seems to be the case during recordings of spinothalamic neurones in the monkey anaesthetized with barbiturate (see Willis, this volume). In the rat, however, either under halothane anaesthesia or non-anaesthetized following spinalization, this does not seem to be the case: as shown in Figure 1 it was found in a systematic study that these neurones increased their discharge rates in relation to the temperature applied to their receptive fields with the highest level being produced by noxious intensities, but a very high level of firing was also evoked by adequate repetitive innocuous mechanical stimuli (Le Bars and Chitour, 1983). Examination of the figures from several laboratories (e.g. Duggan, Headley, Molony) interested in pharmacological studies of WDR neurones indicates that this has been found repeatedly (see El Yassir *et al*, Headley and Parsons, and Hope *et al*, in the present volume).

In any case, there is substantial evidence that a wide spectrum of excitatory and inhibitory influences converge upon dorsal horn neurones involved in the transmission of nociceptive messages, especially with WDR neurones; the degree of polarization of the cell could therefore change for many reasons. Consequently subliminal facilitatory and inhibitory surrounds of receptive fields could be masked or unmasked under certain circumstances. Because of the difficulties associated with intracellular recordings (however see Price *et al*, 1971, Wall and Woolf, and Steedman and Zachary, in this volume), sufficient data about such subliminal inputs are generally lacking. However Zieglgänsberger and Herz (1971) used an approach previously applied to the study of the visual system, i.e. microelectrophoretically administered excitatory amino acids such as glutamate to slightly depolarise the neurone under study. They observed expansions in the sizes of receptive fields of WDR neurones as is shown in Figure 2 for a spino-cervical tract neurone. In some cases, changes in the type(s) of stimuli which were able to activate the cell were also seen. Conversely, the electrophoresis of inhibitory amino acids (glycine, gamma amino-butyric acid), by hyperpolarising the neuronal membrane, elicited marked reductions in the sizes of the receptive fields (see also Yokota and Nishikawa, 1982; Saade et al, 1985; Semba et al, 1985).

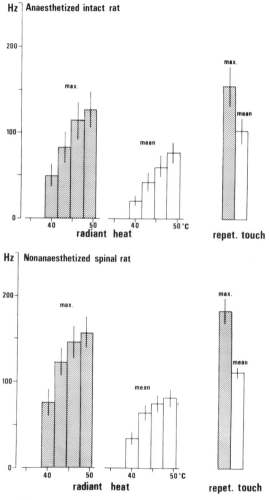

FIGURE 1: Mean firing rates of WDR neurones recorded in the lumbar enlargement of both anaesthetized, intact (upper) and non anaesthetized, spinal rats (lower). Responses evoked by: a) 12 second applications of radiant heat (abscissa: temperature) and b) repetitive light mechanical stimuli. In each case the responses were quantified both in terms of maximal (max: hatched areas) and mean (open areas) levels of firing during stimulation after subtraction of the background activity. Note that these neurones encoded the noxious temperatures but that high levels of firing were achieved when stroking or gently tapping in a rapid, repetitive fashion with a paint brush or a blunt probe (from Le Bars and Chitour, 1983).

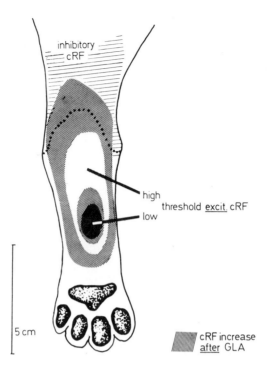

FIGURE 2: Glutamate-induced changes in the excitatory receptive field of a WRD neurone recorded in the lumbar enlargement of a cat. High threshold (white) and low threshold (black) excitatory zones are distinguished. Hatched areas represent the increase in both zones after electrophoretic application of glutamate (from Zieglgänsberger and Herz, 1971, with permission). Using an identical approach in the rat, we (Chitour, Villanueva and Le Bars, unpublished observations) have largely confirmed these findings using D,L-homocysteic (DLH) as the excitatory amino acid. In fact, the increases were sometimes very much greater: for example receptive fields initially restricted to parts of the toes could include the whole limb and part of the tail during the application of a subliminal electrophoretic current. Such observations are not surprising in view of the large dendritic trees of second order cells in the dorsal horn in comparison with their small receptive fields.

In summary, these experiments clearly showed that the properties of the receptive fields of the neurones are highly dependent upon the level of the polarisation of the cell. The factors which potentially have an influence at this level are represented schematically in figure 3. Of course, the depolarizing factors originate mainly from the excitatory receptive field, with all its cutaneous, visceral and muscular inputs, and from the corresponding subliminal fringes (see Lumb and Cervero, Gebhart and Ness, Hylden *et al*, Kniffki, Steedman and Zachary, Willis, and Woolf, in the present volume). Another depolarizing factor could be descending facilitation (see Wall, in this volume). Hyperpolarizing factors are of segmental, propriospinal and supraspinal origins.

Many dorsal horn neurones, particularly WDR neurones, have an adjacent receptive field distinct from the excitatory one (Hillman and Wall, 1969). Most mechanical stimuli applied to this inhibitory field, particularly weak repetitive stimuli, are able to inhibit the neurone's activity. This is illustrated in Figure 4A, where the firing of a convergent neurone, induced by a sustained pinch applied in the centre of its excitatory field, was strongly depressed by light repetitive touch applied within its inhibitory

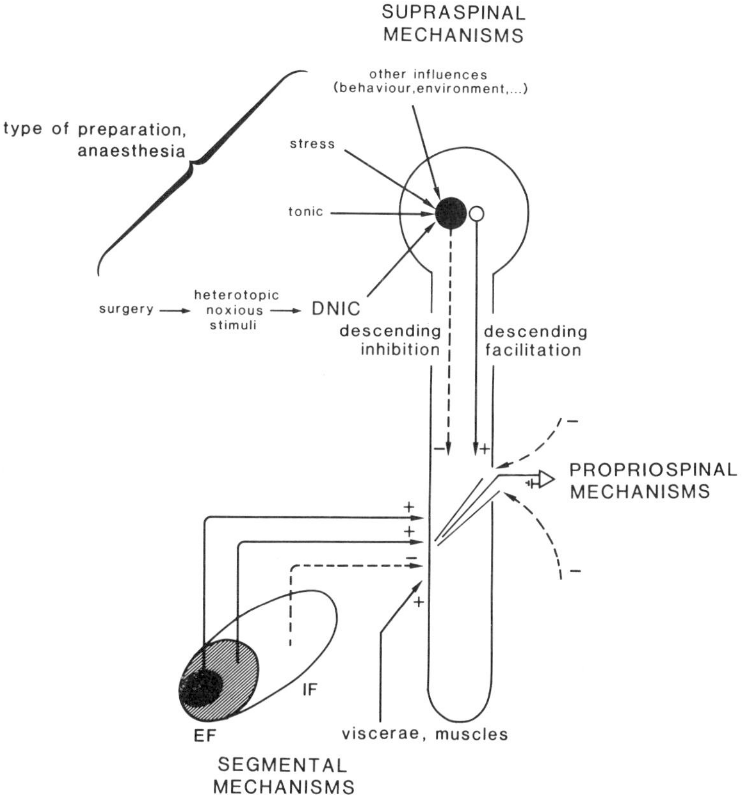

FIGURE 3: Schematic drawing showing the factors that could influence the receptive fields of dorsal horn neurones.

receptive field. This natural stimulation within the cutaneous inhibitory receptive field was equally potent in blocking phasic discharges induced by microelectrophoretic ejection of glutamate (Figure 4B).

In addition to the excitatory and inhibitory influences of segmental origin discussed above, there is evidence that WDR neurones can be inhibited by nociceptive stimuli applied to areas of the body remote from the excitatory and inhibitory segmental fields. These effects involve propriospinal and supraspinal mechanisms. The former can be observed in the dorsal horn of spinal animals (Wagman and Price, 1969; Gerhart *et al*, 1981; Fitzgerald, 1982; Cadden *et al*, 1983 and see Woolf, this volume) while the latter are observed in the intact but not in the spinal animal (Le Bars *et al*, 1979a, b; Gerhart *et al*, 1981; Cadden *et al*, 1983; Morton *et al*, 1987).

It is well known that dorsal horn neurones are under the influence of descending inhibitory controls with supraspinal origins (see Fields and Besson, 1988). Most of the studies devoted to this problem have been carried out by investigating the effects of central electrical stimulation; these have proved the existence of descending inhibitory pathways which are capable of modulating the spinal processing of nociceptive information but have not allowed any conclusions to be reached as to the physiological importance of these controls nor to the circumstances under which they are activated naturally. In fact, the way in which these systems are triggered during such experiments is certainly artificial and involves by-passing parts of a more complex circuit.

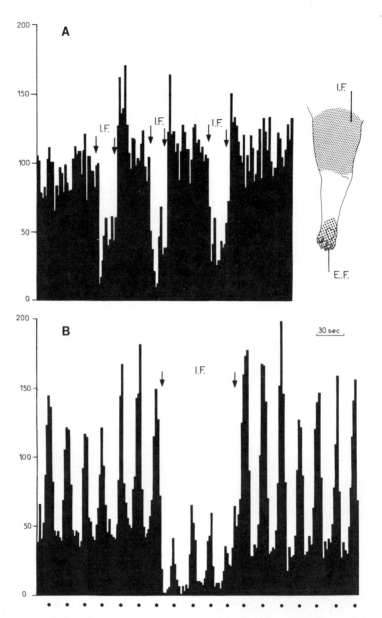

FIGURE 4: Ratemeter records of a lumbar WDR neurone studied in the spinal cat showing synaptically-mediated and chemically-induced firing, which were influenced by natural stimulation within the inhibitory receptive field. The positions of excitatory (EF) and inhibitory (IF) receptive fields on the hindlimb are shown. A: recording showing tonic discharge and the effects of stimulating the inhibitory field (between arrows). B: the effects of stimulating the inhibitory-field (IF) on glutamate-evoked phasic discharges (peaks) on top of the tonic discharge (about 50 spikes/s) induced synaptically by a maintained pinch in the excitatory field. Circles indicate the sequence of periodic injections of glutamate by 10s, 25nA current pulses. (From Besson *et al*, 1974).

Other studies have concluded that tonic descending inhibition exists by means of showing the effects of spinal block on the activities of lumbar neurones in intact and decerebrate animals. Again, it is not known under what physiological circumstances these tonic controls are activated. It has been suggested that stress and environmental conditions can modulate the descending control systems and behaviour has been shown to influence the firing of dorsal horn neurones (Dubner *et al*, 1981; Sorkin *et al*, 1988, and see Collins, this volume).

To date, there is only one circumstance under which descending controls have been

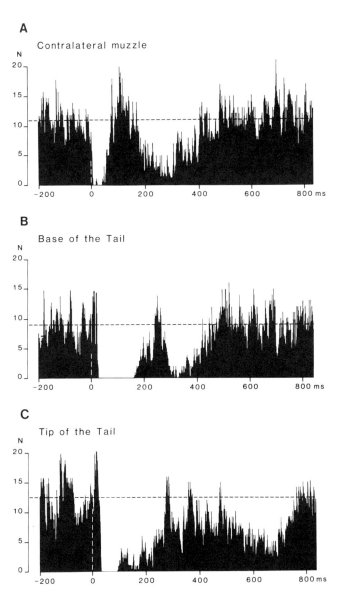

FIGURE 5: Peri-stimulus histograms (bin width: 5 ms) prepared during the continuous electrophoretic application (15 nA) of DLH, onto the membrane of a WDR neurone recorded in the lumbar dorsal horn of an anaesthetized intact rat. Percutaneous electrical stimulation (10 mA; 0.66 Hz; 2 ms duration; 200 ms delay) applied either to the contralateral muzzle (A), the base (B) or the tip (C) of the tail induced a biphasic inhibition. The broken white line shows the time of stimulation while the broken black line represents the mean firing calculated during the prestimulation control period (-200 to 0 ms). Bouhassira, Villanueva and Le Bars, unpublished observations.

unambiguously shown to be activated, viz. when a noxious focus occurs. Indeed, WDR neurones in either the superficial or deeper layers, of the dorsal horn or trigeminal nucleus caudalis are practically all influenced by powerful inhibitory controls. These have been termed Diffuse Noxious Inhibitory Controls (DNIC), because they do not appear to be somatotopically organized (see Le Bars and Villanueva, 1988). The main feature of DNIC is that they can be triggered from any part of the body other than the excitatory receptive field of the neurone under study, provided that the conditioning stimulus is clearly noxious. DNIC cannot be demonstrated in anaesthetized or decerebrate animals in which the spinal cord has been sectioned, the underlying mechanisms cannot therefore be confined to the spinal cord and supraspinal structures must be implicated. In fact, the ascending and descending parts of this loop are confined to the anterolateral quadrants and the dorsolateral funiculi respectively.

In order to investigate the types of peripheral fibres involved in DNIC, one can take advantage of the facts that firstly trigeminal and spinal dorsal horn neurones respond with relatively steady discharges to the electrophoretic application of excitatory amino acids and secondly that DNIC finally act on WDR neurones by a postsynaptic inhibitory mechanism involving hyperpolarization of the neuronal membrane. When trigeminal convergent neurones were directly excited by the electrophoretic application of DL-homocysteate (DLH), the percutaneous electrical application of single square-wave stimuli (10 mA; 2ms) to the tail always induced a biphasic depression of such activity; this depression corresponded to peripheral fibres with conduction velocities in the A-δ and C-fibre ranges, respectively (Bouhassira *et al*, 1987).

Such biphasic inhibitions could be evoked from any part of the body and recorded from any convergent neurones. Figure 5 shows a recording from a superficial lumbar convergent neurone with an excitatory receptive field located on the extremity of the ipsilateral hindpaw; the activity was evoked by DLH and two components of inhibition were induced by the activation of A-δ and C-fibres respectively when a single 2 ms duration shock of 10 mA was applied to the muzzle, the base of the tail or the tip of the tail.

This example illustrates the *whole body inhibitory receptive field* of WDR neurones recorded in intact rats. Indeed these neurones can be excited and inhibited from the segmental excitatory and inhibitory receptive fields and can be inhibited by noxious stimuli applied to the remaining parts of the body. This has several functional consequences, especially regarding the signalling of pain, but since these have been reviewed elsewhere (Le Bars *et al*, 1986; Le Bars and Villanueva, 1988), they will not be considered here. The existence of DNIC could change the properties of the segmental excitatory receptive field. Indeed to reach dorsal horn neurones with micropipettes a laminectomy is required. Any trauma to the bone, especially to the periosteum, constitutes a noxious focus. One can therefore confidently predict that such a surgical wound will trigger DNIC and be a source of descending inhibitory processes that could change the receptive field properties (see also Matthews, 1985).

In summary, 1) the polarisation of the cell and the size of the excitatory receptive field are under the influence of many factors in the case of WDR cells although such factors will obviously be less numerous for nociceptive-specific neurones; 2) if one considers not only the parts of the body which excite WDR neurones but also the parts which inhibit them, then one has to conclude that this type of neurone exhibits a *whole body receptive field* in the intact animal.

The dorsal horn, including the superficial layers, certainly does not work like a telephone network. Unfortunately the power of electrophysiology, although it gives a great deal of information, is very limited by the fact that recordings are made from single units when thousands of other neurones are affected by the *calibrated stimuli* that are applied.

ACKNOWLEDGEMENT

I thank Dr. S. Cadden for advice in the preparation of the manuscript and Miss M. Cayla for secretarial help.

REFERENCES

BESSON, J. M., CATCHLOVE, R. F.H., FELTZ, P. AND LE BARS, D. (1974). Further evidence for postsynaptic inhibitions on lamina V dorsal horn interneurons. *Brain Res.*, **66**, 531-536.

BESSON, J. M. AND CHAOUCH, A. (1987). Peripheral and spinal mechanisms of nociception. *Physiological Reviews*, **67**, 67-186.

BING, Z., VILLANUEVA, L. AND LE BARS, D. (1989) Effects of systemic morphine upon A-δ and C-fibre evoked activities of subnucleus reticularis dorsalis (SRD) neurones in the rat medulla. *Eur. J. Pharmacol.* (in press).

BOUHASSIRA, D., LE BARS, D. AND VILLANUEVA, L.(1987). Heterotopic activation of A-δ and C fibres triggers inhibition of trigeminal and spinal convergent neurones in the rat. *J. Physiol.*, **389**, 301-317.

CADDEN, S. W. (1985). The digastric reflex evoked by tooth-pulp stimulation in the cat and its modulation by stimuli applied to the limbs. *Brain Res.* **336**, 33-44.

CADDEN, S. W., VILLANUEVA, L., CHITOUR, D. AND LE BARS, D. (1983). Depression of activities of dorsal horn convergent neurones by propriospinal mechanisms triggered by noxious inputs: comparison with diffuse noxious inhibitory controls (DNIC). *Brain Res.*, **275**, 1-11.

CLARKE, R. W. (1985). The effects on the jaw-opening reflex evoked by tooth pulp stimulation of surgical trauma, decerebration and destruction of the nucleus raphe magnus, periaqueductal grey matter and brainstem reticular formation in the cat. *Brain Res.* **332**, 231-236.

CLARKE, R. W. AND MATTHEWS, B. (1985). The effects of anaesthetics and remote noxious stimulation on the jaw-opening reflex evoked by tooth-pulp stimulation in the cat. *Brain Res.*, **327**, 105-111.

DUBNER, R., HOFFMAN, D. S. AND HAYES, R. L. (1981). Neuronal activity in medullary dorsal horn of awake monkeys trained in a thermal discrimination task. III. Task-related responses and their functional role. *J. Neurophysiol.*, **46**, 444-464.

FIELDS, H. L. AND BESSON, J. M. (1988). Eds. Pain modulation. *Progress in Brain Research*, vol. **77**, Elsevier.

FITZGERALD, M. (1982). The contralateral input to the dorsal horn of the spinal cord in the decerebrate spinal rat. *Brain Res.*, **236**, 257-287.

GERHART, K. D., YEZIERSKI, R. P., GIESLER, G. J. Jr. AND WILLIS, W. D. (1981). Inhibitory receptive fields of primate spinothalamic tract cells. *J. Neurophysiol.*, **46**, 1309-1325.

HILLMAN, P. AND WALL, P. D. (1969). Inhibitory and excitatory factors influencing the receptive fields of lamina 5 spinal cells. *Exp. Brain Res.*, **9**, 284-306.

LE BARS, D. AND CHITOUR, D. (1983). Do convergent neurones in the spinal dorsal horn discriminate nociceptive from non-nociceptive information? *Pain*, **17**, 1-19.

LE BARS, D., DICKENSON, A. H. AND BESSON, J. M. (1979a). Diffuse noxious inhibitory controls (DNIC). Effects on dorsal horn convergent neurones in the rat. *Pain*, **6**, 283-304.

LE BARS, D., DICKENSON, A. H. AND BESSON, J. M. (1979b). Diffuse noxious inhibitory controls (DNIC). Lack of effect on non-convergent neurones, supraspinal involvement and theoretical implications. *Pain*, **6**, 305-327.

LE BARS, D., DICKENSON, A. H., BESSON, J. M. AND VILLANUEVA, L. (1986). Aspects of sensory processing through convergent neurons. In T. L. Yaksh (ed.), *Spinal afferent processing*, Plenum, pp. 467-504.

LE BARS, D. AND VILLANUEVA, L. (1988). Electrophysiological evidence for the activation of descending inhibitory controls by nociceptive afferent pathways. In H. L. Fields and J. M. Besson (eds.); *Pain modulation Progress in Brain Research*, vol. **77**, pp. 275-299.

MATTHEWS, B. (1985). Peripheral and central aspects of trigeminal nociceptive systems. *Phil. Trans. Royal Soc. B*, **308**, 313-324.

MENDELL, L. M. (1984). Modifiability of spinal synapses (1984). *Physiological Reviews*, **64**, 260-324.

MORTON, C. R., MAISCH, B. AND ZIMMERMAN, M. (1987). Diffuse noxious inhibitory controls of lumbar spinal neurons involve a supraspinal loop in the cat. *Brain Res.*, **410**, 347-352.

PRICE, D. D., HULL, C. D. AND BUCHWALD, N. A. (1971). Intracellular responses of dorsal horn cells to cutaneous and sural nerve A and C fiber stimuli. *Exp. Neurol.*, **33**, 291-309.

SAADE, N., JABBUR, S. J. AND WALL, P. D. (1985). Effects of 4-aminopyridine, GABA and bicuculline on cutaneous receptive fields of cat dorsal horn neurons. *Brain Res.*, **344**, 356-359.

SEMBA, K., GELLER, H. M. AND EGGER, M. D. (1985). 4-aminopyridine induces expansion of cutaneous receptive fields of dorsal horn cells. *Brain Res.*, **343**, 398-402.

SORKIN, L. S., MORROW, T. J. AND CASEY, K. L. (1988). Physiological identification of afferent fibers and postsynaptic sensory neurons in the spinal cord of the intact, awake cat. *Exp. Neurol.*, **99**, 412-427.

VILLANUEVA, L., BOUHASSIRA, D., BING, Z. AND LE BARS, D. (1988). Convergence of heterotopic nociceptive information onto subnucleus reticularis dorsalis neurons in the rat medulla. *J. Neurophysiol.*, **60**, 980-1009.

WAGMAN, I. H. AND PRICE, D. D. (1969). Responses of dorsal horn cells of M. mulatta to cutaneous and sural nerve A and C fiber stimuli. *J. Neurophysiol.*, **32**, 803-817.

YOKOTA, T. AND NISHIKAWA, N. (1982). Effects of picrotoxin upon response characteristics of wide dynamic range neurons in the spinal cord of cat and monkey. *Neurosci. Lett.*, **28**, 259-263.

ZIEGLGANSBERGER, W. AND HERZ, A. (1971). Changes of cutaneous receptive fields of spino-cervical-tract neurones and other dorsal horn neurones by microelectrophoretically administered amino acids. *Exp. Brain Res.*, **13**, 111-126.

SECTION III

SPINAL AND SUPRASPINAL OUTPUTS FROM THE SUPERFICIAL DORSAL HORN

INTRODUCTION TO SECTION III

The Editors

That the axons of lamina I cells travel towards the brain has been known since Kuru detected their retrograde chromatolytic response following cordotomy. However, it was not until the introduction of modern anatomical methods that the problem of the superficial dorsal horn's connections with the brain could be addressed with precision. We now know that lamina I cells innervate a very large number of targets in the medulla, pons, thalamus (including distinct targets in lateral, medial, and caudal nuclei), hypothalamus, and several regions of the telencephalon. The papers in this section review the progress that has been made in mapping the brain regions that are innervated by superficial dorsal horn cells and present exciting new observations on the development, morphology, and neurochemistry of lamina I cells.

CHARACTERIZATION OF LONG ASCENDING TRACT PROJECTION NEURONS AND NON-TRACT NEURONS IN THE SUPERFICIAL DORSAL HORN (SDH)

John A. Beal, Kailas N. Nandi and David S. Knight

Department of Anatomy, Louisiana State University Medical Center, Shreveport
LA 71130, U.S.A

INTRODUCTION

Using the Golgi technique, Ramón y Cajal (1909) showed that the marginal and substantia gelatinosal (SG) layers of the dorsal horn, now collectively known as the superficial dorsal horn (SDH), contained at least four distinct neuronal cell types; these were the *marginale* of the marginal zone and the *transverseux, limitrophe,* and *centrale* cells of the SG. Several investigators in subsequent Golgi studies have described the morphology of a variety of additional types of cells in the SDH (Pearson, 1952; Scheibel and Scheibel, 1968; Matsushita, 1969; Gobel, 1975, 1978a,b, Sugiura, 1975; Mannen and Sugiura, 1976; Beal and Cooper, 1978; Beal, 1979, 1983; Price *et al*, 1979; Bicknell and Beal, 1981a,b, 1984; Schoenen, 1982; Abdel-Maguid and Bowsher, 1984, 1985; Beal and Bicknell, 1984; Bowsher and Abdel-Maguid, 1984; and Lima and Coimbra, 1986). These studies had been performed on a variety of different species at different levels of the neuraxis and there was considerable disagreement between investigators on the various cell types present and on the terminology used. Also, although it is known that the SDH is comprised of both projection and non-projection neurons, these two groups have never been completely distinguished from one another on a morphological basis.

In light of these incongruities and gaps in our knowledge, recent studies in our laboratory, using the rat spinal cord, have been aimed at devising a general unifying system for distinguishing and classifying SDH neurons based on their projection, morphology and pattern of development. Using the Golgi technique and retrograde neuronal tract tracing techniques, alone, and in combination with tritiated thymidine autoradiography, we have traced the development of different groups of SDH neurons from their period of proliferation through their axonal and dendritic maturation, to their final adult form.

PROLIFERATION

Examination of the development of SDH neurons in the rat began with an analysis of neurogenesis and a determination of neuronal birthdates. In order to distinguish neurons which gave rise to long ascending projections (tract neurons) from those which did not (non-tract neurons), experiments were devised which combined tritiated thymidine autoradiography with Fluoro-Gold (FG) and horseradish peroxidase (HRP) tract tracing techniques. In these experiments pregnant rats were injected with tritiated thymidine (5.0μCi/g body wt., specific activity 6.7 Ci/mmole) on one of embryonic (E) days E13 through E16 when SDH neurons were known to proliferate (Nornes and Das, 1974; Altman and Bayer, 1984; Pendergrast and Beal, 1986). Pups were delivered and allowed to survive until postnatal (P) day P30, then a hemisection was performed on twelve animals at cervical spinal cord segment C3. At the lesion site, 4% Fluoro-Gold (Schmued and Fallon, 1986) or 30% HRP (Sigma Type VI) in phosphate buffered saline was administered topically via a gelfoam pledget which was inserted between the severed ends of the cord. After surgery, FG animals were maintained for ten to fourteen days and were then perfused with 4.0% paraformaldehyde and 0.5% glutaraldehyde in phosphate buffer. Tissue was embedded in paraffin, sectioned at 10 to 15 μm in transverse and sagittal planes, then processed for autoradiography and examined under the fluorescence microscope. For HRP, animals were maintained for 2 to 4 days and then perfused with 1.25% glutaraldehyde and 1.0% paraformaldehyde in 0.1M phosphate buffer at pH 7.4. Tissue was sectioned with a vibratome at 30-40 μm in transverse and sagittal planes, processed for TMB histochemistry according to the method of Mesulam (1978), stabilized with 1.0% osmium tetroxide (Nandi et. al., 1988), then processed for ^{3}H thymidine autoradiography.

In both FG and HRP experiments, double labelled cells, i.e., FG or HRP with tritiated thymidine, were observed only on days E13 and E14, with the largest of these (cell body cross sectional areas greater than 120 μm^2) completing cell division on day E13. These results demonstrated that long tract neurons, *i.e.* those which have axons

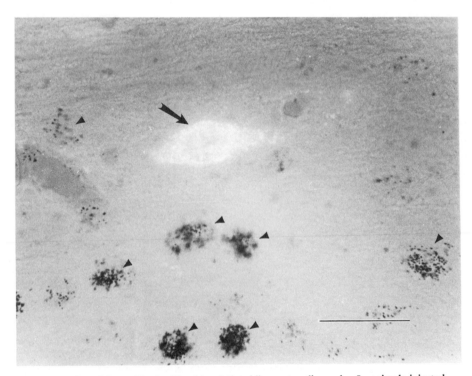

FIGURE 1: FG combined with tritiated thymidine autoradiography. In animals injected with tritiated thymidine on day E15 marginal tract neurons were retrogradely labelled with FG but not tritiated thymidine (arrow). Non-tract neurons were labelled with tritiated thymidine but not FG (arrowheads). Sagittal Section; Scale Bar = 25 μm.

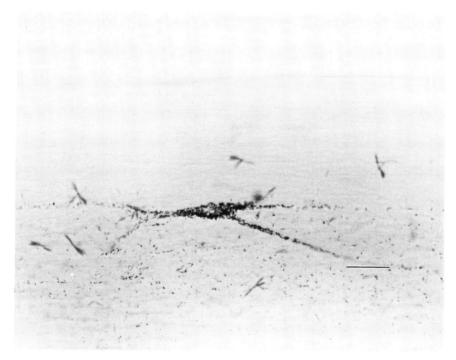

FIGURE 2: Pyramidal shaped marginal tract neuron retrogradely labelled with HRP, demonstrates morphology of cell body and proximal dendritic arbor. Cell displays longitudinal and ventral dendrites. Sagittal section. Scale Bar = 25 μm.

projecting to the upper cervical spinal cord or to more rostral structures, had birthdates prior to day E15. At the same time it showed that all neurons which had birthdates after day E14 were non-tract neurons (Fig. 1).

For the optimal demonstration of retrograde tracers, ten additional animals were labelled with FG or HRP alone and were not processed for autoradiography. In this group, cell body counts of 425 long tract SDH neurons labelled with either FG or HRP, revealed that approximately 90% of the cells were located in the marginal layer, *i.e.* Rexed's (1952) lamina I, and 10% were located in the SG layer, or Rexed's (1952) lamina II.

Since the proximal dendritic tree as well as the cell bodies of these long tract neurons were stained in the FG and HRP retrograde tracing experiments, some of their structural features were also revealed (Fig. 2). Viewed in sagittal sections, the morphology of the cell bodies of FG or HRP stained long tract neurons varied. Cells were large (diameters greater than 25 μm), medium (diameters between 15 and 25 μm), or small (diameters less than 15 μm) and pyramidal, multipolar or fusiform in shape. In the marginal layer, pyramidal or multipolar shaped neurons often exhibited interstitial dendrites which entered the overlying white matter, and/or ventral dendrites which descended into deeper laminae. Fusiform shaped neurons in lamina I gave rise to two or more relatively thick dendrites which ran longitudinally within lamina I parallel to the long axis of the spinal cord. In lamina II, long tract neurons were found, as previously shown by Giesler *et al* (1978) and Willis *et al* (1978), in both the outer (IIo) and inner (IIi) zones of Rexed (1952). Most long tract neurons in lamina II were pyramidal or multipolar in shape. Those in lamina IIo usually exhibited at least one

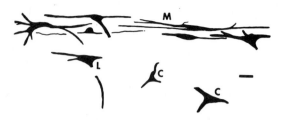

FIGURE 3: Drawings of SDH tract neurons retrogradely labelled with FG or HRP. Marginal (M) neurons of various shapes and sizes are shown. Dendrites ramify in marginal layer, overlying white matter, and ventrally in deeper laminae. Limiting (L) and small (left) and large (right) central (C) cells of the SG are also demonstrated. Taken from sagittal sections. Scale bar = 25 µm.

thick ventral dendrite and some had dendrites which arborized in lamina I. Long tract neurons in lamina IIi were vertically oriented and multipolar or pyramidal in shape (Fig. 3).

MATURATION

The structural maturation of SDH neurons was analyzed using modified Golgi (Adams, 1979) and rapid Golgi (Valverde, 1970) techniques. Tissue was sectioned at 100 to 200 µm in sagittal and transverse planes and drawings of SDH neurons were made with the aid of a light microscope with 100x objective and drawing tube attachment. Over 700 well impregnated SDH neurons were observed and characterized at short interval sequential stages between days E15 and P30. Results showed that cells with the morphological characteristics of long tract neurons underwent axonal and dendritic maturation prior to other types of SDH neurons.

I. Tract Neurons

On day E15 few neurons were impregnated and they were all in very early stages of development. These early neurons exhibited a fine calibre axon and a few stubby primordial dendritic processes. By day E17 the numbers of impregnated neurons had increased and maturation was more advanced. Cell bodies were pyramidal, multipolar, or fusiform in shape. Many had axons which could be traced into the overlying dorsal white matter, the dorsolateral funiculus, or into ventral regions of the gray matter, presumably enroute to ipsi- or contralateral ventrolateral regions of the white matter.

These early neurons gave rise to sparsely branched dendritic arbors which appeared to grow through a simple pattern of elongation which involved the formation of irregularly shaped expansions or growth cones at the growing tips of their dendrites. By day E19, these neurons exhibited distinctive dendritic arbors and displayed many of the characteristics of the tract neurons identified in the HRP and FG tract tracing studies. Many of these early maturing neurons demonstrated the morphological characteristics of the *marginale* cells of the marginal layer and the limiting (*limitrophe*) and central (*centrale*) cells of the SG layer as originally described by Ramón y Cajal (1909). Although some of these neurons acquired spines and other dendritic specializations during the postnatal period, the cell body shape and the basic dendritic pattern was essentially established in the prenatal period. The maturation of these putative tract neurons was followed throughout the postnatal period.

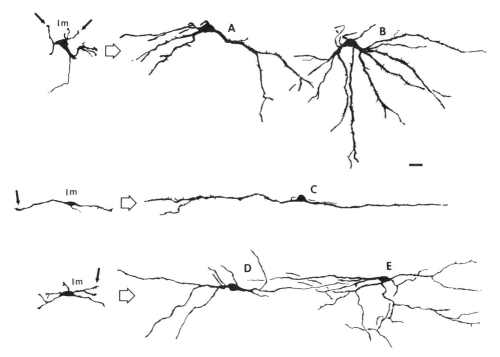

FIGURE 4: Tract neurons in marginal layer undergo dendritic maturation during prenatal period. Immature (Im) neurons (left) display terminal dendritic growth cones (small arrows) and give rise to pyramidal (A and B), fusiform (C) and multipolar (D and E) neurons. Pyramidal and multipolar neurons display dorsal interstitial dendrites and ventral dendrites. Most pyramidal neurons have spiny dendritic arbors while most multipolar neurons display relatively few spines. Drawn from sagittal sections. Scale bar = 25 μm.

A. Marginal Neurons

Marginal (*Marginale*) cells were described by Ramón y Cajal (1909) as long axon cells which were located along the external surface of the SG. Several types of putative tract neurons were observed in the marginal layer of the rat lumbosacral spinal cord. These neurons were similar to those which had been previously described in the spinal nucleus caudalis of the cat (Gobel, 1978a), the lumbosacral spinal cord of the monkey (Groups I, II, and III of Beal *et al*, 1981), and the cervical spinal cord of the rat (Groups II, III and IV of Lima and Coimbra, 1986). These groups included pyramidal, multipolar, and fusiform shaped neurons. Many of these neurons matched the morphology of lamina I neurons which had been shown to project to the midbrain and thalamus as demonstrated via antidromic stimulation and intracellular injection of HRP (Light *et al*, 1981; Hylden *et al*, 1985, 1986).

In the rat we found that a large percentage of these neurons were large to medium but some multipolar and fusiform neurons were in the small size range. Most neurons gave rise to long, sparsely branched dendritic arbors which by day P30 extended longitudinally within the marginal layer and lamina IIo for up to 800 μm . A large number of pyramidal and multipolar neurons also had interstitial and/or ventral dendrites. On some neurons the ventral dendritic arbor was substantial and penetrated as deep as lamina V. Some cells displayed a variety of spines including sessile and some branched and long-necked pedunculated types. In general, spines were distributed along most of the dendritic tree but the density varied from cell to cell; some had numerous spines, others were aspiny. In general, fusiform and multipolar neurons exhibited fewer spines than pyramidal-shaped neurons (Fig. 4).

The axons of putative tract marginal neurons could not be followed in the postnatal period. However, a few neurons exhibited one or two collaterals which ramified in lamina I and, in one instance, a collateral was traced into the deep dorsal horn laminae.

B. SG Neurons

Limiting Cells were described by Ramón y Cajal (1909) as long axon neurons in the external part of the SG. All putative tract neurons described here in the rat in lamina IIo were classified under this general heading. These neurons were medium sized pyramidal to multipolar shaped cells. In most cases these neurons gave rise to a T-shaped dendritic arbor with long rostral and caudal dendrites and one or two large dendritic trunks which fanned out ventrally into laminae II and III. The ventral dendrites gave rise to a variety of different types of spines which were scattered over the mid to distal dendritic tree. The axon most often took origin from the cell body and extended either ventrally through the gray matter or dorsally into the overlying white matter. In the former case, some of the axons gave off collaterals to deep dorsal horn laminae, while in the latter case, some axons gave off collaterals to lamina I.

Those cells with collaterals in lamina I were structurally similar to neurons previously described as stalk cells in the SG (Gobel, 1978b). However, stalk cells have been considered to be non-tract neurons. As will be described later, we found that non-tract neurons with the morphological characteristics of stalk cells had relatively small dendritic arbors. The T-shaped neurons of the present study, on the other hand, had a relatively large dendritic arbor and gave rise to a long ascending axon. For these reasons this cell more closely resembled Ramón y Cajal's (1909) description of the long axon *limiting* cell. Interestingly, a long tract neuron which had been antidromically stimulated and intracellularly injected with HRP was also previously described as having the morphology and position of a lamina II stalk cell; this cell also had a relatively large rostro-caudal (1000 μm) and dorso-ventral (400 μm) dendritic field (Hylden *et al*, 1986).

Central cells were described by Ramón y Cajal (1909) as long axon neurons in the internal portion of the SG. All putative tract neurons described here in lamina IIi were classified under this heading. In the rat, central cells varied considerably in size and shape. The most commonly observed type was a small to medium sized central cell. These neurons were fusiform to multipolar in shape, usually vertically oriented, and gave rise to both a sparsely branched dorsal dendritic arbor which fanned out into laminae I and IIo and a ventral dendritic arbor which extended into lamina III. Dendrites displayed only a few scattered spines.

Large central cells were more rare. These neurons were usually pyramidal in shape and were located in lamina IIi near the lamina III border. These neurons also were vertically oriented and gave rise, from the apex of the pyramid, to a single vertical dendritic trunk that divided into several branches which spread out into the marginal layer. Ventrally these neurons gave rise to two or more large dendritic trunks which spread out obliquely and ventrally and ramified in deeper dorsal horn laminae (Fig. 5).

Transverseux cells, a third group of SG neurons, were originally described by Ramón y Cajal (1909) as fusiform shaped cells with long transverse dendrites which ran medially and laterally across the outer portion of the SG (lamina IIo). We did not find these neurons in the SG layer; however, neurons with this structural pattern were

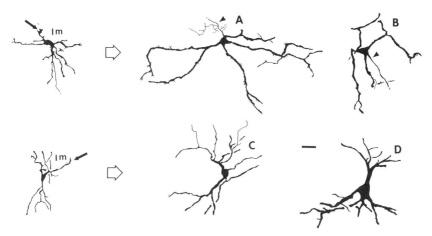

FIGURE 5: Tract neurons in SG layer, like those in marginal layer undergo dendritic maturation during prenatal period. Immature (Im) neurons (left) display dendritic growth cones (small arrows) and give rise to limiting cells (A and B) in lamina IIo and small (C) and large (D) central cells in lamina IIi. Limiting cell A displays dorsal axon (arrowhead) with collaterals in marginal layer while limiting cell B demonstrates ventral axon (arrowhead). Drawn from sagittal sections. Scale bar = 25 μm.

observed in the inner region of the marginal layer near the outer zone of the SG. These neurons were also stained in the FG and HRP experiments which labelled tract neurons.

II. Non Tract Neurons

The remaining neurons of the SDH, the non-tract neurons, underwent dendritic maturation during the postnatal period. Since all neurons did not mature at the same time or rate, it was difficult to pinpoint the exact time when the maturation of a given cell type was initiated. However, as a group, the non-tract neurons in the marginal layer initiated and completed maturation earlier than those in the SG layer.

A. Marginal Neurons

Most marginal neurons had well-formed dendritic arbors by day P10, whereas many SG neurons were still in very early stages of maturation at this time. Putative non-tract neurons were first clearly identified at the time of birth. Most of these *early* non-tract neurons were in the marginal layer and gave rise to several slender delicate dendritic processes which either arborized in the marginal layer or were directed ventrally into the SG layer. Growth cones were not observed on the dendrites of these neurons. Most of these neurons demonstrated axons with local beaded collaterals.

These neurons could be followed throughout the postnatal period and could be grouped into several cell types. Many of these were previously described, in part, in Golgi studies of the lumbosacral spinal cord of the monkey; these were the Type IV neurons of Beal *et al*, (1981). These neurons were also described, in great detail, in the rat cervical spinal cord; these were the neurons in Groups I and IIA of Lima and Coimbra (1986).

In the rat lumbosacral spinal cord, marginal neurons in this group were found to be fusiform to multipolar in shape and could be divided into three types. Using the terminology proposed by Lima and Coimbra (1986) these would be longitudinal fusiform neurons (Type IA), fusiform (Type IB) and multipolar (Type IIA) neurons with ventral dendritic arbors.

187

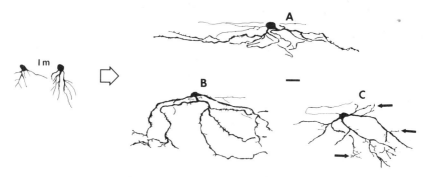

FIGURE 6: Non-tract neurons in marginal layer undergo maturation during early postnatal period. Small fusiform neurons with longitudinal dendrites (A) and fusiform to multipolar (B and C) neurons with ventral dendrites are derived from small immature (Im) stem cells with smooth, slender dendritic processes. Cells A and B, exhibit spiny dendritic arbors while cell C displays many axon-like processes (small arrows). Drawn from sagittal sections. Scale bar = 25 μm.

Longitudinal fusiform neurons formed a longitudinal dendritic field up to 400 μm long that distributed within the marginal layer (Fig. 6A). Dendrites were characterized by regularly arranged short necked spines with prominent round heads. Spines were found on all but the larger proximal dendrites. Axons of these neurons originated from the cell body and divided into several beaded collaterals which distributed within lamina I. Some of these neurons had asymmetrical dendritic arbors, *i.e.* dendrites emanated from only one pole of the cell.

Fusiform and multipolar neurons with ventral dendrites gave rise to fan shaped dendritic arbors which extended ventrally into lamina IIo and IIi, much like that of a lamina II stalk cell (Gobel, 1975, 1978b). These arbors formed a dendritic field approximately 250 μm in the longitudinal plane by 150 μm in the vertical plane. Some of these neurons were characterized by short necked pedunculated spines along the mid to distal dendritic tree and by an axon which distributed beaded collaterals to both laminae I and II. Other neurons in this group displayed a wider variety of dendritic appendages, including sessile and pedunculated spines as well as axon-like processes. Axons of these neurons were found to distribute very fine beaded collaterals to the marginal layer. Some of these neurons also had asymmetrical dendritic arbors (Fig. 6B and C).

B. SG Neurons

Non-tract neurons in the SG layer had a protracted period of maturation. These neurons developed fine axons with intrinsic beaded collaterals similar to those of non-tract marginal neurons. However, the dendritic development of most SG neurons was different from that of the marginal neurons. Immature SG neurons sprouted numerous short beaded dendrites which spread in all directions in a radial or star-like fashion. This pattern of development was first described in the SG of nucleus caudalis in the cat (Falls and Gobel, 1979) and was later described in the SG layer of developing rat spinal cord (Bicknell and Beal, 1984; Beal and Bicknell, 1984). Judging from what appear to be transitional forms in the spinal cord of the rat, star shaped stem cells in the SG underwent a dendritic metamorphosis. This metamorphosis probably involved the lengthening of some beaded processes and the migration of others along the dendritic

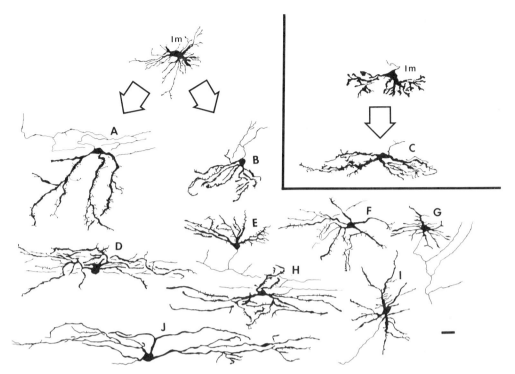

FIGURE 7: Non-tract neurons in SG layer undergo dendritic maturation during postnatal period. Most SG neurons including Type I(A) and II(B) stalk cells, inverted stalk cells (E) arboreal cells (F), star-shaped cells (G), spiny neurons (H), short (D) and long (J) islet cells, and vertical cells (I) are derived from immature (Im) star-shaped stem cells (top left) with numerous beaded dendrites. Insert (upper right) shows an exception to this rule. Type III stalk cell (C) is derived from immature stem cell (Im) with dendrites with large irregular shaped evaginations. Drawn from sagittal sections. Scale bar = 25 μm.

tree (Beal and Bicknell, 1984). The first examples of these neurons were seen at birth. The number of star shaped cells and transitional cell types increased dramatically from birth to day P10 then gradually decreased in number until only a few could be found on day P30.

An analysis of the structure of mature and transitional states of the various types of SDH neurons, as well as the time of their appearance, indicated that most SG interneurons appeared to go through star-shaped transitional stages and then developed into several types of non-tract neurons including stalk, inverted stalk, islet, spiny, arboreal, vertical and adult star-shaped cells (Fig. 7). Of these, stalk and islet cells were the most abundant.

Stalk cells were first described by Gobel (1975) in the spinal nucleus caudalis of the cat and were later depicted in spinal cord of adult monkey (Beal and Cooper, 1978; Price *et al*, 1979) and cat (Bicknell and Beal, 1981). As originally described these neurons were characterized by a fan shaped dendritic arbor which spread both ventrally and longitudinally, *stalk-like* dendritic appendages, and an axon which ramified locally in the overlying marginal layer (Gobel, 1975, 1978b). In the rat, we found three types of neurons which fit the stalk cell category. These cells were characterized by ventral dendritic arbors of different lengths.

Type I stalk cells had a dendritic arbor which extended into lamina III (Fig. 7A).

These neurons matched the morphology of stalk cells which had been iontophoretically filled with HRP and physiologically characterized as *wide dynamic range* neurons in the cat spinal cord (Bennett *et al* 1979, 1980). In the rat, the dendritic arbor of these neurons extended longitudinally for approximately 200 μm and ventrally for approximately 130 μm. The dendrites were characterized by regularly arranged long, medium, and short-necked spines with prominent round heads. The axons of these neurons originated from the cell body or proximal dendritic tree and extended dorsally into the marginal layer where they divided into several longitudinal beaded collaterals with recurrent branches.

Type II stalk cells were small round to fusiform shaped cells (Fig. 7B). They were similar to type I neurons except that these cells had a smaller dendritic arbor which remained within the SG layer. The dendritic field extended longitudinally for approximately 150 μm and ventrally for approximately 75 μm. Dendrites of these cells were characterized by numerous sessile and pedunculated spines and fewer long stalk processes than type I stalk cells. Although predominantly found in lamina IIo, these cells were occasionally found in the marginal layer.

Type III stalk cells were small multipolar shaped cells which had dendritic arbors confined to lamina IIo (Fig. 7C). All of the cells that we observed in this category were found in the lateral half of the SG layer. In correlation with this finding it should be pointed out that type III stalk cells were relatively small and mean cell body areas had been shown to be significantly smaller in the lateral half of the SG layer as compared with neurons in the medial half (Pendergrast and Beal, 1986).

Type III stalk cells gave rise to three or four dendritic trunks which either extended longitudinally or arched ventrally for a short distance then curved rostrocaudally to form a dendritic field which extended longitudinally for 175 to 200 μm and ventrally about 50 μm. The dendrites of type III stalk neurons had craggy irregular contours and often terminated abruptly by giving off one or two short, fine terminal processes. Some neurons in this group displayed asymmetrical dendritic arbors.

The dendritic maturation of type III stalk cells was unique. Analysis of transitional stages suggested that these neurons, unlike most SG interneurons, were not derived from beaded star-shaped transitional forms. Instead, early forms of the type III stalk cell appeared to give rise to large irregularly shaped dendritic evaginations which eventually formed thinner more well defined processes. In conjunction with this observation, it was interesting to note that at day P30 these neurons still had not completely matured as evidenced by the fact that most had few spines or dendritic appendages. It was only when these neurons were observed in older adult animals that the dendrites of these neurons were found to be covered with a variety of short and long necked spines or appendages. These neurons were amongst the last SG neurons to complete dendritic maturation. The axon of type III stalk neurons took origin from the cell body or proximal dendritic tree and distributed collaterals to both lamina I and lamina IIo. The boutons or terminals on these collaterals were relatively large and widely spaced.

Both type II and III stalk cells had dendritic arbors confined to lamina II. Stalk cells with this type of dendritic distribution have previously been filled with HRP and have been physiologically characterized as nociceptive specific neurons in both the cat (Bennett *et al* 1979, 1980; Gobel *et al*, 1980; Light *et al*, 1979, 1981; Light and Kavookjian, 1988) and monkey (Light and Kavookjian, 1988).

Inverted stalk cells in the rat were small round to fusiform-shaped cells located in lamina IIi (Fig. 7E). These neurons had a dendritic arbor that fanned out dorsally giving these cells the profile of a stalk cell which had been turned upside down or inverted. The size of the dendritic field and the dendritic architecture of these cells closely matched that of the type II stalk cell. It is interesting to note that the type II stalk cell and the inverted stalk cell often had dendritic arbors which were in register, *i.e.* the dendritic field of one exactly overlapped the dendritic field of the other as observed in the sagittal plane. The axons of these cells gave off beaded collaterals to both the SG and marginal layers.

Islet cells were first described in depth in Golgi studies in the nucleus caudalis of the cat (Gobel, 1975). Several variations of these neurons in the spinal cord of the cat were filled iontophoretically with HRP and physiologically characterized as nociceptive and non-nociceptive mechanoreceptive (Light *et al*, 1979; Bennett *et al*, 1980; Gobel *et al*, 1980; and as thermoreceptive (Light *et al*, 1979) neurons. Those located in lamina IIo were described as mainly nociceptive specific while those in lamina IIi had longer dendritic arbors and responded mainly to low threshold mechanoreceptors (Light *et al*, 1979; Bennett *et al*, 1980; Gobel *et al*, 1980).

In the rat spinal cord, islet cells were also present in both laminae IIo (Fig.7D) and IIi (Fig. 7J). These neurons were characterized by a narrow rostro-caudal dendritic arbor with recurrent branches and widely scattered dendritic appendages and axon-like processes. Axons of these neurons ramified for the most part in the vicinity of the dendritic tree. However, some neurons in the islet cell category, as also shown in the spinal cord of the cat (Light and Kavookjian, 1988), had collaterals which left the vicinity and entered deeper laminae of the dorsal horn. Cell bodies of islet cells were small to medium in size and the dendritic arbor varied considerably in length (250-700 μm). Some neurons with short dendritic spreads displayed asymmetric dendritic arbors. As also shown in the cat spinal cord (Bennett *et al*, 1980; Gobel *et al*, 1980), islet cells with the longest dendritic arbors were located in lamina IIi. Some of the earliest and some of the latest of the non-tract neurons to undergo dendritic maturation were in the islet cell category. It seems probable that the early islet cells ultimately developed the longest dendritic arbors, since several short islet cells were found to be amongst the last neurons to undergo dendritic maturation.

Spiny cells were found in lamina IIi in the rat spinal cord. Similar cells were found in the spinal nucleus caudalis of the cat (Gobel, 1978b) and in both the monkey (Beal and Cooper, 1978) and human spinal cord (Schoenen, 1982). This type of neuron was originally referred to as a *II-III border cell* by Gobel (1978b). At that time, the SG layer of nucleus caudalis was divided into layer II and III rather than into laminae IIo and IIi which is the standard convention today. Since the name *II-III border cell* is no longer appropriate, we have taken the liberty to shorten the name to *spiny* cell. The spiny cell in the rat had a small fusiform- to polygonal-shaped soma and a dendritic arbor which extended dorsally into lamina IIo and ventrally into lamina IIi (Fig. 7H). Though stellate in its distribution, the major portion of the dendritic arbor extended longitudinally within lamina II for approximately 350-400 μm . The mid to distal dendrites of these cells were covered with numerous sessile and short neck pedunculated spines. The axon usually emanated from a proximal dendrite and distributed some collaterals to the SG. As also observed in the cat (Gobel, 1978b), we found that these cells were relatively rare in the rat. Nonetheless, in the spinal cord of the cat a cell which typified the structure of the spiny cell was filled iontophoretically with HRP and shown physiologically to respond to innocuous tactile stimulation (Light, *et al*, 1979).

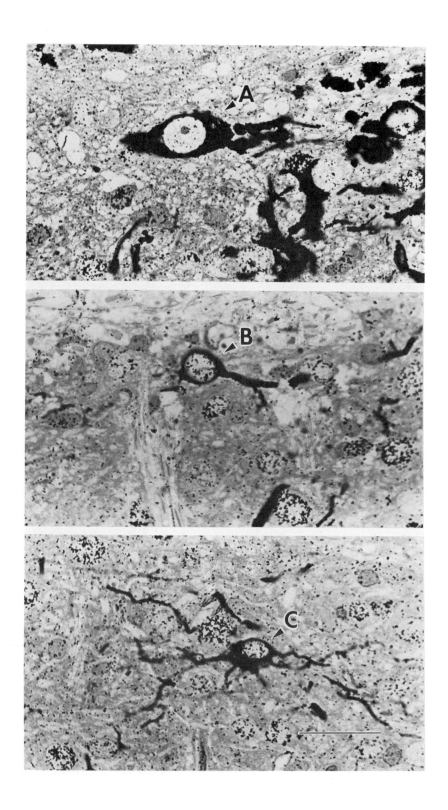

Arboreal cells were first identified by Gobel (1978b) in the SG layer of the cat nucleus caudalis and were so named *because of their tree-shaped dendritic expansions*. We also observed this type of cell in the rat spinal cord. The arboreal cell in the rat had a small round to polygonal-shaped cell body which was located in either the ventral portion of lamina IIo or the dorsal portion of lamina IIi (Fig. 7F). These neurons had four or more primary dendrites which radiated from the cell body in all directions to form a dendritic field approximately 200-250 μm in diameter. Dendrites extended dorsally into lamina IIo and ventrally into the dorsal portion of lamina III. The major portion of the dendritic arbor, however, arborized in lamina IIi. Dendrites gave rise to long and short stalk pedunculated spines, some of which had multiple heads.

Axons of these cells were very fine and usually took origin from a primary dendrite. The complete extent of the axon could not be followed but, like other SG interneurons, these cells gave rise to local collaterals both in the vicinity of their own dendritic tree and beyond. A cell resembling this type had been filled with HRP in the spinal cord of the cat and physiologically characterized as a multireceptive cell (Light and Kavookjian, 1988).

Vertical cells were first described by Bicknell and Beal (1984) in the lumbar spinal cord of the adult rat. These neurons were located in lamina IIi and were characterized by a short, narrow, vertically oriented dendritic arbor that extended dorsally into lamina IIo and ventrally into the dorsal portion of lamina III. Viewed in the sagittal plane, these neurons produced a narrow, sparsely branched dendritic field which was vertically oriented and 150 to 200 μm in length (Fig. 7I). The dendrites were characterized by the presence of both long and short stalked dendritic appendages. Axons of these neurons gave off collaterals which distributed well beyond the extent of the dendritic arbor but, for the most part, remained within lamina II.

Star-shaped cells were first described in the SG of the adult cat spinal cord (Bicknell and Beal, 1981). These cells were designated star-shaped cells because of the radial distribution of their dendritic tree. As in the cat, these neurons were found in both lamina IIo and IIi of the rat. In the sagittal plane, these cells gave rise to as many as 10 primary dendrites which radiated from the cell body in all directions (Fig 7G). The dendritic arbor was sparsely branched and had a characteristic scattered distribution of short stalk and sessile spines. Neurons located in the lateral half of the SG formed a small, roughly radial dendritic field approximately 150 μm in diameter, while neurons located in the medial portion of the SG formed a more longitudinally (200 μm) oriented dendritic arbor. The axon took origin from either the cell body or a dendrite and then extended ventrally into deeper areas of the gray matter. Fine collaterals with very small beads or terminals distributed to lamina III and to lamina II in the vicinity of the cells dendritic tree. The star-shaped appearance of these cells was reminiscent of the star-shaped configuration of immature, developing SG neurons; however, the dendrites of these neurons lacked the varicosities or beads which characterized the immature neurons.

FIGURE 8: Combined Golgi impregnation and tritiated thymidine autoradiographs. In animals injected with tritiated thymidine on day E15, nucleus of putative tract neuron of the marginal layer (A) is unlabelled, while nucleus of non-tract neurons (small spiny neuron (B) in lamina I and stalk cell (C) in lamina IIo) are labelled. Sagittal section. Scale bar = 25 μm.

C. Non-Tract Neuron Verification

In order to verify that the non-tract neurons described in this study were in fact neurons limited to intraspinal connections, we determined the time of origin of several neurons in this group. This was accomplished by using a combined Golgi-autoradiographic technique in which the uptake of tritiated thymidine was examined and measured in Golgi impregnated neurons (Beal *et al*, 1987). Pregnant rats were injected with tritiated thymidine (5.0 mCi/g body wgt., specific activity 6.7 Ci/m mole) on day E15 when only non-tract neurons, as we previously determined, were undergoing neurogenesis. Pups of the dams were delivered and later sacrificed on day P30. Tissue was processed via the Golgi technique of Adams (1979) and impregnated neurons were drawn with the aid of a microscope with drawing tube attachment. Sections were then remounted in JB-4 plastic, sectioned at 2.5 μm , stabilized according to the method of Hitchcock and Hickey (1983), and processed for autoradiography. Several impregnated SDH neurons from the presumptive non-tract group, including small spiny marginal neurons, stalk, islet, and vertical SG cells, were shown to contain radioactive label on day E15, thus verifying their non-tract status (Fig. 8). It must be cautioned however, that these results were limited and did not prove that all neurons with the morphology of the presumptive non-tract neurons demonstrated here were in fact non-tract neurons.

CONCLUSIONS

Results of these studies have provided a general assessment of the projection, morphology, and development of neurons in the SDH of the lumbar spinal cord of the rat. These results have shown that, in general, the same types of neurons described in the SDH of various other species and at other levels of the neuraxis were also present in the lumbar spinal cord of the rat. These neurons can be divided into several groups of morphologically distinct tract and non-tract neurons. Ninety percent of the tract neurons were located in the marginal layer. These included pyramidal, fusiform and multipolar shaped neurons of various sizes. Ten percent of the tract neurons were located in the SG layer. These included limiting cells in lamina IIo and at least two types of central cells in lamina IIi. Non-tract neurons in the marginal layer were divided into longitudinal fusiform neurons and fusiform and multipolar neurons with ventral dendrites. Non-tract neurons in the SG layer were divided into islet, stalk, inverted stalk, arboreal, spiny, vertical and star-shaped cells. On the basis of structure, non-tract neurons, when compared with tract neurons, in most cases, lacked interstitial dendrites, exhibited more intrinsic collaterals, displayed more long stalked appendages and axon-like processes and had smaller dendritic fields.

The development of tract and non-tract neurons was different both structurally and temporally. Tract neurons proliferated prior to day E15 and underwent axonal and dendritic maturation prior to birth. Dendrites developed through a relatively simple mode of dendritic branching and elongation which involved terminal growth cones. Non-tract neurons of the marginal and SG layers proliferated through day E16 and underwent maturation in the postnatal period. Most non-tract neurons in the marginal layer matured early in the postnatal period and dendrites developed as very fine delicate processes which eventually elongated and branched. The maturation period in the SG layer was protracted and most neurons followed a complex pattern of dendritic maturation which involved the formation of numerous beaded dendrites which gradually underwent a reorganization along adult patterns. In general, those cells with the shortest dendritic spread, e.g., type III stalk cells, short islet cells, and vertical cells, were amongst the last neurons to undergo maturation.

ACKNOWLEDGEMENTS

The authors would like to thank Mrs. Wanda Green and Ms. Fala Walker for their excellent technical assistance and Mrs. Gloria Marshall for her many hours of word processing.

REFERENCES

ABDEL-MAGUID, T.E. AND BOWSHER, D. (1984). Classification of neurons by dendritic branching pattern. A categorization based on Golgi impregnation of spinal and cranial somatic afferent and efferent cells in the adult human. *Journal of Anatomy* **138**, 689-702.

ABDEL-MAGUID, T.E. AND BOWSHER, D. (1985). The gray matter of the dorsal horn of the adult human spinal cord, including comparisons with general somatic and visceral afferent cranial nerve nuclei, *Journal of Anatomy* **142**, 33-58.

ADAMS, J.C. (1979). A fast, reliable silver-chromate Golgi method for perfusing fixed tissue. *Stain Technology* **4**, 1947-1951

ALTMAN, J. AND BAYER, S.A. (1984). The development of the rat spinal cord. *Advances in Anatomy Embryology and Cell Biology* **85**, 1-166.

BEAL, J.A. (1979). The ventral dendritic arbor of marginal (lamina I) neurons in the adult primate spinal cord. *Neuroscience Letters* **14**, 201-206.

BEAL, J.A. AND COOPER, M.H. (1978). The neurons in the gelatinosal complex (laminae II and III) of the monkey (Macaca mulatta): A Golgi study. *Journal of Comparative Neurology* **179**, 89-122.

BEAL, J.A., PENNY, J.E. AND BICKNELL, H.R. (1981). Structural diversity of marginal (lamina I) neurons in the adult monkey (Macaca mulatta) lumbosacral spinal cord: A Golgi study. *Journal of Comparative Neurology* **202**, 237-254.

BEAL, J.A. (1983). Identification of presumptive long axon neurons in the substantia gelatinosa of the rat lumbosacral spinal cord: A Golgi study. *Neuroscience Letters* **41**, 9-14.

BEAL, J.A. AND BICKNELL, H.R. (1985). Development and maturation of neurons in the substantia gelatinosa (SG) of the rat spinal cord. In *Development, Organization and Processing in Somatosensory Pathways.*, Ed. W.G. Willis and M.J. Rowe, pp. 23-30. New York: Alan R. Liss, Inc.

BEAL, J.A., KNIGHT, D.S. AND NANDI, K.N. (1987). Determination of the sequence of proliferation of marginal (lamina I) neurons in the spinal cord of the rat. *Neuroscience Abstracts* **13**, 521.

BENNETT, G.J., ABDELMOUMENE, M., HAYASHI, H., AND DUBNER, R. (1980). Physiology and morphology of substantia gelatinosa neurons intracellularly stained with horseradish peroxidase, *Journal of Comparative Neurology* **194**, 809-827.

BENNETT, G.J., HAYASHI, H., ABDELMOUMENE, M., AND DUBNER, R. (1979). Physiological properties of stalked cells of the substantia gelatinosa intracellularly stained with horseradish peroxidase. *Brain Research* **164**, 285-289.

BICKNELL, H.R. AND BEAL, J.A. (1981a). Neurons with dual axons in the substantia gelatinosa (SG) of the adult cat lumbosacral spinal cord, *Experientia* **37**, 1198-1199.

BICKNELL, H.R. AND BEAL, J.A. (1981b). Star shaped neurons in the substantia gelatinosa of the adult spinal cord, *Neuroscience Letters* **22**, 37-41.

BICKNELL, H.R. AND BEAL, J.A. (1984). Axonal and dendritic development of substantia gelatinosa neurons in the lumbosacral spinal cord of the rat. *Journal of Comparative Neurology* **226**, 508-522.

BOWSHER, D. AND ABDEL-MAGUID, T.E. (1984). Superficial dorsal horn of the adult human spinal cord. *Neurosurgery* **15**, 893-899.

FALLS, W. AND GOBEL, S. (1979). Golgi and EM studies of the formation of dendritic and axonal arbors: the interneurons of the substantia gelatinosa of Rolando in newborn kitten. *Journal of Comparative Neurology* **198**, 1-18.

GIESLER, G.T., CANNON, J.T., URCA, G. AND LIEBESKIND, J.C. (1978). Long ascending projections from substantia gelatinosa Rolandi and the subjacent dorsal horn in the rat. *Science* **202**, 84-986.

GOBEL, S. (1975). Golgi studies of the substantia gelatinosa neurons in the spinal trigeminal nucleus. *Journal of Comparative Neurology* **162**, 397-415.

GOBEL, S. (1978a). Golgi Studies of the neurons in layer I of the dorsal horn of the medulla (trigeminal nucleus caudalis). *Journal of Comparative Neurology* **180**, 375-394.

GOBEL, S. (1978b). Golgi studies of the neurons in layer II of the dorsal horn of the medulla (trigeminal nucleus caudalis). *Journal of Comparative Neurology* **180**, 395-414.

GOBEL, S., FALLS, W.M., BENNETT, G.J., ABDELMOUMENE, M., HAYASHI, H. AND HUMPHREY, E. (1980). An EM analysis of the synaptic connections of horseradish peroxidase-filled stalked cells and islet cells in the substantia gelatinosa of adult cat spinal cord, *Journal of Comparative Neurology* **194**, 781-807.

HITCHCOCK, P.F. AND HICKEY, T.L. (1983). A method for combining Golgi impregnation procedures and light microscopic autoradiography. *Journal of Neuroscience Methods* **8**, 149-154.

HYLDEN, J.L.K., HAYASHI, H., BENNETT, G.J., AND DUBNER, R. (1985). Spinal lamina I neurons projecting to the parabrachial area of the cat midbrain. *Brain Research* **336**, 195-198.

HYLDEN, J.L.K., HAYASHI, H., DUBNER, R. AND BENNETT, G.J. (1986). Physiology and morphology of the lamina I spinomesencephalic projection. *Journal of Comparative Neurology* **247**, 505-515.

LIGHT, A.R. AND KAVOOKJIAN, A.M. (1988). Morphology and ultrastructure of physiologically identified substantia gelatinosa (lamina II) neurons with axons that terminate in deeper dorsal horn laminae (III-V). *Journal of Comparative Neurology* **267**, 172-189.

LIGHT, A.R., RETHELYI, M. AND PERL, E.R. (1981). Ultrastructure of functionally identified neurones in the marginal zone and the substantia gelatinosa. In *Spinal Cord Sensation: Sensory Processing in the Dorsal Horn*, ed. Brown, A.G. and Rethelyi, M., pp. 97-106. Edinburgh: Scottish Academic Press.

LIGHT, A.R., TREVINO, D.L. AND PERL, E.R. (1979). Morphological features of functionally defined neurons in the marginal zone and substantia gelatinosa of the spinal dorsal horn. *Journal of Comparative Neurology* **186**, 151-172.

LIMA, D. AND COIMBRA, A. (1986). A Golgi study of the neuronal population of the marginal zone (lamina I) of the rat spinal cord. *Journal of Comparative Neurology* **244**, 53-71.

MANNEN, H. AND SUGIURA, Y. (1976). Reconstruction of neurons of dorsal horn proper using Golgi-stained serial sections. *Journal of Comparative Neurology* **168**, 303-312.

MATSUSHITA, M. (1969). Some aspects of the interneuronal connections in cat's spinal gray matter. *Journal of Comparative Neurology* **136**, 57-80.

MESULAM, M.M. (1978). Tetramethylbenzidine for horseradish peroxidase neurohistochemistry. A non-carcinogenic blue reaction-product with superior sensitivity for visualizing neural afferents and efferents. *Journal of Histochemistry and Cytochemistry* **26**, 106-117.

NANDI, K.N., BEAL, J.A. AND KNIGHT, D.S. (1988). A simple method for combining autoradiography and HRP-TMB histochemistry on the same tissue section. *Journal of Neuroscience Methods*, In Press.

NORNES, H.O. AND DAS, G.D. (1974). Temporal pattern of neurogenesis in spinal cord of rat. I. An autoradiographic study - Time and sites of origin and migration and settling patterns of neuroblasts. *Brain Research* **73**, 121-138.

PEARSON, A.A. (1952). Role of gelatinous substance of spinal cord in conduction of pain. *Archives of Neurology and Psychiatry* **68**, 515-529.

PENDERGRAST, K.R. AND BEAL, J.A. (1986). An autoradiographic and Golgi analysis of the development of neurons in the superficial dorsal horn (SDH) of the rat. *Anatomical Record* **214**, 99A.

PRICE, D.D., HAYASHI, H., DUBNER, R. AND RUDA, M.A. (1979). Functional relationships between neurons of marginal and substantia gelatinosa layers of primate dorsal horn. *Journal of Neurophysiology* **42**, 1590-1608.

RAMÓN Y CAJAL, S. (1909). *Histologie du Systeme Nerveux de l'Homme et des Vertebres*, Vol. I. Madrid: Consejo Superior de Investigaciones Cientificas.

REXED, B. (1952). The cytoarchitectonic organization of the spinal cord in the cat. *Journal of Comparative Neurology* **96**, 415-495.

SCHEIBEL, M.E. AND SCHEIBEL, A.B. (1968) Terminal axonal patterns in cat spinal cord. II. The dorsal horn. *Brain Research* **9**, 32-58.

SCHMUED, L.C. AND FALLON, J.H. (1986). Fluoro-Gold: a new fluorescent retrograde axonal tracer with numerous unique properties. *Brain Research* **377**, 147-154.

SCHOENEN, J. (1982). The dendritic organization of the human spinal cord: The dorsal horn. *Neuroscience* **7**, 2057-2087.

SUGIURA, Y. (1975). Three dimensional analysis of neurons in the substantia gelatinosa Rolandi. *Proceedings of the Japan Academy* **5**, 336-341.

VALVERDE, F. (1970). The Golgi method. A tool for comparative structural analyses. In *Contemporary Research Methods in Neuroanatomy*, ed. Nauta, W.J.H. and Ebbesson, S.O.E., pp. 11-31. New York: Springer-Verlag.

WILLIS, W.D., LEONARD, R.B. AND KENSHALO, D.R. (1978). Spinothalamic tract neurons in the substantia gelatinosa. *Science* **202**, 986-988.

PROJECTIONS AND NEUROCHEMICAL SPECIFICITY OF THE DIFFERENT MORPHOLOGICAL TYPES OF MARGINAL CELLS

Antonio Coimbra and Deolinda Lima

Institute of Histology and Embryology of the Faculty of Medicine and Center of Experimental Morphology of the University of Oporto, Portugal

The importance attributed to lamina I, the marginal zone of Waldeyer, in the transmission of pain and thermal inputs along the somatosensory ascending pathway dates from the anatomo-clinical studies of Foerster and Gagel (1932) and Kuru (1949). A remarkable incidence of retrograde chromatolysis was then described in marginal cells from patients subject to ventrolateral cordotomies which caused contralateral thermal analgesia. The dermatomes affected corresponded to the spinal segments containing retrograde changes in lamina I (Kuru, 1949).

Modern experimental work has confirmed those conclusions. Primary afferent fibers have been identified physiologically as to the modality conveyed and have been filled with HRP: lamina I was the only dorsal horn layer receiving exclusively nociceptive afferents (Brown, 1981; Light and Perl, 1979; Perl, 1984; Sugiura et al, 1986). Although the outer part of the substantia gelatinosa (lamina IIo) shared most of these afferents, it also received some unmyelinated sensitive mechanoreceptors (Sugiura et al, 1986). Incidentally, lamina I has generally been considered the main output relay for the substantia gelatinosa which itself contains few spinofugal neurons (Bennett et al, 1979; Price et al, 1979). Electrophysiological recordings of the responses of spinal cord cells to peripheral stimulation revealed that laminae I and IIo were the only layers in the rat spinal cord containing only nociceptive-specific (NS) and wide-dynamic-range cells (WDR) (Menétrey et al, 1977; Woolf and Fitzgerald, 1983). Lamina I also appears to contain only these two classes in the primate (Ferrington et al, 1987), but in the cat some additional units responding to innocuous cold or deep input (joint and muscle) have been recorded (Craig and Kniffki, 1985).

Projections of lamina I to the thalamus and the mesencephalon have been demonstrated with retrograde labelling in the rat, cat and monkey (Willis, 1985). The role of this lamina as a relay nucleus specialized for nociceptive-thermal long distance transmission does not seem, however, to be entirely true. Antidromic activation from levels above certain spinal segments has disclosed a majority of segmental interneurons (67%) among lamina I cells in the cat (Cervero et al, 1979). Such short-circuit neurons might contain inhibitory transmitters or peptides (Ruda et al, 1986). In fact, after immunostaining lamina I cells with several specific antibodies against such agents in the rat, no accumulation of immunostaining occurred upon dorsal hemisections of the cord above the segments examined (Hunt et al, 1981).

It may be concluded that besides its most recognized function as a projection nucleus the marginal layer is also concerned with modulation of sensory input, a role traditionally ascribed to the substantia gelatinosa (Willis and Coggeshall, 1978; Cervero and Iggo, 1980).

MORPHOLOGY OF LAMINA I CELLS

In view of the diversity of functional types of lamina I cells, efforts have been made to find their morphological counterparts. From one hundred years ago until very recently, the Waldeyer cells observed in coronal sections of the spinal cord appeared to be the sole morphological type. Their characteristic spindle-shaped mediolaterally-extended somata with polar dendrites following the margin of the dorsal horn appeared in numerous descriptions of Golgi preparations (see Cervero and Iggo, 1980, for a review). However, Rexed (1952) using Nissl staining of thick frozen coronal sections, clearly distinguished small- and medium-sized round perikarya from the Waldeyer-like cells. Lately, those two basic morphologies and other cell shapes have been mentioned in retrograde labelling or immunostaining experiments (Table I).

TABLE I

Morphology of lamina I cells, retrogradely labelled or immunostained

Morphology	Staining
Waldeyer-type in coronal sections	HRP from thalamus[1]
	HRP from mesencephalon[2]
	Leu-Enkephalin[3]
	Substance P[4]
Small round cells in coronal sections	HRP from mesencephalon[2]
	GAD[5]
Cells with ventral dendrites (multipolar?) in coronal sections	GAD[5]
Elongated bipolar cells (fusiform?) in longitudinal sections	GAD[5]
Pyramidal cells in longitudinal sections	HRP from mesencephalon[6]
	HRPintracellular in mesenc.-projecting cells[7]
	Leu-Enkephalin[3]

[1]Giesler et al., 1979, [2]Menétrey et al., 1982, [3]Glazer and Basbaum, 1983, [4]Tessler et al., 1981, [5]Barber et al., 1982, [6]Swett et al., 1985, [7]Hylden et al., 1986.

The time seemed ripe for a thorough characterisation of marginal cell structural types, via a study which required cell examinations in the three standard anatomical planes in order to reach a three-dimensional view. This has been attempted with the aid of several Golgi methods in the cat trigeminal spinal nucleus (Gobel, 1978), as well as in the dorsal horn of the monkey (Beal et al, 1981) and the rat (Lima and Coimbra, 1986). This rat study was preceded by another of serial reconstructions of the perikarya and primary dendritic trunks of all cells occurring in semithin coronal epon sections of lamina I (Lima and Coimbra, 1983). Our classification included two types, the pyramidal and the multipolar, already described in the cat (Gobel, 1978), and we added two more types, the fusiform and the flattened neurons.

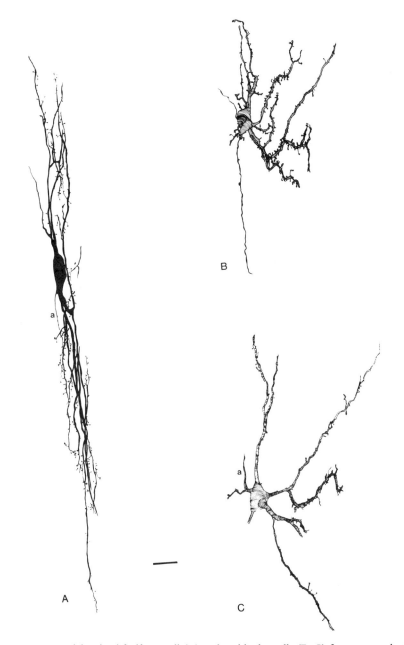

FIGURE 1: Golgi-stained fusiform cell (A) and multipolar cells (B, C) from parasagittal sections. The multipolar cell on top is of the variety with many dendritic branches, that below is a multipolar cell of the variety with a few long dendrites. a = axons. Scale bar = 20 μm.

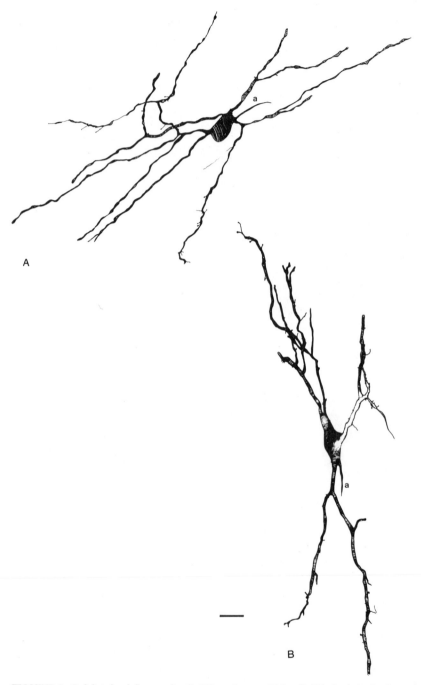

FIGURE 2: Golgi-stained flattened cell (A) and pyramidal cell (B), both in horizontal section. a = axons. Scale bar = 20 μm.

As observed with the Golgi-Rio Hortega method (Lima and Coimbra, 1986), the *fusiform* cells (39% of all marginal cells) had longitudinal spindle-shaped perikarya, bipolar rostrocaudally elongated dendritic trees rich in pedunculated spines and a thin beaded longitudinal axon. These bi-tufted neurons had a profile identical in horizontal and parasagittal views (Fig. 1A) and appeared as roundish small perikarya in coronal view. A subtype occurred with distal dendritic branches inclined ventrally and reaching lamina IIi. Fusiform neurons predominated in the lateral third of the marginal zone (Table II). In all planes the *multipolar* cells (23%) had cuboidal somata from which numerous dendritic trunks arose in all directions; the dorsal one gave rise to very spiny dendritic arbors whose branches were rather sinuous. There were two subtypes, subtype A with many primary dendrites but relatively short dendritic trees (Fig. 1B), and subtype B having fewer but longer dendrites (Fig. 1C) which might reach lamina III and a thick tapering axon (Fig. 1C) of the myelinated type (Condé and Condé, 1973). Multipolar cells were concentrated in the medial third of lamina I (Table II). *Flattened* neurons (13%) were mostly confined to the intermediate third of the mediolateral extent of lamina I (Table II). In horizontal sections, they presented roundish cell bodies from which several scarcely ramified and aspiny dendrites diverged (Fig. 2A). When seen in either sagittal or coronal view, somata were, however, flattened in the dorsoventral direction and the dendrites coursed parallel to the dorsal horn margin. *Pyramidal* neurons (25%) showed rostrocaudally-elongated triangular perikarya (Fig. 2B) in both longitudinal planes with the base always straddling the grey-white matter border. They were also triangular in coronal sections with the wider base facing ventrally. Moderately spiny dendrites arose from the cell angles and ramified mostly longitudinally but also sideways. Dendrites that issued from the angle protruding into the white matter coursed within the latter. Flattened and pyramidal cells reproduced the characteristic profile of the Waldeyer-cells of the old literature when seen in coronal view, and issued axons of the myelinated type.

Our subsequent purpose was to investigate both the projection targets of each structural type by means of retrograde labelling, and their neurochemical features using immunocytochemistry.

SUPRASPINAL TARGETS OF THE DIFFERENT CELL TYPES

Male rats, 270-320 g in weight, were injected with either 30% horseradish peroxidase in 2% DMSO or 1.5% cholera toxin subunit B (CTb) under stereotaxic control in (1) the left thalamus - ventroposterolateral (VPL) and ventroposteromedial (VPM) nuclei (Lima and Coimbra, 1988a); (2) the left half of the caudal mesencephalon - ventrolateral periaqueductal gray (PAG) and/or the cuneiform (Cnf) and the parabrachial nuclei (PBN) (Lima and Coimbra, 1988b); or (3) the left medullary reticular formation - gigantocellular nucleus (Gi) or dorsal reticular formation (DRt) (unpublished observations). To avoid the invasion of the cuneate nucleus by the tracer, some injections in the DRt were performed with the syringe slanted 29° laterally from the vertical plane. Following delays of 48 h for animals injected with free HRP or 72h for those which received CTb, intracardiac perfusions of, respectively, 1000 ml of 1.25% glutaraldehyde and 1% paraformaldehyde, or 500 ml of 4% paraformaldehyde, were performed. Frozen 50 μm sections were cut from HRP labelled material, and 75 μm thick vibratome sections from CTb material. Serial coronal, parasagittal and horizontal sections of segments C1-C8 and T13-L6 were studied after reacting HRP with DAB with metal intensification (Itoh *et al*, 1979), or detecting CTb with a mixture of two monoclonal antibodies followed by the PAP

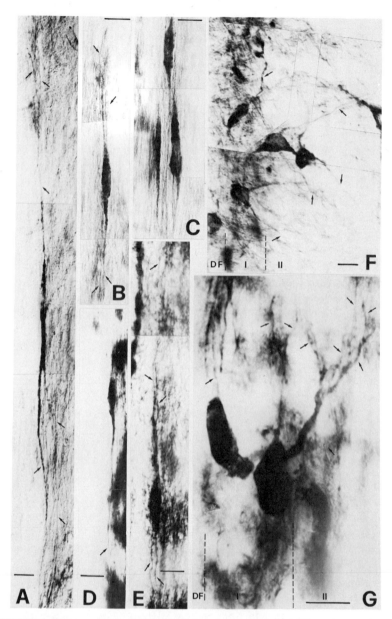

FIGURE 3: Photomontages of CTb-labelled or immunostained fusiform and multipolar cells. In A-C fusiform cells retrogradely labelled from the mesencephalon, in parasagittal (A) and horizontal view (B, C). In D and E, fusiform cells, immunostained for GABA in parasagittal and horizontal views, respectively. In F and G, multipolar cells CTb-labelled from the medulla (F) and stained for GABA (G), both in parasagittal view. Arrows point to distal dendritic branches. Scale bar = 10 μm.

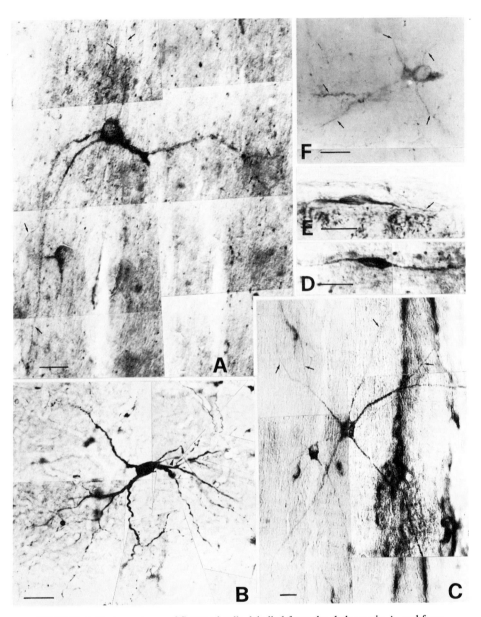

FIGURE 4: Photomontages of flattened cells, labelled from the thalamus in A, and from the medulla in B-D. All cells labelled with CTb, except cell B which was labelled with HRP. A-C fro horizontal, D from coronal sections. Flattened cells immunostained with anti-substance P antibody in E (coronal) and F (horizontal) sections. Arrows point to distal dendrites, arrowhead shows a myelinated axon. Scale bar = 20 μm.

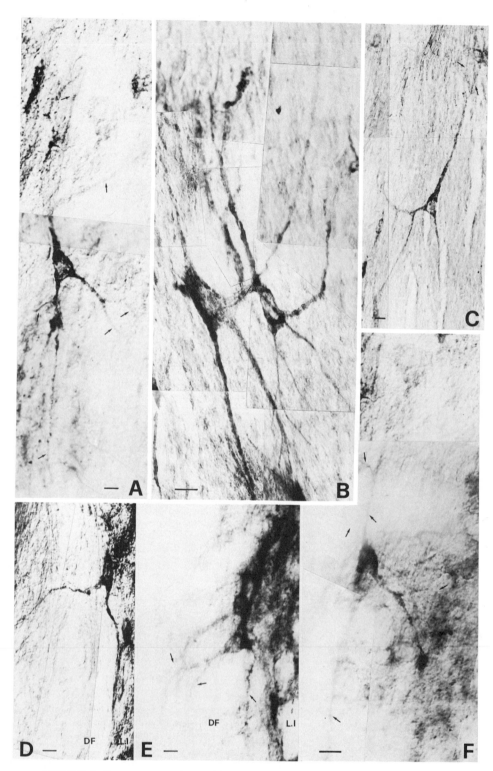

FIGURE 5: Photomontages of pyramidal cells, A-C and F in horizontal view, D and E in parasagittal view. A spinothalamic cell in A, two spinomesencephalic cells in B, a spinobulboreticular cell in C. In D-F, four cells (two in E) which were reacted with enkephalin antibody. DF dorsal funiculus. LI Lamina I. Arrows point to distal dendritic branches. Scale bar = 10 μm.

technique (Ericson *et al*, 1985). All lamina I neurons observed in the three planes of section were drawn with a camera lucida and their positions throughout the mediolateral expanse of the lamina were recorded. Morphometric studies were made of the first 20 drawings in each viewing plane of each morphological lamina I cell type showing solid filling of the dendritic trees by CTb after injections in the thalamus, mesencephalon and DRt, respectively. Perikaryal dimensions and dendritic spreads were measured and a morphometric analysis carried out by the method of the concentric spherical shells (Sholl, 1953) with radii increasing by 20 μm (see Lima and Coimbra, 1986 for details).

Marginal cells labelled with free HRP showed granular staining of perikarya and primary dendritic trunks. CTb labelled many more cells and produced solid filling of dendritic arbors up to third- or fourth-order branches and of the initial portion of the axon. Dendritic spines were not visualized.

Groups or populations of retrogradely labelled cells in the spinal gray were similar to those previously described for the spinothalamic, spinomesencephalic and spinoreticular projections (Chaouch *et al*, 1983; Kemplay and Webster, 1986; Kevetter *et al*, 1982; Menétrey *et al*, 1982; Swett *et al*, 1985) with two important exceptions. Firstly, after free HRP injections in the thalamus, labelling of all spinal groups except the internal basilar column (IBC) were greatly diminished caudal to C2 (Kemplay and Webster, 1986; Lima and Coimbra, 1988a), whereas with CTb the lower cervical and the lumbar segments were also heavily labelled in all groups (Lima and Coimbra, 1988a). Since this tracer is not transported across the synapse in the retrograde direction (Schwab *et al*, 1979; Trojanowski and Schmidt, 1984), these findings permitted us to conclude that the spinothalamic pathway arising from the lower cord was not di-synaptic in the rat as previously claimed on the basis of data obtained with HRP (Kemplay and Webster, 1986). Secondly, considerable labelling of lamina I cells occurred after injections in the DRt. Labelled cells were present in all segments studied after CTb injections but only at C1-C8 after HRP administration with a remarkable decrease in number below C2 (in this case HRP produced some Golgi-like stainings; Fig. 4B). Injection sites with partial inclusion of the cuneate nucleus produced retrograde labelling which was mainly ipsilateral in the medial third of lamina I, IV and V and bilateral in laminae VII and X. After the oblique injections which spared the cuneate nucleus, stained cells occurred in similar numbers in laminae I, VII and X, but staining in laminae IV-V was scarce. Lamina I cells labelled from the thalamus and mesencephalon occurred mostly contralaterally.

The identification of the various structural marginal cell types was based on CTb filling although HRP labelling, despite being confined to perikarya and primary trunks, often allowed cell type recognition. CTb labelled cells exhibited Golgi-like morphologies but the spread of the dendritic trees was shorter, being about 50% of that seen with Golgi staining (Figs 6 and 7). However, the configuration, spatial orientation and branching of the dendritic arbors were similar, as best shown by Sholl's vectograms (Figs. 6 and 7).

As indicated in Table II, flattened (Fig. 4A) and pyramidal cells (Fig. 5A) occurring in the intermediate third of lamina I were labelled from the thalamus. Fusiform cells (Fig. 3A-C), located in the lateral third, and pyramidal cells (Fig. 5B), occurring along the entire mediolateral expanse of lamina I, were labelled from the mesencephalon. The fusiform cells were mainly labelled from the PBN, the pyramidal cells from the PAG. Multipolar cells (Fig. 3F) were only labelled from the medullary DRt and mainly occurred in the medial third. A few pyramidal cells (Fig. 5C) were also labelled from this nucleus and were found in the medial and intermediate thirds. Some flattened cells occurred (Fig. 4B-D) in the intermediate third.

IMMUNOREACTIVITIES OF THE DIFFERENT CELL TYPES

Rats destined for the demonstration of met-enkephalin and substance P in marginal cells were injected intracisternaly with 20 μl of 0.2% colchicine 48 hrs before perfusion with 500 ml of 4% paraformaldehyde in 0.12 M phosphate buffer. Following 2-4 h of postfixation and overnight buffer wash, 50 μm vibratome sections were cut in the three standard anatomical planes at the level of the spinal C1-C2 segments. Material intended for the demonstration of GABA comprised segments C1-C2 and C4-C7; these animals were not injected with colchicine. Floating sections were reacted with each one of three kinds of specific polyclonal antibodies. These were raised in rabbits against met-enkephalin (gift of Dr Nicholas Brecha), substance P (gift of Dr J.Y. Couraud) or GABA (Immunotech). The immunoreactive sites were visualized with the PAP method, and the DAB staining was intensified with osmium or by the method of Adams (1981). Perikarya and dendritic trees were stained up to second- and sometimes third-order branches. Controls were incubations in the absence of the first antibody and pre-adsorption with the corresponding antigens.

Table II

The predominant location in the mediolateral plane of the morphological types of lamina I cells, as revealed by different methods

Types	Golgi and reconstructions	Spinothalamic	Spinomesenc.	Spinobulbar	Immunost.
Fusiform	Lateral		Lateral		GABA (lateral)
Multipolar	Medial			Medial	GABA (medial)
Flattened	Intermediate	Intermediate		Intermediate	Substance P (intermediate)
Pyramidal	Throughout	Intermediate	Throughout	Medial and intermediate	Enkephalin (throughout)

As shown in Table II, fusiform cells (Fig. 3D, E), occurring laterally and multipolar cells (Fig. 3G), occurring medially, reacted with the antibody against GABA. Flattened cells (Fig. 4E-F), located in the intermediate portion, were stained with antibody against substance P. Pyramidal cells (Fig. 5D-F), distributed throughout all lamina I as in the morphological preparations, were stained for met-enkephalin.

POSSIBLE FUNCTIONAL ROLES OF EACH TYPE

These findings suggest a relative specificity of projection target for some structural types of lamina I cells. The fusiform cells, which are the largest marginal neuronal group, projected exclusively to the caudal contralateral mesencephalon and, within it,

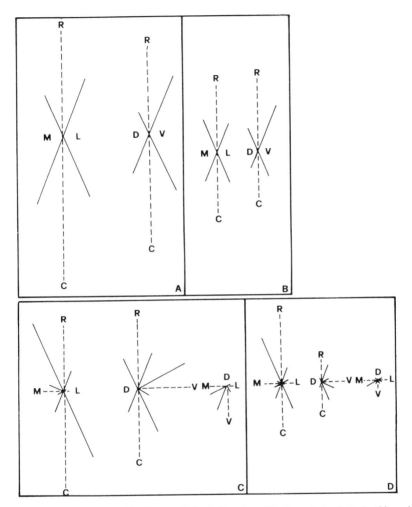

FIGURE 6: Vectograms of fusiform cells in A, B and multipolar cells in C, D. In this and the following figure, the vectograms within each frame are drawn from left to right in horizontal, parasagittal and coronal views (the latter is lacking in A and B). A and C after Golgi staining. B, D after CTb injected in the mesencephalon and in the medullary dorsal reticular formation, respectively. The length of the solid vectors is proportional to the number of dendritic intersections in each octant of the Sholl's grid and the dashed lines are the sum of the two solid vector octants of the rostral (R), medial (M) or lateral (L) quadrants. In fusiform cells (A and B) there are only rostral or caudal vectors in the two longitudinal planes. The spatial orientation of the dendritic arbors is the same, only the number of intersections is much lower in the retrogradely labelled cell (B) than in Golgi-stained material (A) due to the shorter length of the stained dendritic arbors. In C and D, (multipolar cells) vectors of variable length occur in all directions but the dorsal one is lacking. Patterns are similar with both kinds of staining.

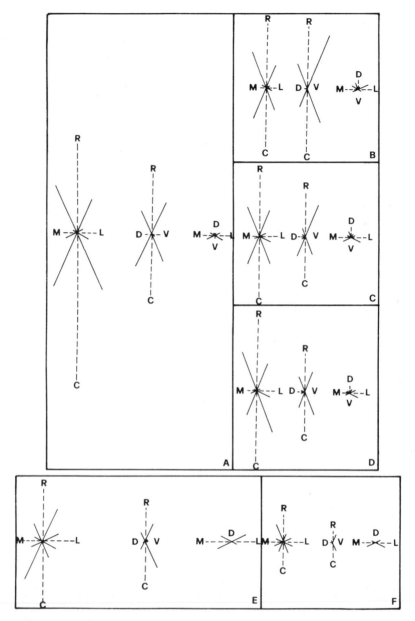

FIGURE 7: Vectograms, constructed as in figure 6, for pyramidal cells in A-D and for flattened cells in E and F. A and E from Golgi stained material, B, F from spinothalamic, C from spinomesencephalic, and D, F from spinobulboreticular-CTb labelled cells. Note the similarity of the vectograms for Golgi and CTb labelled cells in each cell type with shorter lengths in the latter due to the smaller expanses of the CTb filled arbors. Pyramidal cells have larger rostro-caudal than medio-lateral vectors and the medio-lateral vectors are larger than the dorso-ventral ones. Flattened cells have considerable mediolateral vectors which are somewhat shorter than the rostro-caudal ones, and no dorso-ventral vectors.

mainly to the parabrachial nuclei. These nuclei have been proposed to mediate autonomic responses to nociceptive or chemoreceptive input transmitted by spinal and trigeminal marginal cells (Cechetto et al, 1985; Fulwiller and Saper, 1984).

The population of fusiform cells located in the lateral portion of the marginal zone may thus be a subnucleus within the marginal zone endowed with those specific functions. The fact that, according to their morphology in Golgi-stained material, fusiform cells issued unmyelinated axons (Lima and Coimbra, 1986) does not seem an impediment to considering them as projection neurons. Recent experiments in the cat using antidromic activation from the midbrain have shown spinomesencephalic neurons with slow conduction velocities in the unmyelinated range (Hylden et al, 1986).

The multipolar cells are another example of a lamina I cell type with an apparently exclusive supraspinal target, the dorsal reticular formation of the medulla oblongata. Retrograde labelling from this nucleus have, to the best of our knowledge, not been reported before. However, antidromic responses have been obtained in the contralateral lamina I of the rat spinal cord (McMahon and Wall, 1985). Our findings confirm this marginal projection. The classical spinoreticular projection arises in the rat from the outer neck of the dorsal horn (laminae IV-V) and from the ventral horn (VH) end in the ventral pontomedullary reticular formation (Chaouch et al, 1983). This area, namely the gigantocellular reticular nucleus appears to be a relay station transmitting nociceptive spinal input to the intralaminar thalamic nuclei, since the latter are labelled anterogradely from the Gi in the rat (Peschanski and Besson, 1984). We do not know the supramedullary connection of the dorsal reticular formation. However, McMahon and Wall (1985) found lamina I cells excited from both the dorsal medullary reticular formation and the PAG. Such neurones were certainly not multipolar cells which are only labelled from the DRt, but could have been pyramidal cells since this type was labelled from both the DRt and the PAG. One unexpected finding was the visualization with HRP of the commencement of the myelinated portion of some multipolar cell axons (Fig. 4B). This fact and the considerable ventral extension of the dendritic arbors showed that we were dealing with type B multipolar cells (Lima and Coimbra, 1986). Since the dendrites of this subtype reach lamina III (Lima and Coimbra, 1986), medullary projecting multipolar cells may transmit inputs received in the substantia gelatinosa without the interposition of stalked cells functioning as relay neurons (Bennett et al, 1979).

The flattened cells constitute a structurally defined population that is less homogeneous than the fusiform or multipolar populations with respect to specific supraspinal targets, because they were labelled from both the thalamus and, in lesser amounts, from the dorsal reticular formation. In both cases, the cells occurred in the intermediate portion of the marginal zone, and this may support the possibility of double projections from the same neurons. The marginal-dorsoreticular connections reported in the rat by McMahon and Wall (1985) followed a dorsolateral pathway in the lateral funiculus away from the classical ventrolateral position of the spinothalamic tract (Willis and Coggeshall, 1978). However most thalamic projections of lamina I cells have recently been verified to course in the dorsolateral funiculus in the cat (Jones et al, 1985; 1987) and in the primate (Apkarian et al, 1987).

The pyramidal cells are more complex. Those located in intermediate lamina I were mainly labelled from the thalamus, while the medial ones received most from that tracer injected in the medulla. The two groups should thus have different targets despite an identical cell morphology. In addition, a third, larger group of pyramidal cells, occurring throughout the mediolateral expanse of lamina I, was labelled from the mesencephalon. Only experiments with double labelling using distinct tracers may disclose whether this spinomesencephalic contingent contains cells also projecting to the thalamus in the intermediate third, or the medulla in the medial third. The lateral pyramidal cells would be expected to project exclusively to the mesencephalon. It may be remarked that spinomesencephalic pyramidal cells were mainly labelled from the PAG, so that they may be the origin of the ascending branch of the spinal-midbrain loop conveying nociceptive input to the PAG, as proposed by Basbaum and Fields (1984). The descending branch of the loop would consist of PAG neurons sending descending inhibitory input onto the dorsal horn via the nucleus raphe magnus (Basbaum and Fields, 1984).

The presence of some neurochemical agents in cell types with specific projection targets poses other problems. We do not yet know whether retrograde labelling and immunostaining coexisted in the same neurons, or whether different cells of the same structural type were retrogradely labelled in some cases and immunostained in others. If the immunostained cells are local interneurons, as claimed by Hunt et al (1981), then each cell type would have both an interneuronal subset with some inhibitory transmitters or peptides, and a projection subset without them. Recent data however suggest that spinofugal cells may contain these agents. Spreafico et al (1986) observed, in the VB complex of the cat thalamus, large numbers of substance P-reactive terminations which could only be ascribed to a spinal cord origin. Likewise, marginal cells projecting to the thalamus have been shown to contain enkephalin-like immunoreactivity (Coffield and Miletic, 1987). Such findings suggest that our spinothalamic flattened cells of the intermediate third may in fact contain substance P, while the spinothalamic pyramidal cells of the same zone may be enkephalinergic. Coexistence of enkephalin with classical transmitters has been detected in other neural systems (Hökfelt et al, 1984) in which the peptide may regulate receptor binding of the transmitter to pre- or postsynaptic membranes.

Finally, the possible occurrence of GABA in spino-mesencephalic fusiform cells and in spinobulbar multipolar neurons, suggests inhibitory roles for their ascending axons. Some intracellularly-stained lamina I cells have been shown to have long distance axons with local collaterals arborizing in the vicinity of the somata (Bennett et al, 1981). The GABA-staining fusiform and multipolar cells may belong in this category of neurons, functioning as both projection and local circuit-neurons and exerting modulatory inhibition not only in the dorsal horn but also in the midbrain and medulla oblongata.

In summary, the marginal zone contains structural cell types with characteristic morphology, definite mediolateral locations, specific projections and distinct neurochemical properties. These data may be useful in the search for their roles in conveying particular modalities of information, thus clarifying the mechanisms of sensory transmission in the spinal cord and brainstem.

ACKNOWLEDGEMENTS

This research was supported by a Grant of the Stiftung Volkswagenwerk in partnership with the Department of Clinical Neuropharmacology, Max-Planck-Institut für Psychiatrie, Munich (Director - Professor W. Zieglgänsberger), and by Grant No. 87190 (IMU) from JNICT, Lisbon.

REFERENCES

ADAMS, J.C. (1981) Heavy metal intensification of DAB- based HRP reaction product. *Journal of Histochemistry and Cytochemistry*, **29**, 775

APKARIAN, A.V., STEVENS, R.T. AND HODGE, C.J. (1987) The primate dorsolateral spinothalamic pathway. *Soc. Neurosc. Abstr.* **13**: 580

BARBER, R.P., VAUGHN, J.E. AND ROBERTS, E. (1982) The cytoarchitecture of GABAergic neurons in rat spinal cord. *Brain Res.*, **238**: 305-328

BASBAUM, A.I. AND FIELDS, H.L. (1984) Endogenous pain control system: Brainstem spinal pathways and endorphin circuitry. *Ann. Rev. Neurosci.*, **2**: 309-338

BEAL, J.A., PENNY, J.E. AND BICKNELL, H.R. (1981) Structural diversity of marginal (lamina I) neurons in the adult monkey (Macaca mulatta) lumbosacral spinal cord: a Golgi study. *J. Comp. Neurol.*, **202**: 237-254

BENNETT, G.J., HAYASHI, H., ABDELMOUMENE, M. AND DUBNER, R. (1979) Physiological properties of stalked cells of the substantia gelatinosa intracellularly stained with horseradish peroxidase. *Brain Res.*, **164**: 285-289

BENNETT, G.J., ABDELMOUMENE, M., HAYASHI, H., HOFFERT, M.J. AND DUBNER, R. (1981) Spinal cord layer I neurons with axon collaterals that generate local arbors. *Brain Res.*, **209**: 421-426

BROWN, A.G. (1981) *Organization in the spinal cord. The Anatomy and Physiology of Identified Neurones.* Berlin: Springer-Verlag

CECHETTO, D.F., STANDAERT, D.G. AND SAPER, C.B. (1985) Spinal and trigeminal dorsal horn projections to the parabrachial nucleus in the rat. *J. Comp. Neurol.*, **240**: 153-160

CERVERO, F. AND IGGO, A.(1980) The substantia gelatinosa of the spinal cord - a critical review. *Brain*, **103**: 717-772

CERVERO, F., IGGO, A. AND MOLONY, V. (1979) Ascending projections of nociceptor-driven lamina I neurones in the cat. *Exp. Brain Res.*, **35**: 135-149

CHAOUCH, A., MENÉTREY, D., BINDER, D. AND BESSON, J.M. (1983) Neurons at the origin of the medial component of the bulbopontine spinoreticular tract in the rat: An anatomical study using horseradish peroxidase retrograde transport. *J. Comp. Neurol.*, **214**: 309-320

COFFIELD, J.A. AND MILETIC, V. (1987) Enkephalinergic trigeminal and spinal neurons projecting to the rat thalamus. *Soc. Neurosci. Abstr.* **13**: 52

CONDÉ, F. AND CONDÉ, H. (1973) Etude de la morphologie des cellules du noyau rouge du chat par la méthode de Golgi-Cox. *Brain Res.*, **53**: 249-271

CRAIG, A.D. AND KNIFFKI, K.-D. (1985) Spinothalamic lumbosacral lamina I cells responsive to skin and muscle stimulation in the cat. *J. Physiol.*, **365**: 197-221

ERICSON, H., WESTMAN, J. AND BLOMQVIST, A. (1985) Labelling of neuronal connections with monoclonal antibodies against cholera toxin subunit B. *Neurosci. Lett. Suppl.* **22**: S204

FERRINGTON, D.G., SORKIN, L.S. AND WILLIS, Jr., W.D. (1987) Responses of spinothalamic tract cells in the superficial dorsal horn of the primate lumbar spinal cord. *J. Physiol.*, **388**: 681-703

FOERSTER, O. AND GAGEL, O. (1932) Die vorderseitenstrangdurchschneidung beim Menschen. Eine klinisch-patho-physiologisch-anatomische studie. *Z. Ges. Neurol. Psychiat.*, **138**: 1-92

FULWILLER, C.E. AND SAPER, C.B. (1984) Subnuclear organization of the efferent connections of the parabrachial nucleus in the rat. *Brain Res. Rev.*, **2**: 229-259

GIESLER, Jr., G.J., MENÉTREY, D. AND BASBAUM, A.I. (1979) Differential origins of spinothalamic tract projections to medial and lateral thalamus in the rat. *J. Comp. Neurol.*, **184**: 107-126

GLAZER, E.J. AND BASBAUM, A.I. (1983) Opioid neurons and pain modulation: an ultrastructural analysis of enkephalin in the cat superficial dorsal horn. *Neuroscience*, **10**: 357-376

GOBEL, S. (1978) Golgi studies of the neurons in layer I of the dorsal horn of the medulla (trigeminal nucleus caudalis). *J. Comp. Neurol.*, **180**: 375-394

HÖKFELT, T., JOHANSSON, O. AND GOLDSTEIN, M. (1984) Chemical anatomy of the brain. *Science*, **225**: 1326-1334

HUNT, S.P., KELLY, J.S., EMSON, P.C., KIMMEL, J.R., MILLER, R.J. AND WU, J.-Y. (1981) An immunohistochemical study of neuronal populations containing neuropeptides or gamma-aminobutyrate within the superficial layers of the rat dorsal horn. *Neuroscience*, **6**: 1883-1898

HYLDEN, J.L.K., HAYASHI, H., DUBNER, R. AND BENNETT, G. (1986) Physiology and morphology of the lamina I spinomesencephalic projection. *J.Comp. Neurol.*, **247**: 505-515

ITOH, K., KONISHI, A., NOMURA, S., MIZUNO, N., NAKAMURA, Y. AND SUGIMOTO, T. (1979) Application of coupled oxidation reaction to electron microscopic demonstration of horseradish peroxidase: cobalt-glucose oxidase method. *Brain Res.*, **175**: 341-346

JONES, M.W., HODGE Jr., C.J., APKARIAN, A.V. AND STEVENS, R.T. (1985) A dorsolateral spinothalamic pathway in cat. *Brain Res.*, **355**: 188-193

JONES, M.W., APKARIAN, A.V.,STEVENS, R.T. AND HODGE Jr., C.J. (1987) The spinothalamic tract: an examination of the cells of origin of the dorsolateral and ventral spinothalamic pathways in cats. *J. Comp. Neurol.* **260**: 349-361

KEMPLAY, S.K. AND WEBSTER, K.E. (1986) A qualitative and quantitative analysis of the distributions of cells in the spinal cord and spinomedullary junction projecting to the thalamus of the rat. *Neuroscience*, **17**: 769-789

KEVETTER, G.A., HABER, L.H., YEZIERSKI, R.P., CHUNG, J.M., MARTIN, R.F. AND WILLIS, W. (1982) Cells of origin of the spinoreticular tract in the monkey. *J. Comp. Neurol.*, **207**: 61-74

KURU, M. (1949) *Sensory Paths in the Spinal Cord and Brain Stem of Man.* Tokyo: Sogensya

LIGHT, A.R. AND PERL, E.R. (1979) Spinal termination of functionally identified primary afferent neurons with slowly conducting myelinated fibers. *J. Comp. Neurol.*, **186**: 133-150

LIMA, D. AND COIMBRA, A. (1983) The neuronal population of the marginal zone (lamina I) of the rat spinal cord. A study based on reconstructions of serially sectioned cells. *Anat. Embryol.*, **167**: 273-288

LIMA, D. AND COIMBRA, A. (1986) A Golgi study of the neuronal population of the marginal zone (lamina I) of the rat spinal cord. *J. Comp. Neurol.*, **244**: 53-71

LIMA, D. AND COIMBRA, A. (1988a) The spinothalamic system of the rat: structural types of retrogradely labelled neurons in the marginal zone (lamina I). *Neuroscience*, (in press)

LIMA, D. AND COIMBRA, A. (1988b) Morphological types of spinomesencephalic neurons in the marginal zone (lamina I) of the rat spinal cord, as shown after retrograde labelling with cholera toxin subunit B. *J. Comp. Neurol.*, (in press)

MCMAHON, S.B. AND WALL, P.D. (1985) Electrophysiological mapping of brainstem projections of spinal cord lamina I cells in the rat. *Brain Res.*, **333**: 19-26

MENÉTREY, D., GIESLER, Jr., G.J. AND BESSON, J.M. (1977) An analysis of response properties of spinal cord dorsal horn neurones to nonnoxious and noxious stimuli in the spinal rat. *Exp. Brain Res.*, **27**: 15-33

MENÉTREY, D., CHAOUCH, A., BINDER, D. AND BESSON, J.M. (1982) The origin of the spinomesencephalic tract in the rat: an anatomical study using the retrograde transport of horseradish peroxidase. *J. Comp. Neurol.*, **206**: 193-207

PERL, E.R. (1984) Characterization of nociceptors and their activation of neurons in the superficial dorsal horn: First steps for the sensation of pain. In: *Advances in Pain Research and Therapy*, vol. **6**, Neural mechanisms of pain. New York: Raven Press

PESCHANSKI, M. AND BESSON, J.-M. (1984) A spino-reticulo-thalamic pathway in the rat: an anatomical study with reference to pain transmission. *Neuroscience*, **12**: 165-178

PRICE, D.D., HAYASHI, H., DUBNER, R. AND RUDA, M.A. (1979) Functional relationship between neurons of marginal and substantia gelatinosa layers of primate dorsal horn. *J. Neurophysiol.*, **42**: 1590-1608

REXED, B. (1952) The cytoarchitectonic organization of the spinal cord in the cat. *J. Comp. Neurol.*, **96**: 415-495

RUDA, M. A., BENNETT, G. J. AND DUBNER, R. (1986) Neurochemistry and neural circuitry in the dorsal horn. *Prog. Brain Res.* **66**: 219-286

SCHWAB, M.E., SUDA, K. AND THOENEN, H. (1979) Selective retrograde transsynaptic transfer of a protein, tetanus toxin, subsequent to its retrograde axonal transport. *J. Cell Biol.*, **82**: 798-810

SHOLL, D.A. (1953) Dendritic organization in the neurons of the visual and motor cortices of the cat. *J. Anat.*, **87**: 387-406

SPREAFICO, R., BATTAGLIA, G. AND RUSTIONI, A. (1986) Is substance P the marker for a population of spinothalamic neurons? *Soc. Neurosc. Abstr*, **11**: 956

SUGIURA, Y., LEE, C.L AND PERL, E.R. (1986) Central projections of identified, unmyelinated (C) afferent fibers innervating mammalian skin. *Science*, **234**: 358-361

SWETT, J.E., MCMAHON, S.B. AND WALL, P.D. (1985) Long ascending projections to the midbrain from cells of lamina I and nucleus of the dorsolateral funiculus of the rat spinal cord. *J. Comp. Neurol.*, **238**: 401-416

TESSLER, A., HIMES, B.T., ARTMYSHYN, R., MURRAY, M. AND GOLDBERGER, M.E. (1981) Spinal neurons mediate the return of substance P following deafferentation of cat spinal cord. *Brain Res.*, **230**: 263-281

TROJANOWSKI, J.Q. AND SCHMIDT, M.L. (1984) Interneuronal transfer of axonally transported proteins: studies with HRP and HRP conjugates of wheat germ agglutinin, cholera toxin and the B subunit of cholera toxin. *Brain Res.*, **311**: 366-369

WILLIS, W.D. (1985) *The pain system. The neural basis of nociceptive transmission in the mammalian nervous system.* Houston: Karger

WILLIS, W.D. AND COGGESHALL, R.E. (1978) *Sensory Mechanisms of the Spinal Cord.* New York: Plenum Press

WOOLF, C.J. AND FITZGERALD, M.(1983) The properties of neurones recorded in the superficial dorsal horn of the rat spinal cord. *J. Comp. Neurol.*, **221**: 313-328

PROJECTIONS OF THE SUPERFICIAL DORSAL HORN
TO THE MIDBRAIN AND THALAMUS

William D. Willis, Jr.

Marine Biomedical Institute and Department of Anatomy and Neurosciences
University of Texas Medical Branch Galveston, TX 77550, U.S.A.

INTRODUCTION

The mammalian somatosensory system includes a number of projection systems that originate in the spinal cord and terminate in the brainstem and thalamus (Willis and Coggeshall, 1978). Comparable pathways transmit information derived from activity of afferent fibers in the trigeminal and other cranial nerves. Two of the somatosensory tracts from the spinal cord synapse on neurons in the midbrain and thalamus, and so can be designated spinomesencephalic and spinothalamic tracts. However, this simple nomenclature is unlikely to reflect a simple organization, since the synaptic zones are in a number of different nuclei of diverse connectivity and the cells of origin are in all laminae of the spinal cord.

The spinomesencephalic tract (SMT) of the rat, cat and monkey (Fig. 1) terminates in the intermediate and deep layers of the superior colliculus, the intercollicular nucleus, the lateral periaqueductal gray, the cuneiform nucleus, the mesencephalic reticular formation, the red nucleus, the nucleus of Darkschewitz, the anterior and posterior pretectal nuclei and the Edinger-Westphal nucleus (Kerr, 1975; Bjorkeland and Boivie, 1984; Wiberg and Blomqvist, 1984; Wiberg, Westman and Blomqvist, 1987; Yezierski, 1988). The spinothalamic tract (STT) of the rat and monkey (Fig. 2) ends in the ventral posterior lateral (VPL) nucleus, the border zone between the VPL and ventral lateral (VL) nuclei, the medial part of the posterior complex, the central lateral and other intralaminar nuclei and the nucleus submedius (Berkley, 1980; Boivie, 1979; Craig and Burton, 1981; Lund and Webster, 1967; Kerr, 1975; Mehler, Feferman and Nauta, 1960; Peschanski, Mantyh and Besson, 1983). In the cat, only a few STT axons appear to end in the VPL nucleus; instead, there is a projection to a *shell region* (including parts of the posterior complex and the border region between the VPL and the VL nuclei) around the VPL nucleus (Berkley, 1980; Boivie, 1971; Craig and Burton, 1985). Otherwise, STT connections in the cat are similar to those in the rat and monkey.

The SMT and STT are thought to play a key role in pain and at least the STT in temperature sensation and in some aspects of touch. Evidence for this comes chiefly from observations of the effects of spinal cord lesions in humans and in animals (Willis, 1985; Willis and Coggeshall, 1978), as well as from electrophysiological investigations.

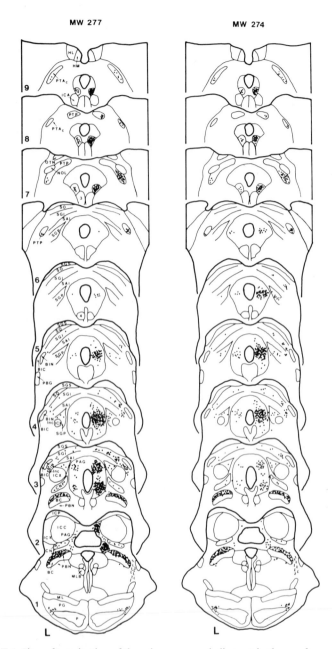

FIGURE 1: Sites of termination of the spinomesencephalic tract in the monkey. Anterograde tracing was done using horseradish peroxidase conjugated with wheat germ agglutinin. The tracer was injected into the lumbar enlargement in the animal whose midbrain is shown in transverse sections at the left and into the cervical enlargement for the experiment at the right. Abbreviations, BC, brachium conjunctivum; BIC, brachium of inferior colliculus; CNF, cuneiform nucleus; ICC, central nucleus of inferior colliculus; ICX, external nucleus of inferior colliculus; PAG, periaqueductal gray; PBN, parabrachial nucleus; PTP, PTAc, pretectal nuclei; SGS, SO, SGI, SAI, SGP, layers of superior colliculus (From Wiberg *et al*, 1987.).

ANATOMY OF SMT AND STT PROJECTIONS FROM SUPERFICIAL DORSAL HORN

The SMT and STT originate at least in part from the superficial layers of the dorsal horn of the spinal cord (Fig. 3), as shown by experiments using retrogradely transported horseradish peroxidase to label the projection neurons (Carstens and Trevino, 1978; Giesler, Menétrey and Basbaum, 1979; Hayes and Rustioni, 1980; Kemplay and Webster, 1986; Jones, Apkarian, Stevens and Hodge, 1987; Liu, 1983; Mantyh, 1982; Menétrey, Chaouch and Besson, 1980; Swett, McMahon and Wall, 1985; Trevino, 1976; Trevino and Carstens, 1975; Wiberg and Blomqvist, 1984; Wiberg et al, 1987; Willis, Kenshalo and Leonard, 1979). Most of the SMT and STT neurons in the superficial dorsal horn are in lamina I, although a few are in laminae II or III (Hayes and Rustioni, 1980; Jones et al, 1987; Menétrey, Chaouch, Binder and Besson, 1982; Wiberg and Blomqvist, 1984; Willis et al, 1979). Other SMT and STT neurons are located in the deep layers of the dorsal horn, the intermediate region and the ventral horn.

Some studies have quantitated the contributions of different laminae to the SMT and STT. Table I shows that in the rat and cat a substantial number of SMT and STT neurons are located in lamina I (Carstens and Trevino, 1978; Craig and Burton, 1981; Harmann, Carlton and Willis, 1988; Jones et al, 1987; Kemplay and Webster, 1986; Swett et al, 1985; Wiberg and Blomqvist, 1984). Similarly, in the monkey a large fraction of both the SMT (54%) and STT (53% of the cells projecting to the lateral thalamus and 16% of those projecting to the medial thalamus) were reported to originate from cells of lamina I (Willis et al, 1979). However, caution is needed in taking the latter figures too literally. The counts were generally based on the number of cells observed in transverse sections, but serial reconstructions were not done. Since many of the projection neurons of lamina I are oriented longitudinally, it is possible that a given neuron was counted more than once, resulting in an overestimate of the proportion of lamina I cells in the population of labelled SMT and STT cells. This criticism would not apply to cells in deep laminae of the spinal cord since neurons in these layers tend to be oriented transversely.

Particular targets of lamina I SMT cells include the lateral periaqueductal gray and adjacent cuneiform nucleus (Harmann et al, 1988; Swett et al, 1985; Zhang, Carlton, Sorkin, Harmann and Willis, 1987). Lamina I STT cells in the monkey terminate laterally in the VPL nucleus (Applebaum, Leonard, Kenshalo, Martin and Willis, 1979; Willis et al, 1979 and medially in the nucleus submedius, at least in the cat (Craig and Burton, 1981).

The similarity in the distribution of SMT and STT cells projecting to the lateral thalamus in the monkey (Fig. 3) led to the hypothesis that a large fraction of these neurons might project to both targets (Willis et al, 1979). Double labelling experiments in the rat (Harmann et al, 1988) and in the monkey (Zhang et al, 1987) have demonstrated collateral projections of some neurons of lamina I (and lamina V) to both the lateral periaqueductal gray and the VPL nucleus. The proportion of neurons having such collateral projections is low (in the rat, only 1.4% of the sampled population of STT cells and 6.2% of SMT cells were found to project to both the VPL nucleus and the lateral periaqueductal gray), but this is likely to be an underestimate, since the injections were restricted to avoid spread of the marker.

Most of the projections of lamina I SMT and STT cells are to the contralateral side of the brain (Table I; Fig. 3). This is shown by counts of the numbers of cells on each side of the spinal cord following injection of HRP into the midbrain or thalamus on one side. For example, in the rat, 82% of the lamina I SMT cells labelled in the spinal cord

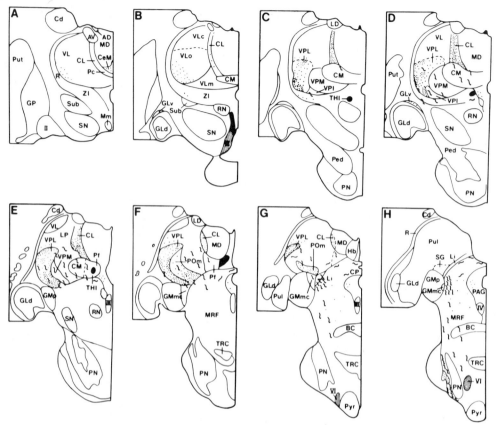

FIGURE 2: Sites of termination of the spinothalamic tract in the monkey. Anterograde tracing was by the silver method for axonal degeneration. Terminal fields are shown by stipple and axons of passage by wavy lines. The lesion was at the midcervical level, well below the lateral cervical nucleus. Abbreviations: CL, central lateral nucleus; GMmc, medial geniculate nucleus; MD, medial dorsal nucleus; POm, medial part of posterior nucleus; Pul, pulvinar; VPL, ventral posterior lateral nucleus; VPM, ventral posterior medial nucleus; VL, VLo, ventral lateral nucleus. (From Boivie, 1979.)

were contralateral to the injection site (Swett *et al*, 1985). In the cat, about 80% of SMT cells (Wiberg and Blomqvist, 1984) and 80-90% of lamina I STT cells project to the contralateral side (Craig and Burton, 1981; Jones *et al*, 1987). Similarly, in the monkey about 92% of SMT cells, 95% of lamina I STT cells projecting to the lateral thalamus and 90% of those projecting to the medial thalamus were found in the lumbosacral enlargement contralateral to the injection site (Willis *et al*, 1979).

Until recently, it has been thought that the SMT and STT ascend together in the ventrolateral quadrant of the spinal cord (cf, Bjorkeland and Boivie, 1984; Boivie, 1971; Willis, 1985). However, several studies in the rat have now demonstrated that the component of the SMT that originates from lamina I ascends in the dorsal part of the lateral funiculus (DLF; McMahon and Wall, 1983; Zemlan, Leonard, Kow and Pfaff, 1978). Likewise, the part of the STT that arises from lamina I ascends in the DLF, at least in the cat (Fig. 4; Jones, Hodge, Apkarian and Stevens, 1985; 1987) and monkey (Apkarian, Stevens and Hodge, 1987). In the cat, the component of the STT ascending in the DLF represents about 25% of the total population of STT cells (Jones *et al*, 1987).

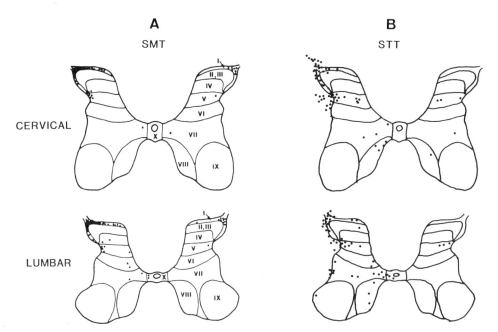

A

SMT

B

STT

CERVICAL

I
II, III
IV
V
VI
VII
VIII   IX

LUMBAR

I
II, III
IV
V
VI
VII
VIII   IX

FIGURE 3: Cells of origin of the spinomesencephalic and spinothalamic tracts in the monkey as demonstrated by retrograde labelling with horseradish peroxidase. The left column shows the locations of retrogradely labelled spinomesencephalic tract cells in the cervical (upper) and lumbar (lower) enlargements following injection of HRP into the region of the periaqueductal gray and cuneiform nucleus. (From Wiberg *et al*, 1987.) The right column shows the distribution of spinothalamic tract cells in the cervical and lumbar enlargements following a large injection of HRP into the contralateral thalamus (unpublished observations).

The axons of lamina I SMT and STT neurons presumably decussate in the spinal cord near the level of the cell body. Evidence for this includes antidromic activation of rat lamina I neurons projecting to the midbrain following stimulation of the contralateral DLF within a few millimetres rostral to the recording site (McMahon and Wall, 1985) and the observation of labelled axons in the cat DLF ipsilateral to the site of injection of horseradish peroxidase into the thalamus (Jones *et al*, 1985).

FUNCTIONAL PROPERTIES OF LAMINA I SMT CELLS

SMT and STT neurons in lamina I can be identified in electrophysiological experiments by antidromic activation using electrodes inserted into the appropriate midbrain or thalamic target zones (Dilly, Wall and Webster, 1968; Price, Hayes, Ruda and Dubner, 1978; Trevino, Coulter and Willis, 1973; Yezierski, Sorkin and Willis, 1987). Recording sites can be estimated from the recording depth or determined by marks placed by passing current through the tip of the microelectrode. However, the actual location of a cell from which recordings are made can only be determined by a mark made during intracellular recording. Unfortunately, only 1 study has as yet been reported in which lamina I SMT or STT cells have been labelled intracellularly (Hylden, Hayashi, Dubner and Bennett, 1986). Most of the evidence concerning the functional properties of these neurons is based on extracellular recordings. Thus, some of the neurons may have been located outside lamina I. However, given the

Table I

SPINOMESENCEPHALIC TRACT

Animal	Segments	% Contra	I-III	IV-VI	VII-X	Reference
Rat (PAG)	All	82	771	?	?	Swett et al. 1985
Rat (PAG)	C6-8 L3-5		52 11	25 6	1 1	Harmann et al. 1988
Cat	C6 & 7 L6 & 7	78 82	63 75	33 17	4 8	Wiberg & Blomqvist, 1984
Monkey	L5-S1	92	911	531	206	Willis et al. 1979
Monkey	C6 & 7 L6 & 7	82 79	165 149	30 47	5 6	Wiberg et al. 1987

SPINOTHALAMIC TRACT

Animal	Segments	% Contra	I-III	IV-VI	VII-X	Reference
Rat	C6-C8 L4-L6	100 100	I-V: 9 I-V: 3	VI: 4 VI:28	? 8	Kemplay & Webster, 1986*
Rat (PAG)	C6-8 L3-5		127 50	115 115	25 20	Harmann et al. 1988
Cat	C7 & 8 L6 & 7		180 60	170 50	140 340	Carstens & Trevino, 1978
Cat	C6-T1 L5-S1	85 to 90	82 253	135 244	30 345	Jones et al. 1987
Cat (Sub-medius)	C6-8 L6-S1	95 80	47 36	2 0	16 24	Craig & Burton 1981
Monkey (Lat.) (Med.)	L5-S1 L5-S1	95 90	403 98	221 209	121 306	Willis et al. 1979

---

* The locations of retrogradely labeled STT neurons in the rat were not reported by laminae, but rather as in the head and neck of the dorsal horn, the *internal basilar column*, the intermediate grey zone or the ventral horn. The equivalent laminae are indicated here.

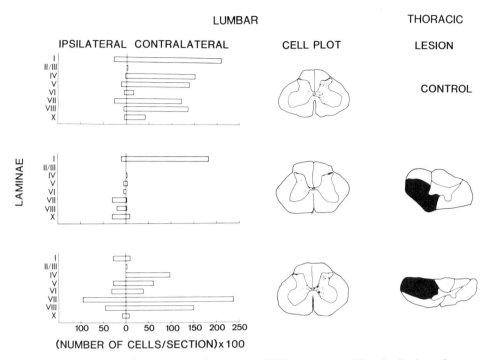

FIGURE 4: Dorsolateral spinothalamic tract (STT) in the cat. The distribution of retrogradely labelling STT cells in the lumbar spinal cord following HRP injection into the thalamus is shown in the upper part of the figure. The middle part shows that the majority of the labelled cells is restricted to lamina I in an animal that had the anterolateral quadrant interrupted prior to the injection of HRP. Conversely, the lower part shows that few cells of lamina I label after interruption of the dorsolateral funiculus. (From Jones *et al*, 1987.)

preponderance of SMT and STT cells in lamina I versus the nearby laminae II and III, it is likely that most of the recordings were in fact from cells of lamina I (assuming that the configurations of the unfiltered action potentials correctly indicated that recordings were from soma-dendritic membranes and not from axons or distal dendrites).

Several electrophysiological studies of lamina I SMT cells have been done in the rat (McMahon and Wall, 1985; Menétrey *et al*, 1980). The sites from which antidromic activation could be produced included the lateral periaqueductal gray and the cuneiform nucleus. The SMT cells were contralateral to the antidromic activation site. Axonal conduction velocities were relatively slow (ranging from 3 to 19 m/s, mean 7.1 m/s, for 13 cells reported by McMahon and Wall, 1985), indicating that the ascending axons were finely myelinated. Excitatory receptive fields for mechanical stimulation of

TABLE I: Counts of cells of origin of the spinomesencephalic and spinothalamic tracts in rat, cat and monkey. The cells were labelled retrogradely following HRP injections. In some cases, the injection site is indicated in the first column (e.g., PAG, nucleus submedius or the lateral vs. medial thalamus). The second column shows the level of the spinal cord analyzed, and column 3 the percentage of the cells that were observed to be contralateral to the injection site. The numbers of labelled cells found in laminae I-III (superficial dorsal horn), IV-VI and VII-X are shown in columns 4-6. The last column gives the sources of the data.

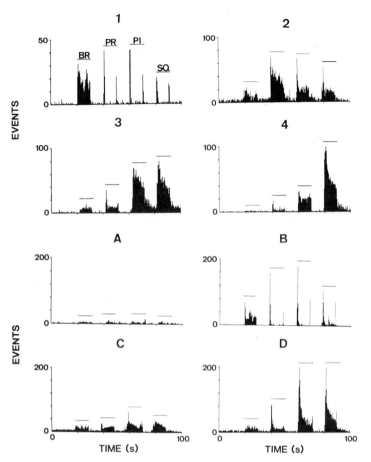

FIGURE 5: Response profiles of different classes of STT cells. In the upper part of the figure are shown the responses to brushing, pressure (marginally painful compression with a large arterial clip), pinch (distinctly painful compression with a small arterial clip) and squeeze (damaging compression with serrated forceps) of STT neurons classified as types I-IV. In the lower panels are the responses of STT cells categorized as types A-D. (From Surmeier *et al*, 1988.)

the skin were generally medium to large in size (Menétrey *et al*, 1980), and the response class was either the *wide dynamic range* (WDR) type (excited by innocuous mechanical stimuli but maximally by noxious intensities) or the *high threshold* (HT) type (activated by mechanical stimuli of only noxious intensities).

At least two studies have been done in which the properties of lamina I SMT cells have been examined in the cat. Hylden *et al*, (1986) recorded from 89 lamina I SMT neurons. The axons terminated in the lateral periaqueductal gray/cuneiform nucleus region on the contralateral (44 cases) or ipsilateral (40 cases) side or both (5 cases). Eight of the cells could also be activated antidromically from the thalamus. Conduction velocities ranged from 1 to 18 m/s (mean of 6.9 m/s), indicating that some of the SMT axons were unmyelinated and others were finely myelinated. The receptive fields of 62 of the SMT cells were characterized. Most (92%) were of the HT type, but 5 SMT neurons were of the WDR type. The receptive fields were small, ranging from a surface area of less than a digit to that of part of the hindpaw. Volleys in peripheral nerve fibers were used to examine inputs from different sizes of afferent fibers. None of the SMT cells responded to volleys restricted to A beta fibers. Most responded to volleys in A delta fibers; 20% of the cells responded to volleys in both A delta and C fibers; 2 cells were activated only by volleys in C fibers. In 19 cases, intracellular labelling showed the location of the cell body to be in lamina I. The dendritic trees of 11 lamina I SMT neurons could be reconstructed. The axons of several had local collaterals.

The other investigation of cat SMT cells was that of Yezierski and Schwartz (1986). Most of the cells examined were located in the deep layers of the dorsal horn or in the ventral horn. However, some were in lamina I. The conduction velocities of the lamina

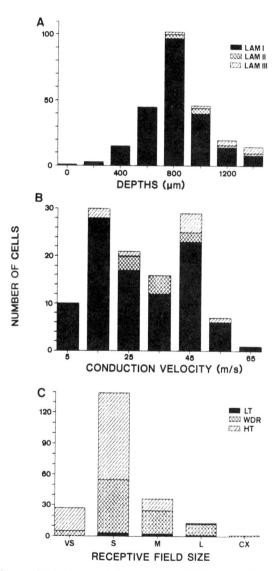

FIGURE 6: Characteristics of a population of primate STT cells in the superficial dorsal horn. In A are shown the depths of recording sites for STT cells of the superficial dorsal horn. Laminae I-III are distinguished as shown. B is a histogram of the conduction velocities of the axons of STT cells of the superficial dorsal horn. Cells in different laminae are indicated. In C are plotted the numbers of STT cells of the superficial dorsal horn with very small, small, medium sized, large or complex receptive fields.

I SMT cells averaged 14.1 m/s. Two of the cells were of the WDR type with a receptive field located on the ipsilateral hindlimb. Two other lamina I SMT cells were of the HT type; one of these had a restricted receptive field on the ipsilateral hindlimb, whereas the other had a complex receptive field involving other parts of the body.

A limited amount of work has been done on lamina I SMT cells in the monkey (Price et al, 1978; Yezierski et al, 1987). Some SMT cells also projected to the ventral posterior lateral (VPL) nucleus of the thalamus, whereas others appeared to project just to the midbrain in the region of the lateral periaqueductal gray (Price et al, 1978; Yezierski et al, 1987). Axonal conduction velocities for 13 monkey lamina I SMT cells were considerably faster (mean of 46 m/s) than those of rat or cat lamina I SMT cells (Yezierski et al, 1987). The excitatory receptive fields of primate lamina I SMT cells were medium or large in size, and the cells were either of the WDR or HT type. Inputs were also observed from muscle, and inhibitory receptive fields could often be demonstrated. All of the units tested responded to noxious heat pulses (Yezierski et al, 1987).

Recently, our laboratory has developed an approach to the classification of somatosensory neurons based on a k means cluster analysis, a multivariate statistical procedure (Chung, Surmeier, Lee, Sorkin, Honda, Tsong and Willis, 1986; Surmeier et al, 1988). The analysis depends upon the responses of a population of cells to a standard series of mechanical stimuli, including a clearly innocuous stimulus (brushing) and three grades of compressive stimuli, ranging from marginally painful (pressure) to distinctly painful (pinch) and finally to overtly damaging (squeeze). A reference population of 318 primate STT cells serves as the basis for assignment of newly observed STT cells or to other types of somatosensory neurons to the response classes of the STT reference population. Two types of analysis have been used. In the first (*within neuron analysis*), the responses of a given neuron to the four standard stimuli are normalized with respect to the maximum response (Surmeier et al, 1988). The pattern of such normalized responses is then compared across the population of individual neurons. Four classes (I-IV) are recognized: Characteristic response profiles are shown in Fig. 5 (upper). The second approach (*across neuron analysis*) involves a comparison of the responsiveness of a given neuron to the mean for the population to each of the four standard stimuli. A given neuron can then be said to respond more or less vigorously to each stimulus than the average cell in the population. Again four response classes could be recognized: types A-D. Response characteristic of these classes are shown in Fig. 5 (lower).

The lamina I SMT cells that were examined (Yezierski et al, 1987) can be assigned to the response categories of STT cells using discriminant analysis. All of the neurons fell into classes 3 or 4 (best response to distinctly painful or overtly damaging mechanical stimuli) and types A (poorly responsive) or D (activated more vigorously than average by noxious mechanical stimuli).

FUNCTIONAL PROPERTIES OF STT CELLS IN LAMINA I

Recordings have been reported for only 2 lamina I STT cells in the rat (Giesler, Menétrey, Guilbaud and Besson, 1976). These cells were activated antidromically from the contralateral thalamus. The receptive field of one of these was of the WDR type and of the other the HT type.

In the first study of the STT using antidromic activation, Dilly et al, (1966) recorded from a single lamina I STT cell in the cervical spinal cord of the cat. This cell responded to brush and touch, but not to more intense mechanical stimulation in a small receptive field on one toe.

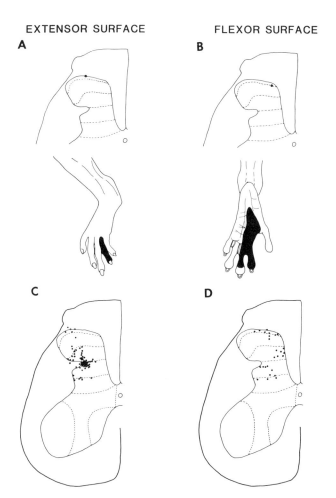

EXTENSOR SURFACE   FLEXOR SURFACE

A   B

C   D

FIGURE 7: Somatotopic organization of STT cells in laminae I and IV, but not V. The locations of two lamina I STT cells and their receptive fields are shown in A and B. The distribution of STT cells with receptive fields on the extensor surface are plotted in C and on the flexor surface in D. (From Willis *et al*, 1974.)

Recently, Craig and Kniffki (1985) recorded from 218 lamina I STT cells in the cat lumbosacral spinal cord. The neurons were activated antidromically from an array of electrodes placed across the contralateral thalamus. Resolution of the destination of the axons was limited to lateral versus medial thalamus. The conduction velocities of the axons were slow, ranging from 1.1 to 16.7 m/s (mean of 3.7 m/s). Thus, many of the cells had axons that must have been unmyelinated. Nearly half of the cells (47%) were activated only from the medial thalamus; 19% were activated only from the lateral thalamus; and 26% were activated from both (the other 8% were activated from *mid-thalamus*).

Electrically evoked volleys were used to determine what classes of peripheral afferent fibers activated cat lamina I STT cells (Craig and Kniffki, 1985). Eighteen cells were excited only by A delta fibers, 46 by A delta and C fibers, and 11 just by C fibers.

Craig and Kniffki (1985) characterized the receptive fields of 47 of the cat lamina I STT cells in their sample. Nineteen of the cells had cutaneous receptive fields and were of the HT class. Six of these responded to noxious heat but not to noxious mechanical stimuli. Most projected to the medial thalamus only (8) or both to medial and lateral thalamus (9); only 2 projected just to the lateral thalamus. Six of the cells were specifically thermoreceptive, responding best to cooling of the skin. These thermo-receptive cells usually projected to the medial (4 cases) or medial and lateral (1 case) thalamus, rather than just to the lateral thalamus (1 case). This observation raises the possibility that thermal sensation depends upon a relay in the medial thalamus. Alternatively, the medial projection of thermoreceptive STT cells in the cat may relate to thermal regulation. Three of the cells had only subcutaneous receptive fields of the HT type. The remaining lamina I STT cells were either *multireceptive*, responding to various combinations of noxious cutaneous or deep stimulation or cold (13 cells) or were unresponsive (6 cells).

Lamina I STT cells have also been examined in the monkey. Price *et al*, (1978) recorded from 9 such neurons (plus 6 lamina I cells that projected also or instead to the midbrain). The STT cells were activated antidromically from the contralateral VPL nucleus. The classifications of the cells were equivalent to WDR (6 cells) or to HT (3 cells) neurons.

In our laboratory, we recorded from 255 STT cells located in the superficial dorsal horn of the primate spinal cord between 1971 and 1985. The activity of these cells has been described in a number of publications (e.g, Applebaum *et al*, 1979; Ferrington, Sorkin and Willis, 1987; Surmeier, Honda and Willis, 1988; Trevino *et al*, 1973; Willis, Trevino, Coulter and Maunz, 1974). Antidromic activation sites included the PO region just medial to the medial geniculate nucleus (34 cells) and the VPL nucleus (221 cells). All but 1 of the cells were activated from the contralateral side (the exception was a cell backfired from the ipsilateral PO region); however, recordings were rarely made on the side ipsilateral to the antidromic stimulating electrode, and so the one positive observation should be regarded as no more than confirmation of the anatomical evidence that some lamina I STT neurons project ipsilaterally (Table I; Willis *et al*, 1979).

Of 255 STT cells in the superficial dorsal horn, it was judged that at least 226 were likely to have been in lamina I, 13 in lamina II and 16 in lamina III. For lamina I, this was based on the following criteria: a mark placed at the recording site (47 cases), reconstruction of the recording site from microelectrode depth and histological identification of the microelectrode track (83 cases) and a depth of 1000 micrometers or less (the remainder). For laminae II and III, location was determined either from marks (13 cases) or histological reconstruction (remaining cases). The distribution of the STT cells of the superficial layers of the dorsal horn in our sample according to depth and by lamina is shown in Fig. 6A. Since the recording sites for a number of lamina I STT cells were found by marks or histological reconstruction to be at depths greater than 1000 micrometers, it is evident that our arbitrary cut-off of 1000 micrometers meant excluding some lamina I STT cells from the population that was analyzed.

The conduction velocities of the STT cells that we studied in the superficial dorsal horn ranged from 6 to 66 m/s (mean of 29.2 m/s). Thus, none of the STT cells in our sample had unmyelinated axons. The distribution of conduction velocities was bimodal, as shown in Fig. 6B. One mode was around 15 m/s, and the other around 45 m/s. We have reported that STT cells in lamina I include both small (89% of the retrogradely labelled population) and large (Waldeyer type: 11%) neurons (Willis *et al*, 1979), and so we can presume that the more numerous cells with slowly conducting axons correspond to the small lamina I STT cells and that the smaller number of ones with more rapidly

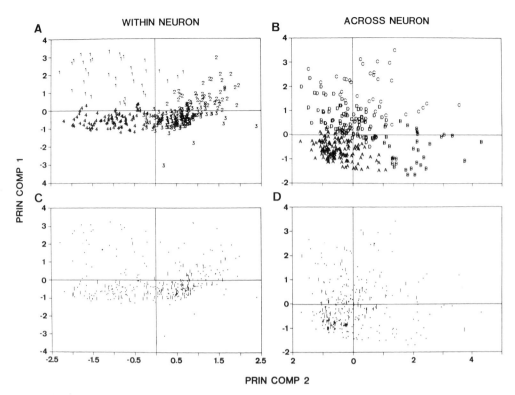

FIGURE 8: Classification of STT cells of the superficial dorsal horn by k means cluster analysis. A and B show the distribution of the responses of types I-IV and A-D STT cells on the plane of the first two principal components. C and D are the same distributions, except that the cells located in the superficial dorsal horn are indicated by I. In A and C, for principal component 1, there is a large positive weighting for responses to brushing and a large negative weighting for responses to squeeze. For principal component 2, responses to intermediate intensities of stimuli are given positive weighting and to the extremes of stimulus intensity negative weighting. In B and D, the intense stimuli give large positive weighting for principal component 1 and the weak stimuli large positive weighting for principal component 2.

conducting axons correspond to the Waldeyer cells. However, this speculation needs to be confirmed by recordings from neurons that are labelled intracellularly, since judgements of neuronal size were made in transverse sections, yet the major axis of most lamina I STT cells is longitudinal. Thus, the dimensions of a given lamina I STT cell need to be measured after three-dimensional reconstruction.

The receptive fields of STT cells in the superficial dorsal horn of the primate spinal cord tend to be very small (covering a surface equivalent to that of a single digit or less) or small (an area less than that of the foot). Figure 6C shows a breakdown of the receptive field sizes of 216 of these cells. A total of 27 cells (12.5%) had very small receptive fields; 139 (64.4%) had small receptive fields. Only 36 cells (16.7%) had medium sized receptive fields (area greater than the foot, but less than the leg below the knee), and 13 (6.0%) had large receptive fields (area greater than the part of the leg below the knee). One cell had a complex receptive field (extending over more than a single limb). Thus, about 77% of the STT cells in the superficial dorsal horn of the monkey had very small or small receptive fields.

There appears to be a somatotopic arrangement of the receptive fields of STT cells

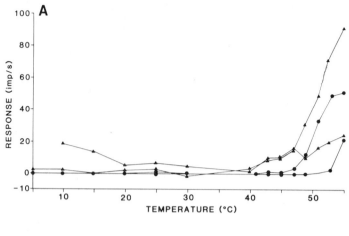

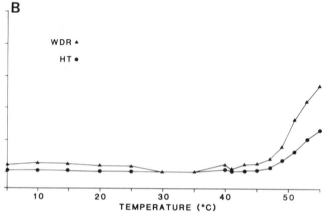

FIGURE 9: Responses of lamina I STT cells to graded thermal stimuli. The graph in A shows the responses of 2 WDR and 2 HT STT cells to thermal stimuli. B shows the mean responses of 12 WDR and 9 HT STT cells to thermal stimuli. WDR cells indicated by filled triangles and HT cells by filled circles. (From Ferrington *et al*, 1987.)

in lamina I (Willis *et al*, 1974). Neurons with fields on the extensor surface tend to be located laterally and those with fields on the flexor surface medially in lamina I (Fig. 7). This arrangement is consistent with the somatotopic organization of the dorsal horn in the cat described by Brown and Fuchs (1975). By contrast, the cell bodies of STT cells in lamina V do not seem to have a distinct somatotopic organization, perhaps because they typically have dendrites that spread throughout much of the cross section of the dorsal horn (Surmeier *et al*, 1988).

In our sample of responses of lamina I STT cells in the monkey, only a few (6 or 2.8%) were of the low threshold (LT) type (responding best to innocuous stimulation of the skin). Most of the STT cells were of the WDR (91, 42.1%) or the HT (119, 55.1%) types.

As discussed above, our laboratory has begun to classify primate STT cells in a different manner, based on a k means cluster analysis of the responses of the cells to a series of 4 standard mechanical stimuli. The distribution of all of the reference set of primate STT cells as classified using a *within neuron analysis* on a plot of the first two principal components is shown in Fig. 8A and for an *across neuron analysis* in Fig. 8B. The classifications of 62 lamina I STT cells are indicated in Fig. 8C and D. Most of the cells belonged to classes 3 (55%) or 4 (29%) and A (53%) or C (31%). Thus, based on the *within neuron analysis* the responses of at least 84% of lamina I STT cells to cutaneous stimulation reflect predominantly an input from nociceptors. Only 1 cell in our sample of lamina I STT cells was classified as type 1 (and B) and so was likely to transmit tactile information.

Since many lamina I STT cells in the monkey can be excited weakly by brushing the skin, an attempt was made to determine if lamina I STT cells could contribute to flutter sensation (Ferrington *et al*, 1987). Vibratory mechanical stimuli were applied to the receptive fields of 14 lamina I STT cells. Although 7 of the neurons could follow indentation of the skin by vibratory stimuli at rates of 1 to 30 Hz, the responses were weak and poorly entrained. It was concluded that lamina I STT cells were unlikely to contribute substantially to flutter.

Lamina I STT cells in the monkey were generally responsive to thermal stimuli (Ferrington *et al*, 1987). For example, Fig. 9A shows the responses of 2 individual WDR and 2 HT cells to thermal stimuli in the range of 5 to 55o C. One of the WDR cells responded to cooling, and all were excited by noxious heating. The stimulus-response curves in Fig. 9B were the mean responses for 12 WDR and 9 HT lamina I STT cells. The WDR cells had steeper stimulus-response curves for heating than did the HT cells. A series of noxious heat stimuli caused sensitization of the skin, resulting in a lowered threshold for noxious heat and an increased responsiveness for a second series of noxious heat stimuli (at least for the lower intensities of noxious heat). Furthermore, noxious heat sensitized the skin to at least the weaker intensities of mechanical stimuli.

DISCUSSION AND CONCLUSIONS

Cells in the superficial dorsal horn, especially in lamina I, are of considerable interest because of their potential role in the processing of information relating to pain and temperature sensations (Cervero, Iggo and Ogawa, 1976; Christensen and Perl, 1970; Price, Hayashi, Dubner and Ruda, 1979). The possibility of an additional contribution to tactile sense should also be kept in mind. Part of the information leading to pain and temperature sense is generally believed to be conveyed to the brain by way of the spinothalamic tract, but it is likely that a contribution to pain is also made by the SMT and other pathways. A substantial proportion of both the SMT and the STT originates from cells of lamina I (although a major contribution is from lamina V and some from all other laminae of the spinal cord gray matter).

Targets of the lamina I SMT projection include the lateral part of the periaqueductal gray and the adjacent cuneiform nucleus (Harmann *et al*, 1988; Swett *et al*, 1985; Zhang *et al*, 1987). It is unclear what functional role is served by these projections. Stimulation in the periaqueductal gray (PAG) can result in nocifensive behavior in animals (Skultety, 1963; Spiegel, Kletzkin and Szekely, 1954) and pain or a feeling of *fear and death* in man (Nashold, Wilson and Slaughter, 1969; 1974). Alternatively or additionally, stimulation in the PAG can produce *analgesia* (Mayer and Liebeskind, 1974; Reynolds, 1969; Rees and Roberts, 1986). It is possible that activity in the lamina I cells of the SMT contributes both to the sensation of pain (by way of ascending connections of the PAG) and to modulation of nociceptive pathways (by way of descending connections of the PAG). However, the relatively large receptive fields of many of these cells, at least in the monkey (Yezierski *et al*, 1987), argue against a role in stimulus localization. Furthermore, the pain experienced by human subjects during electrical stimulation of the PAG is referred to the central part of the body whereas that produced by stimulation in the lateral region of the midbrain containing the STT is referred to the contralateral side. Perhaps the SMT contributes more to the motivational-affective component of pain than to the sensory-discriminative component (cf., Melzack and Casey, 1968). A confounding problem is that electrical stimulation in the PAG can be expected to activate the collaterals of STT cells and thus provide an input to the lateral thalamus through an *axon reflex*.

Lamina I STT cells terminate in both lateral and medial parts of the thalamus. Specific targets include the VPL nucleus (at least in the monkey; Applebaum et al, 1979; Willis et al, 1979) and the nucleus submedius (at least in the cat; Craig and Burton, 1981).

The receptive field properties of the lamina I STT cells that project to the VPL nucleus appear to be suited to signal some of the sensory-discriminative aspects of pain, including stimulus location. The receptive fields of lamina I STT cells tend to be very small or small (Ferrington et al, 1987), and they appear to be somatotopically organized (Willis et al, 1974). The responses of lamina I STT cells to cutaneous stimulation are dominated by input from nociceptors. For example, most lamina I STT cells in the primate are activated strongly by intense compressive cutaneous stimuli (pinching the skin with a small arterial clip or squeezing the skin with serrated forceps) and only weakly or not at all by weak mechanical stimuli such as brushing. Similarly, most STT cells in lamina I respond to noxious heat and some to noxious cold (Ferrington et al, 1987). Lamina I STT cells are poorly entrained by vibratory stimuli and thus seem unlikely candidates to signal flutter (Ferrington et al, 1987).

Another probable function of lamina I STT cells is to signal thermal sensation. We have observed responses to cooling in at least 1 lamina I STT cell in the monkey (Ferrington et al, 1987); however, the same neuron was activated much more vigourously by noxious mechanical and thermal stimuli, and so we concluded that such cells were unlikely to contribute importantly to specific thermoreception (Ferrington et al, 1987). Craig and Kniffki (1985) found that some lamina I STT cells in the cat behaved like specific thermoreceptors, but more of these neurons projected towards the medial thalamus than to the lateral thalamus. It is possible that the target zone in the medial thalamus (or hypothalamus?) is involved in thermal regulation rather than thermal sensation.

The lamina I STT cells that project to the nucleus submedius are more likely to play a role in the motivational-affective than the sensory-discriminative aspects of pain, since the nucleus submedius projects to the orbitofrontal cortex, rather than to the somatosensory cortex (Craig et al, 1982).

A surprising recent finding is that the lamina I STT cells (at least of the cat and monkey; Apkarian et al, 1987; Jones et al, 1985; 1987) project to the thalamus by way of the dorsal part of the lateral funiculus (DLF), rather than through the ventral quadrant of the spinal cord, as had previously been believed. It will be of considerable interest to know if the lamina I SMT and STT cells in the human project through the DLF, since anterolateral cordotomies in patients are quite effective in relieving pain, at least for a period of months (Foerster and Gagel, 1932; White and Sweet, 1969), and often permanently, yet such lesions presumably would leave intact most or all of the projections of lamina I to the midbrain and thalamus. Conversely, a lesion that interrupted all of the spinal cord except for one anterolateral quadrant failed to disrupt pain sensation (Nordenboos and Wall, 1976). Behavioral evidence from experiments on rats (Peschanski, Kayser and Besson, 1986) and monkeys (Vierck and Luck, 1979) is consistent with the human clinical studies. Evidently, tracts ascending in the anterolateral quadrant are both necessary and sufficient for the mediation of pain in humans and possibly in rats and monkeys.

It is possible that pain relief might also be produced by a lesion of the DLF. Such a procedure is normally avoided in humans because of the presence of the lateral corticospinal tract in that quadrant. However, there is some evidence that a cordotomy extending into the DFL can produce analgesia (Moossy, Sagone and Rosomoff, 1967). Another consideration is the spinoreticular (SRT) tract in the anterolateral quadrant. Interruption of the SRT by anterolateral cordotomy might disrupt attentional and arousal mechanisms, producing much more of a deficit than that resulting just from loss of the components of the SMT and STT originating from deep layers of the dorsal horn (cf., Frommer, Trefz and Casey, 1977).

It is concluded that lamina I gives rise to a substantial fraction of the SMT and STT projections in the rat, cat and monkey. The physiological responses of these cells are consistent with the traditional view that these tracts contribute to the transmission of nociceptive (and thermoreceptive) information and that these cells are likely to be important for pain (and for thermal sensation and/or regulation). A special contribution by lamina I STT cells to stimulus localization is suggested by the small receptive fields of these neurons and a somatotopic organization.

ACKNOWLEDGEMENTS

The author thanks his colleagues for their contributions to the experiments done in his laboratory and described here, Grizelda Gonzales for her help with the illustrations and Margie Watson for typing the manuscript. The work in the author's laboratory was supported by NIH research grant NS 09743, program project grant NS 11255 and training grant NS 07185.

REFERENCES

APKARIAN, A.V., STEVENS, R.T. AND HODGE, C.J. (1987). The primate dorsolateral spinothalamic pathway. *Society for Neuroscience Abstracts* **13**, 580.

APPLEBAUM, A.E., LEONARD, R.B., KENSHALO, D.R., Jr., MARTIN, R.F. AND WILLIS, W.D. (1979). Nuclei in which functionally identified spinothalamic tract neurons terminate. *Journal of Comparative Neurology* **188**, 575-586.

BERKLEY, K.J. (1980). Spatial relationships between the terminations of somatic sensory and motor pathways in the rostral brainstem of cats and monkeys. I. Ascending somatic sensory inputs to lateral diencephalon. *Journal of Comparative Neurology* **193**, 283-317.

BJORKELAND, M. AND BOIVIE, J. (1984) The termination of spinomesencephalic fibers in cat, an experimental anatomical study. *Anatomy and Embryology* **170**, 265-277.

BOIVIE, J. (1971). The termination of the spinothalamic tract in the cat. An experimental study with silver impregnation methods. *Experimental Brain Research* **12**, 331-353.

BOIVIE, J. (1979). An anatomical reinvestigation of the termination of the spinothalamic tract in the monkey. *Journal of Comparative Neurology* **186**, 343-370.

BROWN, P.B. AND FUCHS, J.L. (1975). Somatotopic representation of hindlimb skin in cat dorsal horn. *Journal of Neurophysiology* **38**, 1-9.

CARSTENS, E. AND TREVINO, D.L. (1978). Laminar origins of spinothalamic projections in the cat as determined by the retrograde transport of horseradish peroxidase. *Journal of Comparative Neurology* **182**, 151-166.

CERVERO, F., IGGO, A. AND OGAWA, H. (1976). Nociceptor-driven dorsal horn neurones in the lumbar spinal cord of the cat. *Pain*, **2**, 5-24.

CHRISTENSEN, B.N. AND PERL, E.R. (1970). Spinal neurons excited by noxious or thermal stimuli, marginal zone of the dorsal horn. *Journal of Neurophysiology* **33**, 293-307.

CHUNG, J.M., SURMEIER, D.J., LEE, K.H., SORKIN, L.S., HONDA, C.N., TSONG, Y. AND WILLIS, W.D. (1986). Classification of primate spinothalamic and somatosensory thalamic neurons based on cluster analysis. *Journal of Neurophysiology* **56**, 308-327.

CRAIG, A.D. AND BURTON, H. (1981). Spinal and medullary lamina I projection to nucleus submedius in medial thalamus, a possible pain center. *Journal of Neurophysiology* **45**, 443-466.

CRAIG, A.D. AND BURTON, H. (1985). The distribution and topographical organization in the thalamus of anterogradely-transported horseradish peroxidase after spinal injections in cat and raccoon. *Experimental Brain Research* **58**, 227-254.

CRAIG, A.D. AND KNIFFKI, K.D. (1985). Spinothalamic lumbosacral lamina I cells responsive to skin and muscle stimulation in the cat. *Journal of Physiology* **365**, 197-221.

CRAIG, A.D., WIEGAND, S.J. AND PRICE, J.L. (1982). The thalamo-cortical projection of the nucleus submedius in the cat. *Journal of Comparative Neurology* **206**, 28-48.

DILLY, P.N., WALL, P.D. AND WEBSTER, K.E. (1968). Cells of origin of the spinothalamic tract in the cat and rat. *Experimental Neurology* **21**, 550-562.

FERRINGTON, D.G., SORKIN, L.S. AND WILLIS, W.D. (1987). Responses of spinothalamic tract cells in the superficial dorsal horn of the primate lumbar spinal cord. *Journal of Physiology* **388**, 681-703.

FOERSTER, O. AND GAGEL, O. (1932). Die Vorderseitenstrangdurchschneidung beim Menschen. Eine klinisch-patho-physiologisch-anatomische *Studie. Zeitschrift ges. Neurol. Psychiat.*, **138**, 1-92.

FROMMER, G.P., TREFZ, B.R. AND CASEY, K.L. (1977). Somatosensory function and cortical unit activity in cats with only dorsal column fibers. *Experimental Brain Research* **27**, 113-129.

GIESLER, G.J., MENÉTREY, D. AND BASBAUM, A.I. (1979). Differential origins of spinothalamic tract projections to medial and lateral thalamus in the rat. *Journal of Comparative Neurology* **184**, 107-126.

GIESLER, G.J., MENÉTREY, D., GUILBAUD, G. AND BESSON, J.M. (1976). Lumbar cord neurons at the origin of the spinothalamic tract in the rat. *Brain Research* **118**, 320-324.

HARMANN, P.A., CARLTON, S.M. AND WILLIS, W.D. (1988) Collaterals of spinothalamic tract cells to the periaqueductal gray, a fluorescent double-labelling study in the rat. *Brain Research* **441**, 87-97.

HAYES, N.L. AND RUSTIONI, A. (1980). Spinothalamic and spinomedullary neurons in macaques, a single and double retrograde tracer study. *Neuroscience*, **5**, 861-874.

HYLDEN, J.L.K., HAYASHI, H., DUBNER, R. AND BENNETT, G.J. (1986). Physiology and morphology of the lamina I spinomesencephalic projection. *Journal of Comparative Neurology* **247**, 505-515.

JONES, M.W., APKARIAN, A.V., STEVENS, R.T. AND HODGE, C.J. (1987). The spinothalamic tract, an examination of the cells of origin of the dorsolateral and ventral spinothalamic pathways in cats. *Journal of Comparative Neurology* **260**, 349-361.

JONES, M.W., HODGE, C.J., APKARIAN, A.V. AND STEVENS, R.T. (1985). A dorsolateral spinothalamic pathway in cat. *Brain Research* **335**, 188-193.

KEMPLAY, S.K. AND WEBSTER, K.E. (1986). A qualitative and quantitative analysis of the distributions of cells in the spinal cord and spinomedullary junction projecting to the thalamus of the rat. *Neuroscience*, **17**, 769-789.

KERR, F.W.L. (1975). The ventral spinothalamic tract and other ascending systems of the ventral funiculus of the spinal cord. *Journal of Comparative Neurology* **159**, 335-356.

LIU, R. (1983). Laminar origins of spinal projection neurons to the periaqueductal gray of the rat. *Brain Research* **264**, 118-122.

LUND, R.D. AND WEBSTER, K.E. (1967). Thalamic afferents from the spinal cord and trigeminal nuclei. An experimental anatomical study in the rat. *Journal of Comparative Neurology* **130**, 313-328.

MANTYH, P.W. (1982). The ascending input to the midbrain periaqueductal gray of the primate. *Journal of Comparative Neurology* **211**, 50-64.

MAYER, D.J. AND LIEBESKIND, J.C. (1974). Pain reduction by focal electrical stimulation of the brain, an anatomical and behavioral analysis. *Brain Research* **68**, 73-93.

MCMAHON, S.B. AND WALL, P.D. (1985). Electrophysiological mapping of brainstem projections of spinal cord lamina I cells in the rat. *Brain Research* **333**, 19-26.

MEHLER, W.R., FEFERMAN, M.E. AND NAUTA, W.J.H. (1960). Ascending axon degeneration following anterolateral cordotomy. An experimental study in the monkey. *Brain*, **83**, 718-751.

MELZACK, R. AND CASEY, K.L. (1968) Sensory, motivational, and central control determinants of pain. In, *The Skin Senses*, ed. Kenshalo, D.R., pp. 423-439. Springfield, Thomas.

MENÉTREY, D., CHAOUCH, A. AND BESSON, J.M. (1980). Location and properties of dorsal horn neurones at origin of spinoreticular tract in lumbar enlargement of the rat. *Journal of Neurophysiology* **44**, 862-877.

MENÉTREY, D., CHAOUCH, A., BINDER, D. AND BESSON, J.M. (1982). The origin of the spinomesencephalic tract in the rat, an anatomical study using the retrograde transport of horseradish peroxidase. *Journal of Comparative Neurology* **206**, 193-207.

MOOSSY, J., SAGONE, A. AND ROSOMOFF, H.L. (1967). Percutaneous radiofrequency cervical cordotomy, Pathologic anatomy. *Journal of Neuropathology and Experimental Neurology* **26**, 118.

NASHOLD, B.S., WILSON, W.P. AND SLAUGHTER, D.G. (1969). Sensations evoked by stimulation in the midbrain of man. *Journal of Neurosurgery* **30**, 14-24.

NASHOLD, B.S., WILSON, W.P. AND SLAUGHTER, D.G. (1974). The midbrain and pain. *Advances in Neurology* **4**, 191-196.

NOORDENBOS, W. AND WALL, P.D. (1976). Diverse sensory functions with an almost totally divided spinal cord. A case of spinal cord transection with preservation of part of one anterolateral quadrant. *Pain*, **2**, 185-195.

PESCHANSKI, M., KAYSER, V. AND BESSON, J.M. (1986). Behavioral evidence for a crossed ascending pathway for pain transmission in the anterolateral quadrant of the rat spinal cord. *Brain Research* **376**, 164-168.

PESCHANSKI, M., MANTYH, P.W. AND BESSON, J.M. (1983). Spinal afferents to the ventrobasal thalamic complex in the rat, an anatomical study using wheat-germ aaglutinin conjugated to horseradish peroxidase. *Brain Research* **278**, 240-244.

PRICE, D.D., HAYASHI, H., DUBNER, R. AND RUDA, M.A. (1979). Functional relationships between neurons of marginal and substantia gelatinosa layers of primate dorsal horn. *Journal of Neurophysiology* **42**, 1590-1608.

PRICE, D.D., HAYES, R.L., RUDA, M. AND DUBNER, R. (1978). Spatial and temporal transformations of input to spinothalamic tract neurons and their relation to somatic sensations. *Journal of Neurophysiology* **41**, 933-947.

REES, H. AND ROBERTS, M.H.T. (1987). Anterior pretectal stimulation alters the responses of spinal dorsal horn neurones to cutaneous stimulation in the rat. *Journal of Physiology* , **385**, 415-436.

REYNOLDS, D.V. (1969). Surgery in the rat during electrical analgesia induced by focal brain stimulation. *Science* **164**, 444-445.

SKULTETY, F.M. (1963). Stimulation of periaqueductal gray and hypothalamus. *Archives of Neurology* **8**, 608-620.

SPIEGEL, E.A., KLETZKIN, M. AND SZEKELY, E.G. (1954). Pain reactions upon stimulation of the tectum mesencephali. *Journal of Neuropathology and Experimental Neurology* **13**, 212-220.

SURMEIER, D.J., HONDA, C.N. AND WILLIS, W.D. (1988). Natural groupings of primate spinothalamic neurons based upon cutaneous stimulation. Physiological and anatomical features. *Journal of Neurophysiology* **59**, 833-860.

SWETT, J.E., McMAHON, S.B. AND WALL, P.D. (1985). Long ascending projections to the midbrain from cells of lamina I and nucleus of the dorsolateral funiculus of the rat spinal cord. *Journal of Comparative Neurology* **238**, 401-416.

TREVINO, D.L. (1976). The origin and projections of a spinal nociceptive and thermoreceptive pathway. In *Sensory Functions of the Skin in Primates, With Special Reference to Man*, ed. Zotterman, Y., pp. 367-376. Oxford, Pergamon Press.

TREVINO, D.L. AND CARSTENS, E. (1975). Confirmation of the location of spinothalamic neurons in the cat and monkey by the retrograde transport of horseradish peroxidase. *Brain Research* **98**, 177-182.

TREVINO, D.L., COULTER, J.D. AND WILLIS, W.D. (1973). Location of cells of origin of spinothalamic tract in lumbar enlargement of the monkey. *Journal of Neurophysiology* **36**, 750-761.

VIERCK, C.J. AND LUCK, M.M. (1979). Loss and recovery of reactivity to noxious stimuli in monkeys with primary spinothalamic cordotomies, followed by secondary and tertiary lesions of other cord sectors. *Brain* **102**, 233-248.

WHITE, J.C. AND SWEET, W.H. (1969). *Pain and the Neurosurgeon*. Springfield, Thomas.

WIBERG, M. AND BLOMQVIST, A. (1984). The spinomesencephalic tract in the cat, its cells of origin and termination pattern as demonstrated by the intraaxonal transport method. *Brain Research* **291**, 1-18.

WIBERG, M., WESTMAN, J. AND BLOMQVIST, A. (1987). Somatosensory projection to the mesencephalon, an anatomical study in the monkey. *Journal of Comparative Neurology* **264**, 92-117.

WILLIS, W.D. (1985) *The Pain System. The Neural Basis of Nociceptive Transmission in the Mammalian Nervous System*, 347 pp. Basel, Karger.

WILLIS, W.D. AND COGGESHALL, R.E. (1978). *Sensory Mechanisms of the Spinal Cord*, 485 pp. New York, Plenum Press.

WILLIS, W.D., KENSHALO, D.R., Jr. AND LEONARD, R.B. (1979). The cells of origin of the primate spinothalamic tract. *Journal of Comparative Neurology* **188**, 543-574.

WILLIS, W.D., TREVINO, D.L., COULTER, J.D. AND MAUNZ, R.A. (1974). Responses of primate spinothalamic tract neurons to natural stimulation of hindlimb. *Journal of Neurophysiology* **37**, 358-372.

YEZIERSKI, R.P. (1988). Spinomesencephalic tract, projections from the lumbosacral spinal cord of the rat, cat, and monkey. *Journal of Comparative Neurology* **267**, 131-146.

YEZIERSKI, R.P. AND SCHWARZ, R.H. (1986). Response and receptive-field properties of spinomesencephalic tract cells in the cat. *Journal of Neurophysiology* **55**, 76-96.

YEZIERSKI, R.P., SORKIN, L.S. AND WILLIS, W.D. (1987). Response properties of spinal neurons projecting to midbrain or midbrain-thalamus in the monkey. *Brain Research* **437**, 165-170.

ZEMLAN, F.P., LEONARD, C.M., KOW, L.M. AND PFAFF, D.W. (1978). Ascending tracts of the lateral columns of the rat spinal cord, a study using the silver impregnation and horseradish peroxidase techniques. *Experimental Neurology* **62**, 298-334.

ZHANG, D., CARLTON, S.M., SORKIN, L.S., HARMANN, P.A. AND WILLIS, W.D. (1987). Collaterals of spinothalamic tract (STT) neurons to the PAG, a double labelling study in the monkey. *Society for Neuroscience Abstracts* **13**, 113.

DISCUSSION ON SECTION III

Rapporteur: Jens Schouenborg

Department of Physiology and Biophysics, University of Lund, Sölvegatan 19, S-223 62
Lund, Sweden

In this session some of the recent advances regarding the highly divergent output from the superficial dorsal horn (laminae I-II) were reviewed. In addition, several new findings on the morphology and the development of the projection neurones were reported.

DEVELOPMENT OF PROJECTION NEURONES

Beal showed that, in the rat, projection neurones in laminae I-II are generally formed prior to the intrinsic non projection neurones and that they mature earlier than them. Immature laminae I-II projection neurones and non projection lamina I neurones have short dendritic trees that grow simply by elongation and thus look like miniatures of their adult form. By contrast, intrinsic non projection neurones in lamina II appear to pass through an intermediate starshaped stage before developing into one of the several different types of lamina II neurones. It has recently been shown by Fitzgerald (1985) that in the rat the C fibre terminals and the response properties of nociceptive dorsal horn neurones mature during the first postnatal week. A pertinent question raised by Woolf was therefore whether there is a relationship between the maturation of dendrites in laminae I-II and the ingrowth and maturation of primary afferent fibre terminals. Beal responded that this is not the case for projection neurones, but probably is for intrinsic non projection neurones.

Hunt questioned whether the lamination of the superficial dorsal horn could be distinguished in the prenatal rat. Beal answered that it is difficult to distinguish the dorsal border of lamina II in such rats whereas lamina III neurones can be identified.

Iggo inquired about the proportion of projection and non projection neurones in laminae I-II. Beal answered that probably less than 1% of lamina II neurones are projection neurones, whereas about 50% of lamina I neurones are.

MORPHOLOGICAL AND NEUROCHEMICAL SPECIFICITY OF LAMINA I PROJECTION NEURONES

Coimbra and Lima have previously described four types of lamina I neurones in the rat, on the basis of their three-dimensional structure: fusiform, multipolar, flattened and pyramidal cells. These different types of neurones are partly segregated within lamina I. Coimbra reported that these morphologically different types of neurones have partly different projections to the brain, as revealed by retrograde labelling with choleratoxin subunit B. These neurones also contain different neurotransmitters (GABA, met-enkephalin or substance P). The finding that there are distinct classes of neurones in lamina I have different projections and transmitter substances suggests that the function of lamina I neurones is related to their morphology. However, it should be kept in mind that previous attempts by different laboratories to correlate the morphology of lamina I neurones with their classification (based on their cutaneous input) have not been successful (i.e. when using the Wide Dynamic Range (WDR) or Nociceptive Specific (NS) terminology which was the most frequently used in the workshop).

The finding that some of the projection neurones contain GABA or met-enkephalin in their cell bodies, prompted a comment by Duggan regarding the previous lack of reports on long ascending inhibitory paths from the spinal cord. Hunt cautioned that the results of Coimbra and Lima did not necessarily reflect the transmitter content in the axonal terminals, only that the cell bodies contain these substances. Perl further suggested that GABA might be contained in the dendritic vesicles that are known to exist in some lamina I neurones. However, it should be remembered that inhibitory spinoreticular paths to the lateral reticular nucleus have previously been demonstrated, by Ekerot and Oscarsson (1975).

Basbaum inquired about the relative efficiency of choleratoxin subunit B as a retrograde tracer as compared to horseradish peroxidase. Coimbra replied that choleratoxin subunit B is transported better. It also retrogradely fills dendritic branches of up to the third or fourth order, thus allowing a classification of the morphological types of the projection neurones. Coimbra also mentioned that choleratoxin subunit B is transported trans-synaptically in the anterograde direction, but apparently not in the retrograde direction.

PROPRIOSPINAL PROJECTIONS

Steedman reported that some of the lamina II neurones do project to ventral laminae, possibly to deeply located WDR neurones. Thus this ventral projection could be part of the nocifensive spinal reflex circuits or of other segmental reflex circuits (Schouenborg and Sjölund, 1983).

PROJECTIONS FROM LAMINA I TO THE RETICULAR FORMATION OF THE MEDULLA OBLONGATA

In a poster Coimbra and Lima demonstrated a novel projection from lamina I, mainly through the ipsilateral dorsal funiculus, to the bulbar reticular nuclei located just ventral to the dorsal column nuclei. The physiological properties of this pathway were not studied.

PROJECTIONS FROM LAMINA I TO THE MIDBRAIN AND THE THALAMUS

Willis reviewed the results from his research group on the characteristics of the projection in the macaque monkey from lamina I to midbrain nuclei and to the ventral posterior thalamic nuclei. The spinothalamic and spinomesencephalic lamina I neurones studied by Willis and associates had much higher conduction velocities than those reported in similar systems in the cat by Craig and Kniffki and by Hylden and collaborators (this volume). Furthermore, a much larger percentage of the spinothalamic neurones reported by Willis were WDR neurones as compared to the situation in the cat. These discrepancies prompted a discussion on what possible sources of bias there might be. Willis suggested that the relatively large glass micropipettes containing a carbon microfilament used in his studies might have biased the sample against larger neurones. Furthermore the stimulus pulse should be longer than that used; in spontaneously active neurones the antidromic spike might be missed due to collision; and there might be failure of antidromic invasion at branch points.

A further possible explanation for the discrepancies between the results is related to the well known differences in the organization of the spinothalamic tracts between the monkey and the cat. In his presentation, Kniffki mentioned that the projection from lumbosacral lamina I is to the ventral periphery of the ventrobasal nucleus in the cat, whereas the lamina I projection in the monkey is known to be to the central core of the ventrobasal nucleus. Neurones in the ventral periphery of the ventrobasal nucleus were found by Kniffki to project to area 3a in the cat, whereas neurones in the central core of the ventrobasal nucleus are known to project to cortex area 3b/1 in the monkey. Hence, it is possible that the lamina I projections to the lateral thalamus in the cat and monkey are not functionally equivalent.

ON THE DIVERGENCE OF LAMINA I PROJECTIONS

It has been demonstrated previously that some spinothalamic neurones issue axon collaterals to nuclei in the medulla oblongata or in the midbrain (cf. Kevetter and Willis, 1983). Hylden and associates now reported that in the rat an average of 80% of lamina I spinothalamic neurones give off collaterals to the midbrain nuclei parabrachialis, n. cuneiformis and the periaqueductal grey; conversely up to 50% of the lamina I neurones projecting to these midbrain nuclei also project to the thalamus. The degree of collateralization revealed by the study of Hylden et al is much higher than was known previously. It can be concluded that the same nociceptive information is distributed to many nuclei.

ON THE FUNCTION OF LAMINA I PROJECTION NEURONES

The ventrolateral funiculi have long been assumed to contain the most important ascending nociceptive path, mainly because of the profound analgesia which, in humans, follows ventrolateral cordotomy. It is generally agreed that lamina I NS neurones are involved in distributing specific nociceptive information to many supraspinal nuclei. However, it has recently been claimed that lamina I spinomesencephalic and spinothalamic neurones project mainly through the *dorsolateral* funiculus in the rat, cat and monkey (Jones et al, 1985a,b; Hylden et al, this volume), a pathway which is not considered necessary for conscious discrimination of noxious stimuli in humans. For this reason it was suggested by Hylden that these NS neurones are involved in aspects of pain mechanisms other than sensory discriminative, such as autonomic, affective or modulatory mechanisms. Nevertheless, Willis suggested that the lamina I neurones projecting to the ventrobasal thalamic nucleus do indeed subserve the sensory discriminative aspects of pain, whereas the projection to the midbrain might be involved in many different functions, for a variety of responses can be evoked by electrical stimulation of this area. Willis pointed out that cordotomy interrupts several ascending nociceptive tracts such as spinoreticular paths. This could alter the control exerted by brainstem nuclei on the activity of the remaining ascending nociceptive paths so that it is difficult to assess the function of the remaining ascending nociceptive paths under these conditions. Furthermore, following a cordotomy in humans pain sensitivity often returns after a variable interval of months to years, indicating alternative ascending paths for nociception. Cervero also recalled that lesions of the dorsolateral funiculus interrupt several *descending* inhibitory systems, thereby changing the level of activity in other ascending nociceptive paths.

Wall suggested in a later session that NS neurones are part of an antinociceptive system and that they do not contribute directly to nociception. However, since many lamina I neurones project to several nuclei in the medulla, midbrain and thalamus, it can be inferred that a given NS neurone is capable of participating in several different functions.

ON THE THERMAL INFORMATION CARRIED TO THE THALAMUS

It was noted by Kniffki that in the population of primate spinothalamic neurones presented by Willis there were no cold-specific neurones among those projecting to the ventrobasal nucleus: this was similar to his own findings in the cat. Kniffki further suggested that such a projection in the primate might be to medial thalamic nuclei, as was found in the cat.

PROJECTIONS TO THE HYPOTHALAMUS AND TELENCEPHALIC NUCLEI

Giesler and associates have recently found, in the rat, a direct projection to the medial and lateral hypothalamus, the septal nuclei, the n. accumbens and the basal forebrain from lamina I and more ventral laminae in the spinal cord. Studies using retrograde tracer techniques in the rat revealed that some 10,000 neurones projected to this area of the brain from the spinal cord; of these some 10% originated in lamina I. Twenty-eight spinohypothalamic tract (SHT) neurones had been characterized with regard to their cutaneous input; about 75% were WDR neurones and 10% were NS neurones. Since many of the SHT neurones originated in areas of the spinal cord receiving a visceral input Cervero pointed out that a possible visceral input to these SHT neurones should be investigated. Giesler suggested that since the target nuclei of these projections are believed to participate in the expression of a large number of emotional behaviours, some of these projections may participate in the generation of the emotional aspects of pain.

In summary, neurones in the superficial dorsal horn project to spinal as well as numerous supraspinal regions. It is clear that these projection neurones are heterogeneous with regard to morphology and function, although a large proportion of them appear to transmit specific nociceptive information. The significance of the highly divergent projections from lamina I is probably related to the complex motor and autonomic responses, as well as to the complex sensory and emotional experiences, which may be evoked by noxious stimulation of the body.

ACKNOWLEDGEMENTS

Supported by Swedish Medical Research Council (Project no.8138) and the Medical Faculty of Lund, Sweden.

REFERENCES

EKEROT, C.-F. AND OSCARSSON, O.(1975) Inhibitory spinal paths to the lateral reticular nucleus. *Brain Research* **99**, 157-161.

FITZGERALD, M.(1985) The post-natal development of cutaneous afferent fibre input and receptive field organization in the rat dorsal horn. *Journal of Physiology* **364**, 1-18.

JONES, M.W., APKARIAN, A.V., STEVENS, R.T., AND HODGE, C.J. Jr.(1985a) A dorsolateral spinothalamic pathway in squirrel monkey. *Society of Neuroscience Abstracts* **11**, 577.

JONES, M.W., HODGE, C.J. Jr., APKARIAN, A.V. AND STEVENS, R.T.(1985b) A dorsolateral spinothalamic pathway in cat. *Brain Research* **335**, 188-193.

KEVETTER, G.A. AND WILLIS, W.D. (1983) Collaterals of spinothalamic cells in the rat. *Journal of Comparative Neurology* **215**, 453-464.

SCHOUENBORG, J. AND SJÖLUND, B.H. (1983) Activity evoked by A- and C-afferent fibers in rat dorsal horn and its relation to a flexion reflex. *Journal of Neurophysiology* **50**, 1108-1121.

SECTION IV

DEVELOPMENT AND PLASTICITY IN THE SUPERFICIAL DORSAL HORN

INTRODUCTION TO SECTION IV

Allan Basbaum

Department of Anatomy and Physiology, University of California San Francisco,
San Francisco, CA 94143, USA

WHAT DO WE MEAN BY PLASTICITY?

In the following several articles, different examples of plasticity within the spinal cord will be presented. In most cases, what will be described are changes that follow various types of nerve injury. Although the observations are not questioned, and the evidence of plasticity is impressive, several questions must be asked: What is the relevance of such plastic changes to the animal? Must the resultant changes be beneficial or do they merely indicate that changes occur in the presence of relatively significant injury? Does plasticity include all examples in which central nervous system connections are altered? What are the general principles of nervous system function that can be learned from an analysis of the modifiability of nervous system connections? For example, does the process of plasticity that is observed in the dorsal horn recapitulate developmental processes?

If it were demonstrated that the changes observed could compensate for the damage that was produced by the original injury, then we would clearly have gone beyond phenomenology. There is no question, for example, that the size of the representation of digits changes after peripheral nerve section or after digit amputation (Merzenich *et al*, 1983). The changes that occur are orderly; that suggests that the reorganization is not random. But what does the animal experience as a result of this reorganization, and is it an adaptive reorganization? One possibility is that we are dealing with phenomena that come into play not so much after injury, but perhaps during development and learning. Merzenich and colleagues have, in fact, proposed that the generation of somatotopic, topographic maps reflects use-dependent development of connections. Their studies of the consequences of fusing two digits are particularly instructive; they indicate that the temporal and spatial coincidence of stimuli on the two fingers results in the appearance of cells in the somatosensory cortex which have receptive fields that span the two digits. Importantly, cells with receptive fields on both digits persisted for a period after the fingers were separated (Clark *et al*, 1988). These results are quite different from our own studies which demonstrated that cells developed dual receptive fields (on the flank and toe) when the large expanse of tissue between the fields was removed by deafferentation (Basbaum and Wall, 1976). Clearly the flank and toe are not used in unison. Based on those results it appears to be possible that much more aberrant, non-adaptive reorganization, can occur after very extensive injury.

These comments do not bear on the mechanisms that underlie the reorganization that has been demonstrated in many parts of the somatosensory system. Perhaps the two most significant questions are the time course of the changes and the relative contribution of anatomical reorganization *vs* physiological strengthening of pre-existing contacts. The anatomical question is difficult to resolve. Collateral sprouting clearly exists, but over what distances the changes can occur is not established. Local reorganization of synaptic contacts is probably a more common occurrence; for example, when the peripheral branches of the axons are cut, there are significant cytochemical changes in the terminals of primary afferent fibers in the superficial dorsal horn (Tessler *et al*, 1984). To what extent anatomical reorganization underlies the physiological changes that have been seen is, however, not known. The alternative hypothesis is that the modification of the strength of pre-existing connections is critical in the reorganization. In particular it has been suggested that regulation of GABAergic inhibitory controls may result in rapid changes in receptive field sizes (Dykes *et al*, 1984). Recent studies have indicated that there are remarkably large numbers of GABAergic synapses at all levels of the neuraxis; we have counted percentages of immunoreactive GABA boutons in the midbrain periaqueductal gray and the medullary nucleus raphe magnus and have found that up to forty per cent are GABAergic (Cho, Reichling and Basbaum, unpublished observations). Thus the data indicating that bicuculline iontophoresis can produce immediate shifts in receptive fields sizes are not surprising. There would be a very significant loss of GABAergic inhibitory controls that contribute to the size of receptive fields.

In summary, plasticity can mean different things to different people. Documenting the modifiability of central nervous system connections is just the first step; our goal must be to understand the significance of reorganization capabilities.

REFERENCES

BASBAUM, A.I. AND WALL, P.D. (1976) Chronic changes in the response of cells in adult cat dorsal horn following partial deafferentation: The appearance of responding cells in a previously non-responsive region. *Brain Research*, **116**, 181-204.

CLARK, S.A., ALLARD, T., JENKINS, W.M. AND MERZENICH, M.M. (1988) Receptive fields in the body-surface map in adult cortex defined by temporally correlated inputs. *Nature*, **332**, 444-445.

DYKES, R.W., LANDRY, P., METHERATE, R. AND HICKS, T.P. (1984) Functional role of GABA in cat primary somatosensory cortex or anesthetized or paralyzed cats and rats. *Brain Research*, **440**, 133-143.

MERZENICH, M.M., KAAS, J.H., WALL, J.T., NELSON, R.J., SUR, M. AND FELLEMAN, D. (1983) Topographic reorganization of somatosensory cortical areas 3b and 1 in adult monkeys following restricted deafferentation. *Neuroscience* **8**, 33-55.

TESSLER, A., HIMES, B.T., SOPER, K., MURRAY, M., GOLDBERGER, M.E. AND REICHLIN, S. (1984) Recovery of substance P but not somatostatin in the cat spinal cord after unilateral lumbosacral dorsal rhizotomy: a quantitative study, *Brain Research*, **305**, 95-102.

THE SIGNIFICANCE OF PLASTIC CHANGES IN LAMINA 1 SYSTEMS

Stephen B. McMahon and Patrick D. Wall

Sherrington School of Physiology, St. Thomas's Hospital Medical School, London SE1
and Department of Anatomy and Developmental Biology, University College London,
London WC1E 6BT, U.K.

There has been, for very good reasons, a growing interest in the cells of lamina 1 ever since 1970 when Christensen and Perl identified the lamina as the site of a particularly high concentration of nociceptive specific cells. The interest has been further increased by the confirmation of the area as the site of termination of fine afferents, as the site of many powerful chemicals and as the site of origin of large projecting systems. These discoveries have led to precise proposals on the function of the nociceptive specific cells in relation to pain. Perl (1985) writes: *In my view, selective nocireceptive projections have much to do with both the recognition and localization of tissue-damaging stimuli as pain sensation.* It is further proposed that these cells represent a stable component of the nocireceptive projections. Laird and Cervero have emphasised altered responsiveness of multireceptive deep dorsal horn cells following noxious stimulation and concluded: *This shows fundamental differences in the processing of nociceptive information by Multireceptive and Nocireceptive cells* (Laird and Cervero, 1988) and: *These results suggest that the system of the nocireceptive neurones in the superficial dorsal horn is functionally hard-wired* (Cervero and Laird, 1988). These statements with which many other workers agree, are clearly of considerable practical importance as well as being summaries of experimental observations. They therefore deserve particularly careful examination. This paper will review the available data and will conclude that the quoted statements are too strong and that alternative proposals should be entertained.

RESPONSE CHARACTERISTICS OF LAMINA 1 CELLS

These responses are listed in Table I in order of the percent nociceptive specific cells discovered.

All those authors agree that lamina 1 contains large numbers of nocireceptive specific cells and small numbers, or no cells, which respond only to light mechanical stimuli. However, it is apparent that these and other authors report a rather wide scatter of the proportion of nociceptive specific cells discovered in individual types of experiments. A detailed examination of the papers reveals no obvious reason for this scatter. It is clearly not possible to discuss this problem from the results of those authors who, for their own good reasons, have selected cells with particular response properties. In the crucial source paper which triggered this subject, Christensen and

Perl (1970) intentionally rejected those cells which responded to A-β afferents and those cells which habituated. If that criterion had been applied to the rat lamina I projection cells recorded by McMahon and Wall (1983) 45% of the cells would have been rejected. Most of the authors report on all of the observed cells in their particular conditions and yet there remains considerable variation in the same species with the same projection target.

TABLE I

Animal	Projection	No	LT	% WDR	NS	Authors
Cat	Thalamus	218	0	0.5	99.5	Craig and Kniffki, 1985
Cat	PBA and Thalamus	58	0	9	91	Light et al, 1988
Cat	PBA and Thalamus	163	2	10	88	Hylden et al, 1986
Monkey	ALQ at C1	14	0	14	86	Price et al, 1975
Cat	15% to C2	95	0	24	76	Hylden et al, 1987
Cat	Not tested	46	0	24	76	Cervero et al, 1976
Cat	Not tested	10	20	20	60	Light et al, 1986
Cat	Not tested	12	8	33	58	Cervero, 1983
Monkey	Thalamus	255	0	45	55	Willis, 1988
Cat	Not tested	54	15	33	52	Cervero and Tattersall, 1987
Rat	Not tested	151	0	49	51	Woolf and Fitzgerald, 1983
Monkey	Thalamus	15	0	53	47	Price et al, 1978
Monkey	Thalamus	21	0	57	43	Ferrington et al, 1987
Rat	DLF at C2	35	3	54	43	McMahon and Wall, 1983
Rat	DLF at C2	101	4	53	40	McMahon and Wall, 1984
Monkey	Midbrain and Thalamus	15	0	87	13	Yezierski et al, 1987
Cat	Not tested	84	Selected, some warm, most NS			Christensen and Perl, 1970

Abbreviations: ALQ = Anterolateral quadrant of the spinal cord. DLF = dorsolateral funiculus. LT = low threshold only. NS = nocireceptive specific. PBA = parabrachial area. WDR = wide dynamic range.

It is of course very likely that cells which project to a particular target differ from those which do not. For example, Craig and Kniffki (1985) who find the highest proportion of nociceptive specific cells projecting from lamina 1 to cat thalamus, report a large number of non-projecting cells as having responses to low intensity as well as to high intensity stimuli, i.e. WDR cells. However an inspection of types of stimuli, of species, of targets or of recording methods fails to reveal a single factor which explains the various results. It is true that most preparations were anaesthetised and that this factor can bias the response in both directions. Light anaesthesia can decrease inhibition so that some mechanoreceptive cells now respond to a nociceptive input (Collins and Ren, 1987). Further anaesthesia might again decrease the effective input and it could be that cells that are wide dynamic range under light anaesthesia (Dickhaus et al, 1985) become nociceptor specific under conditions of medium anaesthesia.

It is possible that further work will reveal among the various results that a population of hard-wired, line-labelled, dedicated projection cells exist. However we must also examine the alternative possibility that the response properties of these cells are variable and depend on the circumstances under which individual cells are examined. It is the evidence for this plasticity of response which we will now report.

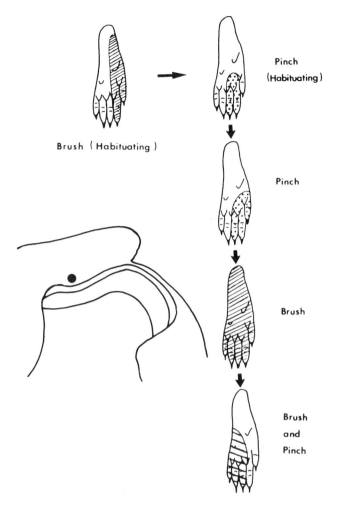

FIGURE 1: Spontaneous variation of response properties. A cell close to lamina 1 as indicated in the diagram changed the modality of its response and the size of its receptive field during a period of repeated testing in a decerebrate rat. Reproduced by permission from Woolf and Fitzgerald, 1983.

PLASTICITY OF RESPONSE CHARACTERISTICS OF LAMINA I CELLS

A. Spontaneous

Dubuisson *et al*, (1979) noticed that the size of receptive fields of superficial dorsal horn cells changed slowly on repeated examination over periods of minutes. These amoeboid receptive fields could expand or contract or oscillate. It is crucial to recognize that this phenomenon and most of the samples of plasticity which we shall report only occur in unanaesthetised preparations. Units were examined in unanaesthetised decerebrate cat superficial dorsal horn and their receptive fields were found to vary. Then anaesthesia was induced (30mg/kg pentobarbitone I.V.) and each unit contracted its receptive field which then remained stable over a subsequent 30 min observation period. Anaesthesia can induce the appearance of hard wiring.

Woolf and Fitzgerald (1983) examined this phenomenon in detail using rat decerebrate spinal unanaesthetised preparations to investigate lamina I cells, some identified by intracellular markers. 10 of 72 neurones showed spontaneous variations of their receptive fields not only in terms of area but also of modality. In an illustrated example in this paper, a lamina 1 cell varied over minutes from a nociceptive specific cell which habituated to a cell which responded to brush only to a wide dynamic range cell (Fig. 1). It could be claimed that such results could only be obtained if the recording electrode wandered from one cell to another. In this particular cell, the variation was observed while holding the single cell intracellularly and subsequently marking it. In all cases, the spike shape was monitored throughout to avoid the possibility of recording from different cells.

B. Evoked by peripheral stimulation

Unhappy about the apparently *spontaneous* nature of the variation we set about

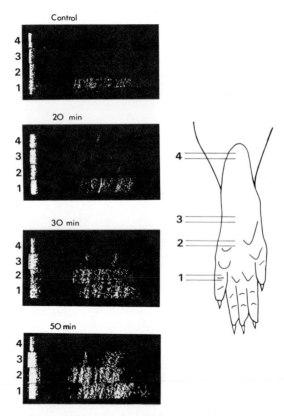

FIGURE 2: Injury induced changes in the responses of a rat lamina 1 cell projecting to C-2 in a decerebrate animal. Four *raster* dot displays each showing the responses of the same unit to percutaneous electrical stimulation applied to four different skin sites (shown on the right hand side of the figure). The responses are shown before (top panel) and at successive times (lower panel) after the creation of a punctate burn between electrodes 3 and 4. In these raster dot displays, each dot represents the occurrence of an action potential and its position on the X axis gives its timing relative to the electrical stimulus, which occurred at the extreme left of the trace. Responses to successive stimuli at 0.2 Hz are shown higher in the figure. The sweep duration was 450 msec. The receptive field was initially limited to the toes but after the injury it slowly expanded to include the lateral and proximal foot. Long latency (C input) responses emerged at some time after the injury. Reproduced with permission from McMahon and Wall, 1984.

seeking what controlled it other than anaesthesia which abolished the variability. Following early observations by Dubuisson (1981) we suspected that injury placed at a considerable distance from the receptive field of a cell might be one way to influence receptive fields (McMahon and Wall, 1984). The cells examined were lumbar lamina I cells projecting in the DLF to C2 in decerebrate rats. Punctate burns were made 5-15 mm distant to the boundaries of the receptive fields. There was a slow increase in the excitability of the cells as seen by an enlargement of receptive field towards the lesion, a decreased mechanical threshold and an increased responsiveness to transcutaneous electrical stimulation applied with needle electrodes both inside and outside the receptive field (Fig. 2). These changes were first seen about 10 minutes after the injury and persisted. Local anaesthetic injected at the site of the injury produced only a partial and slow reversal of the excitability increases. 15 of the 20 cells treated expanded their receptive fields towards the burn and 11 decreased their von Frey hair threshold. Even under anaesthesia, Cervero and Laird (1988) report a small increase in receptive field size in 5 of 10 nociceptive specific neurons after noxious mechanical stimulation. They also state: *This contrasts with the known properties of multireceptive neurones which have initially large receptive fields that can increase in size twofold after noxious stimulation (Cervero et al, 1984; Cook et al, 1987).* Wishing to gain more control over the input which evoked these changes in lamina I cells we turned to a phenomenon of long latency long duration heterosynaptic increased excitability which had been described initially by Woolf (1983) and later by Wall and Woolf (1984). Specifically it had been found that 20 C-fibre strength stimuli at 1Hz applied to the nerve to gastrocnemius but not when applied to the sural nerve would evoke a long term enhancement of spinal cord excitability. It had been found that this increased excitability was not produced by changes in afferent fibres or in motoneurones (Cook *et al*, 1986). It was therefore of considerable interest to examine changes in dorsal horn interneurones including lamina I cells which projected in the contralateral DLF to C2 (Cook *et al*, 1987). When and only when C fibres were included in the afferent conditioning volley from the nerve to gastrocnemius, the response of lamina I cells was facilitated for a long period. The receptive fields of the tested cells were on the feet of the rats and did not involve the gastrocnemius from which the conditioning volley was generated. The receptive field size of the lamina I cells expanded to reach a maximum of double the original size about 15 minutes after the 20 second conditioning volley. The expanded receptive fields declined to their preconditioned size after about 55 minutes. In three of ten neurons that originally responded only to noxious cutaneous mechanical stimulation, the gastrocnemius-soleus conditioning stimulus altered their responsiveness so that they began to respond to low threshold (brush and touch) stimuli as well (Fig. 3). It is apparent that lamina I cells may signal new locations and types of stimuli towards the brain after brief and distant conditioning stimuli.

There are several chapters in this book which report changes of chemistry (such as of C-fos and endogenous opioid and other peptide levels) and changes of physiology with peripheral stimuli with peripheral nerve lesions and with induced arthritis.

C. Evoked by stimulation of descending impulses

We have examined the effect of stimulating descending fibres in the ipsilateral dorsolateral funiculus (DLF) on the response of projecting lamina I cells (McMahon and Wall, 1988).

In agreement with the results of Cervero and Wolstencroft, (1984); Dubuisson and Wall,(1980); Haber *et al*, (1980); Giesler *et al*, (1981); and Tattersall *et al*, (1986), we

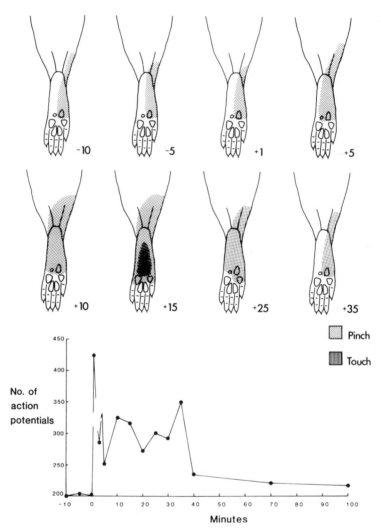

FIGURE 3: Response variation induced in lamina 1 projecting cells by peripheral conditioning stimuli. A lamina 1 cell projecting to C2 was recorded in a decerebrate rat. The pinch-only receptive field was tested at -10 and -5 minutes before a 20s 1Hz A and C fibre conditioning stimulus was applied at time 0 to the nerve to the gastrocnemius muscle. The subsequent changes in the receptive field size and in the effective stimulus are shown at 1, 5, 10, 15, 25 and 35 min after the twenty second conditioning volley. The receptive field expanded and the nociceptive specific cell became a wide dynamic range cell. The lower graph shows the total number of impulses evoked in the cell by a standardised mild pressure stimulus before and after the conditioning volley. Reproduced by permission from Cook *et al*, 1987.

found both excitatory and inhibitory effects of descending volleys. The result of brief trains of DLF stimuli (0.5 or 2 sec at 50Hz) are presented in Table II.

TABLE II

	Excitation % Duration	Inhibition % Duration	No Effect %
Ongoing Activity	36 5-300s	12 4-25s	52
Peripherally Evoked Responses	38 10-300s	54 5-25s	34

	Enlarged % Duration	Decreased % Duration	No Effect %
Receptive Fields	30 <300s	6 <240s	64

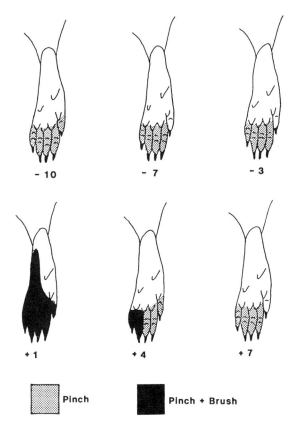

FIGURE 4: Increased excitability of a lamina 1 projecting cell provoked by stimulation of descending volleys. A lamina 1 cell was recorded in a decerebrate rat; it projected in the contralateral DLF to C2. The receptive field was repeatedly tested as shown -10, -7 and -3 minutes and was found to be nociceptive specific. Then a 50Hz 2 second stimulus was applied through a microelectrode in the ipsilateral DLF. At +1 and +4 minutes after the descending conditioning 20 second stimulus, the receptive field had expanded and the cell had been converted from a nociceptive specific unit to one responding to a wide range of pressure stimuli. Reproduced with permission from McMahon and Wall,1988.

The major short-term effect of DLF stimulation on lamina I cells was inhibitory. In contrast, there were long latency long duration effects which were predominantly facilitatory. The cells with expanded receptive fields showed the effect for 2-5 minutes and the area increase was more than 100%. In half of these cells the pressure thresholds for excitation dropped so that nociceptive specific cells became wide dynamic range cells as is shown in Fig. 4.

D. Evoked by block of tonic descending control pathways

In a decerebrate animal, the brain stem generates a steady descending barrage which affects the excitability of spinal cord cells. The effect of this barrage on the excitability of 10 lamina I cells was tested by blocking the cord at C2 (McMahon and Wall, 1988). Three cells were unaffected and 2 increased their excitability. However, 5 became less excitable with a reduction of the receptive field area and of their response to pressure stimuli. Fig. 5 shows an example of such a cell which was converted from a wide dynamic range cell to a nociceptive specific cell. In 3 of these 5 cells, the reduction of excitability was so strong that their normal response to electrical stimulation of C fibres disappeared completely.

E. Evoked by peripheral nerve lesions

As reported elsewhere in this book, Hylden et al, (1987) showed that some cat lamina I cells change their receptive fields after chronic sciatic nerve section. We had previously examined this phenomenon in deeper cells in cat and rat (Devor and Wall, 1981a, 1981b) and furthermore had shown that many of these centrally induced changes could be attributed to the effect on C fibres alone (Wall et al, 1982). Since the lamina I cells are in particularly close proximity to C fibre central terminations and since the C fibres appeared to have a particularly strong effect on receptive fields after peripheral lesions, we thought it would be most informative to study the effect of C-fibre selective capsaicin lesions rather than the effect of cutting whole nerves. This was done by soaking the sciatic and saphenous nerves of adult rats with capsaicin and then, after 14 days, examining the receptive field properties of lamina I projection cells (McMahon et al, 1984). The results are shown in Table III.

The results contain a number of surprises which suggest that C fibres have central effects beyond the classical excitation of central cells. There was no problem in identifying lamina I cells in normal and capsaicin treated animals by antidromic invasion of their cell bodies by impulses originating from their projecting axons. By comparing the frequency of encountering such cells in normal and in unilaterally capsaicin treated animals, there appeared to be no change in the frequency of cells. However there were gross changes in the properties of the cells which had been chronically deprived of their C input. In the normal animals, 12% of cells responded only to electrical stimulation of C fibres. It would therefore be reasonably expected that up to 12% of cells in the capsaicin treated animals would have no receptive fields if the capsaicin had abolished all C fibre input. The actual figure was 32% of all cells had no receptive fields. This suggests that the presence of C fibres influences the ability of cells to respond to A fibres. The cells which still had receptive fields were also highly abnormal in that 72% of them had grossly expanded receptive fields that averaged over three times the normal size. Finally there were signs of a postsynaptic effect of the peripheral capsaicin since there was a doubling of the number of neurons whose projecting axons conducted at less than 2 m/sec. Evidently peripheral C fibres exert a subtle chronic effect on the properties of lamina I cells.

TABLE III

Effect of Peripheral Nerve Capsaicin on Lamina I Cell Responses

Response Type

		LT%	WDR%	NS%	No RF%
Normal	N = 136	4	53	40	3
Capsaicin	N = 99	3	48	16	32

Afferent Input

		A only	A+C	C only	No Response
Normal	N = 58	26	62	12	0
Capsaicin	N = 35	80	41	0	6

Receptive Field Size

Normal	N = 136	average: 130mm^2 (range 10-325)
Capsaicin	N = 49	expanded: 430mm^2
	N = 32	No RF: 0mm^2
	N = 19	No change: 165mm^2

Conduction Velocity of Cells Axon

Normal	N = 110	84% 3-23 m/sec	16% 0.3-2m/sec
Capsaicin	N = 167	66%	34%

Summary of plastic changes in response properties of lamina I neurones

They are affected by: anaesthesia, brief peripheral inputs, brief evoked descending volleys, ongoing descending activity and peripheral lesions particularly of C fibres.

Given that the response properties of at least some lamina I cells including nociceptive specific cells can be changed, we may now turn to evidence on the significance of the response of these cells. For this we need first to ask about the destination of their axons.

DESTINATION OF PROJECTION AXONS OF LAMINA I CELLS

Since this subject is handled in detail elsewhere in this book by a number of the authors responsible for the major findings, we need here only the briefest summary. It is generally agreed that, with certain important exceptions, lamina I cells project mainly contralaterally by way of the dorsolateral funiculus, DLF. For the rat, McMahon and Wall (1983,1988) made two surveys of the distribution in spinal cord white matter of all detected lumbar lamina I cell axons which projected as far as the C2 segment. In the first they searched all quadrants of the cord. In the second, since it was apparent that most cells projected in the DLF, they searched bilaterally to test which DLF contained axons and whether some cells projected to both DLFs (see Table IV).

The subsequent destination of these axons, also discussed elsewhere in this book, includes caudal medulla, caudal midbrain, thalamus and hypothalamus. Our own contribution to this topic (McMahon and Wall, 1985; Swett *et al*, 1985) showed terminations in caudal medulla and in the ponto-midbrain border and emphasised two problems inherent in the interpretation of these results. First, single fibres may project to more than one target. Second, transport methods have a limited resolution in determining the precise location of terminations. This is particularly important in the caudal midbrain and pons where a galaxy of different small sutures crowd together.

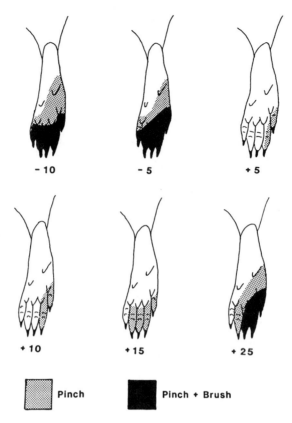

- 10 - 5 + 5

+ 10 + 15 + 25

▨ Pinch   ■ Pinch + Brush

FIGURE 5: Change of response properties of a lamina 1 projecting cell induced by a block of the tonic descending impulses in a decerebrate rat. A single lumbar lamina 1 cell projecting in the contralateral DLF was recorded in a decerebrate rat and the receptive field was repeatedly tested at -10 and -5 minutes before a block was initiated at C3-4 to prevent tonic impulses descending from the brainstem into the spinal cord. At 5, 10, 15 and 25 minutes after the complete onset of the block, the size of the receptive field had decreased and the response modality of the cell had been converted from a wide dynamic range cell to a nociceptive specific cell. Reproduced with permission from McMahon and Wall, (1988).

TABLE IV

Cells projecting to:		Contra DLF	Ipsi DLF	Both DLFs	Contra V	Ipsi V
All quadrants searched	N:136	82%	9%	NT	10%	2%
Only DLFs searched	N:131	85%	8%	8%		

However complex and puzzling may be the final destination of impulses from lamina I cells, we should be able to exploit two related and undoubted facts about these cells in determining their significance. The first is that they are specialised with respect to their anatomy, physiology and pharmacology. They differ from any other known cells in the spinal cord and therefore it is reasonable to predict that some specialised response should disappear if a selective lesion of these cells could be achieved. The second fact is that all agree that these cells project primarily by way of the contralateral dorsolateral funiculus. Putting these two facts together, one might reasonably predict that there would be some disturbance of behaviour specific to lesions of the DLF. Since the cells respond preferentially to noxious inputs, it would be particularly interesting to examine responses to noxious stimuli.

EFFECTS OF DLF SECTION ON BEHAVIOUR PROVOKED BY ACUTE STIMULI

In assessing the results reported in this extensive literature, it is important to differentiate between the effects of contralateral and ipsilateral lesions. Clearly the DLF is a mixed pathway which on the contralateral side carried the bulk of the ascending axons in which we are interested along with others; it also contains a descending component. The ipsilateral DLF is particularly dominated by descending components with a smaller fraction of ascending fibres. Because of the contemporary interest in descending controls, many experiments have been directed at this component; the DLF has been sectioned ipsilaterally or bilaterally. Since the contralateral DLF contains the majority of the ascending axons from lamina 1 cells which carry nociceptive information, one might reasonably predict a hypoalgesia following contralateral DLF section. Since the bulk of the ipsilateral descending fibres are inhibitory, it would seem reasonable to predict a hyperaesthesia after ipsilateral DLF lesions. We will now describe the results of DLF lesions in various species.

(1) The Rat

To say the least, the array of impressively negative results shown in Table V, with contralateral or bilateral lesions, is disappointing. The results of Ryan *et al* (1985) indicated that there might by a slight hyperalgesia to the formalin test that did not reach a significant level. We therefore made unilateral DLF lesions in 5 rats and the formalin test was applied on separate weeks to either foot by Dr. A. Tasker of the Department of Psychology, McGill University, Montreal, Canada. He was not aware of the side of the lesion. Like Ryan *et al* (1985) he found no significant difference in the response to formalin in either the ipsilateral foot or the contralateral foot or in intact controls.

TABLE V

Section	Test	Result	Authors
Bilateral	Pinch	No effect	Basbaum *et al*, 1977
Bilateral	Tail Flick	No effect	Hayes *et al*, 1978
Bilateral	Tail Flick	No effect	Barton *et al*, 1980
Bilateral	Tail Flick	No effect	Rydenhag and Andersson, 1981
Bilateral	Tail Flick	No effect	Watkins *et al*, 1982
Bilateral	Tail Flick	No effect	Watkins *et al*, 1984
Bilateral	Formalin	No effect	Ryan *et al*, 1985
Contra	Heat	No effect	Davies *et al*, 1983
Ipsi	Heat	Hyperalgesia	Davies *et al*, 1983

It could be proposed that this series of acute tests did not measure the affective-motivational aspects of responses to the acute stimuli. This is particularly relevant in view both of the demonstration of hypothalamic terminations described at this meeting by Giesler and of the existence of the amygdala as a secondary target of terminations in the parabrachial region (Bernard *et al*, 1986). We therefore examined three rats with bilateral DLF lesions in a shock escape and avoidance test. This was done with the help of Prof. I. Steele-Russell of University College London using his standard equipment (Plotkin and Steele-Russell, 1969). A start and goal box were separated by a 5ft alley with an electrified grid in the alley and start box providing the unconditioned stimulus from which the operated animals learned to escape with the same alacrity as controls. A conditioning stimulus, a buzzer, provided the animals with the opportunity to learn to avoid the unconditioned stimulus. The lesioned animals learned to avoid the onset of shocks with the same rapidity as controls. Since the shocks were delivered to all four feet and we do not know if C2 DLF lesions interrupt the lamina 1 projection pathways from the forelimbs, these experiments were repeated such that the unconditioned stimulus was a toothed forceps pinch to the hind feet. Three more bilateral C2 DLF lesioned animals learned as rapidly as controls to escape from this stimulus and to use the conditioning stimulus to avoid the pinch.

We must therefore regrettably face the fact that there are eight papers in the literature plus our own three different types of trial in which the effects of contralateral or bilateral DLF lesions did not affect the response of rats to acute noxious stimuli. The one positive result (Davies *et al*, 1983) refers to ipsilateral lesions which produce a hyperalgesia that may reasonably be attributed to the effect of interrupting descending inhibitory pathways.

(2) Cats

The literature on cats is not as extensive as on rats and is complicated by the presence of the pyramidal tract in the DLF in this and other species. Kennard (1954) reported a brief hypoalgesia in a study which could not be repeated by Casey and Morrow (1988) who found thermal hyperalgesia in response to a bilateral lesion. Thermal hyperalgesia in a cat tail flick test was also reported by Hayes *et al*, (1984) following bilateral lesions. Norsell (1983) testing the ability to detect warmth found no change with an ipsilateral lesion but an increased threshold contralaterally. Therefore on balance the cat literature suggests a hyperalgesia.

(3) Monkeys

We have discovered only four papers relevant to this subject in monkeys and find them difficult to interpret. Vierck *et al*, (1971) report that ipsilateral to a DLF lesion there was no change of threshold but an increased force used to arrest the test shock. In the same paper they report a contralateral hypoalgesia. However, Vierck and Luck (1979) examined monkeys that had recovered from a ventrolateral quadrant lesion which had initially produced the expected contralateral analgesia. In an attempt to find the remaining pathways responsible for the reactions to noxious stimuli, they added a dorsolateral lesion and found no changes in the animals response. Levitt and Levitt (1981) were primarily searching for the origin of the dysaesthesia which follows ventral lesions in monkeys. However, with two of their monkeys, CP-1 and WK, inspection of the lesion diagrams suggests that the lesions were primarily in the thoracic dorsolateral white matter. Both these animals began to rub scratch and bite the opposite leg within 8 days suggesting some hyperalgesia which was also seen with much more extensive lesions and with ventral lesions. Christiansen (1966) report on monkeys that:

appreciation of pinch (pupillary dilatation, facio vocal reactions and generalized agitation) was unaltered by posterior funiculus or quadrant lesions.

(4) Man

There is a natural reluctance to make DLF lesions in man, and probably an even greater reluctance to report them if they are made unintentionally, because of the inevitable ipsilateral spasticity which result. Moffie (1975) reports on two such cases and in his summary states: *In two of the cases the lesion was placed (unintentionally) in the posterior quadrant of the spinal cord with good results as to the abolishing of pain.* However, on examining what is written on these two crucial cases the results are not so clear. In his case 3, it is not possible to assess arm sensation since there was carcinomatous infiltration of the brachial plexus; but the leg had normal pin and temperature sensitivity. In his case 4 in which there was an extensive ventral lesion as well as the dorsal destruction there was normal leg sensitivity 18 months after the cordotomy. In the two cases of cord stab wounds reported by Wall and Noordenbos (1977) the patients had a *negative* cordotomy i.e only one ventral quadrant was intact. Both these patients had normal pinprick and temperature sensitivity on the leg contralateral to the intact ventral quadrant. However case 2 with the most severe bilateral dorsal quadrant lesions had a hyperpathia on repeated pinpricks. Both patients had the expected analgesia and thermoanaesthesia in the leg contralateral to the sectioned ventral quadrant.

Summary

What is scientifically correct is not decided by majority vote. The analgesia that might be expected on cutting a nociceptive pathway is not reported by the great majority of the 19 studies. There are reasons to doubt the minority of three who report analgesia. On the contrary signs of hyperalgesia have been noted in all four species studied.

It has been traditional to dismiss unwelcome negative results by such phrases as redundant parallel processing of sensory information. This would assume that exactly equivalent information is transmitted to the brain by different systems so that destruction of one fails to deprive the brain of specific information. Yet many of the papers in this book emphasise those unique properties of the lamina I projection system that it does not share with other projections such as the ventral spinothalamic tract. Therefore section of the bulk of the projecting axons should evoke some change in the animals ability. It is possible that the reason for the mainly negative results is that the animals have been challenged with an irrelevant stimulus. For example it could be that the system is specialised to handle slow chronic inputs rather than acute abrupt inputs. For this reason we have turned to challenge the system with the slow disturbance induced by peripheral nerve lesions (Wall *et al*, 1988).

EFFECT OF DLF SECTIONS ON BEHAVIOUR PROVOKED BY PERIPHERAL NERVE SECTION

When peripheral nerves are cut and ligated, a neuroma forms. A sequence of changes begins in the region of the cut axons (reviewed by Devor, 1988) and sweep centrally to involve the dorsal root ganglia and the spinal cord (reviewed by Wall ,1988). These changes involve the anatomy, physiology and chemistry not only of the cut afferents but also of post-synaptic structures within the cord. Eventually a highly abnormal behaviour starts in rats and in other species in which they attack the

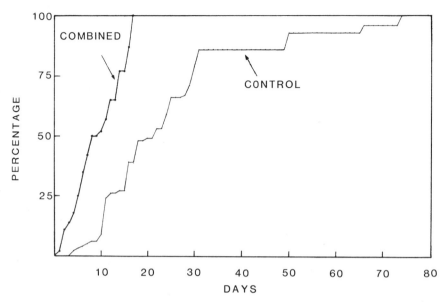

FIGURE 6: The time course of autotomy in 14 control animals and in 13 animals with DLF lesions. The degree of autotomy was observed each day after section and ligation of the sciatic and saphenous nerves on one side. Each day each animal was given an autotomy score of 1-5 if 1-5 nails had been trimmed. When the animal extended the attack onto the toes it was given a score of 10 and was immediately sacrificed. The 100% score on the graph shows the day on which all animals had reached the criterion score of 10. The results show a highly significant acceleration of autotomy in rats with DLF lesions. Reproduced with permission from Wall *et al*, (1988).

anaesthetic area (Rodin and Kruger, 1984). The onset of this autotomy represents some slow central reaction to the existence of peripheral injury. Since DLF lesions had been shown to produce no effect or small and equivocal effects on responses to acute stimuli we decided to investigate their effect on the onset of autotomy.

In 14 control rats the sciatic and saphenous nerves were ligated so that the feet became anaesthetic and neuromata formed in the periphery. Autotomy in these animals began at a mean of 22.4 days after the nerve lesion. DLF sections were made in 13 animals and the sciatic and saphenous nerves were cut and ligated 14 days later. They began autotomy at a mean interval of 8.1 days after the nerve lesion. There was evidently a highly significant acceleration of autotomy with DLF lesions (Fig. 6.).

The nature of this DLF section induced acceleration was studied by further investigation of the effect of ipsilateral or contralateral or bilateral DLF sections. There was no significant difference between the effect of these three operations. Ipsilateral, contralateral and bilateral lesions produced nerve section induced autotomy at mean intervals of 7.3, 9.0 and 7.3 days.

EFFECT OF LESIONS OF TARGETS OF LAMINA 1 PROJECTING AXONS

Section of the DLF, particularly the contralateral DLF, cuts the majority of the projecting axons of the lamina I cells but it obviously also cuts many other axons. These include other ascending axons such as the dorsal spinocerebellar tracts and most importantly descending systems. Having shown a positive effect of DLF section, it was necessary to proceed further in an attempt to define which component was producing the effect. It was decided to attack individual targets of the ascending systems. As

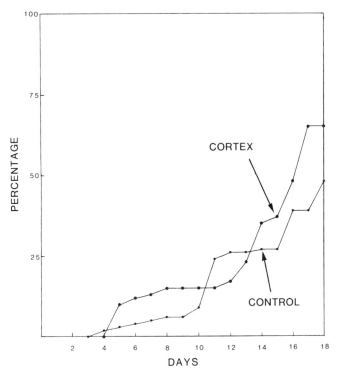

FIGURE 7: The time course of autotomy in 6 rats with cortical lesions and in 14 control rats during the 18 days following section of sciatic and saphenous nerves on the side contralateral to the cortical lesions. Autotomy score as in Fig. 6. There is no significant different between the two groups of animals. Reproduced with permission from Wall *et al*, (1988).

shown by a number of authors in this book, lamina I cells project to several brain stem end stations. The thalamus and the pontine-mesencephalic junction have received particular attention and might be considered likely to affect reactions to injury.

Terminations in the thalamus of lamina I cells have been described in this book to extend to both medial and lateral thalamus. Lesions of all such areas would have been so extensive that it was not felt that interpretation of the results would have been meaningful. Therefore it was decided to make extensive cortical lesions of the contralateral sensory-motor cortex and frontal and parietal cortex which would not only eliminate secondary projection areas of the thalamus but would induce retrograde atrophy in those thalamic cells which projected to the cortex. In 6 animals, suction lesions were made to remove the full depth of the cortex on the right side from the frontal pole to the mid-parietal cortex. After fourteen days, the left sciatic and saphenous nerves were cut and ligated and the onset of autotomy was observed. These animals showed no significant difference in their behaviour from the control animals (Fig. 7).

We then turned to the caudal midbrain target. Recognising that electrolytic lesions could produce confusing results because they would interrupt tracts passing through the region as well as killing local cells, we used instead local injections of the cytotoxic compound ibotenic acid. Examination of these lesions after 5 weeks showed a local loss of nerve cells in an ovoid area without substantial glial infiltration. Given the relatively

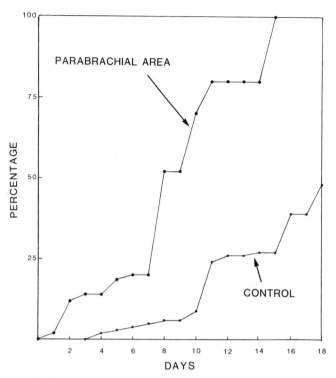

FIGURE 8: The time course of autotomy in rats 1-5 with ibotenic acid lesions in the parabrachial area. There is a highly significant acceleration of autotomy. Reproduced from Wall *et al*, (1988).

large number of end stations reported even in this small area of caudal midbrain, we decided to centre the lesions on the cuneiform nucleus where we had found the highest concentration of lamina 1 axon projecting terminals (McMahon and Wall, 1985; Swett *et al*, 1985). Lesions were made successfully in this area on the right side in five rats and after two weeks the sciatic and saphenous nerves were cut and ligated. Autotomy in these animals began at an average of 5.8 days in contrast to 22.4 days in controls. All animals had reached criterion by 15 days (Fig. 8). Thus the small lesion in the area of the cuneiform and parabrachial nuclei had an accelerating effect on autotomy which did not significantly differ from the result of the DLF lesions.

DISCUSSION ON THE EFFECTS OF CENTRAL LESIONS

We have already summarised the effect of DLF lesions on animal and human responses to acute stimuli. There is only one paper of which we are aware in which the effect of lesions in rats was examined with more prolonged stimulation. Basbaum (1974) made bilateral cervical rhizotomies and showed that this operation was followed after a delay by autotomy of the anaesthetic areas. He also investigated if central lesions would modify this abnormal behaviour. Clearly these experiments differ from ours both in that the root lesions were bilateral and in that the section was of roots rather than of peripheral nerves. In the case of root lesions, cord cells are directly deafferented and there is no peripheral neuroma which could be contributing to the disorder. The onset of autotomy was symmetrical and occurred at an average of 18.5 days. However with right dorsal quadrant lesions there was an acceleration of left sided attacks to 10.5 days and a delay of ipsilateral attacks. It could be that this is a similar phenomenon to the one reported here. In a paper by Dardick *et al*, (1986) the progress of reaction to adjuvant induced polyarthritis in rats was shown to be reduced by ventral quadrant lesions. In a personal communication Basbaum informs us that dorsal quadrant lesions were also produced and did not affect morbidity.

Our results suggest that DLF lesions may accelerate the effect of chronic disturbances while having small effects on the results of acute inputs. Even the response to acute stimuli is on balance exaggerated rather than diminished. This raises the question of the chronic effects of DLF lesions by themselves. In one of three animals with a single DLF lesion, a minor attack on two innervated toes was observed at 30 days even though the peripheral nerves were intact. Basbaum in a personal communication informs us that he too has observed this contralateral effect. As we have already written, Levitt and Levitt (1981) may be interpreted as having observed contralateral chronic signs of increased sensitivity following dorsal lesions in monkeys although their major observations of this phenomenon relate to ventral lesions.

The effect of midbrain lesions on sensitivity other than those directed at the lemniscal systems is sparsely reported in the literature. Nashold *et al*, 1977 reported on the effect of such lesions in man but it must be emphasised that they refer only to lesions which are far rostral and dorsal to the area in the caudal midbrain in which termination of lamina I afferents have been reported. They state: *A small therapeutic lesion confined to this area, although it does not produce any analgesia, resulted in marked calming of the patient and relief of his suffering*, and: *The degree of analgesia after mid brain lesions is often difficult to delineate clinically and it is not related to the degree of pain relief.* While extremely interesting, it seems unlikely that these lesions relate directly to the question of the effect of interrupting lamina I projection and they conclude: *The clinical effects of these midbrain lesions closely resemble those noted after cingulotomy.* There is however a paper in the animal literature which may be highly relevant. Melzack *et al*, (1958) made lesions in cats directed at the central tegmental fasciculus in exactly the caudal midbrain area now said to contain lamina I projection terminals. They reported both a hyperresponsiveness to thermal and mechanical stimuli and guarding behaviour. When the lesions included both this area and the central gray, the animals did not differ from controls. What then might be the mechanisms of the increased response to peripheral events following central lesions to structures involving lamina I projections as we report here from our own results and from the literature. Denervation sensitization of deafferented cells is the explanation favoured by Levitt and Levitt (1981) although this phenomenon is most marked with ventral lesions which all agree produce obvious signs of analgesia but which was not apparent with the lesions reported here. Next the lesions might be producing their action by a direct destruction of descending inhibitory pathways. There is no doubt that such pathways exist (reviewed in Basbaum and Fields, 1988). However these pathways are predominantly ipsilateral. Therefore while the ipsilateral effects reported could well be produced by section of such pathways, it is less likely as an explanation of contralateral effects. Ipsilateral but not contralateral hyperalgesia has been reported in rats (Davies *et al*, 1983) and in monkeys (Vierck *et al*, 1971) following DLF lesions. Similarly there are many reports of provoked descending inhibitions (reviewed in Basbaum and Fields, 1988) running in ipsilateral pathways while contralateral lesions have no effect or a minor effect. We are therefore left with the problem of how to explain the results both of contralateral DLF lesions and of the contralateral caudal midbrain lesions.

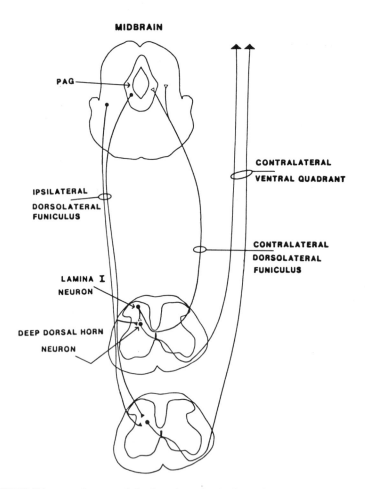

MIDBRAIN

PAG

CONTRALATERAL
VENTRAL QUADRANT

IPSILATERAL
DORSOLATERAL
FUNICULUS

CONTRALATERAL
DORSOLATERAL
FUNICULUS

LAMINA I
NEURON

DEEP DORSAL HORN
NEURON

FIGURE 9: Diagram of proposed slowly acting spino-bulbar-spinal circuit. Lamina 1 cells project mainly by way of the contralateral DLF to a variety of targets in the brain. One of these targets lies in the caudal midbrain. When these midbrain cells are excited by a chronic input, descending influences to the spinal cord are activated. For clarity the descending path is shown as a single unbroken axon, but it is recognised that these pathways have relays in the brainstem. The descending impulses excite the lamina 1 cells, thereby increasing the activity in the ascending arm of the loop. At the same time the descending impulses inhibit deeper dorsal horn cells and thereby decrease behavioural responses to chronic inputs. The circuit reacts with a long latency and long duration and does not influence reactions to abrupt acute inputs.

SUMMARY OF POSSIBLE ROLES OF LAMINA I PROJECTION SYSTEMS

Any theory of the role(s) subserved by lamina I projection cells must take into account a number of pieces of experimental evidence. The most important of these are:
   a) The vast majority of cells receive nociceptive inputs.
   b) The cells project to many areas including the midbrain, terminating in the parabrachial, cuneiform and PAG region - a region where stimulation can have profound effects on nociception.
   c) The axons of the cells ascend mostly in the contralateral DLF.
   d) Section of the DLF in man and animals has only minor effects on nociceptive thresholds when judged acutely.

e) Lesions of the DLF or of known midbrain targets of lamina I projections change the response of animals to chronic nerve section.

f) The lamina I cells have different descending controls compared with deep dorsal cells.

We would like to propose that this population of cells does not function as a simple sensory relay for nociceptive information (*cf.* point d) above), but forms the afferent limb of a spino-bulbo-spinal loop which functions to regulate the excitability or gain of other spinal neurones concerned with the transmission of nociceptive information. A schematic representation of the basic features of this proposal is shown in Fig. 9. Thus the following stages, each of which has some experimental support and each of which suggests further experiments, is proposed:

1) When nociceptors are activated they will excite the somatotopically appropriate lamina I cells. Axon collaterals of lamina I cells may relay impulses to deeper dorsal horn cells. Repetitive activation, especially when C afferents from deep tissues are excited, produces a long lasting increase in the excitability in lamina I cells. This too may be relayed to local dorsal horn cells. The result, following injury, is an acute discharge followed by a slowly augmenting rise of excitability and discharge.

2) Impulses in the lamina I cells are transmitted by way of the contralateral DLF to midbrain targets, especially n. cuneiformis and the PAG.

3) Cells in the caudal midbrain excite other cells in the region which project via the ipsilateral DLF to the spinal cord. These descending projections have a strong regulatory effect on superficial and deep dorsal horn cells in many spinal segments.

4) Thus, the short-term effect of activation of ascending lamina I projection is a rapid inhibition of deep dorsal horn cells while the lamina I cells increase their excitability.

5) The system is unlikely to affect brief responses to brief stimuli.

6) When challenged with a tonic input the effectiveness of the system slowly rises with a positive feed back to exaggerate lamina I responsiveness and a coincident rise of inhibition of deep cells. The development of activity in these feed back loops is slow to mature so that their presence is not apparent in the usual test methods which examine the consequences of acute stimuli.

REFERENCES

BARTON, C., BASBAUM, A.I. AND FIELDS, H.L. (1980) Dissociation of supraspinal and spinal actions of morphine a quantitative evaluation. *Brain Research*, **188**: 487-498.

BASBAUM, A.I. (1974) Effects of central lesions on disorders produced by multiple dorsal rhizotomy in rats. *Experimental Neurology*, **42**: 490-501.

BASBAUM, A.I. AND FIELDS, H.L. (1988) Endogenous pain control mechanisms. In, *Textbook of Pain*, 2nd edition eds. P.D. Wall and R. Melzack, Churchill Livingstone, Edinburgh.

BASBAUM, A.I., MARLEY, N.J.E., O'KEEFE, J. AND CLANTON, C.H. (1977) Reversal of morphine and stimulus-produced analgesia by subtotal spinal cord lesions. *Pain*, **3**: 43-56.

BERNARD, J.F., MA, W., BESSON, J.M. AND PESCHANSKI, M. (1986) A monosynaptic spino-ponto-amygdaline pathway possibly involved in pain. *American Neuroscience Society Abstracts*, **12**: 13-5.

CASEY, K.L. AND MORROW, T.J. (1988) Supraspinal nocifensive responses of cats: Spinal cord pathways, monoamines, and modulation. *Journal of Comparative Neurology*, **270**: 591-605.

CERVERO, F. (1983) Somatic and visceral inputs to the thoracic spinal cord of the cat: effects of noxious stimulation of the bilary system. *Journal of Physiology*, **337**: 51-67.

CERVERO, F., IGGO, A. AND OGAWA, H. (1976) Nociceptor-driven dorsal horn neurones in the lumbar spinal cord of the cat. *Pain*, **2**: 5-24.

CERVERO, F. AND LAIRD, J.M.A. (1988) Nociceptive neurones in the dorsal horn of rat spinal cord: receptive field properties before and after prolonged noxious mechanical stimulation. *Journal of Physiology*, in press.

CERVERO, F., SCHOUENBORG, J., SJÖLUND, B.H. AND WADDELL, P.J. (1984) Cutaneous inputs to dorsal horn neurones in adult rats treated at birth with capsaicin. *Brain Research*, **301**: 47-57.

CERVERO, F., AND TATTERSALL, J. (1987) Somatic and visceral inputs to the thoracic spinal cord of the cat: marginal zone (lamina I) of the dorsal horn. *Journal of Physiology*, **388**: 383-395.

CERVERO, F. AND WOLSTENCROFT, J. (1984) A positive feedback loop between spinal cord nociceptive pathways and antinociceptive areas of the cat's brain. *Pain*, **20**: 125-138.

CHRISTENSEN, B.N. AND PERL, E.R. (1970) Spinal neurons specifically excited by noxious and thermal stimuli: marginal zone of the spinal cord. *Journal of Neurophysiology*, **33**: 293-307.

CHRISTIANSEN, J. (1966) Neurological observations of macaques with spinal cord lesions. *Anatomical Record*, **154**: 330.

COLLINS, J.G. AND REN, K. (1987) WDR response profiles of spinal dorsal horn neurones may be unmasked by barbiturate anaesthesia. *Pain*, **28**: 369-378.

COOK, A.J., WOOLF, C.J. AND WALL, P.D. (1986) Prolonged C-fibre facilitation of the flexion reflex in the rat is not due to changes in afferent terminal or motoneurone excitability. *Neuroscience Letters*, **70**: 91-96.

COOK, A.J., WOOLF, C.J., WALL, P.D. AND McMAHON, S.B. (1987) Expansion of cutaneous receptive fields of dorsal horn neurones following C-primary afferent fibre inputs. *Nature*, **325**: 151-153.

CRAIG, A.D. AND BURTON, H. (1981) Spinal and medullary lamina I projections to nucleus submedius in medial thalamus. *Journal of Neurophysiology*, **45**: 443-466.

CRAIG, A.D. AND KNIFFKI, K.D. (1985) The multiple representation of nociception in the spinothalamic projection of lamina 1 cells in the cat. In, *Development, organization and processing in somatosensory pathways.* Eds. M. Rowe and W.D. Willis, Neurology and Neurobiology, vol. **14**, Liss, New York.

DARDICK, S.J., BASBAUM, A.I. AND LEVINE, J.D. (1986) The contribution of pain to disability in experimentally induced arthritis. *Arthritis and Rheumatism*, **29**: 1017-1022.

DAVIES, J.E., MARSDEN, C.A. AND ROBERTS, M.H.T. (1983) Hyperalgesia and the reduction of monoamines resulting from lesions of the dorsolateral funiculus. *Brain Research*, **261**: 59-68.

DEVOR, M. (1988) The Pathophysiology of Damaged Nerve. in *The Textbook of Pain*, 2nd edition, Eds. P.D. Wall and R. Melzack, Churchill Livingstone, Edinburgh.

DEVOR, M. AND WALL, P.D. (1981a) The effect of peripheral nerve injury on receptive fields of cells in the cat spinal cord. *Journal of Comparative Neurology*, **199**: 277-291.

DEVOR, M. AND WALL, P.D. (1981b) Plasticity in the spinal cord sensory map following peripheral nerve injury in rats. *Journal of Neuroscience*, **1**: 679-684.

DICKHAUS, H., PAUSER, G. AND ZIMMERMANN, M. (1985) Tonic descending inhibition affects intensity coding of nociceptive responses of spinal dorsal horn neurones in the cat. *Pain*, **23**: 145-160.

DUBUISSON, D. (1981) The descending control of substantia gelatinosa, *Ph.D Thesis*, University of London.

DUBUISSON, D., FITZGERALD, M. AND WALL, P.D. (1979) Ameboid receptive fields of cells in laminae 1,2 and 3. *Brain Research*, **177**: 376-378.

DUBUISSON, D. AND WALL, P.D. (1980) Descending influences on single units in laminae 1 and 2 of cat spinal cord. *Brain Research*, **199**: 283-298.

FERRINGTON, D.G., SORKIN, L.S. AND WILLIS, W.D. (1987) Responses of spinothalamic tract cells in the superficial dorsal horn of the primate lumbar spinal cord. *Journal of Physiology*, **388**: 681-703.

GIESLER, G.J., GEBHART, K.D., YEZIERSKI, R.P., WILCOX, I.K., AND WILLIS, W.D. (1981) Postsynaptic inhibition of primate spinothalamic neurons by stimulation in nucleus raphe magnus. *Brain Research*, **204**: 184-188.

HABER, L.H., MARTIN, R.F., CHUNG, J.M., AND WILLIS, W.D. (1980) Inhibition and excitation by primate spinothalamic tract neurons by stimulation in the region of nucleus reticularis gigantocellularis. *Journal of Neurophysiology*, **43**: 1578-1593.

HARMANN, P.A., CARLTON, S.M. AND WILLIS, W.D. (1988) Collaterals of spinothalamic tract cells to the periaqueductal gray: a fluorescent double labelling study in the rat. *Brain Research*, **441**: 87-97.

HAYES, R.L., KATAYAMA, Y., WATKINS, L.R. AND BECKER, D.P. (1984) Bilateral lesions of the dorsolateral funiculus of the cat spinal cord: effects on basal nociceptive reflexes and nociceptive suppression produced by cholinergic activation of the pontine parabrachial region. *Brain Research*, **311**: 267-280.

HAYES, R.L., PRICE, D.D., BENNETT, G.J., WILCOX, G.L. AND MAYER, D.J. (1978) Differential effects of spinal cord lesions on narcotic and non narcotic suppression of nociceptive reflexes. *Brain Research*, **155**: 91-101.

HYLDEN, J.L.K., HAYASHI, H., DUBNER, R., AND BENNETT, G.J. (1986) Physiology and morphology of the lamina I spinomesencephalic projection. *Journal of Comparative Neurology*, **247**: 505-515.

HYLDEN, J.L.K., NAHIN, R.L. AND DUBNER, R. (1987) Altered responses of nociceptive cat lamina I spinal dorsal horn neurons after chronic sciatic neuroma formation. *Brain Research*, **411**: 341-350.

KENNARD, M.A. (1954) The course of ascending fibres in spinal cord of cat essential to the recognition of painful stimuli. *Journal of Comparative Neurology*, **100**: 511-524.

LAIRD, J.M.A, AND CERVERO, F. (1988) Receptive field plasticity of dorsal horn cells: a Comparison between multireceptive and nocireceptive neurones. *Society for Neuroscience Abstracts*, **14**: 913.

LEVITT, M. AND LEVITT, J.H. (1981) The deafferentation syndrome in monkeys: dysaesthesia of spinal origin. *Pain*, **10**: 129-147.

LIGHT, A.R., CASALE, E.J. AND MENÉTREY, D.M. (1986) The effects of focal stimulation in the nucleus raphe magnus and periaqueductal gray on intracellularly recorded neurones in spinal laminae I and II. *Journal of Neurophysiology*, **56**: 555- 571.

LIGHT, A.R., CASALE, E. AND SEDIVEC, M. (1988) The physiology and anatomy of spinal lamina 1 and 2 neurons antidromically activated by stimulation in the parabrachial region of the midbrain and pons. In, *Fine afferent nerve fibres and pain*, Eds. R.F. Schmidt, H.G. Schaible and C. Vahle-Hinz, VCH, Weinheim, New York.

MCMAHON, S.B. AND WALL, P.D. (1983) A system of rat spinal cord lamina I cells projecting through the contralateral dorsolateral funiculus. *Journal of Comparative Neurology*, **214**, 217-223.

MCMAHON, S.B. AND WALL (1984) Receptive fields of rat lamina I projection cells move to incorporate a nearby region of injury. *Pain*, **19**: 235-247.

MCMAHON, S.B. AND WALL (1985) Electrophysiological mapping of brainstem projections of spinal cord lamina I cells in the rat. *Brain Research*, **333**: 19-26.

MCMAHON, S.B. AND WALL (1988) Descending excitation and inhibition of spinal cord lamina I projection neurones. *Journal of Neurophysiology*, **59**: 1204-1219.

MCMAHON, S.B. WALL, GRANUM, S. AND WEBSTER, K.E. (1984) The chronic effects of capsaicin applied to peripheral nerves on responses of a group of lamina I cells in rats. *Journal of Comparative Neurology*, **227**, 393-400.

MELZACK, R., STOTLER, W.A. AND LIVINGSTONE, W.K. (1958) Effects of discrete brain stem lesions in cats on perception of noxious stimulation. *Journal of Neurophysiology*, **21**: 353-367.

MOFFIE, D. (1975) Spinothalamic fibres, pain conduction and cordotomy. *Clinical Neurology and Neurosurgery*, **78**, 261-268.

NASHOLD, B.S., SLAUGHTER, D.G., WILSON, W.P. AND ZORUB, D. (1977) Stereotactic mesencephalotomy. In, Krayenbuhl, H., Maspes, P., Sweet, W.H. (eds) *Progress in Neurological Surgery*, **8**, p. 35, Karger, Basel.

NORSELL, U. (1983) Unilateral behavioural thermosensitivity after transection of one lateral funiculus in the cervical spinal cord of the cat. *Experimental Brain Research*, **53**: 71- 80.

PERL, E.R. (1985) Unravelling the Story of Pain. *Advances in Pain Research and Therapy*, **9**: 1-30, eds. H.L. Fields, R. Dubner and F. Cervero, Raven Press, New York.

PLOTKIN, H.C. AND STEELE-RUSSELL, I. (1969) Quantitative adjustment in magnitude of the hemidecorticate learning deficit by CS duration manipulation. *Physiology and Behaviour*, **4**: 709- 721.

PRICE, D.D. AND MAYER, D.J. (1975) Neurophysiological characterization of the anterolateral quadrant neurones subserving pain in m. mulatta. *Pain*, **11**: 59-72.

PRICE, D.D., HAYES, R.L., RUOA, M.A. AND DUBNER, R. (1978) Spatial and temporal transformations of input to spinothalamic tract neurones and their relation to somatic sensations. *Journal of Neurophysiology*, **41**: 933-947.

RODIN, B. AND KRUGER, L. (1984) Deafferentation in animals as a model for the study of pain: an alternative hypothesis. *Brain Research Reviews*, **7**: 213-228.

RYAN, S.M., WATKINS, L.R., MAYER, D.J. AND MAIER, S.F. (1985) Spinal pain suppression mechanisms may differ for phasic and tonic pain. *Brain Research*, **334**: 172-175.

RYDENHAG, B. AND ANDERSSON, S. (1981) Effect of DLF lesions at different spinal levels on morphine induced analgesia. *Brain Research*, **212**: 239-242.

SWETT, J.E., MCMAHON, S.B. AND WALL, P.D. (1985) Projection of lamina I cells to the midbrain of the rat. *Journal of Comparative Neurology*, **238**: 401-416.

TATTERSALL, J.E.H., CERVERO, F., AND LUMB, B.M. (1986) Viscerosomatic neurones in the lower thoracic spinal cord of the cat: excitations and inhibitions by afferent volleys and by stimulation of brainstem nuclei. *Journal of Neurophysiology*, **56**: 785-796.

VIERCK, C.J., HAMILTON, D.N. AND THORNBY, J.I. (1971) Pain reactivity of monkeys after lesions to the dorsal and lateral columns of the spinal cord. *Experimental Brain Research*, **13**: 140-158.

VIERCK, C.J. AND LUCK, M.N. (1979) Loss and recovery of reactivity to noxious stimuli with primary spinothalamic cordotomies followed by secondary and tertiary lesions of other cord sectors. *Brain*, **102**: 233-248.

WALL, P.D. (1988) The introduction, and The dorsal horn, in, *The Textbook of Pain*, eds. P.D. Wall and R. Melzack, 2nd edition, Churchill Livingstone, Edinburgh.

WALL, P.D., BERY, J. AND SAADÉ, N. (1988) Effects of lesions to lamina I cell projection pathways on reactions to acute and chronic noxious stimuli. *Pain*, **35**, 327-339.

WALL, P.D., FITZGERALD, M., NUSSBAUMER, J.C., VAN DER LOOS, H. AND DEVOR, M. (1982) Somatotopic maps are disorganised in adult rodents treated with capsaicin as neonates. *Nature*, **295**: 691- 693.

WALL, P.D. AND NOORDENBOS, W. (1978) Sensory functions which remain in man after complete transection of dorsal horns. *Brain Research*, **100**: 641-653.

WALL, P.D. AND WOOLF, C.J. (1984) Muscle but not cutaneous C- afferent input produces prolonged increases in the excitability of the flexion reflex in the rat. *Journal of Physiology*, **356**: 443-458.

WATKINS, L.R., COBELLI, D.A. AND MAYER, D.J. (1982) Opiate *vs* non-opiate foot shock-induced analgesia (FSIA): descending and intraspinal components. *Brain Research*, **245**: 97-106.

WATKINS, L., FARIS, P.L., KOMISARUK, B.R. AND MAYER, D. (1984) DLF and intraspinal pathways mediate vaginal stimulation induced suppression of nociceptive responding in rats. *Brain Research*, **294**: 59-65.

WOOLF, C.J. (1983) Evidence for a central component of post- injury pain hypersensitivity. *Nature*, **306**: 686-688.

WOOLF, C.J. AND FITZGERALD, M. (1983) The properties of neurones recorded in the superficial dorsal horn in rat spinal cord. *Journal of Comparative Neurology*, **221**: 313-328.

YEZIERSKI, R.P., SORKIN, L.S. AND WILLIS, W. (1987) Response properties of spinal neurones projecting to midbrain or midbrain-thalamus in the monkey. *Brain Research*, **437**: 165-170.

MOLECULAR EVENTS IN THE SPINAL CORD FOLLOWING SENSORY STIMULATION

S. Williams[1] , A. Pini[2] , G. Evan[3] and S.P. Hunt[1]

MRC Molecular Neurobiology Unit[1] and Ludwig Institute for Cancer Research[3] Cambridge CB2 2QH, UK; Department of Physiology[2] , Columbia University, New York, USA

The proto-oncogene *c-fos* belongs to a class of genes which is rapidly activated in fibroblast and peripheral neuronal cell lines following various forms of stimulation. Of particular relevance are the observations that *c-fos* transcription in PC12 cells followed minutes after stimulation by incubation with either nerve growth factor (Curran and Morgan, 1985, Greenberg *et al*, 1985, Kruijer *et al*, 1985, Milbrandt, 1986) or with second messenger candidates such as cAMP, or depolarisation with high potassium concentrations (Greenberg and Ziff, 1984) sufficient to activate voltage-dependent calcium channels (Morgan and Curran, 1986), or with incubation with acetylcholine (Greenberg *et al*, 1986). It was suggested that *c-fos* induction could be related to the establishment of long-term changes in the central nervous system (Berridge, 1986, Goelet *et al*, 1986). However, attempts to correlate *c-fos* expression with long-term potentiation in the hippocampus or with controlled synaptic stimulation within the forebrain proved negative (Bliss *et al*, 1988). Expression of the protein was demonstrated only by relatively extreme procedures such as treatment with convulsant drugs or direct electrical stimulation (Morgan *et al*, 1987, Dragunow and Robertson, 1987, Bliss *et al*, 1988, Kaczmarek *et al*, 1988).

Within the spinal cord, however, the situation is dramatically different. Hunt *et al*, (1987) showed that activation of small-diameter cutaneous afferents by noxious heat or by chemical stimuli resulted in the rapid appearance of *c-fos* protein within neurons of the superficial laminae of the dorsal horn (Fig. 1A). However, activation of low-threshold cutaneous afferents resulted in fewer labelled cells with a different laminar distribution. No *c-fos* induction was seen in dorsal root ganglia, gracile nuclei or motoneurons, suggesting that large-diameter non-nociceptive fibres did not mediate the post-synaptic event.

Three questions will be addressed in this chapter: (a) what is the relationship between the stimulus and the pattern of *c-fos* positive neurons within the spinal cord? (b) what is the sequence of biochemical events which leads to the appearance of the phosphoprotein? and (c) what are the consequences of *c-fos* protein induction for the neuron?

Male Sprague-Dawley rats (180-250 g) were deeply anaesthetized with Equithesin (4 ml/kg) i.p. before stimulation and perfusion [Equithesin is sodium pentobarbitone 4.8 g; chloral hydrate, 21.25 g; magnesium sulphate, 10.63 g; propylene glycol 198.0 ml;

ethanol, 50.00 ml; to 500 ml with distilled water]. 2 - 24 hours after stimulation, the animals were perfused intracardially with 100 ml sodium phosphate buffered saline (0.1 M, pH 7.4; PB) followed by 300 ml 4% paraformaldehyde in phosphate buffer (0.1 M, pH 7.4; PH). The spinal cord with attached dorsal root ganglia was postfixed for 12 hours and washed overnight in PH containing 30% sucrose. 40-micron frozen sections were incubated overnight in rabbit antiserum to a synthetic 16-residue peptide with a sequence common to the N-terminal regions of all known c-fos and v-fos proteins, prepared and characterised as described in Hunt et al, (1987), diluted 1:10,000 in 0.1 M Tris buffer containing 9.5 g/1 sodium chloride and 0.3% Triton X-100. Sections were then washed in PB for 1 hour and incubated for 2 hours with biotinylated goat anti-rabbit serum (Vector) diluted 1:200, rewashed and incubated for 1 hour with avidin-biotin-horseradish peroxidase complex (Vector) diluted 1:100. Tissue from nerve-lesioned animals was processed with the addition at this stage of HRP-conjugated isolectin B4 (Bandeireia simplicifolia, Sigma) at 1 μg/ml, and incubated for two hours. This lectin selectively labels the population of small-diameter primary afferents containing the enzyme fluoride-resistant acid phosphatase (FRAP) and terminating almost exclusively within the substantia gelatinosa (Silverman and Kruger 1988). Sections were washed for 1 hour in PB and were incubated in diaminobenzidine 100 μg/ml distilled water with 0.01% hydrogen peroxide for 5 min before being washed in PB and mounted on gelatin-subbed glass slides. After drying the stain was fixed by 5 seconds immersion in 0.01% osmic acid followed by a distilled water wash, dehydration in graded alcohols, clearing in Histoclear and mounting in DPX mountant.

In order to investigate the effects of intensity, spatial localisation, timecourse and developmental age on c-fos induction, various single and repeated stimuli were employed as follows. All animals were anaesthetized for the period of stimulation. Thermal stimulation was delivered by immersing the hind-paw in gently stirred water at 40-52° C for 5-20 seconds, and chemical stimulation by coating the paw with 10% mustard oil in liquid paraffin, left undisturbed in an impermeable dressing until the animal was perfused two hours later. Localized noxious chemical stimulation was produced by subcutaneous injections of 5 μl 5% formalin in normal saline. Pinch was delivered, to a fold of skin over the mid-dorsum of the hind-paw, with mosquito forceps closed to the first stop for ten seconds; this produced no visible tissue damage. Non-

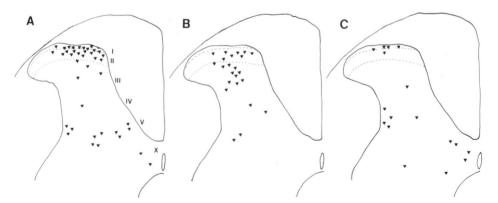

FIGURE 1: Camera lucida drawing of the differential patterns of p55$^{c\text{-}fos}$-like immunoreactivity in rat lumbar spinal cord following (a) heat stimulation (52° C) of the foot; (b) low-threshold stimulation of the hind-limb; (c) intramuscular injection of 5% mustard oil. Each triangle represents three labelled neurons. (From Hunt et al, 1987)

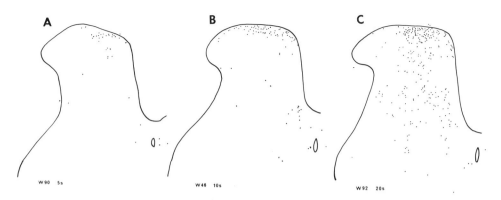

FIGURE 2: Patterns of p55$^{c\text{-}fos}$-like immunoreactivity in the dorsal horn of the rat lumbar spinal cord after immersion of the hind-paw in water at 52° C for (a) 5 seconds, (b) 10 seconds, and (c) 20 seconds.

noxious stimulation of the skin with soft brushes and gentle manipulation of the joints of the hind-limb for 15 minutes was designed to activate low-threshold mechanoreceptors (LTM). 10 μl of 5% mustard oil in liquid paraffin was introduced into the knee joint-space. Trials with dye in the vehicle showed that this was best done by injection through the patellar tendon. 10 μl of 5% mustard oil was injected transcutaneously into the medial belly of the gastrocnemius muscle. 24-48 hour old rat pups were anaesthetized with chloroform vapour and were given subcutaneous injections of 50 mg/kg capsaicin in normal saline, and were then perfused after 2 hours as with the adults.

Many of the above stimuli were applied to the hind-feet of rats following chronic (four weeks) or acute (two days) lesions of the sciatic nerve in the upper thigh. Under Equithesin anaesthesia, the nerve was divided distal to a tight silk ligature and the wound closed with silk sutures.

Fifty ng substance P, or neurokinin A (NKA), in 20 μl saline was injected over 1 minute via a polyethylene cannula into the sub-arachnoid space (Yaksh and Rudy 1976), with a 2-hour survival time.

The intensity of staining of laminae I, II, V and X following immersion of the foot depended on the temperature of the water and the length of immersion. At temperatures of 40-46° C there was little response. In contrast, even brief immersion in water at 52° C elicited a strong signal in the area of foot representation of the cord, particularly in the superficial laminae I and II. Immersion for 10-20 seconds at this temperature produced an increased signal in almost all areas, particularly in lamina II (Fig. 2). Coating of the foot with 10% mustard oil resulted in a consistent pattern of immunoreactivity in laminae I, II, V, and X. 5% mustard oil produced a similar pattern, although fewer immunoreactive nuclei were revealed and fewer of them were densely stained. A stimulus that produced extravasation in the skin was invariably followed by the appearance of dense immunoreactivity in a high proportion of nuclei in a segment of lamina II, and a more diffuse pattern in the deeper cord. When a similar intensity of inflammation had been produced in two rats by mustard oil and water immersion, as judged by the degree of oedema, the pattern of immunocytochemical staining was very similar. There was no p55 c-fos-like immunoreactivity in the spinal cords of animals allowed to survive twenty-four hours or more after stimulation with formalin or heat.

Stimulation by pinch produced a very localised response over less than 1mm of the L3 segment, with the same laminar distribution as the above. Following non-noxious stimulation there was light nuclear labelling of scattered neurons in laminae II to IV, but rarely any in I V (Fig. 1B).

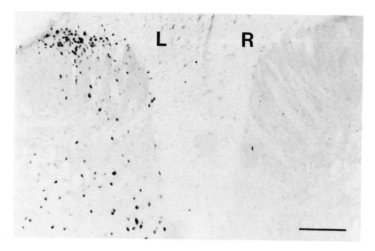

FIGURE 3: Immunoreactive nuclei in transverse section of rat lumbar spinal cord following formalin injection of a digit. L = 2 hours post-injection, R = 24 hours post injection. Scale bar = 200 μm.

Formalin injection produced immunoreactivity in a high proportion of the neuronal nuclei in localised areas of laminae I and II, many of which were densely stained, and scattered nuclei in III - VIII and X (Fig. 3). In horizontal sections through lamina II, the area of signal following injection of a toe-pad widely overlapped the area representing adjacent toes, although the area representing the lateral toe signal was fairly distinct, and the medial toe signal extended rostrally more than the others (Fig. 4). The length of immunoreactive lamina II following injection of two adjacent toes was less than twice the length seen after single toe stimulation (n=4). When two adjacent toes were injected, the apparent density of immunoreactive nuclei was increased in the deeper laminae, though not in I and II.

Following joint stimulation with mustard oil (n=3), there was strong *c-fos* staining in about 20 cells per section from L2 to L6, predominantly in lamina I, with scattered nuclei in V (Fig. 5). Injection of mustard oil into the medial belly of gastrocnemius (n=3) evoked a response largely in laminae I, IV to VIII, and X of segments L4 and L5 (Fig. 1C).

Areas of chronically denervated grey matter in nerve-lesioned animals were revealed by lectin staining of primary afferent terminals in intact dorsal horn. After four weeks, the cords from 12 sciatic-lesioned rats developed a gap in the lectin stain from L2 to L5; this gap bifurcated rostrally around a previously described *peninsula* of saphenous nerve representation (Swett and Woolf, 1985). Under the light microscope, lectin-positive fibres could usually be seen approaching the nuclei in lamina II that became immunoreactive post-stimulation.

Following a chronic sciatic nerve lesion and stimulation with mustard (n=3) or heat (n=3), the peninsula of saphenous representation and other areas adjacent to, but not included in, the lesion which remained lectin-positive, were consistently higher in the number and intensity of stained nuclei, compared with an intact or an acutely lesioned side (Fig. 6). Very little p55 *c-fos*-like immunoreactivity was seen in areas of complete lectin loss. Peripheral sensory loss following nerve lesions was confirmed by gently seizing hindlimb digits with forceps while the animal was recovering from the anaesthetic. Immediately after sciatic nerve section, limb withdrawal followed such stimulation of the medial digit only. After 28 days however, there was withdrawal to pinch of the medial three digits.

Intrathecal application of 50 ng substance P (n=3) or NKA (n=3) resulted in the appearance of dense immunoreactivity in superficial laminae of the dorsal horn, and in nuclei of cells nearest the pia in all cord regions including white matter (Fig. 7). At 24 and 48 hours postnatally, subcutaneous injection of capsaicin produced a pattern of p55 c-fos-like-immunoreactive neurons predominantly within laminae I, II and V (Fig. 8).

The distribution of c-fos-positive neurons within the spinal cord was dependent upon the nature and intensity of stimulation, the peripheral structure stimulated and the spatial localization of the stimulus. The density of positive neurons was altered by chronic peripheral nerve section but was not affected by postnatal age.

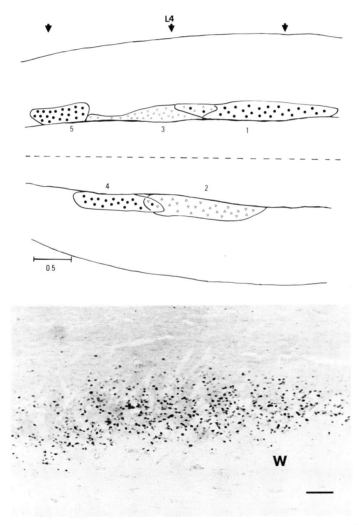

FIGURE 4: Superimposed camera lucida drawings of L3-L5 region of five rat lumbar spinal cords in horizontal section, showing areas of immunoreactivity following injection of each hind-paw digit with 5 μl of 4% formalin. Below, photomicrograph of a horizontal section of the immunoreactive area in lamina II of L4 segment following formalin injection of the medial digit (scale bar = 100 μm).

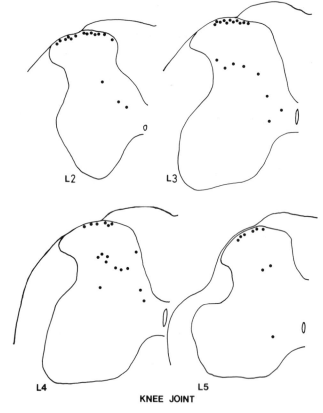

FIGURE 5: Camera lucida drawing of spinal cord segments L2-L5 showing *c-fos* positive nuclei following injection of 10 μl 5% mustard oil into the knee-joint.

The majority of primary afferents are small-diameter C and A-δ fibres. In rat, C-fibres terminate extensively within the superficial dorsal horn, particularly laminae I and II, the substantia gelatinosa and within laminae V and X. A-δ fibres are fewer in number but have an overlapping distribution with C-fibres. Approximately half of the C-fibre population (Hunt and Rossi, 1985), and some A-δ fibres (Lawson *et al*, this volume), contain peptides such as substance P and calcitonin gene-related peptide (CGRP), while the majority of small-diameter sensory neurons respond to noxious stimulation of peripheral tissues (Lynn and Carpenter, 1982). The results of anterograde tracing studies suggest that the termination of sensory fibres within the dorsal horn is dependent upon the type of peripheral tissue innervated. Muscle and joint afferents (Craig and Mense 1983, Schaible *et al*, this volume) terminate extensively within lamina I and deeper laminae including V-VIII and X, but not II to any significant extent, while cutaneous afferents terminate heavily and topographically within lamina II, and also within lamina I and the deeper laminae of the dorsal horn. Stimulation of joint, muscle or skin using discrete noxious stimuli produced a pattern of *c-fos* activation within the dorsal horn that was largely consistent with this differential termination of sensory afferents. Knee and muscle stimulation, for example, produced widespread activation of *c-fos* within lamina I neurons but not in lamina II neurons, while cutaneous stimulation (including stimulation of deep tissues, as with formalin injection into the digit) produced a precise and topographically organized patch of *c-fos*-positive cells

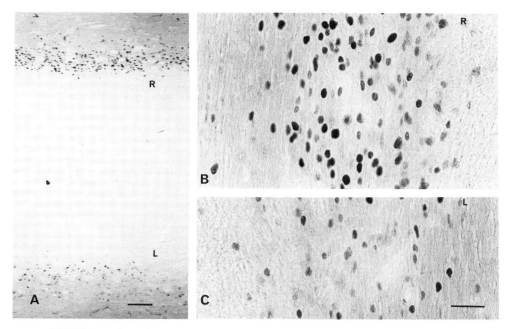

FIGURE 6: Photomicrograph of immunoreactivity in horizontal section of rat lumbar spinal cord following immersion of the hind-foot in water at 52° C for 20 seconds (A, scale bar = 50 μm), where there was a chronic sciatic nerve lesion on the right (R, shown enlarged in B, scale bar = 10 μm) and an acute sciatic nerve lesion on the left (L, shown enlarged in C).

within lamina II. Labelled neurons in laminae I and V were found for considerable distances along the rostrocaudal axis of the spinal cord, with little observable topography. This again would have been predictable from previous studies of the rostrocaudal extent of individually-filled small myelinated fibres within laminae I and V (Light and Perl, 1979).

When using noxious stimuli, the nature of the stimulus applied to the skin appeared to be important only in terms of intensity. Noxious chemical or heat stimulation which led to roughly comparable levels of extravasation and oedema in the stimulated foot produced comparable levels of labelling within the dorsal horn. By reducing the intensity of stimulation, that is by reducing the time of exposure to heat, fewer cells were labelled. This gave the impression of a greater loss of cells from the more sparsely- labelled deeper laminae, but there was a general reduction in the numbers of positive cells throughout both deep and superficial laminae of the dorsal horn. These observations suggest that the summation of synaptic inputs may be important and that the amount of c-fos protein produced is directly related to the degree of synaptic excitation. It may be that more intense stimulation effects polysynaptic changes, as reported by Sagar et al, (1988).

Non-noxious brushing of the foot together with manipulation of the joints produced labelling of neurons within laminae II-IV of the dorsal horn. This may have resulted from the activation of low-threshold, small-diameter fibres although labelling within these laminae was also seen following formalin injection of the digit. *Fixation* of the nerve fibre may have resulted in subsequent injury discharge and c-fos expression within central target cells.

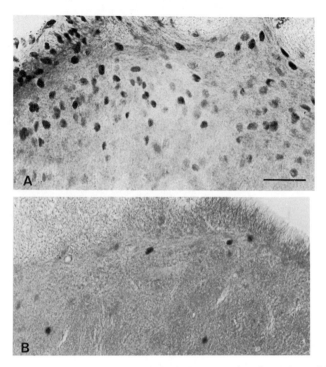

FIGURE 7: Intrathecal perfusion of substance P (SP, 50 ng/50 μl). *C-fos* positive nuclei within SP-perfused (A) but not vehicle-perfused cord (B). Scale bar = 100 μm.

In agreement with other anterograde tracer studies (presented by Molander *et al*, at this Workshop) we were unable to provide any evidence that saphenous nerve terminals significantly invade the adjacent dorsal horn territory 28 days after sciatic nerve section. However, we saw a massive increase in the number of lamina II neurons labelled within the saphenous representation of the dorsal horn, particularly in the area adjacent to sciatic representation where numbers and intensity of labelled cells are usually low. This might reflect local sprouting of primary afferent axons within saphenous territory, perhaps due to increased amounts of a trophic signal, or increased release of neurotransmitter from primary afferents. Deeper laminae of the spinal cord are more difficult to study because of the apparent lack of topography and the extensive rostrocaudal distribution of label from a given stimulus. It is also unclear whether neurons which fire spikes in response to peripheral stimulation are the only neurons that are being labelled by *c-fos* immunocytochemistry. The developmental study reported here indicates that in the 24-48 hour postnatal animal, p55 *c-fos*-like immunoreactivity can be detected following capsaicin treatment, which is thought to act directly on small-diameter primary afferents (Fitzgerald, 1983). It is not until postnatal day 9 that long-latency bursts of spikes follow electrical stimulation of the nerve, suggesting that the subthreshold depolarisation occurring before this time is sufficient to induce *c-fos* protein (Fitzgerald, 1988). This therefore suggests that, in the adult, neurons receiving input from *subliminal* areas of the peripheral receptive field (Woolf, this volume 1988) may be sufficiently depolarised to produce *c-fos* protein but not to generate action potentials.

The induction of the *c-fos* protein within neurons following *physiological* stimulation appears to be an event that is restricted to the spinal cord. It is unclear at present

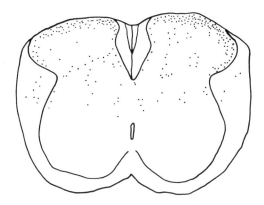

FIGURE 8: Camera lucida drawing of *c-fos* positive nuclei in the spinal cord of a 48-hour rat pup 2 hours after capsaicin treatment (50 μg/kg i.p.).

whether this is due to the release of particular neurotransmitter(s) from primary afferents, to a specialization of the cells themselves, or to a combination of these two possibilities. Substance P or NKA perfused intrathecally into the sub-arachnoid space does result in the generation of p55 *c-fos* in superficial laminae of the dorsal horn, but there are clearly many neurons in laminae VI-VIII which express *c-fos* protein following noxious stimulation of muscle, probably in the absence of a direct peptidergic primary afferent input. Peptide- and FRAP-containing fibres are absent from nerves supplying muscle (McMahon *et al*, 1984). This suggests that there could be a number of effective primary afferent neurotransmitters (beyond the known primary afferent peptides) and perhaps that post-synaptic neurons are specialized to respond in a particular way to depolarization. In PC12 cell lines, the influx of Ca^{++} ions appears to be a key event in the induction of *c-fos* protein (Morgan and Curran 1986). It is of course still necessary to explain why the majority of large-diameter primary afferent targets - motoneurons, gracile nucleus neurons - and the dorsal root ganglion cells do not show *c-fos* protein immunoreactivity following any form of stimulation (Hunt *et al*, 1987). From the data available, a direct monosynaptic connection between small-diameter primary afferents and neurons displaying p55 *c-fos*-like immunoreactivity is strongly suggested, but polysynaptic activation cannot be ruled out (Sagar *et al*, 1988).

As described above, the central distribution of primary afferents from particular peripheral targets matches the pattern of *c-fos*-positive neurons following noxious stimulation of that target, suggesting a close relationship between the primary afferent and the labelled neuron. However, within deeper laminae of the spinal cord, particularly laminae VII and VIII, no direct relationship between small-diameter primary afferents and *c-fos*-positive neurons has been demonstrated and polysynaptic routes may mediate the observed appearance of *c-fos* immunoreactivity.

The significance of the induction of *c-fos* protein is unclear. We suggest that it is a rapid response to injury of peripheral tissue and may contribute to long-term adaptations of these neurons. Recent evidence suggests that *c-fos* phosphoprotein interacts with a 39k protein identified as the product of the jun proto-oncogene. This complex is thought to bind to the transcriptional control elements of other genes containing the AP1 binding-site and to direct gene expression (Rauscher *et al*, 1988). *C-fos* message is detectable within the spinal cord as early as 30 minutes after plantar injection of Freund's adjuvant (R. Dubner, pers. comm.) and the long-term consequences of this treatment are an increased expression of the prodynorphin gene

(Höllt et al, 1987; Ruda et al, 1988), and in the polyarthritic animal, a decreased expression of substance P receptor protein (P.W. Mantyh, pers. comm.).

Whether these early and late genomic events are causally related remains to be demonstrated, but a role for c-fos in the long-term adaptation of neurons to peripheral damage is clearly suggested.

S.W. is supported by the Sir Halley Stewart Trust.

REFERENCES

BERRIDGE, M. (1986) Second messenger dualism in neuromodulation and memory. *Nature* 323: 294-295

BLISS, T.V.P., ERRINGTON, M.L., EVAN, G. AND HUNT, S.P. (1988) Induction of c-fos-like protein in rat hippocampus following electrical stimulation. *J. Physiol.* (in press)

CRAIG, A.D. AND MENSE, S. (1983) The distribution of afferent fibres from the gastrocnemius-soleus muscle in the dorsal horn of the cat, as revealed by the transport of horseradish peroxidase. *Neurosci. Lett.* 41: 233-238

CURRAN, T. AND MORGAN, J. (1985) Superinduction of c-fos by nerve growth factor in the presence of peripherally acting benzodiazepines. *Science* 229: 1265-1268

DRAGUNOW, M. AND ROBERTSON, H.A. (1987) Kindling stimulation induces c-fos protein(s) in granule cells of the rat dentate gyrus. *Nature* 329: 441-442

FITZGERALD, M. (1983) Capsaicin and sensory neurons - a review. *Pain* 15: 109-130

FITZGERALD, M. (1988) The development of activity evoked by fine-diameter cutaneous fibres in the spinal cord of the newborn rat. *Neurosci. Lett.* 86: 161-166

GOELET, P., CASTELLUCCI, V.F., SCHACHER, S. AND KANDEL, E.R. (1986) The long and the short of long-term memory - a molecular framework. *Nature* 322: 419-422

GREENBERG, M.E., GREENE L.A. AND ZIFF, E.B. (1985) Nerve growth factor and epidermal growth factor induce rapid transient changes in proto-oncogene transcription in PC12 cells. *J. Biol. Chem.* 260: 14101-14110

GREENBERG, M.E. AND ZIFF, E.B. (1984) Stimulation of 3T3 cells induces transcription of the c-fos proto-oncogene. *Nature* 311: 433-437

GREENBERG, M.E., ZIFF, E.B. AND GREENE, L.A. (1986) Stimulation of neuronal acetylcholine receptors induces rapid gene transcription. *Science* 234 80-83

HÖLLT, V., HAARMAN, I., MILLAN, M.J. AND HERZ, A. (1987) Prodynorphin gene expression is enhanced in the spinal cord of chronic arthritic rats. *Neurosci. Lett.* 73: 90-94

HUNT, S.P., PINI, A. AND EVAN, G. (1987) Induction of c-fos-like protein in spinal cord neurons following sensory stimulation. *Nature* 328: 632-634

HUNT, S.P. AND ROSSI, J. (1985) Peptide- and non-peptide-containing unmyelinated primary afferents: the parallel processing of nociceptive information. *Phil. Trans. R. Soc. Lond.* B308: 283-289

KACZMAREK, L., SIEDLECKI, J.A. AND DANYSZ, W. (1988) Proto-oncogene c-fos induction in rat hippocampus. *Mol. Brain Res.* 3: 183-186

KRUIJER, W., SCHUBERT, D. AND VERMA, I.M. (1985) Induction of the proto-oncogene c-fos by nerve growth factor. *Proc. Natn. Acad. Sci. U.S.A.* 82: 7330-7334

LIGHT, A.R. AND PERL, E.R. (1979) Reexamination of the dorsal root projection to the spinal dorsal horn including observations on the differential terminations of coarse and fine fibres. *J. Comp. Neurol.* 186: 117-132

LYNN, B. AND CARPENTER, S.E. (1982) Primary afferent units from the hairy skin of the rat hind limb. *Brain Res.* **238**: 29-43

McMahon, S.B., Sykova, E., Wall, P.D., Woolf, C.J. and Gibson, S. (1984) Neurogenic extravasation and substance P levels are less in muscle as compared to skin. *Neurosci. Lett.* **52**: 235-240

Milbrandt, J. (1986) Nerve growth factor rapidly induces *c-fos* mRNA in PC12 rat pheochromocytoma cells. *Proc. Natn. Acad. Sci. U.S.A.* **83**: 4789-4793

Morgan, J., Cohen, D., Hempstead, J. and Curran, T. (1987) Mapping patterns of *c-fos* expression in the central nervous system after seizure. *Science* **237**: 192-197

Morgan, J.I. and Curran, T. (1986) Role of ion flux in the control of *c-fos* expression. *Nature* **322**: 552-555

Rauscher III, F.J., Sambucetti, L.C., Curran, T., Distel, R.J. and Spiegelman,B.M. (1988) Common DNA binding site for fos protein complexes and transcription factor AP-1. *Cell* **52**: 471-480

Ruda, M.A., Iadorola, M.J., Cohen, L.V. and Young III, W.S. (1988) In-situ hybridisation histochemistry and immunocytochemistry reveal an increase in spinal cord dynorphin biosynthesis in a rat model of peripheral inflammation and hyperalgesia. *Proc. Nat. Acad. Sci. U.S.A.* **85**: 622-626

Sagar, S.M., Sharp, F.R. and Curran, T. (1988) Expression of *c-fos* protein in brain: metabolic mapping at the cellular level. *Science* **240**: 1328-1331

Silverman, J.D. and Kruger, L. (1988) Lectin and neuropeptide labelling of separate populations of dorsal root ganglion neurons and associated *nociceptor* thin axons in rat testis and cornea whole-mount preparations. *Somatosensory Res.* **5**: 259-267

Swett, J.E. and Woolf, C.J. (1985) The somatotopic organization of primary afferent terminals in the superficial laminae of the dorsal horn of the rat spinal cord. *J. Comp. Neurol.* **231**: 66-77

Yaksh, T.L. and Rudy, T.A. (1976) Chronic catheterisation of the spinal subarachnoid space. *Physiol. Behav.* **17**: 1031-1036

DENERVATION INDUCED CHANGES IN SOMATOTOPIC ORGANIZATION: THE INEFFECTIVE PROJECTIONS OF AFFERENT FIBRES AND STRUCTURAL PLASTICITY

P.J. Snow and P. Wilson

Mammalian Neurobiology Laboratories, Department of Anatomy, University of Queensland, St. Lucia, Queensland 4067, Australia

> *When I was a child I had a fever,*
> *My hands felt just like two balloons*
> *(Gilmore and Waters, 1979)*

INTRODUCTION

Generally when we speak of plasticity in relation to the nervous system we do not have in our minds only the malleability of structure. We could, for instance, easily be persuaded to consider any phenomenon to which we can attribute alterations of neural circuitry, be they reflected in psychophysical experience or changes in the responsiveness of individual nerve cells. The list of factors that potentially underlie any particular manifestation of plasticity is long and includes mechanisms such as changes in the shape of dendrites (Purves and Hadley, 1985), the effects of transmitter agonists and antagonists (Dykes *et al*, 1984; Zieglgänsberger and Herz, 1971), alteration of the intracellular stores or release of substances that modulate, or potentially modulate, synaptic transmission (Krnjevic and Phillis, 1963; Sillito and Kemp, 1983; Metherate *et al*, 1987; Black *et al*, 1982; Shehab and Atkinson, 1986), and finally, the growth of axons and the formation of new synapses (Goldberger and Murray, 1978; Pubols and Goldberger, 1980; Tsukahara *et al*, 1975; Raisman, 1977).

The phenomenon we know as neural plasticity was probably appreciated long before man had any knowledge of the brain, let alone the existence of nerve cells. Consequently, the repeated demonstration of somatosensory plasticity at the cellular level is only of interest insofar as it might enable us to establish the underlying mechanisms or provide insight into the operation of the intact or damaged somatosensory system. This chapter summarizes a variety of observations that we believe establish a fundamental aspect of nervous organization; an aspect that bestows upon the central nervous system (CNS) the property of structural plasticity.

ORGANIZATION OF TACTILE RECEPTIVE FIELDS AND THE PROJECTIONS OF TACTILE AFFERENTS TO THE DORSAL HORN

Studies of the projections of whole peripheral nerves to the dorsal horn have employed either the transganglionic transport of tracers (Koerber and Brown, 1982;

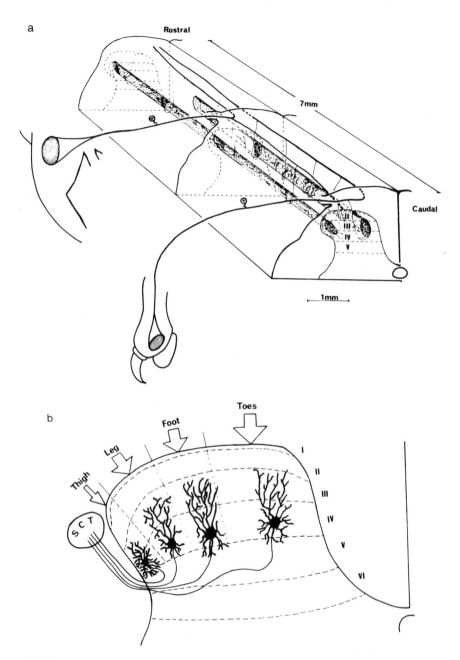

FIGURE 1: The organization within the dorsal horn of the lumbosacral spinal cord, of the collateral arborizations of hair follicle afferent fibres (a) and the dendrites and receptive fields of spinocervical tract neurons (b). (a) Note the columnar organization of the arborizations of single afferents and the restriction of the arborizations of toe and thigh afferents to the medial and lateral regions of the dorsal horn, respectively. (b) Note the mediolateral compartmentalization of the representation of the hindlimb and the position of the dendritic trees of the spinocervical tract neurons. Fig. 1a is modified from Brown *et al*, (1977b).

Molander and Grant, 1986; Nyberg and Blomquist, 1985; Woolf and Fitzgerald, 1986) or the mapping of regions that have been depleted of fluoride resistant acid phosphatase as a consequence of nerve transection (Devor and Claman, 1980). These studies have shown that the afferents of particular nerves have a precise somatotopic organization which is such that nerves supplying the proximal part of a limb project to the lateral dorsal horn while nerves supplying the distal parts project to the medial dorsal horn.

The intraaxonal injection of HRP into single, group II, cutaneous, afferent fibres has been used to establish the organization of their collateral arborizations within the dorsal horn. This work has shown that these arborizations are found in or around Rexed's laminae III and IV where the terminations of the collaterals of a single fibre are contained within a narrow (width 150-400μm), longitudinal column of tissue (Fig 1a) (Brown et al, 1977b, 1978, 1981). In this position these terminations are ideally placed to make synaptic contacts with the dendrites of spinocervical tract (SCT) neurons (Fig. 1b) and other mechanoreceptive dorsal horn neurons (DHNs) (Brown et al, 1977a, 1980a,b; Wilson et al, 1986). Given this organization of afferent terminals it is not surprising to find; (a) that the location of the tactile receptive fields (RFs) of neurons located medially in the dorsal horn are radically different from those of neurons, that in the cat, lie only 1.0 mm away in the lateral region and (b) that there is only a gradual change in RF position between cells displaced along the rostrocaudal axis of the cord (Fig. 2a) (Brown and Fuchs, 1975; Brown et al, 1980; Light and Durkovic, 1984; Wilson et al, 1986).

From these studies on the SCT cell - hair follicle afferent (HFA) system, it was concluded that there existed a clear correlation between the structure and function (Brown et al, 1980b; Brown and Noble, 1981) and while it has since been found that the low threshold RFs of some SCT cells have an excitatory subliminal fringe, it is important to note that input from this fringe *does not* appear to be mediated by group II HFAs (Brown et al, 1987). It is perhaps also important to emphasize that when care is taken to localize the responsive neurons, the area of skin represented by a group of SCT cells is similar to that which is represented by a group of unidentified DHNs recorded across the same region of the dorsal horn. That is to say, in the region of termination of group II cutaneous primary afferent fibres (laminae III and IV) of chloralose anaesthetized cats, there is only a single somatotopic map of tactile input and no somatotopically displaced cells have been located (Wilson, Meyers and Snow, 1986).

As we have noted previously (Wilson et al, 1987) the organization of the terminations of cutaneous afferents seems quite incompatible with the suggestion put forward by Devor and Wall (1981a; 1981b) to explain the mediolateral reorganization of somatotopy in the dorsal horn that they reported followed denervation of the distal hindlimb. These workers suggested that in normal animals tactile afferents innervating the proximal skin of the hindlimb and terminating in the lateral part of the dorsal horn also have ineffective synapses with DHNs in the medial dorsal horn. They further proposed that after transection of the nerves that supply afferents to this medial region, these ineffective synapses somehow become functional. Since then some anatomical evidence has been obtained that collaterals of afferents in thigh nerves may form, in the medial dorsal horn, *en passant* synapses as they sweep laterally from the dorsal columns through the medial dorsal horn (Devor et al,1986), but there is as yet no indication as to which sensory receptors are innervated by these axons. Finally, in evaluating these theories it must be emphasized that the existence of the phenomenon of mediolateral

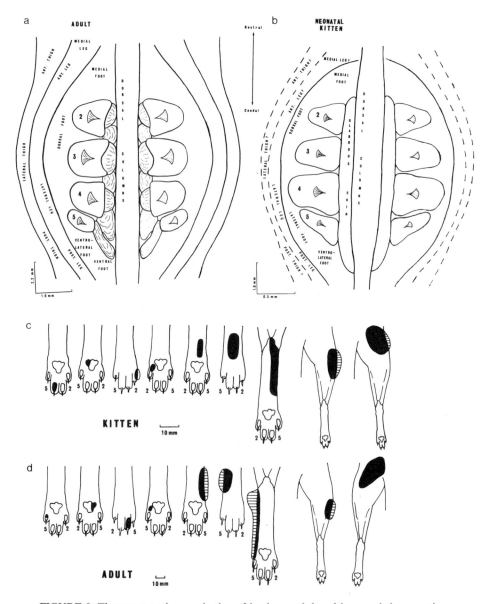

FIGURE 2: The somatotopic organization of lumbosacral dorsal horn and the receptive fields of single neurons in the adult cat and the neonatal kitten. (a) Somatotopic map in the adult based on mapping the receptive fields of single spinocervical tract neurons. (b) Somatotopic map in the neonatal kitten based on mapping the receptive fields of single unidentified dorsal horn neurons in the neonatal kitten. Because of the small size of the dorsal horn the boundaries indicated by the dashed lines were often difficult to confirm precisely. Note in (a) and (b) the similarity in the representation of the toes and the skin of the foot. (c) and (d) The receptive fields of single neurons in the adult cat and the neonatal kitten. Note the similarity in the sizes of the receptive fields in relation to the size of the hindpaw. Figures are modified from Wilson and Snow (1988a).

reorganization has certainly not been unequivocally established (see Brown *et al*, 1984; Pubols, 1984; Wilson, 1987; Wilson *et al*, 1987).

Although the distribution of group II afferent terminals was not compatible with theories concerning a mediolateral reorganization of somatotopy it did not negate the possibility that a single tactile afferent might have ineffective synapses rostral or caudal to its somatotopically appropriate (SA) region; that region of the dorsal horn where its RF is contained within the RFs of DHNs (Fig. 3a). To test this hypothesis we stained single HFA fibres in the dorsal columns intraaxonally and then mapped the RFs of DHNs below the stained segment of axon (Meyers and Snow, 1984). The results showed that at least 42% of the HFA collaterals in the medial part of the dorsal horn projected to somatotopically inappropriate (SIA) regions - regions in which the RFs of the afferents were not represented within the RFs of DHNs (Figs. 3b, 4a and b). Collaterals within the 600 μm length of cord adjacent to the SA regions were normal in appearance but beyond that point collaterals in the SIA region (SIA collaterals) showed very little branching and had few or no boutons. Within the toe representation of normal animals we have observed such collaterals at distances of up to 3 mm from the boundary between the SA and the SIA regions (Fig. 4a; Wilson and Snow, unpublished observations). In terms of somatotopy, this is equal to the length of dorsal horn devoted to the representation of a complete digit (Fig. 2a) (Wilson *et al*, 1986).

It is unlikely that conventional neuroanatomical or neurophysiological techniques could reveal such endings. That this is so may be deduced from a perusal of studies in which central axonal arbors have been labelled transganglionically with HRP or its lectin conjugates. Most authors agree that there is minimal overlap between the central arborizations of afferents in peripheral nerves labelled by these methods, unless the nerves themselves have overlapping cutaneous territories (Koerber and Brown, 1982; Molander and Grant, 1986; Woolf and Fitzgerald, 1986). This is particularly true of overlap in the mediolateral axis of the dorsal horn, but even in cases where some rostrocaudal overlap has been demonstrated, such as between the spinal projections of the palmar digital nerves that supply adjacent digits in the cat (Nyberg and Blomqvist, 1985) the overlap may reflect the overlap of the peripheral fields of the two nerves. It is, however, also possible that the overlap of digit projections simply reflects the length of cord over which DHNs would have RFs on the skin between two adjacent digits. For instance, the figures of Nyberg and Blomqvist (1985) show, when the transganglionic transport of HRP is used to demonstrate the projections of the nerves from two adjacent digits, that the rostrocaudal overlap of these projections is in the order of 1 mm. Clearly this is far less than the 6 mm of overlap that would be expected on the basis of our intraaxonal staining studies of the SIA collaterals of HFAs in the cat (Fig. 4a) (Meyers and Snow, 1984; Wilson and Snow, unpublished observations). Perhaps this discrepancy reflects the fact that such techniques seem to label the terminals of fine afferents far more easily than they do those of larger group II myelinated fibres (Nyberg and Blomqvist, 1985). Collaterals of similar appearance to the SIA collaterals of cat HFA fibres have been observed to issue from single intraaxonally stained cutaneous group II mechanoreceptive afferents in the rat spinal cord (Woolf, 1987) and from single C-fiber afferents in the guinea-pig dorsal horn (Sugiura *et al*, 1986; see also article by Sugiura in this volume), though in neither case was the relationship of the collaterals to the local somatotopy established. Finally it is important to mention that electrophysiological studies (Meyers and Snow, 1986) have shown that, in the cat, at least some of the SIA collaterals are invaded by action potentials.

While it is premature to claim that the SIA collaterals are completely ineffective (ie.

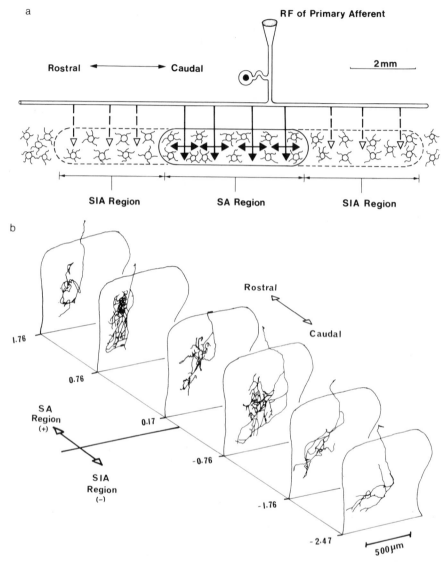

FIGURE 3: (a) Schematic diagram in which a single cutaneous afferent gives rise to ineffective, somatotopically inappropriate (SIA) axonal terminations rostral and caudal to the somatotopically appropriate (SA) region - that region in which the receptive fields of dorsal horn neurons overlap, or include, that of the afferent fibre. (b) The organization of the collateral arborizations of a single hair follicle afferent fibre within the SA and SIA regions of the dorsal horn of a normal adult cat. The positive and negative numbers indicate the distance of the collaterals rostral and caudal, respectively, from the border between the SA and SIA regions. Note the relative simplicity of the arborizations of the two most caudal collaterals in the SIA region.

produce no epsps in DHNs), it must be concluded that, at least under the conditions of our experiments, most of them play no part in the synthesis of the extracellularly determined RFs of DHNs. Certainly most of them could not activate the dendrites of cells within the SA region, for in the medial part of the dorsal horn, the dendrites of even the largest cells extend, along the rostrocaudal axis of the cord, only about 500 μm from the cell body (Proshansky and Egger, 1977; Brown et al, 1977b) - a distance much shorter than the distance between many of the SIA collaterals and the SA region (see Fig. 3b) (Meyers and Snow, 1984). More important, however, are the observations that the arborizations of SIA collaterals are much simpler that those of normal collaterals and that, at least at the level of the light microscope, they appear to be virtually devoid of synaptic boutons. These observations suggest that SIA collaterals have little or no synaptic influence on DHNs. We suggest that, in general, such blind axonal endings might exist in all topographically organized regions of the CNS and that they may represent a hitherto unrecognised but fundamental aspect of brain organization which, as we shall show below, endows the CNS with a the latent potential for structural plasticity.

SOMATOTOPIC MAPS IN ADULT SPINAL CORD

Owing to the predictability of changes in somatotopy with direction, a detailed somatotopic map is not a prerequisite for demonstrating the existence of SIA collaterals. However, a detailed map is an absolute necessity for detecting alterations in the RFs of postsynaptic neurons, alterations that may be attributable to the increases in the effectiveness of afferent input from any particular area of skin. The spatial accuracy of maps depends very much on the precision with which individual cells are localized. This is particularly true in those parts of a map where there is a high somatotopic gradient - i.e. regions where large changes in the positions of RFs occur over small transneural distances. If a set of projection neurons is available then an electrode may be positioned close to single antidromically identified cells. As it is likely that individual cells in such a set will have similar, well defined and somewhat predictable mechanoreceptive properties, the presence of induced alterations of synaptic input is more easily demonstrable than it is among a randomly sampled, unidentified population of neurons. Furthermore, by recording the antidromically evoked spike, a projection neuron can still be accurately localized after the complete or partial loss of its peripheral RF (Brown et al, 1984). In contrast, where the response to cutaneous stimulation is itself used to locate unidentified cells, there is a danger that in an unresponsive region an experimenter might inadvertently accept recordings from responsive neurons that are, in fact, quite distant from the electrode tip (Pubols, 1984; Wilson, 1987). This is particularly true when somatotopic maps are based on recordings of multi-unit activity or what has become known as multiunit hash.

For the above reasons we decided to derive a detailed map of the representation of the hindlimb of the cat from the discharge patterns of SCT cells (Wilson et al, 1986). The resultant map is shown in Figure 2a and is a distal view of the hindlimb in which the toes are represented in a rostrocaudal order from toe 2 to toe 5. The internal details of this map are highly repeatable from animal to animal, and within a single individual the representations of the left and right hindlimb are mirror images. Finally, within the toe representation the RFs of single SCT cells usually cover only a small fraction of the total skin area of a single toe (Fig. 2c, 5a, 6a and 7a). Thus the cells of origin of the SCT provides the experimenter with a precisely organized representation of the hindlimb and its individual digits.

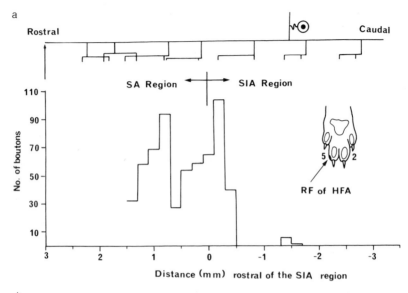

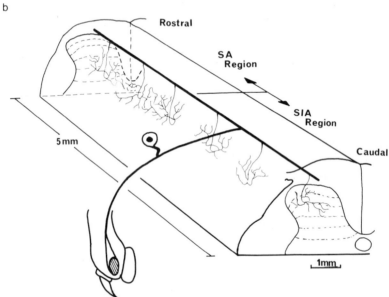

FIGURE 4: (a) The distribution of the collaterals and synaptic boutons of a single hair follicle afferent (HFA) fibre across the border between the somatotopically appropriate (SA) and the somatotopically inappropriate (SIA) regions in a normal adult cat. The positive and negative numbers indicate the distance of the collaterals rostral and caudal, respectively, from the border between the SA and SIA regions. Note that the collaterals that are more that 500μm from the SA region have few boutons compared with those in the SA region. (b) Three dimensional representation of the most caudal 6 collaterals from the HFA axon shown in (a). Note the relative simplicity of the arborizations of the two most caudal collaterals in the SIA region.

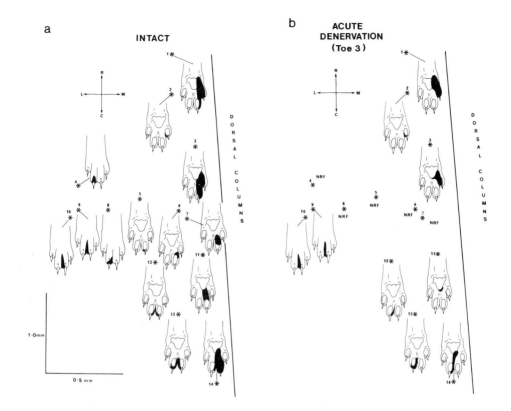

FIGURE 5: The immediate effects of denervation of toe 3 on the receptive fields of single, antidromically identified, spinocervical tract neurons within and around the toe 3 representation of a normal adult cat. (a) The receptive fields of single spinocervical tract neurons before denervation of toe 3. (b) The receptive fields of the same neurons within 3 to 4 hours of denervation of toe 3. Note the absence of receptive fields of neurons in the center of the deprived region and the partial receptive fields of neurons that have receptive fields that formerly were partially on the denervated skin (tracks 3, 9, 10, 11, 12 and 14). NRF - no detectable receptive field.

EFFECTS OF DENERVATING A SINGLE TOE IN ADULT AND NEONATAL ANIMALS

Given the rostral to caudal representation of individual toes, an obvious way of potentially forcing the expression of SIA inputs is to denervate a single digit. In the literature on denervation-induced map changes in adult mammals there are several examples of *immediate* (< 48 h) changes in map boundaries (see below). In the spinal cord the utilization of antidromically identified SCT neurons together with the careful recording of track coordinates enabled us to test unequivocally for any immediate expression of new afferent inputs. To do this we plotted the RFs of single SCT neurons within and close to the representation of toe 3, then denervated that toe and immediately examined the responsiveness of the same SCT neurons to cutaneous stimuli. The results showed that within a few hours of denervation there were no signs of the expression of new cutaneous inputs. Those SCT cells with RFs that extended across the border between denervated and innervated skin simply lost that portion of their RF situated on the denervated skin (cf. Fig. 5a with Fig. 5b). There was little or no change in this situation over the next 20 days (Wilson and Snow, 1986). However, 30 to

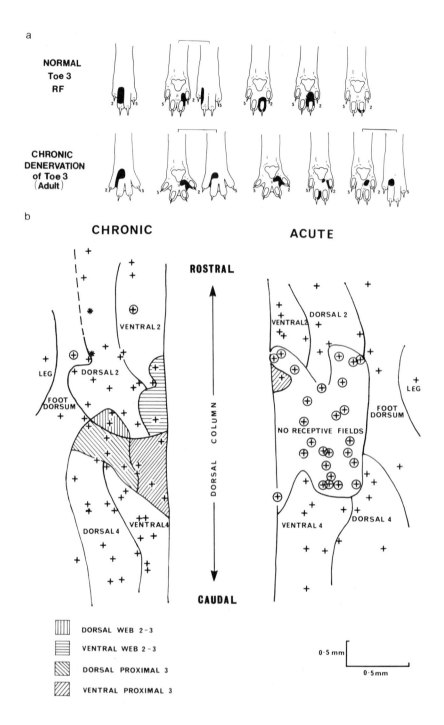

a

NORMAL
Toe 3
RF

CHRONIC
DENERVATION
of Toe 3
(Adult)

b

CHRONIC

ACUTE

ROSTRAL

VENTRAL 2

LEG

DORSAL 2

FOOT
DORSUM

VENTRAL 4

DORSAL 4

DORSAL COLUMN

CAUDAL

VENTRAL 2

DORSAL 2

FOOT
DORSUM

LEG

NO RECEPTIVE FIELDS

VENTRAL 4

DORSAL 4

||||||| DORSAL WEB 2-3

≡≡≡ VENTRAL WEB 2-3

//// DORSAL PROXIMAL 3

//// VENTRAL PROXIMAL 3

0·5 mm

0·5 mm

70 days after denervation many SCT cells in the deprived toe 3 representation had developed new cutaneous RFs on toes 2 or 4 - skin that is normally represented only rostral or caudal of the toe 3 representation (Fig. 6a and b). Although the new RFs were rarely split or abnormally large (Fig. 6a) it was not possible to make any unequivocal statements about the topographical orderliness of the reorganized region other than that toe 2 was represented rostrally and toe 4 caudally (Fig 6b). What is important is that this reorganization is exactly what we would have predicted on the basis of an increase in the effectiveness of those SIA collaterals of toe 2 and toe 4 afferents that normally lie within the toe 3 representation (cf. Fig. 3a with Fig 6b). Furthermore, the rostrocaudal reorganization we have found in the toe representation of the cat is consistent with independent findings of Markus *et al*, (1984), who showed that chronic section of the sciatic nerve in the rat caused a caudal spread of up to 2 mm in the representation of the cutaneous territory of the saphenous nerve, rather than a medial spread of the representation of the proximal skin of the thigh.

In order to determine whether anatomical changes in the pre-existing SIA collateral arborizations might be the basis for the rostrocaudal reorganization of somatotopy we denervated toe 3 or both toes 3 and 4 in neonatal kittens and raised them to adulthood (Wilson and Snow, 1988b). Presumably nerve section at this stage of development would result in a greater mortality (Aldskogius and Risling, 1981) of sensory cells and perhaps more pronounced changes in central circuitry. In most of these animals SCT cells throughout the deprived region had RFs on skin that normally would have been represented rostrally or caudally (Figs. 7a and b). A substantial number (30%) of SCT neurons had multiple RFs, usually one on the rostrally represented intact toe and one on the caudally represented intact toe (Fig. 7a). In order to remove the mechanically sensitive neuromas, the partially regenerated nerves in the operated toe(s) were usually recut acutely in these experiments, but in a few cases where this was not done it was found that some SCT cells were additionally excited by light tactile stimulation of the skin covering a large area of the operated toes. Thus the expression of new inputs is apparently not reversed by the reinnervation of neonatally denervated skin. As in those animals that were exposed to nerve section as adults, the locations of the new RFs were such that they could be accounted for by an increase in the efficacy of the SIA collaterals of intact afferent fibres. In the cases where toes 3 and 4 were denervated SCT cells that were up to 5 mm caudal of the normal representation of toe 2 were found to be activated by light tactile stimulation of the skin of that toe (Fig 7b). This distance represents the longest distance over which denervation induced reorganization has been observed within the somatosensory system.

After mapping the reorganized region in neonatally-denervated adult cats we

---

FIGURE 6: The effects of chronic and acute denervation of toe 3 on the receptive fields of spinocervical tract neurons in and around the toe 3 representation in the adult cat. (a) The receptive fields of spinocervical tract neurons within the toe 3 representation of normal adult cats and the receptive fields of spinocervical tract neurons in this position 30 to 70 days after denervation of toe 3. (b) Somatotopic maps from three single experiments in which the left toe 3 was chronically denervated and the right toe 3 was acutely denervated. The boundaries of the acutely deprived region were used to line up the maps from the three experiments. Proximal toe 3 refers to the proximal skin on toe 3 that remains innervated after section of the digital nerves. The circled crosses indicate the position of tracts in which cells had no light tactile cutaneous receptive field. Modified from Wilson and Snow (1987).

a

NORMAL
TOE 3

NEONATAL
DENERVATION
of Toe 3

b NEONATAL
DENERVATION

ACUTE
DENERVATION

TOE 3
&
TOE 4
REGION

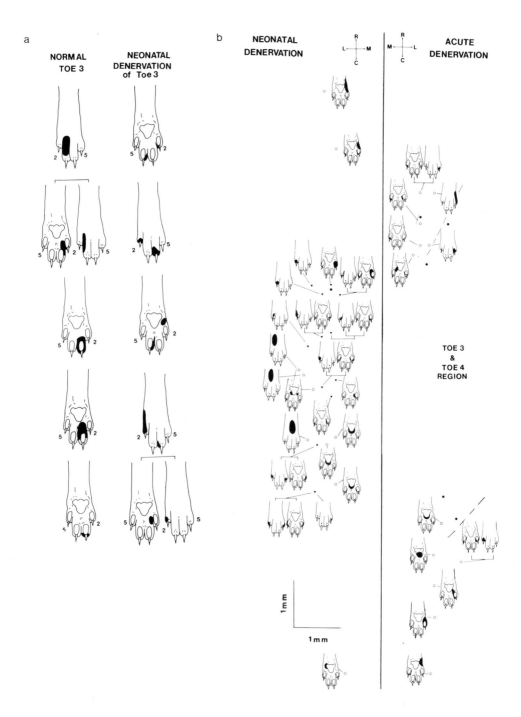

1 mm

1 mm

attempted to impale and to inject, with HRP, single HFA fibres that supplied the toes adjacent to the denervated toes. The axons of such afferents are difficult to find in individual experiments and it was often necessary to accept penetrations which allowed only a relatively short injection period, with the result that only a short length of axon was stained. Thus in order to maximize the staining of SIA collaterals, axons were injected in the dorsal columns at a level that was as close as possible to half way along the somatotopically reorganized region. In each experiment, histological examination of this region showed that it received collaterals from the injected axons. In 3 out of 6 axons, SIA collaterals were found that gave rise to more complex arborizations and bore a variable number of boutons (Fig. 8a and b). In the other cases the SIA collaterals resembled those in normal animals in that they had simple arborizations and lacked boutons.

These results have led us to conclude that within the spinal cord the rostrocaudal reorganization of somatotopy that follows *neonatal* nerve section involves local proliferation of the SIA collateral arborizations of cutaneous afferents. Furthermore, as the dorsal horn of the neonatal kitten shows a normal somatotopic representation of the toes (Fig. 2a and b), we suggest that a similar mechanism underlies the rostrocaudal reorganization of somatotopy that we have observed in the adult cat (Wilson and Snow, 1988a). Thus it would seem that although many SIA collaterals are normally ineffective in activating neurons, they may develop an influence over nearby nerve cells in situations where there is a loss of the normal, dominant input to these cells. The stimulus for proliferation of SIA collaterals might be the same as that which evokes collateral sprouting of C-fibre arborizations in neonatal rat dorsal horn after peripheral nerve section (Fitzgerald and Vrbova, 1985), or which causes myelinated afferents to sprout into lamina II in rats in which C-fibres have been destroyed by neonatally treatment with capsaicin (Nagy and Hunt, 1983). Such morphologically based plasticity may, of course, be augmented by the strengthening of normally weak synaptic inputs from primary afferents which have been shown to exist in SIA regions by electrical stimulation of nerves or by application of drugs to functionally unidentified dorsal horn neurons (Pubols *et al*, 1986; Markus and Pomeranz, 1987).

FIGURE 7: The effects of denervation of toe 3 or toes 3 and 4 in neonatal kittens on the somatotopic organization of spinocervical tract neurons within the toe representation of adult cats. (a) The receptive fields of spinocervical tract neurons within the representation of toe 3 in normal adult cats (left column) and in adult cats in which toe 3 has been denervated in the first week of life (right column). Note the split receptive fields that are much more common in these animals than in cats which were denervated as adults (see Fig. 6a). (b) Somatotopic organization of spinocervical tract cells in an adult cat in which toes 3 and 4 of the left foot were denervated in the first week of life. Toes 3 and 4 of the right foot were denervated acutely in order to establish more easily the normal caudal boundary of the toe 2 representation and the normal rostral boundary of the toe 5 representation. Note that cells in the deprived portion of the representation have developed new receptive fields on toes 2 and 5 (see filled triangles) - areas that are normally represented more than 3mm rostral or caudal to the center of the deprived region. Filled circles show the position of spinocervical tract cells that lack a detectable receptive field. Open circles indicate the position of spinocervical tract cells with receptive fields that were considered to be normal in relation to the position of these cells within the normal the somatotopic representation of the foot and toes.

ORIGIN OF SIA PROJECTIONS

One possible origin of the SIA collaterals is that they represent the remnants of connections that were effective during an earlier developmental stage but were withdrawn during the later formation of precise, topographically matched projections between sets of neurons (Purves and Lichtman, 1980). Unfortunately, there are few useful data concerning this point. On the basis of transganglionic HRP studies the projections of peripheral cutaneous nerves to the dorsal horn appears to be identical in both the neonatal and adult rat (Fitzgerald and Swett, 1983; Smith, 1983). While these data have been taken to indicate that there is no stage of exuberant afferent projections in the developing mammalian somatosensory system (Fitzgerald, 1985) there remain some serious concerns relating to the estimation of the size of the projections zones of peripheral nerves from transganglionic labelling (see section 2 above). Electrophysiologically we have shown that in the cat at the time of birth, both the RFs of single DHNs and the internal organization of the somatotopic map are not detectably different from those seen in the adult (Fig. 2a, b, c and d)(Wilson and Snow, 1988a). Perhaps this is not surprising given the long gestation period of the cat and at birth even the SI cortex already appears to contain an orderly and adult-like representation of the body (Rubel, 1971). Nevertheless, Golgi studies have indicated that the mature pattern of afferent arborizations in the dorsal horn is not yet present at birth (Scheibel and Scheibel, 1969). Alternatively, perhaps both SIA and SA collaterals simply develop to their adult-like state, or perhaps the former lose their efficacy and their synaptic boutons during prenatal development. In the rat, dorsal root afferents grow into the cord at embryonic day 17-18 (Smith, 1983). Large diameter fibres are the first to arrive in the dorsal horn with the finer C-fibre afferents arriving in lamina II around embryonic day 19-20 (Fitzgerald, 1987). While there appears to be a postnatal shrinkage of the RFs of DHNs in the rat this has been attributed to the late formation of synapses by C-fibres and the maturation of interneuronal systems in lamina II, rather than to any change in the projections of the afferents themselves (Fitzgerald, 1985). However, a possible role of changing SIA projections in this maturation of RFs has not been ruled out.

EVIDENCE FOR SIAS AT OTHER LEVELS OF THE NEURAXIS

In SI cortex of the cat there are now two lines of evidence that indicate that thalamo-cortical neurons have SIA projections. Firstly, while the skin of each toe is represented over a tangential area of approximately 1 to 1.5 mm^2 (Felleman et al, 1983), intraaxonal staining has shown that those single thalamo-cortical neurons that receive input from the toe have terminal arborizations that occupy an area of 0.7 to 2.6 mm^2 (Landry and Deschenes, 1981). As the RFs of these thalamocortical neurons covered only about 1/4 to 1/3 of the hairy skin of a single toe SIA projections must exist. Secondly, SIA projections have been demonstrated directly by intracortical terminal microstimulation and the subsequent antidromic activation of single thalamo-cortical neurons from somatotopically identified regions of the toe representation in SI cortex. Using this technique SIA projections could be demonstrated at tangential distances of up to 830 μm from the SA region (Fig. 9) (Snow et al, 1988).

Unlike the SIA projections of primary afferents to the dorsal horn (Meyers and Snow, 1984) there is no evidence that the arborizations of the SIA projections of thalamo-cortical neurons are structurally any different from those of the SA projections (Landry and Deschenes, 1981). This statement is, however, based only on the published

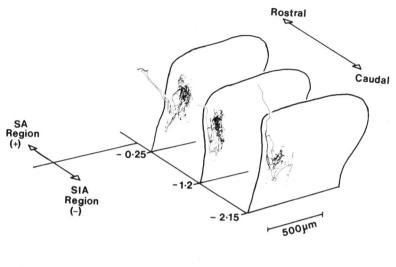

SA Region (+)

SIA Region (−)

Rostral

Caudal

− 0·25

−1·2

− 2·15

500μm

b

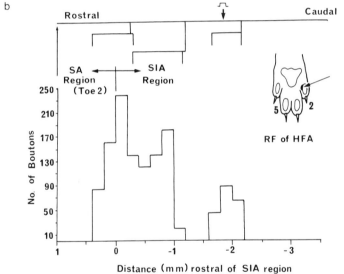

Rostral

Caudal

SA Region (Toe 2)

SIA Region

No. of Boutons

250
210
170
130
90
50
10

RF of HFA

5   2

1   0   -1   -2   -3

Distance (mm) rostral of SIA region

FIGURE 8: (a) The organization of the collateral arborizations of a single hair follicle afferent (HFA) fibre with a receptive field (RF) on toe 2, in an adult cat in which the nerves to toes 3 and 4 were cut and ligated in the first week of life. Mapping the contralateral dorsal horn showed that these collaterals are all within the region of dorsal horn that normally would have contained the representation of toe 3. (b) The distribution of collaterals and the density of boutons of the single HFA shown in (a). Note that although all these collaterals project to the neonatally deprived, SIA region, they still give rise to many boutons, presumably as a result both of local proliferation of the SIA arborizations and of synaptogensis. This figure should be compared with similar data obtained from normal adult cats and plotted in Figure 4a. The positive and negative numbers represent the distance rostral and caudal of the border between the somatotopicaly appropriate (SA) and the somatotopically inappropriate (SIA) regions. The arrow above the axon indicates the site of intraaxonal injection of HRP.

figures (Landry and Deschenes, 1981) of the terminations of thalamo-cortical neurons in which it is not possible to identify either a region of simple branching or which parts of the terminations lie in SA and in SIA cortex. Nevertheless the *immediate* (< 48 h) reorganization of cortical somatotopy observed following peripheral nerve section in the monkey (Merzenich *et al*, 1983a,b), cat (Metzler and Marks, 1979), raccoon (Kelahan and Doetsch, 1984) and rat (Wall and Cusick, 1984) suggests that the SIA projections of thalamo-cortical neurons may be structurally normal but ineffective as a result of tonic inhibitory mechanisms (see Dykes *et al*, 1984; Snow *et al*, 1988). However, structural changes such as the local proliferation of the SIA terminations of thalamocortical fibres might also contribute to somatotopic reorganization for it has been shown in the monkey, raccoon and rat that longer postoperative survival times result in a progressive increase in the influence of intact cutaneous inputs to distances of up to 600 μm from their normal representation (Merzenich *et al*, 1983a,b; Kelahan and Doetsch, 1984; Wall and Cusick, 1984).

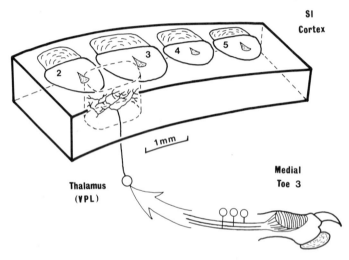

FIGURE 9: The somatotopically inappropriate projections of single thalamo-cortical neurons to the digit representation in the SI cortex of the cat. The figurine of the paw representation is derived from data presented in the figures of Felleman *et al*, (1983) and the projection of the thalamocortical neuron is derived from the data of Landry and Deschenes (1981) and Snow *et al*, (1988).

GENERAL CONCLUSION

The experiments reviewed above show that in the spinal dorsal horn of adult mammals, primary afferent fibres give rise to simple axonal arborizations that do not appear to have synaptic boutons or to excite spinal neurons. In the cat, the removal, early in life, of the normal cutaneous primary afferent input to a restricted area of dorsal horn stimulates branching and synapse formation in some of the simple axonal arborizations of intact afferents that supply skin nearby to the denervated region thus enabling these afferents newly to excite the cells in the deprived region. It has yet to be seen whether, in adult animals, removal of afferent input induces similar microstructural changes in the ineffective SIA terminations.

We have reviewed some evidence for the existence of ineffective axonal endings at higher levels of the somatosensory system. We propose that such endings exist

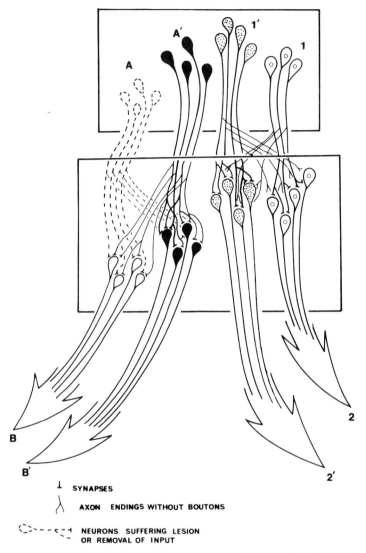

FIGURE 10: Schematic diagram illustrating the proposed distribution of ineffective axonal terminations within the CNS and the effects of removing the excitatory input from, or lesioning, a set of afferent neurons, on the microstructure and the synaptic efficacy these terminations. The two pathways on the left (A to B and A' to B') serve similar, though not identical, functions. The two pathways on the right (1 to 2 and 1' to 2') also serve similar functions but these functions are quite different from those served by the two pathways on the left. Ineffective axonal terminations form a functionally inert, anatomical link between A and B', A' and B, 1 and 2' and 1' and 2. This link does not involve synapses. No such links exist between alphabetically- or numerically-labelled sets of neurons. The removal of input to, or lesion of, A permits the ineffective axonal terminations from A' to proliferate and develop synaptic boutons thereby enabling A' to influence B. Thus B becomes responsive to the same inputs as B' - an output that previously served a closely allied though not identical function to that served by B. No communication is established between the alphabetically-labelled pathways and those labelled numerically. In this model structural plasticity does not violate the localization of function that is such a basic feature of CNS organization

throughout the CNS. That they have not been previously documented might reflect not only the difficulty of identifying them with conventional electrophysiological or neuroanatomical techniques but also a natural inclination for neuroscientists to seek correlations between function and structure.

If ineffective axonal terminations are organized elsewhere in the CNS as they are in the spinal dorsal horn and the SI cortex, then the plasticity they impart to the brain would be spatially constrained. That is to say, depriving an area of its major input would enable inputs that normally excite an adjacent area to assume, in addition, an influence over the deprived area. Both the spatial and directional aspects of this spread of influence require some qualification. Within the mature somatosensory system the influence of intact inputs has been shown to spread up to about 600 μm in the SI cortex and up to 5000 μm in the spinal dorsal horn. However, in relation to the directionality of this spread it seems clear that in the spinal cord such changes occur only along the longitudinal axis of the cord and not in the mediolateral direction. Therefore, we would suggest that the tolerance of this form of plasticity rests in the spatial organization and regionality of function apparent at a particular locus in the CNS. Consider, for instance, a group of nerve cells whose function is closely allied to that of a neighbouring group. This group would be surrounded by a few simple, physiologically ineffective, axonal terminations from afferent neurons that provide strong synaptic connections to the neighbouring group (Fig. 10). Removal of the dominant input to the group of nerve cells would cause these ineffective, afferent terminations to proliferate and form synapses. Thus an input that once drove only the neighbouring group will now drive, in addition, the deprived group, thereby permitting the continued usage of the deprived group for a purpose not vastly different from that which they once served. An important aspect of this model is that although afferents that carry quite different information might activate sets of neurons *nearby* the deprived group, these afferents do not give rise to ineffective axonal projections in the vicinity of the deprived group. Consequently these afferents cannot establish an influence over the deprived group. Thus in this model structural plasticity does not violate the localization of function that is such a basic feature of CNS organization (Fig. 10).

ACKNOWLEDGEMENTS

We wish to thank Ms D. Crook for her technical assistance, Ms K. E. Snow for drawing the figures and Drs A. Bowers and K. Bedi for critically reading the manuscript. This work was supported by the a grant from the Australian NH and the MRC and from the Queensland Brain Research Foundation to the authors.

REFERENCES

ALDSKOGIUS, H. AND RISLING, M. (1981). Effects of sciatic neurectomy on neuronal number and size distribution in the L7 ganglion of kittens. *Experimental Neurology* 74, 597-604.

BLACK, I.B., KESSLER, J.A., ALDER, J.E. AND BOHN, M.C. (1982). Regulation of substance P expression and metabolism *in vivo* and *in vitro*. In: *Substance P in the Nervous System*, CIBA Foundation symposium 91, ed. PORTER, R. and O'CONNOR, M., pp. 107-118, Pitman, London.

BROWN, A.G., FYFFE, R., NOBLE, R., ROSE, P.K. AND SNOW, P.J. (1980a). The density, distribution and topographical organization of spinocervical tract neurones in the cat. *Journal of Physiology* 300, 409-428.

BROWN, A.G., FYFFE, R.E.W., NOBLE, R. AND ROWE, M.J. (1984). Effects of hind limb nerve section on lumbosacral dorsal horn neurones in the cat. *Journal of Physiology* **354**, 375-394.

BROWN, A.G., FYFFE, R.E.W., ROSE, P.K. AND SNOW, P.J. (1981). Spinal cord collaterals from axons of type II slowly adapting units in the cat. *Journal of Physiology* **316**, 469-480.

BROWN, A.G., KOERBER, H.R. AND NOBLE, R. (1987). An intracellular study of spinocervical tract cell responses to natural stimuli and single hair afferent fibres in cats. *Journal of Physiology* **382**, 331-354.

BROWN, A.G. AND NOBLE, R. (1982). Connexions between hair follicle afferent fibres and spinocervical tract neurones in the cat: the synthesis of receptive fields. *Journal of Physiology*, **323**, 77-91.

BROWN, A.G., ROSE, P.K. AND SNOW, P.J. (1977a). The morphology of spinocervical tract neurones revealed by intracellular injection of horseradish peroxidase. *Journal of Physiology* **270**, 747-764.

BROWN, A.G., ROSE, P.K. AND SNOW, P.J. (1977b). The morphology of hair follicle afferent fibre collaterals in the spinal cord of the cat. *Journal of Physiology* **272**, 779-797.

BROWN, A.G., ROSE, P.K. AND SNOW, P.J. (1978). Morphology and organization of axon collaterals from afferent fibres of slowly adapting type I units in cat spinal cord. *Journal of Physiology* **277**, 15-27.

BROWN, A.G., ROSE, P.K. AND SNOW, P.J. (1980b). Dendritic trees and cutaneous receptive fields of adjacent spinocervical tract neurones in the cat. *Journal of Physiology* **300**, 429-440.

BROWN, P.B. AND FUCHS, J.L. (1975). Somatotopic representation of hindlimb skin in cat dorsal horn. *Journal of Neurophysiology* **38**, 1-19.

DYKES, R.W., LANDRY, P., METHERATE, R. AND HICKS, T.P. (1984). Functional role of GABA in cat primary somatosensory cortex: shaping receptive fields of cortical neurons. *Journal of Neurophysiology* **52**, 1066-1093.

DEVOR, M., BASBAUM, A.I. AND SELTZER, Z. (1986). Spinal somatotopic plasticity: possible anatomical basis for somatotopically inappropriate connections. In: *Development and Plasticity in the Mammalian Spinal Cord*, pp. 239-253, ed. GOLDBERGER, M. E., GORIO, A. and MURRAY, M., Padova, Fidia Research Series Vol. 3.

DEVOR, M. AND CLAMAN, D. (1980). Mapping and plasticity of acid phosphatase afferents in rat dorsal horn. *Brain Research* **190**, 17-28.

DEVOR, M. AND WALL P.D. (1981a). Effect of peripheral nerve injury on receptive fields of cells in the cat spinal cord. *Journal of Comparative Neurology* **199**, 277-291.

DEVOR, M. AND WALL P.D. (1981b). Plasticity in the spinal cord sensory map following peripheral nerve injury in rats. *Journal of Neuroscience* **1**, 679-684.

DYKES, R.W., LANDRY, P., METHERATE, R. AND HICKS T.P. (1984) Functional role of GABA in cat primary somatosensory cortex: shaping receptive fields of cortical neurons. *Journal of Physiology* **357**, 1-22

FELLEMAN, D.J., WALL, J.T., CUSICK, C.G. AND KAAS, J. (1983). The representation of the body surface in S-1 of cats. *Journal of Neuroscience* **3**, 1648-1669.

FITZGERALD, M. (1985). The post-natal development of cutaneous afferent fibre input and receptive field organization in the rat dorsal horn. *Journal of Physiology* **364**, 1-18.

FITZGERALD, M. (1987). Prenatal growth of fine-diameter primary afferents into the rat spinal cord: a transganglionic tracer study. *Journal of Comparative Neurology* **261**, 98-104.

FITZGERALD, M. AND SWETT, J. (1983). The termination pattern of sciatic nerve afferents in the substantia gelatinosa of neonatal rats. *Neuroscience Letters* **43**, 149-154.

FITZGERALD, M. AND VRBOVA, G. (1985). Plasticity of acid phosphatase (FRAP) afferent terminal fields and of dorsal horn cell growth in the neonatal rat. *Journal of Comparative Neurology* **240**, 414-422.

GILMORE, D. AND WATERS, R. (1979). Comfortably Numb. In: *The Wall*, Pink Floyd Music Publishers, Ltd. London.

GOLDBERGER, M.E. AND MURRAY, M. (1978). Recovery of movement and axonal sprouting may obey some of the same laws. In: *Neuronal Plasticity*, ed. COTMAN, C.W., pp. 73-96, New York, Raven Press.

KELAHAN, A.M. AND DOETSCH, G.S. (1984). Time-dependent changes in functional organization of somatosensory cerebral cortex following digital amputation in adult raccoons. *Somatosensory Research* **2**, 49-81.

KOERBER, H.B. AND BROWN, P.B. (1982) Somatotopic organisation of hindlimb cutaneous nerve projections to cat dorsal horn. *Journal of Neurophysiology* **48**, 481-489.

KRNJEVIC, K. AND PHILLIS, J.W. (1963). Pharmacological properties of acetylcholine sensitive cells in the cerebral cortex. *Journal of Physiology* **166**, 328-350.

LANDRY, P. AND DESCHENES, M. (1981). Intracortical arborizations and receptive fields of identified ventrobasal thalamocortical afferents to the primary somatic sensory cortex in the cat. *Journal of Comparative Neurology* **199**, 345-371.

LIGHT, A.R. AND DURKOVIC, R.G. (1984). Features of laminar and somatotopic organization of lumbar spinal cord units receiving cutaneous inputs from hindlimb receptive fields. *Journal of Neurophysiology* **52**, 449-458.

MARKUS, H. AND POMERANZ, B. (1987). Saphenous has weak ineffective synapses in sciatic territory of rat spinal cord: electrical stimulation of the saphenous or application of drugs reveal these somatotopically inappropriate synapses. *Brain Research* **416**, 315-321.

MARKUS, H., POMERANZ, B. AND KRUSHELNYCKY, D. (1984). Spread of saphenous somatotopic projection map in spinal cord and hypersensitivity of the foot after chronic sciatic denervation in adult rat. *Brain Research* **296**, 27-39.

MERZENICH, M.M., KAAS, J.H., WALL, J.T., NELSON, R.J., SUR, M. AND FELLEMAN, D. (1983a). Topographic reorganization of somatosensory cortical areas 3b and 1 in adult monkeys following restricted deafferentation. *Neuroscience* **8**, 33-55.

MERZENICH, M.M., KAAS, J.H., WALL, J.T., SUR, M., NELSON, R.J. AND FELLEMAN, D. (1983b). Progression of change following median nerve section in the cortical representation of the hand in areas 3b and 1 in adult owl and squirrel monkeys. *Neuroscience* **10**, 639-665.

METHERATE, R., TREMBLAY, N. AND DYKES, R.W. (1987). Acetylcholine permits long-term enhancement of neuronal responsiveness in cat primary somatosensory cortex. *Neuroscience* **22**, 75-81.

METZLER, J. AND MARKS, P.S. (1979). Functional changes in cat somatic sensory-motor cortex during short term reversible epidural blocks. *Brain Research* **177**, 379-383.

MEYERS, D.E.R. AND SNOW, P.J. (1984). Somatotopically inappropriate projections of hair follicle afferent fibres to the cat spinal cord. *Journal of Physiology* **347**, 59-73.

MEYERS, D.E.R., WILSON, P. AND SNOW, P.J. (1984). Distribution of the central terminals of cutaneous primary afferents innervating a small skin patch: the existence of somatotopically inappropriate projections. *Neuroscience Letters* **44**, 179-185.

MEYERS, D.E.R. AND SNOW, P.J. (1986). Distribution of activity in the spinal terminations of single hair follicle afferent fibres to somatotopically identified regions of the cat spinal cord. *Journal of Neurophysiology* **56**, 1022-1038.

MOLANDER, C. AND GRANT, G. (1986). Laminar distribution and somatotopic organization of primary afferent fibers from hindlimb nerves in the dorsal horn. A study by transganglionic transport of horseradish peroxidase in the rat. *Neuroscience* **19**, 297-312.

NAGY, J.I. AND HUNT, S.P. (1983). The termination of primary afferents within the rat dorsal horn: evidence for rearrangement following capsaicin treatment. *Journal of Comparative Neurology* **218**, 145-158.

NYBERG, G. AND BLOMQVIST, A. (1985). The somatotopic organization of forelimb nerves in the brachial dorsal horn: an anatomical study in the cat. *Journal of Comparative Neurology* **242**, 28-39.

PROSHANSKY, E. AND EGGER, M.D. (1977). Dendritic spread of dorsal horn neurons in cats. *Experimental Brain Research* **28**, 153-166.

PUBOLS, L.M. (1984). The boundary of proximal hindlimb representation in the dorsal horn following peripheral nerve lesions in cats: a reevaluation of plasticity in the somatotopic map. *Somatosensory Research* **2**, 19-32.

PUBOLS, L.M., FOGLESONG, M.E. AND VAHLE-HINZ, C. (1986). Electrical stimulation reveals relatively ineffective sural nerve projections to dorsal horn neurons in the cat. *Brain Research* **371**, 109-122.

PUBOLS, L.M. AND GOLDBERGER, M.E. (1980). Recovery of function in dorsal horn following partial deafferentation. *Journal of Neurophysiology* **43**, 102-117.

PURVES, D. AND HADLEY, R.D. (1985). Changes in the dendritic branching of adult mammalian neurones revealed by repeated imaging *in situ*. *Nature* **315**, 404-406.

PURVES, D. AND LICHTMAN, J.W. (1980). Elimination of synapses in the developing nervous system. *Science* **210**, 153-157.

RAISMAN, G. (1977). Formation of synapses in the adult rat after injury: similarities and differences between a peripheral and a central nervous site. *Philosophical Transactions of the Royal Society of London Series B* **278**, 349-359.

RUBEL, E.W. (1971). A comparison of somatotopic organization in sensory neocortex of kittens and adult cats. *Journal of Comparative Neurology* **143**, 447-480.

SHEHAB, S.A.S. AND ATKINSON, M.E. (1986). Vasoactive intestinal polypeptide increases in areas of the dorsal horn from which other neuropeptides are depleted following peripheral axotomy. *Experimental Brain Research* **62**, 422-430.

SCHEIBEL, M.E. AND SCHEIBEL, A.B. (1969). Terminal patterns in cat spinal cord. III. Primary afferent collaterals. *Brain Research* **13**, 417-443.

SILLITO, A.M. AND KEMP, J.A. (1983). Cholinergic modulation of the functional organization of the cat visual cortex. *Brain Research* **289**, 143-155.

SMITH, C.L. (1983). The development and postnatal organization of primary afferent projections to the rat thoracic spinal cord. *Journal of Comparative Neurology* **220**, 29-43.

SNOW, P.J., NUDO, R.J., RIVERS, W, JENKINS, W.M. AND MERZENICH, M.M. (1988). Somatotopically inappropriate projections from thalamocortical neurons to the S1 cortex of the cat demonstrated by the use of intracortical microstimulation.

Somatosensory Research **5**, 349-370.

SUGIURA, Y., LEE, C.L. AND PERL E.R. (1986). Central projections of identified, unmyelinated (C) afferent fibers innervating mammalian skin. *Science* **234**, 358-361.

SWETT, J.E. AND WOOLF, C.J. (1985). The somatotopic organization of primary afferent terminals in the superficial laminae of the rat spinal cord. *Journal of Comparative Neurology* **231**, 66-77.

TSUKAHARA, N., HULTBORN, H., MURAKAMI, F. AND FUJITO, Y. (1975). Electrophysiological study of formation of new synapses and collateral sprouting in red nucleus after partial denervation. *Journal of Neurophysiology*, **38**, 1359-1372.

WALL, J.T. AND CUSICK, C.G. (1984). Cutaneous responsiveness in primary somatosensory (S-1) hindpaw cortex before and after partial hindpaw deafferentation in adult rats. *Journal of Neuroscience* **4**, 1499-1515.

WILSON, P. (1987). Absence of mediolateral reorganization of dorsal horn somatotopy after peripheral deafferentation in the cat. *Experimental Neurology* **95**, 432-447.

WILSON, P., MEYERS, D.E.R. AND SNOW, P.J. (1986). The detailed somatotopic organization of the lumbosacral enlargement of the cat. *Journal of Neurophysiology* **55**, 604-617.

WILSON, P., MEYERS, D.E.R. AND SNOW, P.J. (1987). Changes of spinal circuitry in response to alterations of input; an evaluation of the development and basis of contemporary theories. In: *Effects of Injury on Trigeminal and Spinal Somatosensory Systems*, pp. 227-238, ed. PUBOLS, L. M. and SESSLE, B. J., Alan R. Liss, Inc., New York.

WILSON, P. AND SNOW, P.J. (1986). The time course of reorganization of spinal somatotopy following denervation of a single digit in the cat. *Proceedings of the Australian Physiological and Pharmacological Society* **17**, 98P.

WILSON, P. AND SNOW, P.J. (1987). Reorganization of the receptive fields of spinocervical tract neurons following denervation of a single digit in the cat. *Journal of Neurophysiology* **57**, 803-818.

WILSON, P. AND SNOW, P.J. (1988a). Somatotopic organization of the dorsal horn in the lumbosacral enlargement of the spinal cord in the neonatal cat. *Experimental Neurology,* **101** 428-444.

WILSON, P. AND SNOW, P.J. (1988b). Reorganization of the receptive fields of spinocervical tract cells following neonatal peripheral nerve transection in the cat. *Proceedings of the Australian Physiological and Pharmacological Society* **19**, 103P.

WOOLF, C.J. (1987) Central terminations of cutaneous mechanoreceptive afferents in the rat lumbar spinal cord. *Journal of Comparative Neurology* **261**, 105-119.

WOOLF, C.J. AND FITZGERALD, M. (1986). Somatotopic organization of cutaneous afferent terminals and dorsal horn neuronal receptive fields in the superficial and deep laminae of the rat lumbar spinal cord. *Journal of Comparative Neurology* **251**, 517-531.

ZIEGLGANSBERGER, W. AND HERZ, A. (1971). Changes of cutaneous receptive fields of spino-cervical-tract neurons and other dorsal horn neurones by microelectrophoretically administered amino acids. *Experimental Brain Research* **13**, 111-126.

PHYSIOLOGICAL AND PHARMACOLOGICAL INDUCTION OF C-FOS PROTEIN IMMUNOREACTIVITY IN SUPERFICIAL DORSAL HORN NEURONES

J.D. Leah, T. Herdegen and M. Zimmermann

II Physiologisches Institut, Im Neuenheimer Feld 326, Universität Heidelberg
Heidelberg, D6900 FRG

INTRODUCTION

Proto-oncogenes are authentic cellular genes involved in replication, growth and differentiation of cells (Weinberg, 1985; Marx, 1987). Proteins encoded by proto-oncogenes can act as receptor proteins, growth factors, phosphotyrosinekinases or as nuclear proteins. The *c-fos* protein has this latter function, binding to specific histone complexes and acting as a start signal for DNA enfolding (Rauscher *et al*, 1988). *C-fos* activity has been studied primarily with *in vitro* systems, especially within undifferentiated or embryonic cell cultures. In contrast, few observations describe the conditions of expression of *c-fos* protein in differentiated neurones *in vivo*. Recently, Hunt *et al* (1987) demonstrated that peripheral noxious and non-noxious stimuli induce *c-fos* protein in spinal neurons. The importance of this lies in its acting as a biochemical link between extracellular signals and the expression of those genes that produce long-term alterations in spinal neuronal functioning and that can give rise to sensory perturbations (Berridge, 1986). We describe here initial *in vivo* results of the induction of the *c-fos* protein in superficial dorsal horn neurones both by activity in primary afferents and by certain neuropeptides and transmitter compounds that are physiologically active in the cord.

METHODS

Experiments were performed on 200-350 g Sprague-Dawley rats anaestethized with pentobarbitone (60 mg/kg, i.p.). In one group the noxious excitant capsaicin (50 μl of 300 μM) was injected into the plantar region of the hindpaw to stimulate n. tibialis which terminates in the medial part of laminae I/II. In others a 3 cm incision of the skin of the dorsal thigh was made to stimulate the n. cutaneous femoris posterior which terminates in the lateral part of laminae I/II (Swett and Woolf, 1985). In a second group the lumbar spinal cord was exposed by laminectomy and the dura reflected. A small pool containing a compound in 50 μl Tyrode solution was placed on the cord surface. The compounds used were the neuropeptides substance P (SP, 0.1nM - 1 μM), neurotensin (NT, 0.1 nM-1 μM), somatostatin (SOM, 1 μM), dynorphin A 1-8 (DYN, 1 μM) and bombesin (BB, 1 μM); the excitatory amino acid transmitter compounds,

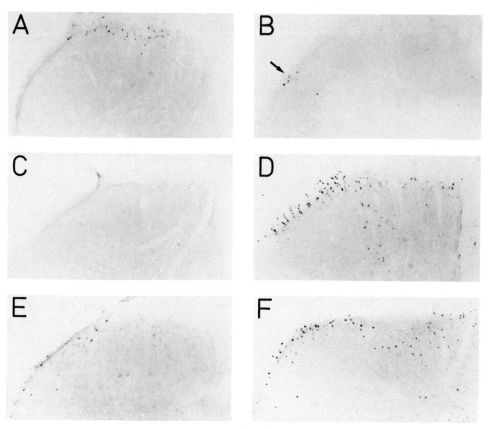

FIGURE 1: A: *c-fos* immunoreactive nuclei in cells in the medial part of the superficial dorsal horn following injection of capsaicin into the ventral area of the hindpaw. B: Immunoreactive nuclei (arrow) in the lateral part of laminae I/II following an incision in the skin of the thigh. C: Absence of *c-fos* staining following exposure of the dorsal spinal cord to 1 μM 3-APS. D: Staining of nuclei due to exposure of the cord to 3 mM NAAG. E: Staining in a few cells induced by 1 μM NMDA. F: Dense *c-fos* labelling caused by 1 μM BB.

D-homocysteic acid (DHC, 3 mM), N-acetyl-aspartylglutamate (NAAG, 1 μM and 3 mM) and N-methyl-D-aspartic acid (NMDA, 1 μM); and the inhibitory amino acid and GABA analogue 3-amino-propanesulphonic acid (3-APS, 1 μM). Tyrode solution alone acted as the control.

After 2.5 hours the animals were perfused through the aorta with 4% paraformaldehyde. The cord was removed, postfixed, cryoprotected in 30% sucrose, and 50 μm sections cut on a cryostat. The free-floating sections were then incubated in primary antiserum against the 151-292 sequence of the *c-fos* protein (a generous gift from Prof. R. Müller, EMBL) for 48 hours. They were then processed using standard avidin-biotin immunochemistry (Vectastain). The numbers of immunoreactive cell nuclei in laminae I/II were screened in an average of 20 sections for each of the compounds.

RESULTS

Capsaicin injected into the ventral hindpaw caused *c-fos* immunoreactivity in numerous nuclei exclusively in the ipsilateral medial laminae I/II. The incision in the thigh caused immunoreactivity exclusively in ipsilateral laminae I/II (Fig. 1 A,B).

No immunoreactive nuclei were seen in exposed spinal cords treated with Tyrode solution alone, or with the inhibitory amino acid 3-APS (Fig. 1C). In contrast, the excitatory amino acids DHC and NAAG at 3mM (Schneider and Perl, 1988) caused 10-20 *c-fos* stained cells in laminae I/II in each section (Fig. 1D). For consistency in quantification stained nuclei were counted only in the medial part of laminae I/II. 1 μM NAAG or NMDA gave 2-5 stained nuclei/section (Fig. 1 E). All the excitatory neuropeptides (Kelly, 1982) at 1 μM (which is approximately the concentration released into the cord following afferent nerve stimulation; Duggan *et al*, 1988) also caused *c-fos* staining in the superficial laminae neurones, but to different extents. Thus BB produced 20-25 intensely stained nuclei/section (Fig. 1F). SP 100 nM and 1 μM similarly caused 15-25 stained nuclei and even at 0.1 and 1 nM this peptide induced weak staining in 2-5 nuclei. NT 100 nM and 1 μM similarly produced weak labelling in 3-6 nuclei, but was not effective at concentrations lower than 100 nM. 1 μM DYN also caused staining in 5-8 cells. In contrast, 1 μM of the predominantly inhibitory peptide SOM induced staining in only 0-1 nuclei/section.

DISCUSSION

These results reiterate the finding of Hunt *et al* (1987) that noxious sensory input causes *c-fos* expression in superficial dorsal horn neurones and further indicate that the expression may be restricted to those cells in the termination region of the particular afferent stimulated (see also this volume). This suggests that *c-fos* expression could be used to map somatotopically activated regions in the spinal cord, a proposal for which there is now further evidence (Sagar *et al*, 1988).

Our results also indicate that neuropeptides and transmitter compounds with excitatory actions in the superficial dorsal horn can induce expression of the *c-fos* oncogene, whereas inhibitory transmitters and peptides are ineffective. It is of interest that SP in concentrations as low as 1 nM was effective in inducing *c-fos*. Thus this and other neuropeptides may be neurochemically active in the superficial dorsal horn at concentrations below those that produce behavioural reactions. Thus the expression of *c-fos* could be used further to examine the activation of superficial spinal neurones by neuroactive compounds.

REFERENCES

BERRIDGE, M. (1986). Second messenger dualism in neuromodulation and memory. *Nature* **323**, 294-295.

DUGGAN, A.W., HENDRY, I.A., MORTON, C.R., HUTCHISON, W.D. AND ZHAO, Z.Q. (1988). Cutaneous stimuli releasing immunoreactive substance P in the dorsal horn of the cat. *Brain Research* **451**, 261-273.

HUNT, S.P., PINI, A. AND EVAN, G. (1987). Induction of *c-fos*-like protein in spinal cord neurones following sensory stimulation. *Nature* **328**, 632-634.

KELLY, J. (1982). Electrophysiology of peptides in the central nervous system. *British Medical Bulletin* **38**, 283-290.

MARX, J.L. (1987). The *c-fos* as a master switch. *Science* **237**, 854-856.

RAUSCHER, F.J., SAMBUCETTI, L.C., CURRAN, T., DISTEL, R.J. AND Spiegelman, B.M. (1988). Common DNA binding site for fos protein complexes and transcription factor AP-1. *Cell* **52**, 471- 480.

SAGAR, S.M., SHARP, F.R. AND CURRAN, T. (1988). Expression of *c-fos* protein in brain: Metabolic mapping at the cellular level. *Science* **240**, 1328-1331.

SCHNEIDER, S.P. AND PERL, E.R. (1988). Comparison of primary afferent and glutamate excitation of neurones in the mammalian spinal dorsal horn. *Journal of Neuroscience* **8**, 2062-2073.

SWETT, J.E. AND WOOLF, C.J. (1985). The somatotopic organization of primary afferent terminals in the superficial laminae of the dorsal horn of the rat spinal cord. *Journal of Comparative Neurology* **231**, 66-77.

WEINBERG, R.A. (1985). The action of oncogenes in the cytoplasm and nucleus. *Science* **230**, 770-776.

MODALITY PROPERTIES AND INHIBITORY RECEPTIVE FIELDS OF DORSAL HORN NEURONS IN CATS WITH DORSOLATERAL FUNICULUS LESIONS

Lillian M. Pubols, Harumitsu Hirata* and Paul B. Brown**

Robert S. Dow Neurological Sciences Institute/Department of Neurosurgery, Good Samaritan Hospital and Medical Center 1120 N.W. 20th Avenue, Portland, OR 97209 U.S.A.

INTRODUCTION

As the contributions to this volume attest, much of the recent interest in the superficial dorsal horn is due to its apparent role in nociception. In a recent report concerning the effects of dorsolateral funiculus lesions on the response properties of dorsal horn neurons (Pubols et al, 1987) we described a number of findings that relate to the role of the dorsal horn in nociceptive transmission. The present paper focusses upon this aspect of the study, and discusses it in the context of previous work on the processing of nociceptive information in the dorsal horn.

METHODS

The subjects for these experiments were normal adult cats (n=10) and adult cats with right T12 dorsolateral funiculus lesions studied at <1 (n=2), 3 (n=2), 14-16 (n=4), and 28-30 (n=5) days postoperatively. Single cell recording was carried out in the right L6 and L7 dorsal horn in animals anesthetized with sodium pentobarbital. A dorsal column electrical stimulus was used to search for cells that were driven either synaptically or antidromically. The excitatory responses of these cells both to natural mechanical stimulation of the skin and to electrical stimulation of A fibers in the sural nerve was noted, as was any spontaneous activity. The low intensity mechanical stimuli were movement of hairs and light touch with a 1 g force. The high intensity stimulus was a noxious but non-damaging pinch (160 g) applied to a skin fold with a pair of hemostatic forceps. Cells that displayed spontaneous activity were also tested for inhibition of this activity by these natural stimuli. The extent of the lesions and the location of recording sites were reconstructed from histologically prepared sections through the appropriate regions of spinal cord. Further details of these methods may be found elsewhere (Pubols et al, 1988).

---

* Present address:Department of Neuroscience, University of Florida College of Medicine, Gainesville, FL 32610, U.S.A.
**Present address: Department of Physiology, West Virginia University Medical Center, Morgantown, WV 25606, U.S.A.

RESULTS

Dorsolateral funiculus lesions were found to alter several properties of dorsal horn neurons in a time-dependent manner. Excitability of the dorsal horn was reduced acutely, in that many electrode penetrations in <1 day animals had no cells responding to peripheral stimuli, and a higher than normal proportion of cells that responded to the dorsal column search stimulus, but not to peripheral stimuli. The percentage of cells that were spontaneously active was significantly greater than normal at 3 and 14-16 days postoperatively (51 and 39%, respectively, *vs.* 24% in normals), returning to normal by 28 days postoperatively (23%). The percentage of cells that responded to sural nerve stimulation was reduced at <1 and 3 days, and increased to a level that was significantly higher than normal at 28-30 days postoperatively (64 *vs.* 31%).

The percentages of cells that responded maximally to low intensity stimuli (LT), only to high intensity stimuli (HT), or differentially to both (MR) were not significantly different from normal at any survival time (Fig. 1). These percentages in normal cats were 44, 22 and 34%, respectively. All three types of cell were found in laminae I-V. The mean dorso-ventral locus of LT cells was at the border of laminae III and IV, while the mean loci for HT and MR were significantly deeper, in the middle of lamina IV.

Approximately 7% of all cells were found to have cutaneous inhibitory receptive

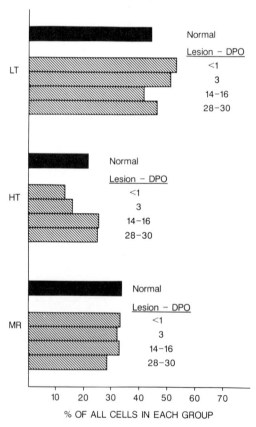

FIGURE 1: Percentage of cells that were LT, HT and MR in normal cats and in cats with lesions examined from <1 to 30 days postoperatively (DPO). The total number of cells in each group was 327, 15, 37, 103, and 101 in the normal, <1, 3, 14-16, and 28-30 DPO groups, respectively.

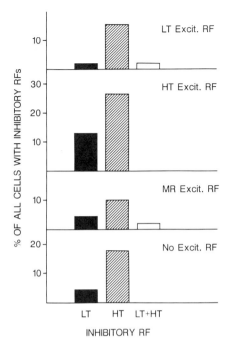

FIGURE 2: Distribution of cells with inhibitory receptive fields with respect to the nature of their excitatory and inhibitory receptive fields (RFs).

fields. There were no obvious differences between the cells with inhibitory receptive fields recorded in normal animals *vs.* those recorded in lesioned animals. Cells with inhibitory fields included LT, HT, and MR, as well as cells with no excitatory receptive fields (Fig. 2). The majority were inhibited by high intensity stimulation, but cells with low threshold inhibitory receptive fields were also observed. Only 2 out of a total of 45 cells with inhibitory receptive fields were found to have *Diffuse Noxious Inhibitory Control* (LeBars *et al*, 1979).

DISCUSSION

Significant, time-dependent changes in spontaneous and some types of evoked activity were noted following DLF lesions, and have been discussed in relationship to various short and long term mechanisms of neural plasticity (Pubols *et al*, 1988). Surprisingly, in view of the extensive evidence for descending inhibition of nociceptive input to the dorsal horn (*e.g.* Fields *et al*, 1977; Willis *et al*, 1977; Duggan and Griersmith, 1979), no change was found in the proportions of LT, HT, and MR neurons as a result of the lesions. Collins and Ren (1987) found that the percentage of wide-dynamic-range neurons was low in the dorsal horn of intact, unanesthetized cats (9% of all cells with low threshold input) but increased significantly following either spinal cord transection or pentobarbital sodium anesthesia (34 and 61%, respectively). In the present study approximately 43% of all cells with low threshold input were MR in anesthetized animals, a percentage that was not significantly increased by a subtotal cord transection. These results are more in accord with those of Jones and Gebhart (1987), who found that lidocaine blockade of the DLF results in non-selective release of descending inhibition. El Yassir and co-workers report in this volume that nociceptive-selective inhibitory effects of serotonin are mediated by $5HT_{1B}$ but not $5HT_{1A}$

receptors in the dorsal horn. Thus, recent studies indicate that conclusions about the specificity of descending inhibition for nociceptive input often depend upon the particular stimulation, blockade, lesion or pharmacological methods employed, and suggest a greater complexity of the descending control systems than was originally envisioned.

As noted above, the superficial dorsal horn is thought to play an important role in nociception. In the present study the superficial dorsal horn was, indeed, found to contain cells with nociceptive input. On the other hand, we found the average location of all HT and MR cells recorded to be in the middle of lamina IV. This is a reminder that the deeper dorsal horn contains a high proportion of cells with nociceptive inputs, and raises again the question of the respective contributions of superficial *vs.* deep regions of the dorsal horn in the processing of nociceptive information.

A relatively small percentage of cells in the present sample were found to have cutaneous inhibitory receptive fields. Since inhibition of spontaneous rather than evoked activity was the criterion employed, and since less than 50% of all cells studied had such activity, this is undoubtedly a somewhat low estimate of the proportion of cells with inhibitory receptive fields. An even smaller percentage (<1%) showed *Diffuse Noxious Inhibitory Control*. In our earlier paper (Pubols *et al*, 1988) it was suggested that this phenomenon might be less common in cats than in rats. However, Morton *et al*, (1988) recently found a greater incidence of cells showing inhibition from stimulation of remote body regions in the cat by measuring the inhibition of evoked, rather than spontaneous, activity.

Neurons showing inhibition were highly diverse with respect to the various possible combinations of excitatory and inhibitory receptive fields. Noxious stimuli were effective in inhibiting dorsal horn cells more often than were non-noxious stimuli, and HT were more likely to have inhibitory receptive fields than were LT. However, these generalizations are clearly only a first approximation in describing these results since many of these cells had low threshold excitatory and/or inhibitory receptive fields.

A high percentage of the cells in the substantia gelatinosa (SG) have been found to have persistent spontaneous activity that is strongly inhibited by low and/or high threshold cutaneous stimulation. These have been called *inverse* cells (Cervero *et al*, 1979). Many of the cells with inhibitory receptive fields in the present study had similar physiological properties, but approximately 80% of them were located in deeper laminae. One can partially distinguish these cells from inverse cells physiologically since a majority of inverse cells are inhibited by both low and high threshold stimuli (Cervero *et al*, 1979), while only 4% of the cells in our sample had this characteristic. Nevertheless, determining that a dorsal horn cell with an inhibitory field is, or is not, an inverse cell of the SG would be difficult on the basis of physiological criteria alone.

ACKNOWLEDGEMENTS

Supported by Research grant NS19523 from the National Institutes of Health

REFERENCES

CERVERO, F., IGGO, A. AND MOLONY, V. (1979) An electrophysiological study of neurones in the substantia gelatinosa Rolandi of the cat's spinal cord. *Quart. J. Exptl. Physiol.* **64**, 297-314.

COLLINS, J.G. AND REN, K. (1987) WDR response profiles of spinal dorsal horn neurons may be unmasked by barbiturate anesthesia. *Pain* **28**, 369-378.

DUGGAN, A.W. AND GRIERSMITH, B.T. (1979) Inhibition of the spinal transmission of nociceptive information by supraspinal stimulation in the cat. *Pain* **6**, 149-161.

FIELDS, H.L., BASBAUM, A.I., CLANTON, C.H. AND ANDERSON, S.D. (1977) Nucleus raphe magnus inhibition of spinal cord dorsal horn neurons. *Brain Res.* **126**, 441-453.

JONES, S.L. AND GEBHART, G.F. (1987) Spinal pathways mediating tonic coeruleospinal, and raphe-spinal descending inhibition in the rat. *J. Neurophysiol.* **58**, 138-159.

LEBARS, D., DICKENSON, A.H. AND BESSON, J.M. (1979) Diffuse, noxious inhibitory control (DNIC). I. Effects on dorsal horn convergent neurones in the rat. *Pain* **6**, 283-304.

MORTON, C.R. HU, H.-J., XIAO, H.-M., MAISCH, B. AND ZIMMERMANN, M. (1988) Inhibition of nociceptive responses of lumbar dorsal horn neurones by remote noxious afferent stimulation in the cat. *Pain* **34**, 75-84.

PUBOLS, L.M., HIRATA, H. AND BROWN, P.B. (1988) Temporally dependent changes in response properties of dorsal horn neurons after dorsolateral funiculus lesions. *J. Neurophysiol.* **60**, in press.

WILLIS, W.D., HABER, L.H. AND MARTIN, R.F. (1977) Inhibition of spinothalamic tract cells and interneurons by brain stem stimulation in the monkey. *J. Neurophysiol.* **40**, 968-981.

DISCUSSION ON SECTION IV

Rapporteur: Gary J. Bennett

Neurobiology and Anesthesiology Branch, National Institute of Dental Research
National Institutes of Health, Bethesda, MD, USA

The presentations in this session, and the discussions that followed, revolved principally around four topics: Do different types of neuron express plasticity to different degrees or in different ways? What are the stimulus conditions necessary to evoke modifications in neuronal responsivity? What are the mechanisms that underlie the various kinds of plasticity? And, what is the function of lamina I projection neurons with regards to pain perception and stimulus-evoked plasticity? It is apparent that definitive answers are not near to hand and that these questions will occupy a great deal of our research efforts in the future.

There is general agreement that the changes in responsivity that are evoked by noxious stimulation are pronounced and relatively easy to produce in wide-dynamic-range (WDR) neurons in the deeper layers of the dorsal horn. However, the results from experiments with lamina I neurons are more complex. Experiments reported by Laird and Cervero (this volume; Cervero and Laird, 1989) indicate that intense noxious stimuli (tail pinches of 8N force and 2 min duration) have relatively small and brief effects on nociceptive specific (NS) lamina I neurons. Receptive field (RF) size was unchanged in 50% of their cases and in the rest was increased only by about 10% for 20 min or less. Mechanical thresholds decreased in only 30% of the cells. The decrease was to 50-75% of the control level (which still does not approach the threshold of low-threshold mechanoreceptors) and lasted for 5-15 min. Such changes are decidedly small and brief when compared to the changes evoked in the deeper WDR neurons by the same stimuli under identical experimental conditions. Wall, however, reviewed observations indicating that in other cases noxious stimuli evoke a distinctly large and prolonged change in lamina I cell responses. For example, Cook and her colleagues (1987) have shown that 20s of a 1 Hz, C-fiber strength tetanus to a muscle nerve causes an increase in the RF size of lamina I projection cells to an average peak of 200% of control for more than 50 min. McMahon and Wall (1984) have reported that a similar long-lasting expansion of RF size and a decrease in sensitivity to mechanical stimuli can be evoked by a small burn placed outside of the lamina I cell's RF and that these changes are dependent upon C fiber input from the injured region. As another example, Hylden, Dubner, and their colleagues (Hylden et al, 1989; Dubner et al, this volume) have found that NS lamina I projection neurons with RFs on a hindpaw that is inflamed and edematous due to an injection of Freund's adjuvant show very dramatic changes. Within hours of the induction of inflammation, the size of RFs that were initially confined to an area on one or two digits expand to include most of the hindpaw.

It is important to note that primary afferent sensitization cannot account for the injury-evoked changes in lamina I cell responsivity and that these changes must thus be due to mechanisms within the CNS (McMahon and Wall, 1984; Cook et al, 1987; Hylden et al, 1989).

It is clear that some forms of noxious stimulation evoke little lamina I cell plasticity while others evoke very pronounced plasticity. What is it about these experiments, or their different forms of noxious stimulation, that accounts for the different effects? It may be of significance that a C-strength tetanus applied to a cutaneous nerve produces relatively small changes (comparable to those seen by Laird and Cervero), whereas C-strength tetani applied to muscle nerves produce relatively large changes (e.g., Wall and Woolf, 1984; Cook et al,1987). Pinches might preferentially activate cutaneous afferents while input from an inflamed paw might include a significant component from nociceptors innervating muscle or other deep tissues. Another possibility is that different kinds of lamina I cells may be differentially plastic. Several observations suggest that future work on lamina I cell plasticity must pay more attention to the heterogeneity of the connectivity of lamina I cells. First, anatomical and physiological analyses indicate that this region includes projection neurons and interneurons of the local circuit or intersegmental type (Beal and Coimbra and Lima, this volume; Cervero et al, 1979). Second, there are clear indications of significant differences in the patterns of primary afferent convergence onto lamina I cells. For example, it has long been known that the cutaneous input (ignoring thermoreceptors) to some lamina I neurons is dominated by myelinated nociceptors while others receive an additional input from unmyelinated polymodal nociceptors (Christensen and Perl, 1970). Moreover, it is now firmly established that some lamina I neurons are WDR cells and receive afferent drive from both nociceptors and low-threshold mechanoreceptors (for reviews see Dubner and Bennett, 1983; Hylden et al,1986). In addition, it has been shown that an even greater diversity of patterns of afferent drive is found if visceral inputs are included in the characterization. Thus, a subset of thoracic lamina I neurons appears to be innervated exclusively by cutaneous nociceptors, while others are innervated by both cutaneous and visceral afferents (Cervero and Tattersall, 1988; Cervero and Lumb,1988). In view of the markedly different effects of conditioning C-strength stimuli applied to cutaneous and muscle nerves (Wall and Woolf, 1984), it is most unfortunate that we have so very little information about the distribution of muscle nociceptors to the various subsets of lamina I cells. Similarly, we know very little about the ability of visceral afferent input to produce plastic changes in lamina I cell responses. The potential importance of this latter point is underscored by two recent observations. First, McMahon (1988) has shown that inflammation of the bladder can produce long-lasting increases in the excitability of dorsal horn neurons and that this plasticity is at least partly due to a change in central processing. Second, Foreman and his colleagues (1988) have demonstrated both excitatory and inhibitory interactions between the effects of visceral and cutaneous stimuli on the responses of neurons with viscerosomatic convergence. Viscerosomatic interactions have heretofore been considered only in regard to their relevance for referred pain. However, the aforementioned work and the recently described differences in the neurochemistry and distributions (laminar and segmental) of the terminals of cutaneous, muscle, and visceral nociceptors (Sugiura et al and Sharkey et al, this volume; Cervero, 1988) suggest that the lamina I system's response to a non-trivial injury might involve a complex constellation of effects evoked by different kinds of afferents from each of several different tissues and that these effects might be expressed differentially in different kinds of lamina I cells (Cervero, 1988). In this regard, it is also unfortunate that no one has systematically examined input from viscera, muscle, and other deep tissues in their characterizations of the afferent drive to lamina I neurons with antidromically-identified input to the various projection targets of the several classes of lamina I cells (see Coimbra and Lima and Willis, this volume).

It seems likely that at least some of the short duration changes that can be induced in lamina I cells may be due entirely to purely functional changes in spinal circuitry. Woolf, for example, has shown (see this volume) that C-fiber input can induce an increase in central excitability that reveals a previously ineffective (*i.e.* subthreshold) polysynaptic input. This sort of mechanism, however, is unlikely to be the sole explanation for long-term effects. Long duration effects seem to call for changes in synaptic connectivity or efficacy that are mediated by actual structural alterations. Snow and Wilson (this volume) have investigated such phenomena by perturbing the somatotopic map expressed between the terminal arbors of A-β low-threshold mechanoreceptors and spinocervical tract neurons in laminae III-IV. This is an especially advantageous system in which to study the determinants of RF boundaries because the map has a relatively fine grain and its normal organization is known in very great detail. In the normal case, the primary afferent arbors extend beyond the region of cells that respond to their activation. This *somatotopically inappropriate* portion of the arbor is identifiable morphologically: it has relatively sparse branching and the terminal branches end bluntly, without forming boutons. In neonatally-denervated adults the map is rearranged and the *inappropriate* portion of the arbor is now richly branched and emits normal boutons. Denervating an adult yields the same rearrangement of the map and it is likely (but not yet demonstrated) that similar morphological changes are responsible. It is conceivable that the denervation-induced changes seen in the RFs of NS lamina I neurons (Hylden *et al*, 1987) are produced by comparable alterations in the terminal arbors of nociceptive primary afferents.

It is nearly certain that changes in neuronal responsivity mediated by structural alterations involve concurrent, non-trivial (*e.g.* not merely increased metabolic demand) changes in neuronal gene expression. However, it is not clear whether short-term changes in responsivity are mediated by purely functional alterations (*re-tuning*) or whether these changes also require significant genetic interactions (for example, see Ruda *et al*, this volume). The exciting possibility that the latter may be true was reviewed in S. Hunt's presentation. He and his colleagues (Hunt *et al*, 1987) have shown that cutaneous stimulation induces the proto-oncogene *c-fos* in spinal neurons (see also Basbaum *et al* and Leah *et al*, this volume). Other cells activated by this stimulation (dorsal root ganglion cells, dorsal column nuclei cells etc) do not reveal *c-fos* induction.

C-fos encodes for a nuclear, DNA-binding protein whose function is poorly understood. It is known, however, that in PC12 and other cell types the induction of *c-fos* is initiated by voltage-sensitive Ca^{++} flux and by other second messenger systems. Neuropeptides and neurotransmitters are known to engage second messenger systems. For example, it is known that substance P causes a dramatic increase in intracellular Ca^{++} in spinal dorsal horn neurons (*e.g.* Womack *et al*, 1988). It is thus possible that primary afferent-evoked synaptic activity may act via intracellular intermediaries to alter, in the postsynaptic cell, the expression not only of *c-fos* but also of other genes and that these genetic effects may underlie many aspects of neuronal plasticity. The laminar distribution of *c-fos* activation may be stimulus specific (Hunt *et al*, 1987; Basbaum *et al*, this volume). Thus, noxious heat is followed by *c-fos* expression in laminae I-II and

IV-V while innocuous mechanical stimulation is followed by expression in laminae III-IV. An apparent exception to the laminar specificity of the effect is found with subcutaneous injection of formalin, which is thought to be a purely noxious stimulus. It was noted, however, that formalin might damage nerve branches and thus evoke an injury discharge in low-threshold mechanoreceptors. These observations suggest that *c-fos* activation might be a useful activity marker, although, as Woolf, Dubner and others pointed out, it may be more strictly accurate in the sense of a marker for monosynaptic primary afferent-evoked depolarization. The exact link between primary afferent input and *c-fos* activation remains to be determined. Nevertheless, *c-fos* activation clearly shows, for the first time, that genetic events may be induced by stimulus-evoked primary afferent activity. Moreover, the *c-fos* work forces us to consider the possibility that there is a continuous interaction between synaptic events and the cell's genome, and that the cell is thus able to regulate the effects of its synaptic input. The time frame of this regulation is of the greatest importance in understanding the changes in neuronal responsivity described above. There is no doubt that it is fast enough to account for effects seen within hours or days of stimulation, but is it fast enough to be involved in the changes that are detected within minutes of stimulation?

Wall's presentation showed that our current knowledge about lamina I cell plasticity suggests an answer to the general question of the function of this system (see McMahon and Wall, this volume). His review of the evidence pertaining to this question stressed three key points. As is usual, most of the evidence for these points is strongest for rat and cat and considerably more problematic for monkey and man. The first point is that a very large majority (about 80% or more, depending on species and, perhaps, target) of lamina I cells projecting to the brain have their axons ascending in the dorsolateral funiculi (DLF). Second, transection of the DLF does not produce any sign of hypoalgesia, in contrast to the well-documented effect that follows transection of the anterolateral quadrant. Third, McMahon and Wall (1988) have recently shown that activation of the descending control system(s) that travel in the ipsilateral DLF evoke (after an initial inhibition) a prolonged excitation and facilitation of the responses of some lamina I projection neurons, whereas WDR neurons in the deeper laminae are only inhibited. Based on these and other observations, McMahon and Wall propose that lamina I projection neurons (particularly those innervating the brain stem centers of descending modulation) function as the ascending leg of a feedback loop that modulates nociception. The descending control acts to inhibit the activity of nocireceptive transmission neurons in the deeper laminae and also to facilitate the activity of its own trigger - the lamina I neurons. As the authors note, if this is indeed a function of lamina I projection neurons, then it is most likely to be apparent in the case of intense/prolonged noxious stimulation. In effect, we are reminded that the nociceptive system has two roles - to detect and analyse noxious events and to respond to noxious states. The organization of the nocireceptive system is undoubtedly integrated, but it may appear to be very different when it is responding to events *vs* states.

It has long been apparent that descending controls are intensified by noxious stimuli. Le Bars and his colleagues, for example, have shown that noxious stimuli engage a descending control system (DNIC) that travels down the DLF and selectively inhibits WDR neurons in the deep laminae without producing any appreciable inhibition of lamina I NS neurons (Le Bars *et al*, 1979). Thus information transmitted by NS cells is continuously available as a trigger for modulating the activity of the deeper cells. However, these workers have found that the ascending leg in the DNIC loop is in the anterolateral quadrants (Villanueva *et al*, 1986). It may be of importance to note that the stimuli used to evoke DNIC have been relatively brief and applied to regions other than the RF of the neuron which is inhibited (*i.e.* heterotopic conditioning stimuli). Thus it is possible that DNIC and the lamina I/DLF-triggered process proposed by McMahon and Wall may be different. If a difference does exist, it may be related to the differences between acute and chronic pain processes; or different systems may be involved in homotopic and heterotopic modulation. Moreover, it is now well known that there are multiple descending control systems and it is possible that they have different ascending legs. For example, it is known that some ventral horn neurons with ascending axons in the anterolateral quadrants are also excited by activation of the descending control pathway (*e.g.* Cervero and Wolstencroft, 1984; Giesler *et al*, 1981). Such observations are not incompatible with the proposed role for lamina I neurons. One can easily imagine that cells such as those in lamina VII participate in related control mechanisms, for example they may have a role in the postural adjustments that are seen after injury.

A key component of the McMahon and Wall proposal is that ipsilateral DLF stimulation produces a relatively long-term facilitation of lamina I projection neurons. This is manifested by an increase in spontaneous discharge, a facilitation of responses to peripheral stimuli, and an expansion of RFs. These effects are very similar to those produced by noxious stimuli themselves (*e.g.*, Cook *et al*, 1987; Woolf and Fitzgerald, 1983; McMahon and Wall, 1984). Thus, it is proposed that the descending control system's response to injury includes an increase in the sensitivity of its input leg. The mechanisms generating this increase seem to be complex and involve, at least in part, segmental circuitry. Changes in lamina I cell responsivity evoked by noxious peripheral stimulation can be seen in spinalized animals (e.g. Cook *et al*, 1987). Experiments by McMahon and Wall (1988) indicate that the effects of ipsilateral DLF stimulation itself may be partly due to the activation of descending axons and partly to the activation of segmental circuitry via antidromic impulses in projections ascending the DLF. The latter might include antidromic activation of the local axonal arbors of lamina I cells.

McMahon and Wall's proposals will no doubt lead to a great deal of experimentation. It is to the authors' credit that their hypothesis generates several non-obvious predictions. For example, the theory predicts that the increased excitability and enlarged RFs seen in lamina I neurons during adjuvant-induced inflammation (e.g., Hylden *et al*, 1989) will be partially decreased or delayed by a transection of the proximal, ipsilateral DLF (the downward leg of the loop that facilitates lamina I cells). In contrast, the same lesion will sever the downward leg of the loop that inhibits deeper cells and this might lead to an increase (disinhibition) of the inflammation-induced increased excitability and enlarged RFs of lamina V WDR cells. Correspondingly, the theory predicts that prolonged DLF stimulation of the contralateral DLF rostral to an unilateral DLF transection should activate descending modulation and evoke facilitation of lamina I cells and inhibition of lamina V cells, even in the absence of peripheral injury.

REFERENCES

CERVERO, F. (1988). Visceral pain. In: *Pain Research and Clinical Management*, eds. Dubner, R., Gebhart, G.F. and Bond, M.R., pp.216-226. Amsterdam: Elsevier.
CERVERO, F., IGGO, A. AND MOLONY, V. (1979). Ascending projections of nociceptor-driven lamina I neurones in the cat. *Experimental Brain Research* 35, 135-149.
CERVERO, F. AND LAIRD, J.M.A. (1989). Nociceptive neurones in the dorsal horn of

rat spinal cord: receptive field properties before and after prolonged noxious mechanical stimulation. *Journal of Physiology*, in press.

CERVERO, F. AND LUMB, B.M. (1988). Bilateral inputs and supraspinal control of viscero-somatic neurones in the lower thoracic spinal cord of the cat. *Journal of Physiology* **403**, 221-237.

CERVERO, F. AND TATTERSALL, J.E.H. (1987). Somatic and visceral inputs to the thoracic spinal cord of the cat: marginal zone (lamina I) of the dorsal horn. *Journal of Physiology* **388**, 383-395.

CERVERO, F. AND WOLSTENCROFT, J.H. (1984). A positive feedback loop between spinal cord nociceptive pathways and antinociceptive areas of the cat's brain stem. *Pain* **20**, 125-138.

CHRISTENSEN, B.N. AND PERL, E.R. (1970). Spinal neurons specifically excited by noxious and thermal stimuli: marginal zone of the spinal cord. *Journal of Neurophysiology* **33**, 293-307.

COOK, A.J., WOOLF, C.J., WALL, P.D. AND MCMAHON, S.B. (1987). Dynamic receptive field plasticity in rat spinal cord dorsal horn following C-primary afferent input. *Nature* **325**, 151-153.

DUBNER, R. AND BENNETT, G.J. (1983). Spinal and trigeminal mechanisms of nociception. *Annual Review of Neuroscience* **6**, 381-418.

FOREMAN, R.D., HOBBS, S.F., OH, U.-T. AND CHANDLER, M.J. (1988). Differential modulation of thoracic and lumbar spinothalamic tract cell activity during stimulation of cardiopulmonary sympathetic afferent fibers in the primate: a new concept for visceral pain? In: *Pain Research and Clinical Management*, eds. Dubner, R., Gebhart, G.F. and Bond, M.R., pp. 227-231, Amsterdam: Elsevier.

GIESLER, G.J., JR., YEZIERSKI, R.P., GERHART, K.D. AND WILLIS, W.D. (1981). Spinothalamic tract neurons that project to medial and/or lateral thalamic nuclei: evidence for a physiologically novel population of spinal cord neurones. *Journal of Neurophysiology* **46**, 1285-1308.

HUNT, S.P., PINI, A. AND EVAN, G. (1987). Induction of *c-fos*-like protein in spinal cord neurons following sensory stimulation. *Nature* **328**, 632634.

HYLDEN, J.L.K., HAYASHI, H., DUBNER, R. AND BENNETT, G.J. (1986). Physiology and morphology of the lamina I spinomesencephalic projection. *Journal of Comparative Neurology* **247**, 505-515.

HYLDEN, J.L.K., NAHIN, R.L. AND DUBNER, R. (1987). Altered responses of nociceptive cat lamina I spinal dorsal horn neurons after chronic sciatic neuroma formation. *Brain Research* **411**, 341-350.

HYLDEN, J.L.K., NAHIN, R.L., TRAUB, R.J. AND DUBNER, R. (1989). Expansion of receptive fields of spinal lamina I projection neurons in rats with unilateral adjuvant-induced inflammation: the contribution of central dorsal horn mechanisms. *Pain*, in press.

LE BARS, D., DICKENSON, A.H. AND BESSON, J.M. (1979). Diffuse Noxious Inhibitory Control (DNIC): II. Lack of effect on non-convergent neurones, supraspinal involvement and theoretical implications. *Pain* **6**, 305-327.

MCMAHON, S.B. (1988). Neuronal and behavioural consequences of chemical inflammation of rat urinary bladder. *Agents and Actions*, in press.

MCMAHON, S.B. AND WALL, P.D. (1984). Receptive fields of rat lamina I projection cells move to incorporate a nearby region of injury. *Pain* **19**, 235-247.

MCMAHON, S.B. AND WALL, P.D. (1988). Descending excitation and inhibition of spinal cord lamina I projection neurons. *Journal of Comparative Neurology* **59**, 1204-1219.

VILLANUEVA, L., PESCHANSKI, M., CALVINO, B. AND LE BARS, D. (1986). Ascending pathways in the spinal cord involved in triggering of Diffuse Noxious Inhibitory Controls in the rat. *Journal of Neurophysiology* **55**, 34-55.

WALL, P.D. AND WOOLF, C.J. (1984). Muscle but not cutaneous C-afferent input produces prolonged increases in the excitability of the flexion reflex in the rat. *Journal of Physiology* **356**, 443-458.

WOMACK, M.D., MACDERMOTT, A.B. AND JESSELL, T.M. (1988). Sensory transmitters regulate intracellular calcium in dorsal horn neurons. *Nature* **334**, 351-353.

WOOLF, C.J. AND FITZGERALD, M. (1983). The properties of neurones recorded in the superficial dorsal horn in rat spinal cord. *Journal of Comparative Neurology* **221**, 313-328.

NEUROTRANSMITTERS AND PEPTIDES IN THE SUPERFICIAL DORSAL HORN

INTRODUCTION TO SECTION V

P. Max Headley

Department of Physiology, University of Bristol, School of Medical Sciences
University Walk, Bristol BS8 1TD, UK

Studies on the identification and synaptic properties of primary afferent neurotransmitters have been concentrated either on the Ia-motoneurone synapse, as a paradigm of CNS neurotransmission, or on the transmission from nociceptive primary afferents in the dorsal horn, for the logical reason that control of transmission at this site would be a potentially highly effective means for eliciting analgesia.

Both substance P (see refs in Hökfelt et al, 1975) and excitatory amino acids (see Curtis and Johnston, 1974 for review) have for many years been proposed as primary afferent transmitters, on mainly neurochemical rather than physiological evidence. The search received a boost in favour of short chain peptides largely as the result of two reports in the mid-1970s; firstly Hökfelt and collaborators (1975) reported that small dorsal root ganglion neurones contain substance P, supporting the postulate that this might be the neurotransmitter at the primary afferent terminals of high threshold afferents. Secondly Otsuka and Konishi (1976) found that substance P could be released from spinal cord following activation of primary afferents and, a year later, Jessel and Iversen (1977), in a frequently cited report, found that release from slices of trigeminal nucleus could be inhibited by opiates.

The largely frustrated search for a specific central role for such peptides needs no review here; the reader is referred to reviews such as those of Hunt (1983), Salt and Hill (1983) and Besson and Chaouch (1987). Suffice it to say that the identification of neuropeptides as primary afferent transmitters is hampered by various problems including questions over the specificity of antibodies used (given the frequent impurity of peptides supplied commercially; see Brown et al, 1986), over the coexistence of different peptides in the same primary afferent, extending even to opioid peptides (eg Weihe et al, 1985), over the finding that 80% of substance P is transported from primary afferent neurones in a peripheral rather than central direction (Harmer and Keen, 1982) and, perhaps most important, the lack of adequately selective receptor antagonists for the proposed transmitter peptides.

That such short chain peptides can be released from the spinal cord has been known for over a decade, but the details of neither the stimulus-dependency nor the site of release have been clear. The technique of antibody microprobes pioneered by Duggan and Hendry (1986) has already provided important insights into these questions, and raises serious doubts as to the anatomical origin of the peptides collected in spinal cord superfusion experiments. The technique promises much; see the contribution by Duggan in this session. His results clearly indicate independent but stimulus-dependent release of substance P and somatostatin consistent with either transmitter or modulator roles for these peptides. An important suggestion of a patho-physiological function for some of these peptides arises from the findings of groups at NIH and Munich that chronic noxious stimuli result in a marked increase in dynorphin-like immunoreactivity in the dorsal horn (eg Millan *et al*, 1986; and see Ruda in this session). That peptide synthesis is increased is consistent with the finding that gene expression can be induced rapidly in response to afferent input, as is the case with the oncogene c-fos, as reported by Hunt and by Basbaum in this volume.

Within the last few years there has been a resurgence of interest in excitatory amino acids (EAA) as primary afferent transmitters, with a mood that the peptides be relegated to the somewhat nebulous position of *neuromodulators*. Indeed such a possibility could have been inferred over a decade ago, for the early EM immunohistochemical investigation of Pickel *et al* (1977) indicated that the visualized substance P-like immunoreactivity was separate from unlabelled clear vesicles which would normally be postulated to contain transmitter (and which may well contain EAA). It has taken longer for histochemical techniques to be developed for the visualization of putative EAA-utilizing neurones. Such techniques have been applied to primary afferent cell bodies. They include firstly the uptake of labelled glutamine (Duce and Keen, 1983), secondly the immunohistochemical localization either of EAA-related enzymes such as glutaminase (Cangro *et al*, 1985) and glutamic oxalacetate transferase (Inagaki *et al*, 1987) or of glutamate itself (Battaglia *et al*, 1987), and thirdly the retrograde labelling of perikarya following the injection of labelled D-aspartate into regions of terminals (Hunt 1983; Barbaresi *et al*, 1985). Unfortunately these techniques, as applied to the dorsal root ganglion and/or primary afferent projections, yield grossly variable results. For none of these techniques is there any direct physiological or pharmacological corroboration in this pathway, although the D-aspartate labelling technique does correlate well with electrophysiological results in those supraspinal pathways investigated to date (Beart *et al*, 1988; Wiklund *et al*, 1988). The paper by Perl and Schneider, which follows, addresses directly the role of excitatory amino acids in mediating afferent inputs onto dorsal horn neurones. Importantly, in such *in vitro* electrophysiological preparations it becomes possible to investigate the distinction between mono- and poly-synaptic connections.

A further important aspect of primary afferent transmitter release concerns the physiological modulation of such release via receptors located on or near the terminals of these afferents. This aspect was not covered by any speakers at this symposium. There is histochemical and neurochemical evidence that spinal binding sites for both opioids and serotonin are reduced following removal of primary afferent fibres, suggesting that such receptors, amongst others, are present on primary afferents. Moreover there have been various physiological investigations of these receptors, the studies addressing either Ia terminals on motoneurones or small diameter afferents in the dorsal horn. Most studies have combined the microelectrophoretic administration of transmitter-related compounds from multibarrel pipettes with antidromic excitability testing of peripherally-recorded afferent fibres, using current pulses delivered via one barrel of the pipette. There are however various important technical difficulties which should be borne in mind when assessing this literature. Whilst in the case of Ia afferents it is possible to gauge the proximity of the pipette tip to the termination (most importantly from the ability of low currents of microelectrophoretic agents to reach and influence synaptically-generated variations in terminal excitability), the same is not the case with dorsal horn afferents. Unmyelinated afferent fibres may have accessible receptors along their length, not just at their terminals (eg Brown and Marsh, 1978). In addition the anodal blocking factor for terminal regions (at least for myelinated afferents; see Curtis and Lodge, 1982) can be substantially lower than for preterminal segments, so that stimuli only slightly supra-threshold will result in block rather than activation of that afferent; the effects of transmitter compounds in such a situation cannot be reliably interpreted (see Curtis and Lodge, 1982). Furthermore any effects of the administered compounds may be mediated indirectly via other cell elements rather than directly on receptors on the terminal under investigation. Thus with Ia terminals the effects of excitatory amino acids are evidently mediated via changes in the extracellular medium consequent on the excitation of local neurones (Curtis *et al*, 1984a); serotonin effects appear to be mediated indirectly following activation of sodium-dependent uptake mechanisms (Curtis *et al*, 1983) and enkephalin affects synaptic primary afferent depolarization by altering the release of GABA at the axo-axonic synapse onto the Ia afferent rather than by affecting the Ia terminal itself (Curtis *et al*, 1984b). The variable results obtained in tests on dorsal horn afferents (see Besson and Chaouch, 1987, for review) are thus not entirely surprising.

In summary, therefore, there is growing but disparate evidence in favour of excitatory amino acids as primary afferent transmitters in the superficial dorsal horn, there is a clarification of the stimuli required for, and the sites of release of, various neuropeptides, and there is a growing realization that the expression of peptides is dynamically responsive to sensory afferent inputs. One can be more optimistic than for many years that clarification of these issues will follow relatively rapidly. The effects mediated by presynaptic receptors on primary afferent terminals in the dorsal horn remain more confused.

REFERENCES

BARBARESI P, RUSTIONI A AND CUÉNOD M (1985). Retrograde labelling of dorsal root ganglion neurons after injection of tritiated amino acids in the spinal cord of rats and cats. *Somatosensory Research* **3**: 57-74.

BATTAGLIA G, RUSTIONI A, ALTSCHULER RA AND PETRUSZ P (1987). Glutamic acid coexists with substance P in some primary sensory neurons. In: *Fine Afferent Nerve Fibres and Pain.* Eds: RF Schmidt, H-G Schaible and C Vahle-Hinz. VCH Press, Weinheim, FRG. pp77-84.

BEART PM, NICOLOPOULOS LS, WEST DC AND HEADLEY PM (1988). An excitatory amino acid projection from ventromedial hypothalamus to periaqueductal gray in the rat: autoradiographic and electrophysiological evidence. *Neuroscience Letters* **85**: 205-211.

BESSON J-M AND CHAOUCH A (1987). Peripheral and spinal mechanisms of nociception. *Physiological Reviews* **67**: 67-186.

BROWN DA AND Marsh S (1978). Axonal GABA-receptors in mammalian peripheral nerve trunks. *Brain Research* **156**: 187-191.

BROWN JR, HUNTER JC, JORDAN CC, TYERS MB, WARD P AND WHITTINGTON AR (1986). Problems with peptides - all that glisters is not gold. *Trends in Neuroscience* **9**: 100-102.

CANGRO CB, SWEETNAM PM, WRATHALL JR, HASER WB, CURTHOYS NP AND NEALE JH (1985). Localization of elevated glutaminase immunoreactivity in small DRG neurons. *Brain Research* **336**: 158-161.

CURTIS DR, HEADLEY PM AND LODGE D (1984a). Depolarization of feline primary afferent fibres by acidic amino acids. *Journal of Physiology* **351**: 461-472.

CURTIS DR AND JOHNSTON GAR (1974). Amino acid transmitters in the mammalian central nervous system. *Ergebnisse Physiologie* **69**: 97-188.

CURTIS DR, LEAH JD AND PEET MJ (1983). Effects of noradrenaline and 5-hydroxytryptamine on spinal 1a afferent terminations. *Brain Research* **258**: 328-332.

CURTIS DR AND LODGE D (1982). The depolarisation of feline ventral horn group Ia spinal afferent terminations by GABA. *Experimental Brain Research* **46**: 215-233.

CURTIS DR, MALIK R AND LEAH JD (1984b). The effects of naloxone, morphine and methionine enkephalinamide on Ia afferent terminations in the cat spinal cord. *Brain Research* **303**: 289-298.

DUCE IR AND KEEN P (1983). Selective uptake of [^{3}H]glutamine and [^{3}H]glutamate into neurons and satellite cells of dorsal root ganglia *in vitro*. *Neuroscience* **8**: 861-866.

DUGGAN AW AND HENDRY IA (1986). Laminar localization of the sites of release of immunoreactive substance P in the dorsal horn with antibody coated microelectrodes. *Neuroscience Letters* **68**: 134-140.

HARMER A AND KEEN P (1982). Synthesis, and central and peripheral axonal transport of substance P in a dorsal root ganglion-nerve preparation *in vitro*. *Brain Research* **231**: 379-385.

HÖKFELT T, KELLERTH JO, NILSSON G AND PERNOW B (1975). Substance P: localization in the central nervous system and in some primary sensory neurons. *Science* **190**: 889-890.

HUNT SP (1983). Cytochemistry of the spinal cord. In: *Chemical Neuroanatomy*. Ed: PC Emson. Raven Press, NY. pp 53-84.

INAGAKI N, KAMISAKI Y, KIYAMA H, HORIO Y, TOHYAMA M AND WADA H (1987). Immunocytochemical localizations of cytosolic and mitochondrial glutamic oxalacetic transaminase isozymes in rat primary sensory neurons as a marker for the glutamate neuronal system. *Brain Research* **402**: 197-200.

JESSEL TM AND IVERSEN LL (1977). Opiate analgesics inhibit substance P release from rat trigeminal nucleus. *Nature* **268**: 549-551.

MILLAN MJ, MILLAN MH, CZLONKOWSKI, A HÖLLT, V PILCHER, CWT HERZ A AND COLPAERT FC (1986). A model of chronic pain in the rat: response of multiple opioid systems to adjuvant-induced arthritis. *Journal of Neuroscience* **6**: 899-906.

OTSUKA M AND KONISHI S (1976). Release of substance P like immunoreactivity from isolated spinal cord of newborn rats. *Nature* **264**: 83-84.

PICKEL VM, REIS DJ AND LEEMAN SE (1977). Ultrastructural localization of substance P in neurons of rat spinal cord. *Brain Research* **122**: 534-540.

SALT TE AND HILL RG (1983). Neurotransmitter candidates of somatosensory primary afferent fibres. *Neuroscience* **10**: 1083-1103.

WEIHE E, HARTSCHUH W AND WEBER E (1985). Prodynorphin opioid peptides in small somatosensory primary afferents of guinea pig. *Neuroscience Letters* **58**: 347-352.

WIKLUND L, BEHZADI G, KALEN P, HEADLEY PM, NICOLOPOULOS LS, PARSONS CG AND WEST DC (1988). Autoradiographic and electrophysiological evidence for excitatory amino acid transmission in the periaqueductal gray projection to nucleus raphe magnus in the rat. *Neuroscience Letters*, In press.

GLUTAMATE AND OTHER PUTATIVE MEDIATORS OF FAST SYNAPTIC ACTION IN THE SUPERFICIAL DORSAL HORN

Edward R. Perl and Stephen P. Schneider

Department of Physiology, University of North Carolina at Chapel Hill, Chapel Hill
NC 27514, U.S.A.

Recently there has been substantial interest in the nature of central synaptic transmitters for the nerve fibers of the dorsal roots. To a large extent, this attention has stemmed from work suggesting peptides as putative synaptic mediators, particularly in the outer laminae of the spinal dorsal horn. Since the first proposals for their involvement in synaptic function, a number of different peptides have been associated with dorsal root ganglion (DRG) cells and their central terminals (Hökfelt *et al.*, 1978; Hunt, 1983). Such peptides are demonstrable by immunohistochemistry in a considerable fraction of the small diameter cells of the dorsal root ganglia which are associated largely with thin, slowly-conducting afferent fibers. Thinly myelinated and unmyelinated dorsal root fibers principally enter the spinal cord through the lateral division of the dorsal roots and are known to terminate heavily in laminae I and II (Edinger, 1889; Ranson, 1913; Light and Perl, 1979b). These observations are consistent with the immunocytochemical staining for peptides of dorsal root fiber origin which is heaviest in the superficial dorsal horn (Hökfelt *et al.*, 1978; Hunt, 1983).

Initial evidence for peptides in the synaptic terminals of primary afferent fibers in the superficial dorsal horn engendered enthusiasm and at first it was presumed that these substances acted in the fashion of well-established synaptic mediators in conveying excitation (Otsuka, *et al.* 1972; Jessell and Iversen, 1977). Subsequently evidence appeared that peptides such as substance P and calcitonin-gene-related-peptide (CGRP) may not have the membrane actions appropriate for impulse-to-impulse transfer of activity across synapses (Murase and Randic, 1984; Ryu *et al.*, 1988). Specifically, direct application of substance P and certain other peptides attributed to DRG neurons have a much longer latency and duration of action than would be expected for mediators of rapid synaptic action. Furthermore, peptides localized to terminals of the superficial dorsal horn by immunocytochemistry appeared in profiles containing both clear round vesicles and larger dense core vesicles (e.g. Leeman *et al.*, 1979) with most observers reporting that antibodies directed against peptides such as substance P appeared to bind only to the dense core vesicles (but see Chan-Palay and Palay, 1977). These considerations led to proposals of coexistence of peptides with other synaptic transmitters and a modulator action for peptides (Krivoy *et al.*, 1979).

Rapid synaptic action has been demonstrated for activity evoked by thin myelinated and unmyelinated primary afferent fibers in neurons of the superficial dorsal horn

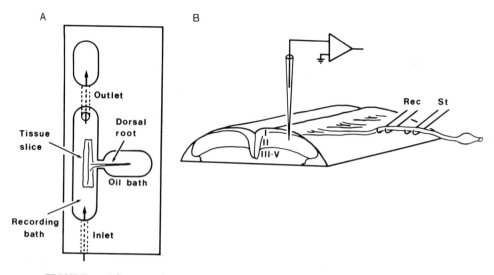

FIGURE 1: Diagram of the *in vitro* experimental chamber and arrangement. Rec: recording electrode. St: stimulating electrode. (Reproduced by permission from Schneider and Perl, 1988)

(Christensen and Perl, 1970; Kumazawa and Perl, 1978; Light *et al*, 1979). If the peptides associated with the central terminals of fine diameter fibers are not responsible for the rapid transmission of synaptic excitation, what mediators are employed for rapid transfer of activity across these synapses?

Amino acids as excitatory transmitters for primary afferent fibers are long established candidates for excitatory synaptic action in the central nervous system. In particular, L-glutamate has been suggested as a transmitter at the central terminals of dorsal root fibers because it is the only amino acid with a known excitatory action, that appears in higher concentration in the dorsal than in the ventral roots (Duggan and Johnston, 1970). Generally, it has been argued that L-glutamate is nonselective in its excitatory action on central nervous system neurons and from this standpoint could be considered as a synaptic transmitter for all dorsal root fibers (Curtis *et al.*, 1960; Zieglgänsberger and Herz, 1971; Zieglgänsberger and Puil, 1973; Galindo *et al.*, 1977; Hill and Salt, 1982). At the same time, there are indications that different DRG neurons vary in affinity for antibodies directed against a glutamate epitope and in the amount of enzyme or metabolic activity associated with glutamate (Cangro *et al.*, 1985; Duce and Keen, 1983; Cuenod *et al.*, 1981; Rustioni and Cuenod, 1982; Battaglia and Rustioni, 1988).

Identification of a chemical mediator at a synaptic junction requires several lines of evidence; these include a presence in presynaptic terminals, release by presynaptic neuronal activity, a postsynaptic action equivalent to that initiated by presynaptic neural activity and block of action by competitive agents also blocking usual synaptic action at the junction. Some of these steps require close control of concentrations of agents and chemical environment which for a neuropil as complex as the dorsal horn of the spinal cord *in vivo* is problematic. Accordingly, we attempted to simplify circumstances by experiments *in vitro* so as to gain better control of the chemical environment of dorsal horn neurons. However, it also appeared essential to retain the inherent organization of the primary afferent fiber relationships to dorsal horn neurons, and so we used a preparation of the mammalian spinal cord in which a slice of the dorsal horn from

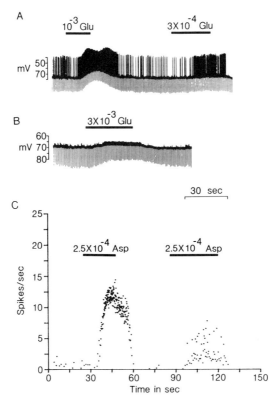

FIGURE 2: Responses of presumed lamina II neurons to indicated concentrations of L-glutamate (GLU) or L-aspartate (Asp). A and B: Intracellular recordings from different neurons. Downward deflections represent constant-current pulses applied through the recording microelectrode to measure neuronal input resistance. Action potential amplitudes are truncated in this and subsequent figures by the display devices. Concentrations of agents in artificial cerebrospinal fluid (ACSF) are given in mM. C: Discharge frequency as a function of time for an extracellularly recorded unit in relation to L-aspartate application. Heavy horizontal bars in this and all subsequent figures mark the time during which superfusion fluid was changed to that containing the indicated substance. (Reproduced by permission from Schneider and Perl, 1985)

young hamsters is made with one or more dorsal roots attached (Schneider and Perl, 1985a,b; 1988).

To maintain the integrity of the dendritic tree of dorsal horn neurons and branches of primary afferent fibers, horizontal slices were prepared of the spinal cord; these were 10-15 mm long and 500 μm thick and contained neurons in laminae I through V. The spinal cord slice was placed into a well through which fluid at room temperature (22-24° C) was circulated; the attached dorsal root and dorsal root ganglion was situated in a separate oil-filled chamber (Fig. 1). The tissue slice was superfused by artificial cerebrospinal fluid (ACSF) equilibrated with 95% O_2 and 5% CO_2 (pH 7.4, 125 mM NaCl, 5 mM KCL, 2.5 mM $CaCl_2$, 1.5 mM $MgSO_4$, 1.25 mM NaH_2PO_4 , 24 mM $NaHCO_3$ and 10 mM glucose) at 22-24° C. A dorsal root placed upon stimulating electrodes 8-10 mm from the spinal cord was used to initiate afferent volleys which were monitored by bipolar recording electrodes placed centrally on the root close to the spinal cord. In spite of short conduction distances, reasonable separation of the A $\alpha\beta$, A δ and the C-fiber components was possible even though conduction velocities in this

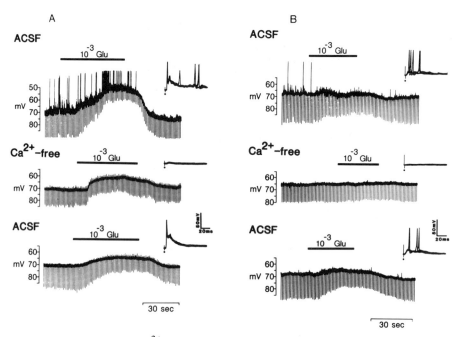

FIGURE 3: Effects of a Ca^{2+} free medium on L-glutamate action and dorsal root volleys. Presumed lamina II neurons. Inserts to the right of each longer record shows the responses evoked by single volleys containing activity in both A and C fibers. Other details as in Fig. 2. (Reproduced by permission from Schneider and Perl, 1985)

species are relatively slower than those of larger mammals and the preparation was below normal body temperature. Extracellular and intracellular recordings were made from neurons of the dorsal horn using pipette microelectrodes with tip diameters under 0.2 μm. The ACSF superfusing the spinal cord exchanged the fluid in the chamber approximately 10 times per minute, making possible rapid changes in the composition of the bathing fluid.

EFFECTS OF APPLIED L-GLUTAMATE AND L-ASPARTATE

In this preparation, neurons from laminae I through V retain responsiveness to dorsal root volleys for 8-10 hours. In early experiments, because of its reputation as a universal excitant of central neurons, L-glutamate was added to the superfusion fluid in various concentrations to test viability of the preparation and excitability of its neurons. Some neurons were readily excited by L-glutamate in the ACSF at concentrations as low as 50-100 μM (Fig. 2A). Excitation by L-glutamate was often evidenced by a membrane depolarization of several millivolts, a decrease in neuronal input resistance and often the appearance of discharges. In other neurons, bath applied L-glutamate produced only a small depolarization and a decrease in input resistance but no discharges (Fig. 2B). L-aspartate was essentially equally potent as an excitant of neurons responsive to glutamate (e.g. Fig. 2C).

Given the ready excitation of some neurons, we were surprised to find that only a fraction of the neurons excited by dorsal root afferent volleys could be activated by either L-glutamate or L-aspartate at concentrations up to 3 mM. Units unresponsive to L-glutamate appeared in the same preparations and physically close to responsive neurons (e.g. Fig. 3B). The method of application of L-glutamate or L-aspartate was not crucial. Iontophoretic application of L-glutamate from micropipettes excited the same extracellularly recorded units that responded to the amino acid in the bathing fluid. Conversely, units unresponsive to one form of the amino acid application were in general unresponsive to the other. In a survey of dorsal horn neurons responding to dorsal root volleys sampled largely by extracellular recordings, only about one third (51 of 160) were excited by either bath or iontophoretically applied L-glutamate or L-aspartate.

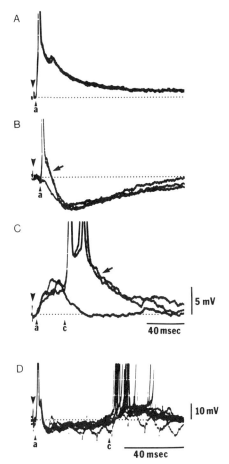

FIGURE 4: Effects of volley composition on responses of different dorsal horn neurons recorded *in vitro*. a: synaptic activity related to A fibers. c: synaptic activity related to C fibers. A: Nucleus proprius neuron whose response was only related to A fibers in afferent volley (Vm =-52mV). B: Superficial dorsal horn neuron: volleys to suprathreshold stimuli for Aδ fibers - arrow; Aαβ fibers alone - no arrow. (Vm = -63 mV). C: Superficial dorsal horn neuron. Responses evoked by volleys in Aδ and C fibers - arrow: Aαβ fibers alone - no arrow. D: Lamina III-IV neurone (Vm = -62 mV). Volleys contained activity in A and C fibers. Downward pulses represent current injected through the recording electrode. (Reproduced by permission from Schneider and Perl, 1988)

A neuron of a complex neuropil containing multiple interconnections between elements may be acted upon by an agent applied extracellularly either directly or indirectly through other neurons. Replacement of Ca^{2+} with Mn^{2+} in the extracellular medium is a reversible method of interfering with synaptic transmission (Llinas and Sugimori, 1980); such a substitution effectively blocks excitation of dorsal horn neurons by dorsal root stimulation (Fig. 3). Systematic substitution of Ca^{2+} by Mn^{2+} (or Co^{2+}) in the superfusion medium for the normal ACSF suggested that when L-glutamate excitation occurred, it often (50% or more of the trials) resulted from direct action upon the element under study since depolarization and a decrease in input resistance persisted after block of synaptic transmission from the dorsal root volleys (Fig.3). For certain neurons (e.g. Fig. 3A) a direct excitation, not dependent upon Ca^{2+} was superimposed upon a presumably synaptically-mediated effect that was dependent upon the presence of Ca^{2+}. Neurons considered unresponsive included those exhibiting a slight increase in baseline membrane noise and a small drop in input resistance that reversibly disappeared in Ca^{2+}-free medium, in the fashion illustrated by Fig. 3B. Masking inhibition appeared unlikely as an explanation for absence of L-glutamate excitation because excitation did not appear after removal of Ca^{2+} and inhibitory processes acting on the neuron under observation should have been suppressed by the low Ca^{2+}. Superfusion of the slice with ACSF containing $1\,\mu M$ tetrodotoxin had effects similar to low Ca^{2+} solutions on the presumed indirect excitatory actions of L-glutamate except that reversal of block of dorsal root synaptic action was difficult to demonstrate. The parallel blockade of L-glutamate action by low Ca^{2+} and tetrodotoxin low Ca^{2+} did not simply change a postsynaptic Ca^{2+} conductance activated by glutamate.

TABLE I

Relationship of afferent volley composition to excitation by aspartate and glutamate

Excitatory components of dorsal root compound potentials for 143 extracellularly recorded dorsal horn units classified according to their responses to aspartate and glutamate (Excited, Not Excited). A: units activated by volleys containing only the A fiber (myelinated) component. C: units activated only by volleys containing activity conducting in the C fiber (unmyelinated) range. Mixed: units activated by both A and C components of dorsal root volleys (Reproduced by permission from Schneider and Perl, 1985a)

Response to dorsal root stimulation

Response to Asp/Glu:	A	C	Mixed
Excited	16	13	19
Not Excited	63	11	21

The responses of dorsal horn neurons relate to components of dorsal root volleys in several ways (Hunt and Kuno, 1959; Christensen and Perl, 1970; Kumazawa and Perl, 1978; Light et al, 1979). Some exhibit excitation related only to input from the more rapidly-conducting (A $\alpha\beta$) myelinated fibers, some either only to that from the more slowly-conducting myelinated fibers (A δ) or unmyelinated (C) afferent fibers, and still others to that from various combinations of myelinated and unmyelinated components of the afferent volleys. In addition, a number of dorsal horn neurons have mixtures of excitation and inhibition evoked by single volleys. Neurons exhibiting dorsal root input primarily or exclusively from the large myelinated fibers typically are located deep to the substantia gelatinosa (laminae II), those with prominent or exclusive input from the unmyelinated fibers tend to be located in laminae II or the laminae I and II interface and those with prominent input from slowly-conducting myelinated fibers (Aδ) tend to be situated in lamina I, the outer part of lamina II (IIo) or deep in the dorsal horn. Neurons with these different characteristics were regularly noted in the slice preparation; examples of intracellular records are shown in Fig. 4.

No exclusive relationship appeared between excitation by a particular afferent volley component and cells excited or not excited by L-glutamate; however, as Table I illustrates, several preferential relationships were noted. In our extracellularly recorded sample, neurons not excited by glutamate were likely to be those receiving demonstrable afferent excitation only from myelinated fibers. In contrast, about one-half of the neurons excited only when C fiber components were present responded to L-aspartate and L-glutamate. A correlation also appeared between the location of neurons and their response to L-glutamate. The bulk of the neurons responsive to extracellularly applied L-glutamate were situated superficially in laminae I or II as illustrated by Fig. 5. Those unresponsive to L-glutamate were distributed throughout the dorsal horn.

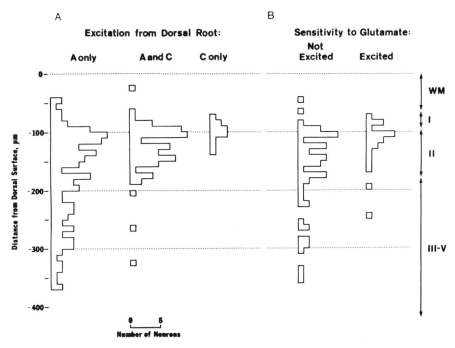

FIGURE 5: Recording locations of neurons in relation to afferent volley excitation (A) and responsiveness to superfusion with 1 mM L-glutamate (B). Approximate limits of Rexed's dorsal horn laminae are indicated on the right. WM: white matter. (Reproduced by permission from Schneider and Perl, 1988)

These data indicated that the response of mammalian dorsal horn neurons to L-glutamate is considerably more selective than has heretofore been suggested. Moreover, this selectivity in response was related to the location of the neurons and to the principal source of primary afferent excitation. Such observations are consistent with the idea that a compound similar to L-glutamate is a transmitter at dorsal horn synapses of some primary afferent neurons; however, it is far from convincing evidence on this point. For this reason, we undertook additional studies aimed at comparing more directly primary afferent and glutamate excitation.

EFFECTS OF EXCITATORY AMINO ACID BLOCKING AGENTS

Pharmacological agents that selectively block synaptic transmission, commonly by competing for the same receptor molecules, are valuable tools for establishing the identity of a chemical mediator agent acting at a synapse. At least three distinct membrane receptors have been identified for L-glutamate excitation; these include receptors most effectively activated by kainate, by quisqualate and by *N*-methyl-D-aspartate (NMDA). Of the compounds readily available, only D(-)2amino-5-phosphonovaleric acid (APV) is reported to be highly selective for a given receptor, acting principally or exclusively at the NMDA receptor (Watkins and Evans, 1981; Perkins and Stone, 1982). Several agents including kynurenic acid block more than one of these receptor sites. Using intracellular recordings so as to make possible the observation both of subthreshold excitatory actions and of inhibitory effects, we compared on 35 dorsal horn neurons the effects of such blocking agents both on dorsal root excitation and on the actions of applied L-glutamate.

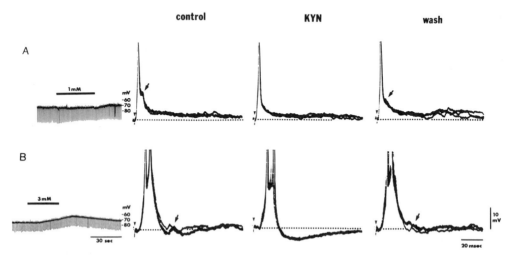

FIGURE 6: Effect of the excitatory amino acid receptor blocking agent, kynurenic acid (KYN), on responses initiated by primary afferent volleys in neurons unresponsive to bath-applied L-glutamate. A: laminae III-IV neuron; B: superficial dorsal horn neuron. Left column: Record showing effect of indicated concentrations of L-glutamate in ACSF. Control - ACSF fluid; KYN - after exposure to ACSF + kynurenic acid 1mM); Wash: 10 min after return to normal ACSF. (Reproduced by permission from Schneider and Perl, 1988)

NMDA receptors are reported to be inactivated by the presence of Mg^{2+} at the concentrations present in our ACSF (1.5 mM). Under our experimental conditions with standard ACSF, rapid excitation of dorsal horn neurons by dorsal root volleys was routine. This was one indication that NMDA receptors may not be crucial for fast synaptic activation from primary afferent fibers. Furthermore, when APV and other strong competitive blockers of NMDA receptors were tested, they were without effect upon rapid excitation by either dorsal root volleys or by bath applied L-glutamate. Kynurenic acid, a non selective excitatory amino acid blocker with a particular affinity for the kainate and quisqualate receptors did not interfere with dorsal root synaptic action on those neurons unresponsive to L-glutamate (Fig. 6). On the other hand, kynurenic acid severely depressed or completely blocked excitation evoked by dorsal root volleys for neurons excited by L-glutamate, e.g., Fig. 7; note in Fig. 7A the parallel reductions by kynurenic acid of excitation by glutamate and by dorsal root volleys for a superficial dorsal horn neuron. In contrast, kynurenic acid regularly left a membrane hyperpolarization evoked by dorsal root volleys unchanged, e.g., Fig. 7A. In other neurons with complex excitatory input, kynurenic acid suppressed discharges or synaptic potentials related to C-fiber components of volleys in neurons while having little effect on the excitatory activity related to A $\alpha\beta$ fibers (Fig. 7B). Similarly, in cells receiving excitation from both fast- and slowly-conducting A fibers, kynurenic acid reduced A δ - related potentials without producing notable changes in A $\alpha\beta$ excitation (Fig. 6) In general, kynurenic acid did not produce a recognizable decrease in fast dorsal root excitation for neurons unresponsive to L-glutamate at concentrations over 1 mM.

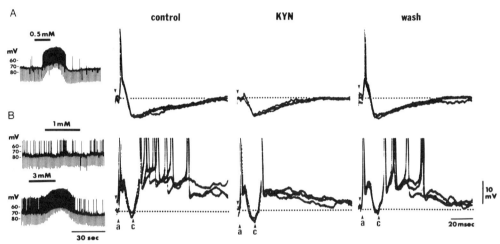

FIGURE 7: Effect of the excitatory amino acid receptor blocking agent, kyurenic acid (KYN), on responses evoked by primary afferent volleys. A: Neuron in superficial dorsal horn. B: Neuron in laminae III - IV. Left: L-glutamate application. Three consecutive traces from oscilloscope showing responses to suprathreshold dorsal root volleys. Control - ACSF; KYN - after addition of 1 mM kynurenic acid. Other notations as in Fig. 2. Note effect of KYN on later components, seemingly related to slower A fiber components. (Reproduced by permission from Schneider and Perl, 1988)

The lack of response of over 50% of our sample of dorsal horn neurons to either L-glutamate or L-aspartate was confirmed in the intracellular observations. Neurons unresponsive to applied L-glutamate were regularly excited by dorsal root afferent volleys. Therefore, the absence of response to L-glutamate was not due to a lack of excitability. Furthermore, neurons unresponsive to L-glutamate were excited by D,L-homocysteate in concentrations of < 1mM in the ASCF. The latter indicated that the bath-applied amino acids reached the neurons being tested and confirmed the cell's capacity to respond to applied agents. The dipeptide N-acetylaspartylglutamate excited neither L-glutamate-responsive nor unresponsive neurons in concentrations reported to be effective elsewhere in the nervous system (Zaczek et al., 1983).

It seems reasonable to deduce from these studies of applied L-glutamate and the use of excitatory amino acid blocking agents that only some dorsal horn neurons have membrane receptors for L-glutamate-like agents. In neurons containing them, such membrane receptors activate ionic channels causing a rapid membrane depolarization. A second point made by our observations is that block of certain excitatory amino acid membrane receptors also interferes with excitation from a subset of primary afferent fibers. In particular, neurons of the superficial dorsal horn receiving excitation from slowly-conducting primary afferent fibers appear likely to have excitatory receptors for L-glutamate and to have excitation from dorsal root fibers obstructed by agents competing for these excitatory receptors. On the other hand, only a part of the dorsal root fiber population exciting superficial dorsal horn neurons does so by receptors activated by L-glutamate. Moreover, some dorsal horn neurons receiving excitation from more rapidly-conducting A $\alpha\beta$ fibers of dorsal root also have that excitation interfered with by competitive antagonists for kainate and quisqualate receptors. Therefore, a glutamate-like substance appears to be utilized for rapid synaptic transmission by primary afferent neurons representing a substantial proportion of those with C and A δ fibers and a smaller fraction of those with larger-diameter myelinated fibers.

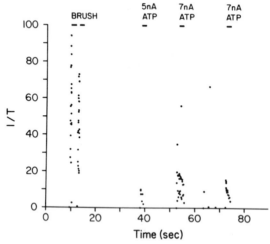

FIGURE 8: A plot of extracellularly recorded discharges of superficial dorsal horn neuron of cat in relation to cutaneous stimulation and iontophoresis of ATP. Each impulse appears as a dot plotted vertically as the reciprocal of interval from the previous impulse (frequency) against time (abscissa). Stimulation periods and periods of iontophoresis are marked by horizontal heavy lines at the top of the graph. The unit was maximally excited by gentle mechanical stimulation of the skin and hairs. It responded to both A fiber and C fiber components of a dorsal root volley. Current used for iontophoresis is indicated. (Reproduced by permission from Fyffe and Perl, 1984)

The conclusion that a glutamate-like agent acts as a synaptic transmitter for a number of thin but not for many larger diameter primary afferent fibers is supported by observations suggesting a special concentration of glutamate or glutamate-synthetic enzymes in the smaller neurons of the dorsal root ganglia. Cangro et al. (1985) described an elevated immunoreactivity for a phosphate-dependent glutaminase in small DRG neurons, an accumulation which may be associated with synthesis of releasable pools of L-glutamate (Kvamme, 1983). Small diameter neurons of the dorsal root ganglia have been found to accumulate far more glutamine, a precursor in the synthesis of glutamate, than do larger diameter neurons (Duce and Keen, 1983). In DRG, antibodies directed against a glutamate epitope bind to many small and intermediate-sized neurons but only to few large neurons (Battaglia and Rustioni, 1988). Some small neurons staining with an antiglutamate antibody are also immunoreactive with antibodies directed against substance P, implying a coexistence of these two agents in certain cells (Battaglia and Rustioni, 1988).

340

PURINERGIC TRANSMISSION BY PRIMARY AFFERENT FIBERS IN THE SUPERFICIAL DORSAL HORN

If some primary afferent fibers do not utilize an agent activating glutamate receptors to excite superficial dorsal horn neurons rapidly, what other substances might be employed for synaptic transmission? One possibility has already been alluded to, an agent activating the receptors that respond to the amino acid D,L-homocysteate. Another candidate was suggested some years ago by Holton and Holton (1954) who proposed adenosine triphosphate (ATP) as a possible central mediator for unmyelinated (C) fibers. This idea was revived by Dodd *et al.* (1983) after they concluded that the fluoride-resistant acid phosphatase (FRAP) concentrated in laminae II and in small diameter dorsal root ganglion cells acted selectively on 5' nucleotides, substrates which implicated the phosphatase in nucleotide metabolism. While Silverman and Kruger (1988) have recently found much less substrate selectivity for FRAP than Dodd *et al.* reported, Jahr and Jessell (1983) followed the earlier lead on 5' nucleotides and showed that when ATP was applied locally it evoked a rapid and brief membrane depolarization in a population of cultured dorsal horn neurons different from those responsive to L-glutamate. This observation, in turn prompted our laboratory to examine the effects of iontophoretically applied ATP on dorsal horn neurons *in vivo* (Fyffe and Perl, 1984).

ATP applied by weak iontophoretic current through recording micropipette electrodes produced a remarkably selective excitation of a subpopulation of cat neurons, principally located in the superficial dorsal horn. As illustrated by the graphs of Fig. 8 and 9, iontophoretic application of ATP evoked vigorous excitation of extracellularly-recorded units which were also activated by gentle mechanical stimuli or sudden cooling. Such neurons were located largely in lamina II or outer lamina III. As shown in Table II, neurons activated by innocuous mechanical stimuli and receiving

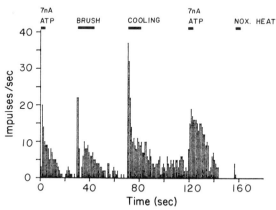

FIGURE 9: Discharges evoked from a superficial dorsal horn neuron by iontophoresis of ATP and by various cutaneous stimuli. Impulses for each sec are indicated by the height of the vertical lines. The unit was maximally responsive to innocuous mechanical disturbance of the skin and hair and was excited by both A and C fiber components of dorsal root volleys. The current used for ATP iontophoresis is indicated. Brush: a light stroke with a soft brush to the receptive field. Cooling: mixed mechanical and cooling stimulus produced by spraying ethyl chloride on the receptive field. Nox. Heat: noxious heat produced by a radiant source sufficient to sear the hair and the skin. (Reproduced by permission from Fyffe and Perl, 1984)

excitation from C-fibers with receptive fields on hairy skin were regularly excited by iontophoretic application of ATP. In contrast, selectively nocireceptive neurons of the same segments, whether or not receiving excitatory input mediated by C afferent fibers, were almost never responsive to ATP. On the other hand, multireceptive neurons, those excited by both innocuous mechanoreceptive primary afferent units with thin fibers and also receiving excitation from nociceptors, on occasion responded vigorously to ATP. The excitatory action of ATP did not appear to be related to its chelating action since strong chelators among ATP breakdown products such as pyrophosphate did not have the same selective excitatory action.

TABLE II

Neurons tested by ATP iontophoresis

	Innocuous mechanoreceptive (n=58)			Multireceptive (n=34)		Nocireceptive (n=28)		
	A only	A&C	C only	A only	A&C	A only	A&C	C only
Repeated trials	4/36	8/11	3/4	1/17	3/12	0/11	1/12	0/2
One trial only	1/4	2/2	1/1	2/2	1/3	1/2	---	0/1
Total	5/40	10/13	4/5	3/19	4/15	1/13	0/12	0/3
	(13%)	(77%)	(80%)	(16%)	(27%)	(8%)	(0%)	(0%)

Effectiveness of ATP iontophoresis in activating neurons classified according to the nature of their peripheral excitation. A only: neurons only responsive to the A fibers in afferent volleys; A&C: neurons responsive to both A and C fibers of afferent volleys; C only: neurons evidencing responses only to C-fiber component of afferent volleys. Repeated trials used graded currents from 2 to 40 nA. The results in which only one series or a single positive trial could be done should be considered questionable and are presented to minimize selection of data. Observations on 23 units were not included because the neurons either showed signs of injury at a crucial state in the test or evidenced characteristics of a recording from an axon. Responses counted as positive appeared at 2-5 nA, with maximal excitation occurring at <15nA. Negative trials were those in which no activation appeared with iontophoretic currents of 20-40 nA. (Reproduced with permission from Fyffe and Perl, 1984).

Unfortunately, at present there are no established specific antagonists for the action of ATP upon membrane receptors. Moreover, experiments are further complicated both by the rapid degradation of ATP and by the difficulty of interpreting results using it in bath application because of its potent metabolic action. Therefore, definitive analysis of ATP or other purinergic excitation of spinal neurons is difficult and awaits further exploration.

CONCLUSIONS AND SUMMARY

Taking into account the results of the studies described here as well as information from the literature, it appears likely that membrane receptors for relatively small molecules, L-glutamate or a similar amino acid and a purinelike substance such as ATP, are associated with the rapid activation of superficial (laminae I and II) dorsal horn neurons by primary afferent input. The primary afferent transmission by activation of glutamate-like receptors appears to be from a different set of primary afferent fibers than those associated with purine excitation. An ATP related agent, at least in the cat, appears to be a candidate transmitter for a class of cutaneous sense organs with thin afferent fibers that are maximally excited by innocuous mechanical stimuli. By elimination, primary afferent excitation of the commonlyencountered lamina I and II neurons that are selectively nocireceptive or thermoreceptive may use L-glutamate-like agents as mediators. A glutamate-like agent appears to be the mediator of fast synaptic action for more types of primary afferent fibers than employ an ATP synergist and the glutamate-utilizing population includes some fibers projecting more deeply in the spinal cord gray matter. Nonetheless, both types of agents appear to be related to rapid synaptic activation by the small diameter primary afferent fibers that terminate heavily in the superficial dorsal horn.

ACKNOWLEDGEMENTS

We thank Ms Sherry Derr for assistance in preparing the manuscript. Supported by a grant, NS10321, from the NINCDS of the U.S. Public Health Service

REFERENCES

BATTAGLIA, G. AND RUSTIONI, A. (1988). Co-existence of glutamate and substance P in dorsal root ganglion neurons of rat and monkey. *Journal of Comparative Neurology*, In press.

CANGRO, C.B., SWEETNAM P.M., WRATHALL J.R., HASER W.B., CURTHOYS, N.P. AND NEALE J.H. (1985). Localization of elevated glutaminase immunoreactivity in small DRG neurons. *Brain Research* **336**, 158-161.

CHAN-PALAY, V. AND PALAY, S.L. (1977). Ultrastructural identification of substance P cells and their processes in rat sensory ganglia and their terminals in the spinal cord by immunocytochemistry. *Proceedings of the National Academy of Sciences USA* **74**, 4050-4054.

CHRISTENSEN, B.N. AND PERL, E.R. (1970). Spinal neurons specifically excited by noxious or thermal stimuli: marginal zone of the dorsal horn. *Journal of Neurophysiology* **33**, 293-307.

CUENOD, M., BAGNOLI P., BEAUDET A., RUSTIONI A., WIKLUND, L. AND STREIT, P. (1981). Transmitter specific retrograde labeling of neurons. In *Cytochemical Methods in Neuroanatomy*, ed. Chan-Palay, V. and Palay, S.L., pp. 17-44. New York: Alan R. Liss.

CURTIS, D.R., PHILLIPS, J.W. AND WATKINS J.C. (1960). The chemical excitation of spinal neurones by certain acidic amino acids. *Journal of Physiology* **150**, 656-682.

DODD, J., JAHR, C.E., HAMILTON, P.N., HEATH, M.J., MATTHEW, W.D. AND JESSELL, T.M. (1983). Cytochemical and physiological properties of sensory and dorsal horn neurons that transmit cutaneous sensation. *Cold Spring Harbor Symposia on Quantitative Biology* **48**, 685-695.

DUCE, I.R. AND KEEN, P. (1983). Selective uptake of [^{3}H]glutamine and [^{3}H]glutamate into neurons and satellite cells of dorsal root ganglia *in vitro*. *Neuroscience* **8**, 861-866.

DUGGAN, A.W. AND JOHNSTON, G.A.R. (1970). Glutamate and related amino acids in cat spinal roots, dorsal root ganglia and peripheral nerves. *Journal of Neurochemistry* **17**, 1205-1208.

EDINGER, L. (1889). Über die Fortsetzung der hinteren Rückenmarkswurzeln zum Gehirn. *Anat. Anzeiger* **4**, 121-128.

FYFFE, R.E.W. AND PERL, E.R. (1984). Is ATP a central synaptic mediator for certain primary afferent fibers from mammalian skin? *Proceedings of the National Academy of Sciences* **81**, 6890-6893.

GALINDO, A., KRNJEVIC, K. AND SCHWARTZ, S. (1977). Microiontophoretic studies on neurones in the cuneate nucleus. *Journal of Physiology* **192**, 359377.

HILL, R.G. AND SALT, T.E. (1982). An iontophoretic study of the responses of rat caudal trigeminal nucleus neurones to non-noxious mechanical sensory stimuli.

Journal of Physiology **327**, 65-78.

HÖKFELT, T., ELDE, R., JOHANSSON, O., LJUNGDAHL, A., SCHULTZBERG, M., FUXE, K., GOLDSTEIN, M., NILSSON, G., PERNOW, B., TERENIUS, L., GANTEN, D., JEFFCOATE, S., REHFELD, J. AND SAID, S. (1978). Distribution of Peptide-containing Neurons. In *Psychopharmacology: A Generation of Progress* , ed. Lipton, M.A., DiMascio, A. and Killam, K.F., pp. 39-66. New York: Raven Press.

HOLTON, P. AND HOLTON, F.A. (1954). The capillary dilator substances in dry powders of spinal roots; a possible role of adenosine triphosphate in chemical transmission from nerve endings. *Journal of Physiology* **126** , 124-140.

HUNT, C.C. AND KUNO, M. (1959). Background discharge and evoked responses of spinal interneurones. *Journal of Physiology* **147**, 364-384.

HUNT, S.P. (1983). Cytochemistry of the Spinal Cord. In *Chemical Neuroanatomy* , ed. Emson, P.C., pp. 53-84. New York: Raven Press.

JAHR, C.E. AND JESSELL, T.M. (1983). ATP excites a subpopulation of rat dorsal horn neurons. *Nature* **304** , 730-733.

JESSELL, T.M. AND IVERSEN, L.L. (1987) Opiate analgesics inhibit substance P release from rat trigeminal nucleus. *Nature,* **268**, 549-551.

KRIVOY, W.A., COUCH, J.R., HENRY, J.L. AND STEWART, J.M. (1979). Synaptic modulation by substance P. *Federation Proceedings* **38**, 2344-2347.

KUMAZAWA, T. AND PERL, E.R. (1978). Excitation of marginal and substantia gelatinosa neurons in the primate spinal cord: indications of their place in dorsal horn functional organization. *Journal of Comparative Neurology* **177** , 417-434.

KVAMME, E. (1983). Glutaminase (PAG). In *Glutamine, glutamate, and GABA in the Central Nervous System* , ed. Hertz, L., Kvamme, E., McGeer, E. and Schousboe, A., pp. 51-67. New York: Alan R. Liss.

LEEMAN, S.E., BARBER, R.P., VAUGHN, J.E., SLEMMON, J.R., SALVATERRA, P.M. AND ROBERTS, E. (1979). The origin, distribution and synaptic relationships of substance P axons in rat spinal cord. *Journal of Comparative Neurology* **184** , 331-351.

LIGHT, A.R. AND PERL, E.R. (1979b). Reexamination of the dorsal horn projection to the spinal dorsal horn including observations on the differential termination of coarse and fine fibers. *Journal of Comparative Neurology* **186** , 117-132.

LIGHT, A.R., TREVINO, D.L. AND PERL, E.R. (1979). Morphological features of functionally defined neurons in the marginal zone and substantia gelatinosa of the spinal dorsal horn. *Journal of Comparative Neurology* **186** , 151-172.

LLINAS, R. AND SUGIMORI, M. (1980). Electrophysiological properties of *in vitro* Purkinje cell somata in mammalian cerebellar slices. *Journal of Physiology* **305** , 171-195.

MURASE, K. AND RANDIC, M. (1984). Actions of substance P on rat spinal dorsal horn neurones. *Journal of Physiology* **346** , 203-217.

OTSUKA, M., KONISHI, S. AND TAKAHASHI, T. (1972) A further study of the motoneuron-depolarizing peptide extracted from dorsal roots of bovine spinal nerves. *Proceedings of the Japanese Academy* **48**, 747-752.

PERKINS, M.N. AND STONE, T.W. (1982). An iontophoretic investigation of the actions of convulsant kynurenines and their interaction with the endogenous excitant quinolinic acid. *Brain Research* **247** , 184-187.

RANSON, S.W. (1913). The course within the spinal cord of the non-medullated fibers of the dorsal roots: a study of Lissauer's tract in the cat. *Journal of Comparative Neurology* **23** , 259-281.

RANSON, S.W. (1914). The tract of Lissauer and the substantia gelatinosa Rolandi. *American Journal of Anatomy* **16** , 97-126.

RUSTIONI, A. AND CUENOD, M. (1982). Selective retrograde transport of D-aspartate in spinal interneurons and cortical neurons of rats. *Brain Research* **236** , 143-155.

RYU, P.D., GERBER, G., MURASE, K. AND RANDIC, M. (1988). Actions of calcitonin gene-related peptide on rat spinal dorsal horn neurons. *Brain Research* **441** , 357-361.

SCHNEIDER, S.P. AND PERL, E.R. (1985a). Selective excitation of neurons in the mammalian spinal dorsal horn by aspartate and glutamate *in vitro*: correlation with location and excitatory input. *Brain Research* **360** , 339-343.

SCHNEIDER, S.P. AND PERL, E.R. (1985 b). Kynurenic acid antagonizes synaptic and amino acid excitation of hamster spinal dorsal horn neurons in vitro . *Society of Neuroscience Abstracts* **11** , 217.

SCHNEIDER, S.P. AND PERL, E.R. (1988). Comparison of primary afferent and glutamate excitation of neurons in the mammalian spinal dorsal horn. *Journal of Neuroscience* **8** , 2062-2073.

SILVERMAN, J.D. AND KRUGER, L. (1988). Acid phosphatase as a selective marker for a class of small sensory ganglion cells in several mammals: Spinal cord distribution, histochemical properties, and relation to fluoride-resistant acid phosphatase (FRAP) of rodents. *Somatosensory Research* **5** , 219-246.

WATKINS, J.C. AND EVANS, R.H. (1981). Excitatory amino acid transmitters. *Annual Review of Pharmacology and Toxicology* **21** , 165-204.

ZACZEK, R., KOLLER, K., COTTER, R., HELLER, D. AND COYLE, J. (1983). *N*-acetylaspartylglutamate: An endogenous peptide with high affinity for a brain *glutamate* receptor. *Proc. Natl. Acad. Sci. USA* **80** , 116-1119.

ZIEGLGANSBERGER, W. AND HERZ, A. (1971). Changes of cutaneous receptive fields of spino-cervical-tract neurones and other dorsal horn neurones by microiontophoretically administered amino acids. *Experimental Brain Research* **13**, 111-126.

ZIEGLGANSBERGER, W. AND PUIL, E. (1973). Actions of glutamic acid on spinal neurones. *Experimental Brain Research* **17**, 35-49.

PERIPHERAL STIMULI RELEASING NEUROPEPTIDES IN THE DORSAL HORN OF THE CAT

A.W. Duggan, C.R. Morton*, I.A. Hendry* and W.D. Hutchison*

Department of Preclinical Veterinary Sciences, University of Edinburgh, EH9 1QH, U.K.
and *Department of Pharmacology, Australian National University PO Box 341, ACT
Australia

For a compound to be accepted as a transmitter of information from one neurone to another it is sufficient to show that it is released by impulses in the presynaptic element, that it has effects on the postsynaptic element identical with those associated with physiological transmission and that the amounts released are adequate to produce these effects. While newer *in vitro* methods have enabled more detailed analysis of the actions of suspected transmitters on postsynaptic membranes, the demonstration of release of compounds from nerve terminals in the central nervous system has proved more difficult to refine (Mitchell, 1975; Marsden, 1984). Analysis of voltammetry traces obtained using carbon fibre microelectrodes gives information on release of monoamines in the brain (Marsden, 1984) but this technique appears not to be suitable for neuropeptides. The push pull cannula continues to be used to measure release (Kuraishi *et al*, 1985; Hirota *et al*, 1985; Oku *et al*, 1987) despite its relatively large diameter (circa 600 μm). Intracranial dialysis employs smaller diameter tubing (200 μm), but requires a loop to pass right through the area of interest (Ungerstedt, 1984; Brodin *et al*, 1987; Westerlink *et al*, 1987, Sorkin *et al*, 1988). This method has the advantage of limiting the size of molecules collected from the area perfused.

A newer approach to release has been to immobilize antibodies to a compound of interest to the outer surfaces of glass microelectrodes and to use such microprobes to bind molecules released from discrete sites within the central nervous system. After use in the brain or spinal cord, microprobes are incubated in a solution containing a radiolabelled form of the neuropeptide being studied and sites of release are detected on autoradiographs as zones of inhibition of binding of the labelled peptide (Duggan and Hendry, 1987, Duggan *et al*, 1987, 1988a,b).

Studies of neuropeptide release are of particular importance in attempting to assign functional significance to the complexities revealed by histochemical studies of the neuropeptides contained within dorsal root ganglion cells and of their central terminations in the spinal cord (Gibson *et al*, 1981; Hökfelt *et al*, 1976, 1977; Jessell, 1982; Leah *et al*, 1985a, 1985b; Price, 1985). The questions which need to be answered include: (a) is there a chemical coding of dorsal root ganglion cells such that particular functional types release particular peptides?; (b) where are these compounds released? and does co-existence of necessity mean co-release or do changes in peripheral stimuli produce changes in what is released centrally?

The anatomical approach to the functional significance of neuropeptides contained within dorsal root ganglion cells suffers from an inability to identify structures functionally when examining sections of either peripheral nerve or dorsal root ganglion cells. Thus while approximately 70% of peripheral primary afferent fibres in dorsal roots of the rat are unmyelinated (Gasser, 1955), only 15-20% of dorsal root ganglion cells contain substance P (SP) (Hökfelt et al, 1976). It is probable that this means that not all nociceptors contain SP and indeed, based on estimates of the proportion of nociceptors contained within peripheral nerve, Hunt and Rossi (1984) have proposed parallel inputs from the periphery of peptide-containing and nonpeptide-containing primary afferent nociceptors. A methodological improvement on strictly anatomical methods has been to combine physiological characterization of defined dorsal root ganglion cells with subsequent immunohistochemical determination of contained neuropeptides (Leah et al, 1985b). Such experiments assume that peptides demonstrated by immunohistochemistry are released by the stimuli used to characterize the neurones studied. This is not unreasonable but there are results from experiments on peripheral tissue indicating that the patterning of impulses can influence what is released from nerve terminals containing more than one releasable compound (Stjärne, 1986; Lundberg et al, 1986). Thus there is a need to determine whether a defined stimulus, applied to the peripheral receptive field of a primary afferent neurone, results in release of a neuropeptide (or neuropeptides) from its central terminals. It is not currently possible to do this at the level of a single neurone. Hence, even if a particular stimulus causes the detection of more than one neuropeptide in the spinal cord, it is not possible to differentiate between co-release and release from different populations of primary afferent fibres. Nevertheless there is now a convincing body of data that natural peripheral stimuli do cause a central release of neuropeptides and the results to date suggest that subdivisions exist within nociceptors in terms of substances released. The present account will deal only with release of substance P and somatostatin.

RELEASE OF IMMUNOREACTIVE SUBSTANCE P (IRSP) IN THE SPINAL CORD

Because of the presence of irSP in many small diameter dorsal root ganglion cells, most investigators have examined release of irSP following either electrical stimulation of unmyelinated primary afferents or noxious peripheral stimuli; these latter stimuli have been exclusively cutaneous. Nothing is known of the ability of deep somatic or visceral stimuli to release irSP in the spinal cord.

(a) Spinal Cord Perfusion

Perfusion of the surface of the spinal cord of the anaesthetized cat has shown a release of irSP following electrical stimulation of high threshold primary afferents (Yaksh et al, 1980). In subsequent experiments (Go and Yaksh, 1987) intense heat (metal plates at 75°C applied to the hind limbs intermittently for 30 minutes) produced small increases in irSP in the spinal perfusate. Now that there is evidence that peripheral noxious stimulation causes a release of irSP from pial nerves (Duggan et al, 1988b) and it appears that such release is exaggerated by inflammation, the significance of release into a spinal perfusate is less certain. The proportion of irSP in a spinal perfusate which is actually derived from the spinal cord requires extended examination.

(b) Push pull cannulae and microdialysis

The most extensive studies using push pull cannulae to measure irSP release have come from Kuraishi and his colleagues. They found in rabbits that noxious mechanical, but not thermal, stimuli produced a 10-fold increase in irSP in a perfusate of the dorsal horn (Kuraishi *et al*, 1985a) and that this release was reduced by topical application of morphine (Hirota *et al*, 1985) and noradrenaline (Kuraishi *et al*, 1985b). The thermal stimulus used was a focused light bulb and the temperatures attained were measured with a subcutaneous thermocouple. The maximum temperature used was 48.5°C and it was stated that subdermal temperatures of 44°C were exceeded for more than 11 minutes of the 20 minute stimulus period. These temperatures are probably of considerable significance as will be discussed with the antibody microprobe results. Subdermal temperatures of 50°C and higher were not used. The combined results of experiments on somatostatin and SP release led to the proposal that SP is released in the spinal cord by noxious mechanical stimuli and somatostatin by noxious thermal stimuli. It follows that polymodal nociceptors release neither peptide since these neurones fire impulses in response to either stimulus. The precise location of the end of the push pull cannula was not stated in these experiments but with diameters of 600 μm such cannulae cannot locate a site of release with any precision. The push pull cannula has also been used in the spinal cord of the rat (Oku *et al*, 1987). With normal rats, flexing the ankle did not increase irSP release over basal values whereas with polyarthritic rats, eight fold increases were observed.

Microdialysis tubing can be reduced to 200 μm diameter (Westerlink *et al*, 1987; Sorkin *et al*, 1988) but the only study of irSP release from the spinal cord has used tubing of 500 μm diameter (Brodin *et al*, 1987). It was found that electrical stimulation of unmyelinated fibres of the sciatic nerve of the cat produced a release of irSP but the site of release was not localized more precisely than showing that release was greater in the lower than in the upper lumbar segments.

(c) Antibody Microprobes

Initial results with antibody microprobes showed that, in the anaesthetized spinal cat, electrical stimulation of large diameter primary afferents of the tibial nerve did not produce release of irSP within the spinal cord but that increasing the stimulus strength to include unmyelinated (C) fibres resulted in release in the region of the substantia gelatinosa of the ipsilateral dorsal horn (Duggan and Hendry, 1986). Such a result is shown in Figure 1. These experiments indicated that a zone of irSP release also appeared at the spinal cord surface although the significance of this was not apparent. No systematic study was made of the patterning of impulses needed in C fibres to produce irSP release. Most commonly a continuous tetanus of 0.3 ms pulses at 10-31 Hz was used for 15 to 20 minutes. Unlike perfusion methods, antibody microprobes detected release of irSP in the absence of prior injection of protease inhibitors.

The sensitivity of the microprobes used in these and subsequent experiments was such that prior incubation in synthetic substance P with concentrations of 10^{-7} M or greater produced at least 50% inhibition of the binding of radiolabelled SP. These initial experiments estimated inhibition of binding semi-quantitatively from inspection of photographic enlargements of X-ray film images of microprobes (Figure 1). Thus it was not possible to measure accurately the increases over basal release produced by nerve stimulation, as can be done, for example, with perfusion methods. Analysis of subsequent experiments employed a computer-assisted image density analysis which

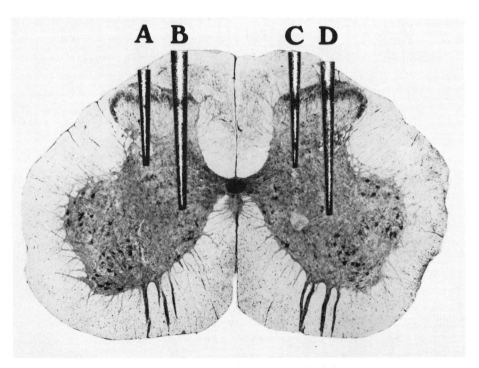

FIGURE 1: Release of immunoreactive substance P (irSP) in the dorsal horn measured with antibody microprobes. Photographic enlargements of X-ray film images of microprobes are superimposed on a spinal cord section image. Microprobe A represents no peripheral stimulation (20 minutes in the spinal cord), microprobe B was 30 minutes in the cord during electrical stimulation of large myelinated afferents of the ipsilateral tibial nerve. Microprobes C and D were 20 and 30 minutes respectively in the spinal cord during electrical stimulation of unmyelinated fibres of the ipsilateral tibial nerve. Microprobes B and D were inserted 3mm into the spinal cord. Reproduced (with permission) from Duggan and Hendry (1986).

prepared graphs of the optical density of x-ray film images of microprobes with respect to depth in the spinal cord. The analysis was in 16 μm steps. Importantly, results from defined experimental and control groups of microprobes could be averaged and statistical estimates of significance assigned to differences between the two groups (Hendry *et al*, 1988). Examples are shown in Figures 2 and 4.

When using noxious peripheral stimuli, a release of irSP was produced both in the region of the substantia gelatinosa and at the cord surface following noxious thermal, mechanical and chemical stimuli (Duggan *et al*, 1987, 1988a,b). With noxious heat the hind paw was immersed in a water bath and, although temperatures of 45°-48°C are generally regarded as painful both in man (Chery-Croze, 1983), and cats (Zimmerman, 1976) a bath temperature of 50°C was needed to produce release of irSP in the dorsal horn. The noxious mechanical stimulus was pinching of the skin of digital pads with small alligator clips, these being applied for 2 minutes and then removed for one minute, the cycle being repeated for 15 to 30 minutes. Thus the mechanical stimulus was not quantitatively graded in the way that noxious heat was. Non-noxious mechanical stimulation (a brass weight applied to the hind paws) did not result in irSP release. The noxious chemical stimulus was painting the skin of digital pads with methylene chloride (Adriaensen *et al*, 1980) and thus it also was not a graded stimulus. Methylene chloride produced considerable swelling of the hind paws. With all types of noxious stimuli a stimulus duration of at least 15 minutes was needed to produce release consistently. Figure 2 illustrates a significant release of irSP in the substantia gelatinosa following heating of the hind paw to 52°C, but not when using stimulus temperatures of 46° and 48°C.

These results with microprobes were interpreted as indicating that polymodal nociceptors contain and release substance P, although an associated release from

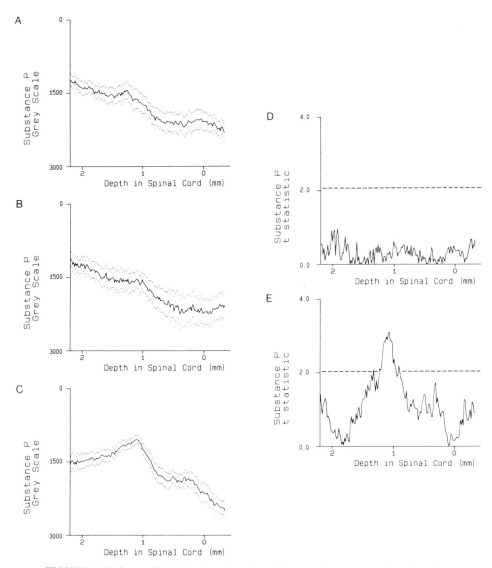

FIGURE 2: Release of irSP in the substantia gelatinosa and at the spinal cord surface following a noxious thermal stimulus. The graphs are mean image density analyses of defined groups of microprobes. Optical density (in arbitrary units, see Hendry and Duggan, 1988) is plotted with respect to depth in the spinal cord in 16 μm intervals. A: the mean of 14 microprobes inserted into the spinal cord with the ipsilateral hind paw in water of 36°-44°C. B: The mean of 10 microprobes, water temperature of 46°-48°C. C: The mean of 20 microprobes, water temperature 52°C. D: A plot of the t-statistics derived for the differences between A and B. E: A plot of the t-statistics for the differences between A and C.

specialised nociceptors could not be excluded. The long stimulus times needed to detect release and the failure to measure release with noxious thermal stimuli of 45°-48°C were believed to result from a relative insensitivity of the microprobe technique. Perfusion methods also commonly require collection times of 20 to 30 minutes to measure significant release of a variety of peptides. Subsequent studies of somatostatin release however, have shown that, for an assay procedure which had a similar *in vitro* sensitivity to that used with substance P, prolonged stimulus times were not needed to elicit a release of somatostatin in the spinal cord. Either relatively massive amounts of somatostatin are released relative to substance P, or the high noxious heat temperatures and prolonged times used with substance P have physiological significance.

Cutaneous thermal stimuli in the range 45° to 48°C are painful and both with microprobes and push-pull cannulae these temperatures failed to produce a release of irSP. Higher temperatures (50° and 52°C) used for longer times will damage the skin and produce sensitization of nociceptors (Bessou and Perl, 1969; Perl *et al*, 1974; Lynn, 1977; Fitzgerald, 1979). Such sensitization occurs in the injured area and in the zone of hyperalgesia which develops around a site of injury and which is dependent on the integrity of nerves supplying the injured and adjacent areas (Lewis, 1935, 1942). Hyperalgesia is believed to result from the release of compounds from afferent nerve endings in the skin (Lewis, 1935; King *et al*, 1976; Fitzgerald, 1979) and several mechanisms have been proposed for the spread of hyperalgesia beyond the injured areas. These include: (a) each peripheral branch of a nociceptor acting equally as an afferent and an efferent. This was first proposed by Bayliss (1901) as the basis of axo-axonic reflexes. Lewis (1935) however denied this mechanism since he believed that nerves were essential for the spread of hyperalgesia beyond an injured area, and the area to which pain can be localised is smaller than the associated area of hyperalgesia: (b) different branches of nociceptors have different functions: some are afferents and some are efferents; (c) the proposal of Lewis (1935, 1942) that a subset of nerves, nocifensors, was responsible for the spread of hyperalgesia. Nocifensors were proposed as having large territories encompassing the receptive fields of more than one nociceptor.

The results on central release of SP are consistent with release from a set of primary afferents which are not active with the lower noxious thermal temperatures (45°-48°C) but which become active under conditions of high temperatures for relatively prolonged periods, when sensitization of receptors and spreading hyperalgesia are almost certainly operative. It is possible that central release of SP is detected only when normal peripheral nociceptors are sensitized in areas of tissue damage. This explanation is not favoured by studies in the monkey, however, since heating the skin above 51°C resulted in increased firing of small myelinated nociceptors but reduced responsiveness of unmyelinated nociceptors (Campbell *et al*, 1979; LaMotte, 1984). Substance P is believed to be contained mainly within unmyelinated primary afferents of the cat (Leah *et al*, 1985a,b). Lewis (1935) first proposed a system of nerves active only with inflammation, and recent studies of joint afferents have come to a similar conclusion (Schaible and Schmidt, 1988). Thus acute chemical arthritis of the cat knee joint resulted in sensitization of high threshold mechanosensitive fine diameter afferents but in addition mechanosensitivity was induced in a population of afferent fibres previously unresponsive to noxious or non-noxious joint stimulation. It is possible these cutaneous *nocifensors* contain and release substance P.

It is appropriate to mention here that much of the interest in attempting to identify the compounds which, when released from peripheral nerve terminals, produce vasodilatation and hyperalgesia, was due to the belief that such compounds should also be released at central terminals and would thus be likely transmitters of nociceptive information (Dale, 1935). What evidence is there that only high threshold nociceptors or nocifensors produce peripheral vasodilatation and hyperalgesia? The most direct experiments are those of Kenins (1981) who isolated filaments of peripheral nerve from which only single C fibre action potentials could be recorded, characterised them physiologically, and stimulated them electrically. Only polymodal nociceptors were found to produce increased cutaneous vascular permeability when electrically stimulated. The noxious thermal stimulus used to characterize receptors was, however, an undescribed probe at 50°C. Although this was described by Kenins as non-damaging to the skin, it still remains to be determined if nociceptors excited by skin temperatures of 45°-48°C produce cutaneous hyperalgesia and vasodilatation.

The proposal that a subset of primary afferent fibres, active under conditions of tissue damage and hyperalgesia, release substance P centrally is, however, consistent with some puzzling histochemical observations. As cited previously, only 20-30% of small diameter dorsal root ganglion cell bodies contain SP (Hökfelt et al, 1975). In addition in the experiments of Leah et al (1985), of 15 physiologically identified nociceptors, only 2 were subsequently shown to contain substance P. Of 10 unidentified cells with axons conducting in the C fibre range, 7 contained substance P. The noxious heat stimulus in these experiments was touching the skin with a brass rod at 60°C and there may not have been time for hyperalgesia to develop. These observations and inferences do not associate substance P with normal nociceptors. If released SP is indeed a transmitter of information from a system of fibres signalling peripheral damage sufficient to produce hyperalgesia, then impulses in these fibres may not ultimately result in the perception of pain. That may be the province of nociceptors activated by less damaging stimuli.

The finding of a noxious stimulus-evoked release of irSP at the spinal cord surface has important implications for the structure and function of primary afferent nociceptors. Analysis of the conditions necessary to produce such release (Duggan et al, 1988b) led to the proposals that :

(a)The irSP was contained within an inflammatory exudate derived from pial vessels and nerves at the edge of the area of spinal cord cleared of pia mater so as to permit entry of microprobes into the spinal cord. It is known that irSP is released into inflammatory exudates within blisters produced by damaging thermal cutaneous stimuli (Helme et al, 1986; Jonsson et al, 1986).

(b)The presence of irSP at the cord surface was initially noxious stimulus dependent but with gradual accumulation of the exudate the peptide was continually present.

The noxious stimulus dependency of release at the cord surface implies a branch of primary afferent nociceptors innervating the pia mater. This could enter via the dorsal roots or the ventral roots. Langford and Coggeshall (1979) found a 20-30% excess of fibres contained within dorsal roots over cell bodies in dorsal root ganglia of the rat. Many of these supernumerary fibres could be destined for the pia mater and not the spinal cord. Dalsgaard et al (1982) have proposed that many of the SP- containing fibres of the ventral roots innervate pial structures. Figure 3 illustrates two possible modes of innervation of pial vessels by branches of primary afferents.

SP-containing nerve fibres have been reported in the pia mater of the brain and spinal cord (Uddman et al, 1981; Edvinsson et al, 1981; Dalsgaard et al, 1982; Liu-Chen et al, 1983) where they have been associated with blood vessels and particularly with arteries. Substance P has been shown to produce a dose dependent relaxation of the cat middle cerebral artery contracted by prostaglandin $F_{2\alpha}$ (Edvinsson *et al*, 1981). Moskowitz *et al* (1983) have shown a high potassium stimulated release of SP from an *in vitro* preparation of bovine pia arachnoid. It is possible therefore that the function of SP released from the central branches of nociceptors is to control cerebral and spinal blood flows. Thus impulses initiated by damaging noxious peripheral stimuli, when propagated into all the central terminals, will result in transmission of nociceptive information to neurones of the dorsal horn but also in alterations of central nervous blood flow. There is a need to measure segmental cord blood flow before and after damaging peripheral stimuli.

A In dorsal root

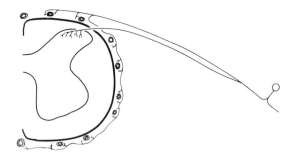

B In ventral root

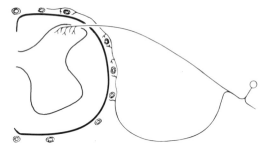

FIGURE 3: Innervation of pial vessels by branches of primary afferent fibres entering by the dorsal roots (A) or ventral roots (B). Although the branch is shown from the central process of a dorsal root ganglion cell, it could equally come from the peripheral process.

This hypothesis has the implication that not all of the central branches of a primary afferent neurone have the same function. If this is so then different transmitters may be needed at the different types of endings. This may be the real significance of coexistence of more than one peptide within primary afferent neurones. Neuropeptides are synthesized predominantly in the cell bodies of neurones and are transported thence to the terminals (Scharrer, 1987). If no mechanism is available to segregate a particular compound (or compounds) into one group of terminals then all will be synthesized in the cell body and transported to all terminals. It is probable therefore that all will be released with the arrival of an impulse in a terminal but not all will necessarily have a postsynaptic action. This is not an economical use of transmitter molecules but it may be the only way that a neurone can have terminals with differing functions. This hypothesis, to be tested, requires extended experiments with antagonists of released compounds to see which are necessary for transmission of information. There are several instances, however, where a released compound has had no detectable effect on the target tissue (Campbell, 1987).

RELEASE OF IMMUNOREACTIVE SOMATOSTATIN (IRSS) IN THE SPINAL CORD

The tetradecapeptide somatostatin (SS) has a similar anatomical distribution to SP, being localized by immunoreactive techniques in small diameter DRG neurones and in the superficial laminae of the dorsal horn of several species (Hökfelt *et al*, 1975; Forssman *et al*, 1979; Ho and Berelowitz, 1984; Leah *et al*, 1975a; Krukoff *et al*, 1986; Tessler *et al*, 1986). Fewer DRG cells contain irSS than contain irSP: in the cat about 5% of these neurones contain irSS (Leah *et al*, 1985a).

Release of irSS has been less extensively studied than release of irSP.

(a) In Vitro Preparations

A calcium-dependent release of irSS has been evoked from *in vitro* preparations of rat spinal cord by superfusion with solutions containing high concentrations of potassium ions or capsaicin (Sheppard *et al*, 1979; Gamse *et al*, 1981). More recently Bonnano *et al*, (1988) have reported irSS release from cerebral cortical slices following electrical field stimulation. Such studies are of limited value in identifying the neuronal origin of the released peptide and cannot address the physiology of the release.

(b) Push-pull cannula

Kuraishi *et al*, (1985a) have measured irSS release in the rabbit spinal cord in response to cutaneous stimuli. The noxious thermal stimulation employed (described above) evoked irSS release within the ipsilateral dorsal horn but noxious mechanical stimulation was ineffective. As discussed previously, these experiments did not localize the site(s) of release more precisely than to the dorsal horn.

(c) Antibody microprobes

To investigate possible irSS release in the spinal cord, antibody microprobes have been used in the lumbar dorsal horn of anaesthetized cats. Such microprobes have revealed a basal release of irSS in the absence of peripheral stimulation, centered 1.1-1.2 mm from the dorsal cord surface, in the region of the substantia gelatinosa (Morton *et al*, 1988a). There was also release of irSS at the surface of the cord.

The basal release of irSS in the substantia gelatinosa region was readily detected on microprobes placed in the cord for only 5 min, and was much more prominent than that observed for irSP in the same spinal region under similar conditions (Duggan *et al*, 1987, 1988b). It was considered that this release of irSS might result from continuous firing of thermoreceptors. Such receptors are activated by stimulus temperatures in the range 30°-40°C but the most effective stimulus is around 43°C (Kenshalo, 1976). With microprobes however, it was found that following immersion of the hind limbs into water of temperatures between 15° and 31°C, the irSS release in the substantia gelatinosa region was similar to basal levels (Morton *et al*, 1988b). This release of irSS was increased when the stimulus temperature was noxious. Figure 4 illustrates irSS release in the substantia gelatinosa during innocuous thermal stimulation of the ipsilateral hind paw with a continuously-stirred water bath. With a stimulus

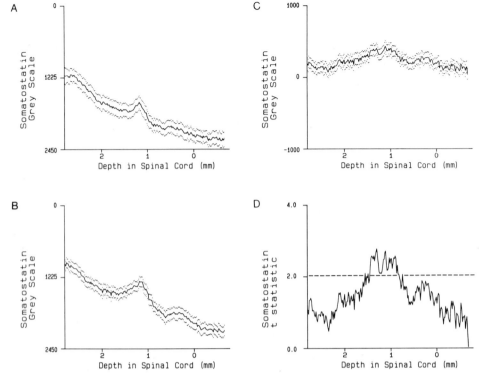

FIGURE 4: Release of irSS in the substantia gelatinosa following cutaneous thermal stimulation. The graphs are mean image density analyses of defined groups of microprobes. Ordinate; optical density (in arbitrary units, see Hendry *et al*, 1988). Abscissa: depth of microprobe insertion in the spinal cord in 16 μm intervals. A: the mean of 21 microprobes inserted into the dorsal horn with ipsilateral hindpaw in water at 15°C or 41°C. B: the mean of 15 microprobes, water temperature 52°C. C: the differences between groups A and B. D: a plot of the t-statistics derived from the differences shown in C. The broken line is the t-value indicating significance at P = 0.05.

temperature of 52°C this release of irSS was significantly increased.

Although both irSP and irSS were released by noxious skin heating the release patterns of these two peptides differed for mechanical stimulation. Thus, using the noxious mechanical stimulation previously found adequate to evoke irSP release (alligator clips to the digital pads), no increase in irSS release in the substantia gelatinosa region was recorded (Morton *et al*, 1988b).

Compared with SP, the basal irSS release was unexpectedly high. Such release could have originated from the central terminals of primary afferents since irSS is localized within cat DRG neurones (Leah *et al*, 1985a; Tessler *et al*, 1986). The stimulus for this release is unknown but, in this *in vivo* preparation, the primary afferent input via the posterior primary rami to the spinal segments studied would have been considerable since extensive surgery was needed to expose the spinal cord. Activity in hind paw thermoreceptors was probably excluded as a source since warming or cooling the hind paw did not significantly alter the basal irSS release.

In addition, irSS could be released from local interneurones of the upper dorsal horn. While a proportion of the irSS in laminae I and II is of primary afferent origin, experiments examining the results of dorsal rhizotomy and capsaicin treatment have shown that intrinsic spinal neurones contribute significantly to the intraspinal pool of irSS (Jancso et al, 1981; Nagy et al, 1981; Priestley et al, 1982; Gibson et al, 1982; Tessler et al, 1986). The results of the microprobe experiments with noxious heat would still require that these neurones be selectively excited by noxious thermal, but not mechanical afferent input.

The specificity of irSS release in relation to the type of noxious stimulus evoking release makes it unlikely that this peptide is released from polymodal nociceptors. A more probable source is some form of specialized heat nociceptor which has been described in the hind paw skin of the cat (Iggo, 1959; Beck et al, 1974). It is not known if such nociceptors contain irSS. In the experiments of Leah et al, (1985b) in the cat, of 6 DRG neurones containing irSS, one was a polymodal nociceptor, one responded only to noxious mechanical stimulation, one was activated by innocuous mechanical stimulation and cutaneous cooling, while the remaining 3 C-fibres could not be excited by such stimuli. The interpretation of these findings is complicated not only by the co-existence of other peptides such as SP and cholecystokinin in these cells, but by species differences. In the rat, irSS and irSP occur in separate populations of DRG neurones (Hökfelt et al, 1976) while in the cat, most of the irSS-containing cells also contain irSP but not vice versa (Leah et al, 1985a). Thus in the cat, it is tempting to speculate that the subset of DRG neurones containing both irSS and irSP might be specialized heat nociceptors, while those devoid of irSS but containing irSP (and possibly other peptides) have another function, perhaps as nocifensor neurones. In the experiments of Kuraishi et al, (1985a), the noxious heat stimulus used was inadequate to evoke irSP release but irSS release was detected, suggesting that irSS release can be produced by lower stimulus temperatures that irSP release. With antibody microprobes, release of irSS was readily detected after noxious heating for 5 min, which is probably too soon for any hyperalgesic effect to have developed. Both these observations support the proposal for separate neuronal sources for these two peptides.

Further evidence for the involvement of SP and SS in spinal nociceptive transmission comes from studying behavioural responses following direct application of these peptides to the spinal cord. In unanaesthetized rats, intrathecal administration of SP or SS has elicited a characteristic caudally-directed scratching behaviour which has been interpreted as indicative of pain perception (Seybold et al, 1982; Wiesenfeld-Hallin, 1985).

In addition, SP potentiated the excitability of spinal flexion reflexes to both mechanical and thermal noxious stimuli, whereas SS had this effect only with thermal stimuli (Wiesenfeld-Hallin, 1986). This is in accord with the antibody microprobe experiments, in which noxious skin heating evoked release of both peptides in the substantia gelatinosa region of the dorsal horn but noxious mechanical stimulation was selective for irSP release. It is thus possible that SP is generally involved in the spinal transmission of information indicating tissue damage from any source while SS has a more circumscribed role for noxious thermal information.

Both irSP and irSS were detected at the spinal cord surface. With both peptides the amount measured was minimized or prevented by regular suction of the base of the pial opening, suggesting that both were contained within an inflammatory exudate possibly derived from pial structures. The detection of both irSP and irSS at this site raises the possibility that a number of neuropeptides are released from pial nerves to regulate the blood flow to the CNS. In support of this concept are observations that, as well as SP, cerebrovascular nerves contain vasoactive intestinal polypeptide and calcitonin gene-related peptide, both potent dilators of cephalic arteries (Larsson *et al*, 1976; Edvinsson *et al*, 1980; Bevan *et al*, 1986; Hanko *et al*, 1985; McCulloch *et al*, 1986). There are no reports of irSS occurring in pial nerves but a possibly relevant observation is that human pia mater possesses a higher density of SS binding sites (Reubi *et al*, 1986).

These experiments on neuropeptide release are in their infancy but already they are suggesting wider functions for primary afferent neurones than previously described. Whether a chemical coding (in functional terms) will apply to these neurones cannot yet be decided. Apart from the exteroceptive information which impinges on human consciousness, a host of other sensory information from visceral and deep somatic sources is conveyed by dorsal root ganglion cells and a complete study of neuropeptide release from the central terminals of these neurones needs to consider these other types of stimuli. The proposal that substance P release is not simply related to nociceptors which signal pain but rather appears to be related to tissue damage, is an example of chemical coding not readily linked to a sensation perceived consciously. The problems of co-existence and co-release remain, but release studies have suggested that different terminals of primary afferents can have different functions and this diversity of function may be the real reason for co-existence.

REFERENCES

ADRIAENSEN, H., GYBELS, J., HANDWERKER, H.O. AND VAN HEES, J. (1980) Tendencies of chemically evoked discharges in human cutaneous nociceptors and of the concurrent subjective sensations. *Neuroscience Letters*, **20**, 55-59.

BAYLISS, W.M. (1901) On the origin from the spinal cord of the vaso-dilator fibres of the hind limb, and on the nature of these fibres. *Journal of Physiology*, **26**, 173-209.

BECK, P.W., HANDWERKER, H.O. AND ZIMMERMANN, M., (1974) Nervous outflow from the cat's foot during noxious radiant heat stimulation. *Brain Research*, **67**, 373-386.

BESSOU, P. AND PERL, E.R. (1969) Response of cutaneous sensory units with unmyelinated fibers to noxious stimuli. *Journal of Neurophysiology*, **32**, 1025-1043.

BEVAN, J.A., BUGA, G.M. MOSKOWITZ, M.A. AND SAID, S.I. (1986) In vitro evidence that vasoactive intestinal peptide is a transmitter of neuro-vasodilation in the head of the cat. *Neuroscience*, **19**, 597-604.

BONNANO, G. RAITERI, M. AND EMSON, P.C. (1988) *In vitro* release of somatostatin from cerebral cortical slices: characterization of electrically evoked release. *Brain Research*, **447**, 92-97.

BRODIN, E., LINDEROTH, B., GAZELIUS, B. AND UNGERSTEDT, U. (1987) *In vivo* release of substance P in cat dorsal horn studied with microdialysis. *Neuroscience Letters*, **76**, 357-362.

CAMPBELL, G. (1987) Co-transmission. *Annual Review of Pharmacology and Toxicology*, **27**, 51-70.

CAMPBELL, J.N., MEYER, R.A. AND LAMOTTE, R.H. (1979) Sensitization of myelinated nociceptive afferents that innervate monkey hand. *Journal of Neurophysiology*, **42**, 1669-1679.

CHÉRY-CROZE, S. (1983) Painful sensation induced by a thermal cutaneous stimulus. *Pain*, **17**, 109-137.

DALE, H.H. (1935) Pharmacology and nerve endings. *Proceedings of Royal Society of Medicine*, **28**, 319-332.

DALSGAARD, C.-J., RISLING, M. AND CUELLO, C. (1982) Immunohistochemical localization of substance P in the lumbosacral spinal pia mater and ventral roots of the cat. *Brain Research*, **246**, 168-171.,

DUGGAN, A.W. AND HENDRY, I.A. (1986) Laminar localization of the sites of release of immunoreactive substance P in the dorsal horn with antibody coated microelectrodes. *Neuroscience Letters*, **68**, 134-140.

DUGGAN, A.W., HENDRY, I.A., GREEN, J.L., MORTON, C.R. AND HUTCHISON, W.D.(1988a) The preparation and use of antibody microprobes. *Journal of Neuroscience Methods*, **23**, 241-248.

DUGGAN, A.W., HENDRY, I.A., MORTON, C.R., HUTCHISON, W.D. AND ZHAO, Z.Q.(1988b) Cutaneous stimuli releasing immunoreactive substance P in the dorsal horn of the cat. *Brain Research*, **451**, 261-273.

DUGGAN, A.W., MORTON, C.R., ZHAO, Z.Q. AND HENDRY, I.A. (1987) Noxious heating of the skin releases immunoreactive substance P in the substantia gelatinosa of the cat; a study with antibody microprobes. *Brain Research*, **403**, 345-349.

EDVINSSON, L., FAHRENKRUG, J., HANKO, J., OWMAN, C., SUNDLER, F. AND UDDMAN, R. (1980) Vasoactive intestinal peptide (VIP)- containing nerves of intracranial arteries in mammals. *Cell Tissue Research*, **208**, 135-142.

EDVINSSON, L., MCCULLOCH, J. AND UDDMAN, R. (1981) Substance P: immunohistochemical localization and effect upon cat pial arteries *in vitro* and *in situ*. *Journal of Physiology*, **318**, 251-258.

FITZGERALD, M. (1979) The spread of sensitization of polymodal nociceptors in the rabbit from nearby injury and by antidromic nerve stimulation. *Journal of Physiology*, **297**, 207-216.

FORSSMAN, W.G., BURNWEIT, C., SHEHAB, T. AND TRIEPEL, J. (1979) Somatostatin-immunoreactive nerve cell bodies and fibers in the medulla oblongata et spinalis. *Journal of Histochemistry and Cytochemistry*, **27**, 1391-1393.

GAMSE, R., LACKNER, D., GAMSE, G. AND LEEMAN, S.E. (1981) Effect of capsaicin pretreatment on capsaicin-evoked release of immunoreactive somatostatin and substance P from primary sensory neurons. *Naunyn-Schmiedeberg's Arch. Pharmacology*, **316**, 38-41.

GASSER, H.S. (1955) Properties of dorsal root un-medullated fibres on the two sides of the ganglion. *Journal of Gen. Physiology*, **38**, 709-728.

GIBSON, S.J., MCGREGOR, G., BLOOM, S.R., POLAK, J.M. AND WALL, P.D. (1982) Local application of capsaicin to one sciatic nerve of the adult rat induces a marked depletion in the peptide content of the lumbar dorsal horn. *Neuroscience*, **7**, 3153-3162.P6

GIBSON, S.J., POLAK, J.M., BLOOM, S.R. AND Wall, P.D. (1981) The distribution of nine peptides in rat spinal cord with special emphasis on the substantia gelatinosa and on the area around the central canal (lamina X). *Journal of Comparative Neurology*, **201**, 65-74.

GO, V.L.W. AND YAKSH, T.L. (1987) Release of substance P from the cat spinal cord. *Journal of Physiology,* **391**, 141-167.

HANKO, J., HARDEBO, J.E., KAHRSTROM, J., OWMAN, C. AND SUNDLER, F. (1985) Calcitonin gene-related peptide is present in mammalian cerebrovascular nerve fibres and dilates pial and peripheral arteries. *Neuroscience Letters*, **57**, 91-95.

HELME, R.D., KOSCHORKE, G.M. AND ZIMMERMANN, M. (1986) Immunoreactive substance P release from skin nerves in the rat by noxious thermal stimulation. *Neuroscience Letters*, **63**, 295-299.

HENDRY, I.A., MORTON, C.R. AND DUGGAN, A.W. (1988). Analysis of antibody microprobe autoradiographs by computerized image processing. *Journal of Neuroscience Methods*, **23**, 249-256.

HIROTA, N., KURAISHI, Y., HINO, U., SATO, Y., SATOH, M. AND TAKAGI, H.(1985) Met-enkephalin and morphine but not dynorphin inhibit noxious stimulus-induced release of substance P from rabbit dorsal horn *in situ*. *Neuropharmacology*, **24**, 567-570.

HO, R.H. AND BERELOWITZ, M. (1984). Somatostatin 28_{1-14} immunoreactivity in primary afferent neurons of the rat spinal cord. *Neuroscience Letters*, **46**, 161-166.

HÖKFELT, T., LJUNDAHL, A., TERENIUS, L., ELDE, R. AND NILSSON, G. (1977) Immunohistochemical analysis of peptide pathways possibly related to pain and analgesia: enkephalin and substance P. *Proceedings of the National Academy of Science, USA.*, **74**, 3081-3085.

HÖKFELT, T., ELDE, R., JOHANSSON, O., LUFT, R. AND ARIMURA, A. (1975) Immunohistochemical evidence for the presence of somatostatin, a powerful inhibitory peptide, in some primary sensory neurons. *Neuroscience Letters*, **1**, 231-235.

HÖKFELT, T., ELDE, R., JOHANSSON, O., LUFT, R., NILSSON, G. AND ARIMURA,A. (1976) Immunohistochemical evidence for separate populations of somatostatin-containing and substance P-containing primary afferent neurons in the rat. *Neuroscience*, **1**, 131-136.

HUNT, S.P. AND ROSSI, J. (1985) Peptide and non-peptide containing unmyelinated primary afferents: the parallel processing of nociceptive information. In: *Nociception and Pain* (Eds. A.Iggo, L.L.Iversen and F.Cervero) pp. 65-72. The Royal Society, London.

IGGO, A. (1959) Cutaneous heat and cold receptors with slowly-conducting (C) afferent fibres. *Quarterly Journal of Experimental Physiology*, **44**, 362-370.

JANCSO, G., HÖKFELT, T., LUNDBERG, J.M., KIRALY, E., HALASZ, N., NILSSON, G., TERENIUS, L., REHFELD, J., STEINBUSCH, H., VERHOFSTAD, A., ELDE, R., SAID, S. and BROWN, M. (1981) Immunohistochemical studies on the effect of capsaicin on spinal cord medullary peptide and monoamine neurons using antisera to substance P, gastrin/CCK, somatostatin, VIP, enkephalin, neurotensin and 5-hydroxytryptamine. *J. Neurocytology*, **10**, 963- 980.

JESSELL, T.M. (1982) Substance P in the nociceptive sensory neurons. In:*Substance P in the Nervous System*. Ciba Foundation Symposium, **91**, 225-248.

JONSSON, C.-E., BRODIN, E., DALSGAARD, C.-J. AND HAEGERSTRAND, A. (1986) Release of substance-P-like immunoreactivity in dog paw lymph after scalding injury. *Acta Physiol. Scand.*, **126**, 21-24.

KENINS, P., (1981) Identification of the unmyelinated sensory nerves which evoke plasma extravasation in response to antidromic stimulation. *Neuroscience Letters*, **25**, 137-141.

KENSHALO, D.R. Correlations of temperature sensitivity in man and monkey, a first approximation. In Zotterman, Y. ed. *Sensory Functions of the Skin in Primates*, Pergamon Press, Oxford, 1976, pp. 305-330.

KING, J.S., GALLANT, P., MEYERSON, V. AND PERL, E.R. (1976) The effects of anti-inflammatory agents on the responses and sensitization of unmyelinated (C) fiber polymodal nociceptors. In: *Sensory Functions of the Skin in Primates*. Vol. 2. (Ed. Y. Zotterman) pp. 463-470. Pergamon Press , Oxford.

KRUKOFF, T.L., CIRIELLO, J. AND CALARESU, F.R. (1986). Somatostatin-like immunoreactivity in neurons, nerve terminals, and fibers of the cat spinal cord. *Journal of Comparative Neurology,* **243**, 13-22.

KURAISHI, Y., HIROTA, N., SATO, Y., HINO, Y., SATOH, M. AND TAKAGI, H. (1985a) Evidence that substance P and somatostatin transmit separate information related to pain in the spinal dorsal horn. *Brain Research,* **325**, 294-298.

KURAISHI, Y., HIROTA, N., SATO, Y., KANETO, S., SATOH, M. AND TAKAGI, H.(1985b) Noradrenergic inhibition of the release of substance P from primary afferents in the rabbit spinal dorsal horn. *Brain Research* **359** 177-182

LAMOTTE, R.H. (1985) Cutaneous nociceptors and pain sensation in normal and hyperalgesic skin. In *Neural Mechanisms of pain* Advances in Pain Research and Therapy. Vol. **6**, (Ed. L.Kruger and J.C.Leibeskind) pp. 69-82, Raven Press, New York.

LANGFORD, L.A. AND COGGESHALL, R.E. (1979) Branching of sensory axons in the dorsal root and evidence for the absence of dorsal root efferent fibres. *Journal of Comp. Neurology,* **184**, 193-204.

LARSSON, L.I. EDVINSSON, L., FAHRENKRUG, J., HAKANSON, R., OWMAN, C., Schaffalitzky de Muckadell, O. and Sundler, R. (1976) Immunohistochemical localization of vasodilator polypeptide (VIP) in cerebrovascular nerves. *Brain Research,* **113**, 400-404.

LEAH, J.D., CAMERON, A.A., KELLY, W.L. AND SNOW, P.J. (1985a) Coexistence of peptide immunoreactivity in sensory neurons of the cat. *Neuroscience,* **16**, 683-690.

LEAH, J.D., CAMERON, A.A. AND SNOW, P.J. (1985b) Neuropeptides in physiologically identified mammalian sensory neurones. *Neuroscience Letters* **56** 257-264.

LEWIS, T., (1935) Experiments relating to cutaneous hyperalgesia and its spread through somatic nerves. *Clinical Science,* **2**, 373- 423.

LEWIS, T., (1942) *Pain.* Macmillan Press, London.

LIU-CHEN, L.-Y., HAN, D.H. AND MOSKOWITZ, M.A. (1983) Pia arachnoid contains substance P originating from trigeminal neurons. *Neuroscience,* **9**, 803-808.

LUNDBERG, J.M., RUDEHILL, A., SOLLEVI, A., Theodorsson-Norheim, E. and Hamberger, B. (1986) Frequency- and reserpine- dependent chemical coding of sympathetic transmission: differential release of noradrenaline and neuropeptide Y from pig spleen. *Neuroscience Letters,* **63**, 96-100.

LYNN, B., (1977) Cutaneous hyperalgesia. *British Medical Bulletin,* **33**, 103-107.

MCCULLOCH, J., UDDMAN, R., KINGMAN, T.A. AND EDVINSSON, L. (1986) Calcitonin gene-related peptide: functional role in cerebrovascular regulation. *Proceedings of the National Academy of Science USA,* **83** 5731-5735.

MARSDEN, C.A. (1984) Measurement of neurotransmitter release *in vivo.*In: *Methods in the Neurosciences,* Vol. **6**. IBRO Handbook Series. Wiley Interscience Publication.

MITCHELL, J.F. (1975) Collection techniques. In: *Methods in Brain Research,* (Ed. P.B.Bradley), John Wiley, London, pp. 295- 332.

MORTON, C.R. HUTCHISON, W.D. AND HENDRY I.A. (1988a) Release of immunoreactive somatostatin in the spinal dorsal horn of the cat. Submitted for publication.

MORTON, C.R. HUTCHISON, W.D., HENDRY, I.A. AND DUGGAN, A.W. (1988b) Physiological stimuli releasing immunoreactive somatostatin in the spinal cord: a study with antibody microprobes. Submitted for publication.

MOSKOWITZ, M.A., BRODY, M. AND LIU-CHEN, L.Y. (1983) *In vitro* release of immunoreactive substance P from putative afferent nerve endings in bovine pia arachnoid. *Neuroscience*, **9**, 809-814.

NAGY, J.I., HUNT, S.P., IVERSEN, L.L. AND EMSON, P.C. (1981) Biochemical and anatomical observations on the degeneration of peptide-containing primary afferent neurons after neonatal capsaicin. *Neuroscience*, **6**, 1923-1934.

OKU, R., SATOH, M. AND TAKAGI, H. (1987) Release of substance P from the spinal dorsal horn is enhanced in polyarthritic rats. *Neuroscience Letters*, **74**, 315-319.

PERL, E.R., KUMAZAWA, T., LYNN, B. AND KENINS, P. (1974) Sensitization of high threshold receptors with unmyelinated (C) afferent fibres. In: *Somatosensory and Visceral Receptor Mechanisms*. (Eds. A.Iggo and G. Ilinsky) Progress in Brain Research, 43, 263-278.

PRICE, J. (1985) An immunohistochemical and quantitative examination of dorsal root ganglion neuronal subpopulations. *Journal of Neuroscience*, **5**, 2051-2059.

PRIESTLEY, J.V., BRAMWELL, S., BUTCHER, L.L. AND CUELLO, A.C. (1982) Effect of capsaicin on neuropeptides in areas of termination of primary sensory neurones. *Neurochemistry International*, **4**, 57-65.

REUBI, J.C., MAURER, R. AND LAMBERTS, S.W.J. (1986) Somatostatin binding sites in human leptomeninx. *Neuroscience Letters*, **70**, 183-186.

SCHAIBLE, H.G. AND SCHMIDT, R.F. (1988) Direct observation of the sensitization of articular afferents during an experimental arthritis. In: *Proceedings of the Vth World Congress on Pain*, (Eds. R. Dubner, G. Gebhart and M.A. Bond), Elsevier Science Publications, 44-50.

SCHARRER, B. (1977) Neurosecretion: beginnings and new directions in neuropeptide research. *Annual Review of Neuroscience*, **10**, 1- 18.

SEYBOLD, V.S., HYLDEN, J.L.K. AND WILCOX, G.L. (1982) Intrathecal substance P and somatostatin in rats: behaviors indicative of sensation. *Peptides*, **3**, 49-54.

SHEPPARD, M., KRONHEIN, S., ADAMS, C. AND PIMSTONE, B. (1979) Immunoreactive somatostatin release from rat spinal cord *in vitro*. *Neuroscience Letters*, **15**, 65-70.

SORKIN, L.S., STEINMAN, J.L., HUGHES, M.G., WILLIS, W.D. AND McADOO, D.J.(1988) Microdialysis recovery of serotonin released in spinal cord dorsal horn. *Journal of Neuroscience Methods*, **23**, 131- 138.

STJARNE, L. (1986) New paradigm: sympathetic transmission by multiple messengers and lateral interaction between monoquantal release sites. *Trends in Neuroscience*, **9**, 547-548.

TESSLER, A., HIMES, B.T., GRUBER-BOLLINGER, J. AND REICHLIN, S. (1986) Characterization of forms of immunoreactive somatostatin in sensory neuron and normal and deafferented spinal cord. *Brain Research*, **370**, 232-240.

UDDMAN, R., EDVINSSON, L., OWMAN, C. AND SUNDLER, F. (1981) Perivascular substance P: occurrence and distribution in mammalian pial vessels. *Journal of Cerebral Blood Flow and Metabolism*, **1**, 227-232.

UNGERSTEDT, V. (1984) Measurement of neurotransmitter release by intracranial dialysis. In: *Measurement of Neurotransmitter Release in vivo*. (Ed. C.A. Marsden) pp 81-105, Wiley, Chichester.

WESTERLINK, B.H.C., DAMOMA, G., ROLLEMA, H., DE VRIES, I.B. AND HORN, A.S.(1987) Scope and limitations of *in vivo* brain dialysis: a comparison of its application to various neurotransmitter systems.

WIESENFELD-HALLIN, Z. (1985) Intrathecal somatostatin modulates spinal sensory and reflex mechanisms: behavioral and electrophysiological studies in the rat. *Neuroscience Letters*, **62**, 69-74.

WIESENFELD-HALLIN, Z. (1986) Substance P and somatostatin modulate spinal cord excitability via physiologically different sensory pathways. *Brain Research*, **372**, 172-175.

YAKSH, T.L., JESSELL, T.M., GAMSE, R., MUDGE, A.W. AND LEEMAN, S.E. (1980) Intrathecal morphine inhibits substance P release from mammalian spinal cord *in vivo*. *Nature*, **286**, 155-156.

ZIMMERMAN, M. (1976) Neurophysiology of nociception. In: *International Review of Physiology*, Vol. 10, (Ed. R.Porter) Neurophysiology II. University Park Press, Baltimore, pp. 179-221.

SOMATIC, ARTICULAR AND VISCERAL NOXIOUS-STIMULUS EVOKED EXPRESSION OF C-FOS IN THE SPINAL CORD OF THE RAT: DIFFERENTIAL PATTERNS OF ACTIVITY AND MODULATION BY ANALGESIC AGENTS

Allan I. Basbaum, Robert Presley, Daniel Menétrey, Shu-Ing Chi and Jon D. Levine

Departments of Anatomy, Physiology, Medicine and Anesthesiology, University of California San Francisco, San Francisco, CA 94143 and INSERM U-161, 2, rue d'Alésia 75014 Paris, France

Recent years have seen a remarkable increase in our understanding of the anatomical circuitry through which noxious stimuli are presumed to access spinal cord, brainstem and thalamic structures. Many studies of the anatomy of pain processing mechanisms have addressed the distribution of primary afferent fibers, including the differential central projection of single nociceptive fibers which have been identified electrophysiologically. Those studies have demonstrated that there is a very dense projection to the superficial dorsal horn from Aδ and C fibers. Other studies have used retrograde tracing techniques to characterize the organization of ascending projection systems that arise from the dorsal and ventral horns. Still other studies have focused on the cytochemistry of the primary afferent and second order neurons and on the descending control systems that modulate their firing. Largely because of the high concentration of peptidergic cells and terminals in the superficial dorsal horn, EM immunocytochemical studies of peptide circuits have focused in that region. (For reviews see Basbaum and Fields, 1984; Besson and Chaouch, 1987)

What is missing is direct evidence that these neurons are indeed involved in the processing of nociceptive information that relates to pain behavior. The fact that electrophysiological studies have implicated cells in the superficial dorsal horn in the transmission of nociceptive messages is not sufficient to conclude that those neurons contribute to the pain behavior one sees in awake animals. As a corollary of that statement, such electrophysiological studies cannot provide information about the changes that occur when analgesic drugs are administered in animals that are experiencing pain. Electrophysiological studies of spinal neurons are typically performed in anesthetized or decerebrate-spinal preparations. To overcome that problem, some authors have attempted to study spinal cord nociceptive neurons in the awake animal. That approach, however, is extremely time consuming and the yield of neurons is very small, but preliminary results suggest that there are significant differences between the responses of neurons in the anesthetized and awake animals (Bromberg and Fetz, 1987; Collins, 1987; Duncan *et al*, 1987; Sorkin *et al*, 1988).

Single cell analysis cannot reveal the Gestalt of the pattern of activity that is generated in the spinal cord when an awake, freely moving animal experiences a noxious stimulus. What is needed is a method to monitor the activity of large numbers of neurons in the freely moving animal. Although the 2-deoxyglusose method (Sokoloff *et al*, 1977) has proven useful for monitoring metabolic changes in large regions of the brain, the results from studies in the spinal cord have been somewhat disappointing (Ciriello *et al*, 1982; Abram and Kostreva, 1986; Juliano *et al*, 1987). The technique is very limited in its spatial resolution; moreover, it is both complicated and time consuming. The cytochrome oxidase method, although offering single cell resolution, has not yet been used to monitor changes in activity in the cord. In part, this is because most cells have a relatively high baseline level of cytochrome oxidase staining (Wong-Riley and Kageyama, 1986); it is thus difficult to detect small increases in enzyme activity.

The *c-fos* proto-oncogene is the normal mammalian homologue of the *c-fos* oncogene found in the FBJ and FBR murine osteogenic sarcoma viruses. It encodes a nuclear protein, Fos, that binds to DNA *in vitro* and is thought to affect transcription or mRNA processing, but its function is largely unknown. Early investigations explored its possible role as a regulator of mitogenesis and cell differentiation. *C-fos* can be induced by a variety of hormones, growth factors, tumor promoters such as phorbol ester, and cellular second messengers including cAMP, diacylglycerol, and calcium ions (Kriujer *et al* 1984, 1985). In non-dividing, neuronally differentiated PC12 cells, *c-fos* is rapidly transcribed in response to nicotinic and muscarinic stimulation of acetylcholine receptors; this response shows a dose-response relationship and is abolished by treatment with specific nicotinic and muscarinic antagonists (Greenberg *et al*, 1984, 1985, 1986).

Induction of *c-fos* activity in the intact adult mammalian CNS has been described in response to drug-induced seizures, with pronounced *c-fos* expression noted in areas of the cortex, hippocampus, and limbic system (Dragunow and Robertson, 1988; Morgan *et al*, 1987). In these experiments, treatment with antiepileptics such as benzodiazepines (diazepam, midazolam) and pentobarbital completely abolished the *c-fos* response. Thus, expression of the *c-fos* gene may serve as a useful marker of neuronal activity.

Recently, Hunt *et al* (1987) reported that by monitoring the expression of the proto-oncogene, *c-fos*, it is also possible to provide such a marker of *activity* in the spinal cord. Details of their studies are described in this volume. In our studies, we monitored the expression of the *c-fos* nuclear protein, under conditions of noxious stimulation, in the presence or in the absence of analgesic agents. This has allowed us to correlate *c-fos* in the spinal cord with pain behavior. Our studies emphasize the contribution of anesthetics to modulation of nociceptive information in *pain* studies and provide evidence that the responsiveness of different populations of nociceptive spinal neurons varies over time. Of particular relevance to the topic of this symposium is that our results suggest that previous studies, in anesthetized animals, have underemphasized the contribution of nociceptive neurons in the deeper part of the spinal gray to the generation of pain.

NOXIOUS STIMULUS-EVOKED *C-FOS* EXPRESSION IN THE RAT SPINAL CORD

The original study by Hunt and colleagues (1987) was performed in Equithesin (chloral hydrate/barbiturate) anesthetized animals. We, however, were interested in correlating the *activity* of spinal cord neurons (assessed by the expression of *c-fos*) with the pain behavior of the rat. This required that we study the animals under conditions in which their behavior could be monitored. To evaluate the effect of anesthesia on the ability of spinal neurons to express *c-fos* we compared the pattern of noxious stimulus-evoked expression of *c-fos* in anesthetized and unanesthetized rats. The model of pain which we chose for those studies involved formalin injection into a single paw (Dubuisson and Dennis, 1977). This is a particularly useful model because it evokes a short-lived *acute* pain behavior followed about twenty minutes later by a more prolonged pain behavior that is considered to result from the experience of pain of a more persistent nature. The latter is important because we are interested in evaluating the spinal cord cells that process information that is more clinically relevant. There is also a relatively large body of literature on the analgesic effects of narcotics in the formalin test; the data provide a valuable basis for our subsequent studies of opiate-induced changes in *c-fos* expression (see below).

In our study, one group of rats was anesthetized with pentobarbital (10 to 80mg/kg, ip); formalin (5%, 50μl) was then injected into the plantar surface of the paw in anesthetized rats that were maintained under anesthesia for the duration of the experiment. A second group of rats received no anesthetic during the experiments. At varying times after injection of the formalin, all rats were deeply anesthetized and perfused with a 4% paraformaldehyde fixative. Frozen fifty micron sections through the lumbar and rostral sacral spinal cord were cut and immunostained with an antiserum directed against *c-fos*. We used two different antisera. One was a polyclonal antiserum that was raised in the rabbit (kindly provided by Dr Dennis Slamon of the Departments of Haematology and Oncology at UCLA); it was raised against an *in vitro* translated *c-fos* gene. We also used a mouse monoclonal antiserum that was directed against a synthetic peptide located at the N terminal of the *c-fos* protein (Microbiological Associates Inc., Bethesda, Md.). The pattern of staining with the two antibodies was comparable. Although we could not perform absorption controls with the polyclonal antiserum, we did establish that the staining with the monoclonal antiserum was completely abolished when the antibody was incubated with the N-terminal peptide fragment, but not with other synthetic fragments of the *c-fos* molecule.

Our studies demonstrated that there are important differences in the pattern of noxious stimulus-evoked expression of *c-fos* in anesthetized and in unanesthetized rats (Presley *et al*, 1988b). The most intense and widespread staining is found in the unanesthetized rats. Consistent with the overall distribution described by Hunt *et al* (1987) we found large numbers of labelled cells in the superficial dorsal horn, (laminae I and outer II) in the neck of the dorsal horn (lamina V) and in the dorsal part of lamina VII (Figure 2). The labelling was almost exclusively ipsilateral to the stimulated side; it extended throughout the lumbar spinal cord and into the rostral sacral segments. Only in the unanesthetized rat, was there staining of cells in the ventral horn (ventral lamina VII and lamina VIII). Interestingly, there was bilateral labelling in lamina VIII. Somwehat surprisingly, we also found considerable numbers of labelled neurons just ventral to the SG, *i.e.* in laminae III and IV, regions traditionally associated with the transmission of non-nociceptive information. These appear to be specifically produced by formalin injection; Hunt did not find similar staining with mustard oil and we never found labelled cells in laminae III and IV with other inflammatory stimuli which we have used (*e.g.* Freund's adjuvant, see below).

These early studies were the first clue that activity of neurons in the more ventral parts of the spinal gray may be particularly important in the processing of pain of a tonic nature. Our next series of studies was directed at the time course of the expression of *c-fos* in animals injected with formalin into a single paw. Again, consistent with Hunt's early report, we found that there was extensive labelling of cells within one hour of peripheral stimulation. The labelled cells, however, were concentrated in the dorsal horn; only at two and four hours after formalin injection did we detect *c-fos* immunoreactive neurons in the ventral horn, in particular in laminae VIII. At eight and sixteen hours after formalin injection we noticed a clear reduction in the numbers of cells and in the intensity of staining.

There are several possible explanations for the delayed appearance of *c-fos* immunoreactive cells in the ventral horn. Conceivably, the expression of *c-fos* in the ventral horn requires temporal summation of activity. The establishment of persistent

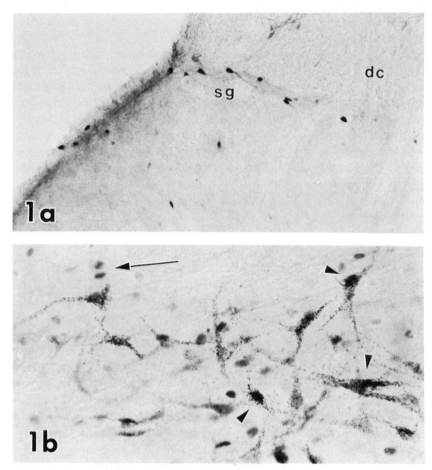

FIGURE 1: a: Photomicrographs illustrating *c-fos*-immunoreactive neurons in the marginal layer of the lumbar spinal cord of the rat. The noxious stimulus which generated this pattern of staining was an injection of complete Freund's adjuvant into the hindpaw. The rat survived for sixteen hours (dc: dorsal columns; sg: substantia gelatinosa). b: Photomicrograph of a horizontal section through the marginal layer of the lumbar spinal cord of the rat illustrating cells that were retrogradely labelled after an injection of WGA-apoHRP-Au. The section was silver enhanced to make the retrogradely labelled cells visible at the light microscopic level. The section was also immunostained to identify neurons which expressed *c-fos*-immunoreactivity (arrows) in response to injection of Freund's adjuvant into the hindpaw. Several double-labelled cells (*i.e.* *c-fos*-immunoreactive projection neurons) can be seen in this photomicrograph (arrowheads). These cells have a black (*c-fos*-immunoreactive) nucleus and contain punctate, silver precipitate in the cytoplasm.

activity in the spinal cord after peripheral injury is, in fact, thought to contribute to changes in nociceptive threshold that can be detected in a limb opposite to the one which is injured (Woolf, 1983). Thus, the delayed changes in the expression of c-fos in the ventral horn may provide a way to monitor spinal cord activity that underlies centrally-mediated hyperalgesic states. By blocking the peripheral input with local anesthetic one hour after the formalin is administered, we are trying to determine whether the delayed expression of c-fos in neurons of the ventral horn requires maintained peripheral input. There is also evidence that the activity of neurons in the ventral horn requires the activation of excitatory spinobulbospinal loops (Giesler et al 1981; Cervero and Wolstencroft, 1984.) Studies from several laboratories have suggested that spinobulbospinal loops contribute to the response properties of spinoreticular neurons in the ventral horn of the spinal cord. This bulbospinal excitatory drive may contribute to the expression of c-fos in ventral horn neurons.

Having established that the noxious stimulus produces a very extensive distribution of labelled neurons in awake animals, we next addressed the differential patterns of activity produced in different models of pain. Three pain models were tested, subcutaneous inflammation produced by intraplantar injection of Freund's adjuvant (Ruda et al, 1988); periarticular inflammation produced by ankle injection of urate crystals (Otsuki et al, 1986; Coderre and Wall, 1987) and noxious visceral stimulation, produced by intraperitoneal injection of acetic acid (Taber et al, 1969). The first two of these studies were performed in the unanesthetized animal; the rats were perfused sixteen hours after the injections. The visceral stimulation studies were performed in barbiturate anesthetized rats; the rats were perfused one hour after the visceral stimulus was administered.

Freund's adjuvant injection into the plantar surface of foot produced the most extensive c-fos labelling. Several features of the labelling characterize this model. First, there was a very marked difference in the rostro-caudal extent of the labelling in different laminar regions of the cord. Although the greatest number of cells and the most intense labelling was found in the superficial dorsal horn, the rostrocaudal extent of neurons in that region was limited. Marginal neurons were concentrated at the L4/L5 junction and extended rostrally through L3 (Figure 1a). At the L4/L5 junction, c-fos immunoreactive neurons were also found in the outer part of the substantia gelatinosa. The largest rostro-caudal distribution of labelled cells was found in lamina V, VII and VIII. These were located at all levels of the lumbar cord. Urate crystal injection into the ankle produced a very similar labelling pattern in the lumbo-sacral cord. The major difference was that there were far fewer cells seen in after ankle inflammation in all laminae. This observation correlates with the fact that animals injected with adjuvant have higher pain scores than animals injected with urate crystals, i.e. the intensity of pain correlates with the numbers of labelled neurons.

The pattern of labelling after noxious visceral stimulation was very different from that seen in other models. The labelling was bilateral and symmetric; this is presumably due to the intraperitoneal spread of the injected acetic acid. There was also a much greater rostrocaudal spread of the labelling; we recorded cells from the cervical to the sacral cord. The greatest number of cells was found at segments near the thoracolumbar junction. The cells were concentrated in lamina I, the neck of the dorsal horn (near lamina V) and lamina X. Very few cells were recorded in the outer part of the substantia gelatinosa. In contrast to the pattern of labelling after subcutaneous or ankle inflammation, we found that marginal neurons, rather than neurons in laminae V, VII and VIII) had the greatest rostrocaudal spread. In fact, in acetic acid injected rats, the labelled cells in the neck of the dorsal horn and lamina X were restricted to the thoracolumbar junction.

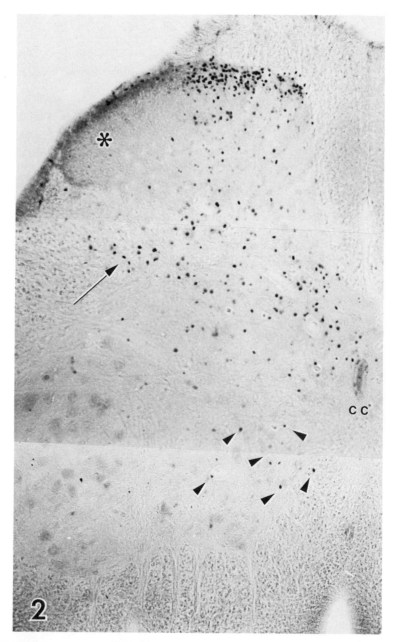

FIGURE 2: Low power photomicrograph illustrating the overall distribution of *c-fos*-immunoreactive neurons in the lumbar spinal cord of a rat which received an injection of formalin into the ipsilateral hindpaw. The rat was killed two hours after injection of the formalin. There is very dense labelling in the superficial dorsal horn, in the lateral part of the neck of the dorsal horn (arrow) and around the central canal (cc). Since this experiment was performed in the unanesthetized rat, labelled cells can also be detected in lamina VIII (arrowheads). Note the absence of staining in the lateral part of the upper dorsal horn (asterisk), a region which does not receive input from the hindpaw.

FIGURE 3: Low power photomicrograph illustrating the effect of 10mg/kg morphine (sc) on the noxious-stimulus (formalin injection-evoked) expression of *c-fos* in the lumbar spinal cord of the rat. There is a profound reduction in the numbers of cells which express *c-fos* and in the intensity of staining of those which are labelled. It is only in the superficial dorsal horn (laminae I and outer II; arrowheads) where labelled cells can be detected in significant numbers. The magnification is the same as in Figure 2 but there was somewhat more section shrinkage in tissue from this rat. Symbols as in Fig. 2.

Based on anatomical studies of the central projection of small diameter primary afferents (Devor and Claman, 1980; Molander and Grant, 1985; Swett and Woolf, 1985) it is our impression that the majority of superficial dorsal horn neurons which express *c-fos* in response to noxious stimulation are located within the terminal field of the

371

afferent fibers from the inflamed foot. At more rostral segments (away from the L4/L5 segments) there is a progressive medial shift in the distribution of c-fos immunoreactive neurons, corresponding to the medial shift in the distribution of afferent terminals labelled by transganglionic transport of wheatgerm agglutinin-horseradish peroxidase. This is compatible with the hypothesis that many of the neurons which express c-fos in the superficial dorsal horn are driven monosynaptically by small diameter, presumed nociceptive primary afferent fibers from the injured paw. The results with visceral stimulation provide further evidence in support of this hypothesis. Thus, Sugiura reported at this meeting that visceral afferent fibers (of small diameter) have a very extensive rostrocaudal spread in the spinal cord, much greater than is seen after injection of single small diameter, nociceptive, somatic afferents. In addition, the visceral afferents terminate predominantly in laminae I, V and X, precisely where we found neurons which expressed c-fos after intraperitoneal injection of acetic acid. On the other hand, since small diameter primary afferents project minimally, if at all, to the ventral horn, we believe that the expression of c-fos in those regions probably was secondary to activity generated over polysynaptic pathways.

The functional significance of the labelling pattern, however, is unclear. Hunt et al, (1987) reported that there was a differential pattern of staining when different stimulus intensities were used. Thus non-noxious stimulation produced labelling in laminae III and IV, which is consistent with those laminae containing neurons which respond exclusively to non-noxious stimulation (Besson and Chaouch, 1987). Since noxious stimulation produces labelling that is focused in regions that predominantly contain nociceptive neurons, as demonstrated in electrophysiological studies (Besson and Chaouch, 1987) it is likely many of the c-fos positive neurons located in our experiments are indeed nociresponsive. We can say little, however, about neurons which are not labelled. They may not have responded to the noxious stimulus, or may only express c-fos in amounts too low to be detected by immunocytochemistry, or there may be a time-dependent expression of the protein. The fact that a cell is labelled also provides no assurance that the particular cell was transmitting the nociceptive message rostrally.

C-FOS IMMUNOREACTIVE PROJECTION NEURONS IN THE RAT SPINAL CORD

It is, however, possible to provide some information concerning the target of some of the labelled cells. In particular we can examine whether c-fos immunoreactive neurons are at the origin of ascending projections. To this end, we performed double-label studies in which spinal projection neurons were labelled by retrograde transport of a protein gold complex and the c-fos neurons were immunostained with a peroxidase reaction product (Hsu et al, 1981). Since the retrograde tracer is predominantly located in cytoplasmic organelles and the c-fos product is localized in cell nuclei, it was very easy to recognize double-labelled neurons (Figure 1b). The tracer used was one which we recently developed. It consists of wheatgerm agglutinin coupled to an enzymatically inactive horseradish peroxidase (apoHRP). This protein complex is then coupled to 10nm colloidal gold (Menétrey, 1985; Basbaum and Menétery, 1987). The tracer is particularly useful in these studies because it persists in labelled neurons for long periods and thus the injection can be made long before the c-fos inducing noxious stimulus is presented. With that approach, there is no unintentional induction of c-fos by the surgical procedure used to inject the tracer. In these double-label studies, we used injection of Freund's adjuvant as the noxious stimulus. Several days after the retrograde tracer was injected, adjuvant was injected into the plantar surface of the paw.

Sixteen hours later the rat was anesthetized and perfused. The retrograde tracer was detected in frozen sections by a silver intensification procedure which makes the colloidal gold visible at the light microscopic level. This was followed by the *c-fos* immunostaining protocol.

There are five major sources of spinal ascending pathways that originate in the lumbosacral cord of the rat. (Giesler *et al*, 1979; Menétrey *et al*, 1983, 1984a,b; Menétrey, 1987). These include the spinothalamic tract, terminating in the medial and lateral thalamus; the spinomesencephalic tract, terminating in the midbrain PAG, parabrachial nuclei and nucleus cuneiformis; the spinoreticular tract, terminating in the medullary and pontine reticular formation; and the spinosolitary tract (Menétrey and Basbaum, 1987). To label the largest number of ascending projection neurons, we made multiple injections into all of these brainstem and thalamic targets. In some animals the retrograde tracer was injected contralateral to the injured paw; in others it was injected ipsilaterally. This allowed us to separately analyze the contribution of *c-fos* immunoreactive neurons to contralaterally and ipsilaterally projecting ascending spinal pathways.

We found considerable overlap in the location of retrogradely labelled cells and *c-fos* immunoreactive cells. Although most of the retrogradely labelled and *c-fos* positive cells were singly labelled, we found considerable numbers of double-labelled neurons. The double-labelled neurons were distributed in four major regions of the lumbo-sacral cord. The majority were located in the marginal layer (Figure 1b). In fact, almost 37% of the total population of double-labelled cells were located in the superficial dorsal horn. In a very few sections we noted double-labelled neurons in the outer part of the substantia gelatinosa. It is our impression that these are displaced marginal neurons. Other cells were found in the lateral part of the neck of the dorsal horn, and in laminae VIII and X.

Double-labelled neurons were found after retrograde tracer injections contralateral or ipsilateral to the injured paw. The relative proportion of contralaterally and ipsilaterally projecting neurons, however differed in the four different regions. In the marginal layer, contralaterally projecting *c-fos* immunoreactive neurons predominated; in the lateral part of the neck of the dorsal horn there were more ipsilaterally projecting cells. In laminae VIII and X, the contralaterally and ipsilaterally projecting cells were approximately equally divided. Interestingly, all of the double-labelled cells in lamina VIII were located contralateral to the injured paw. Note that other areas of the gray matter, for example, the medial part of the neck of the dorsal horn and lamina VII, contained many retrogradely labelled and *c-fos* immunoreactive cells, but few double-labelled neurons. Recently, we repeated these double-label studies in animals which received the visceral noxious stimulus. In those animals we also found many double-labelled neurons, however these were only found in the marginal layer. Our data corroborate other anatomical and electrophysiological studies which have implicated the marginal zone in the central transmission of information from nociceptive visceral afferents in the rat. (Jansco and Maggi, 1987; Cervero and Tattersall, 1987; Ness and Gebhart, 1987).

These data indicate that at least some of the cells which express *c-fos* in response to peripheral noxious stimulation have axons that project into the major ascending spinal pathways. Since the location of the majority of the double-labelled cells corresponds to those regions of spinal cord which contain neurons responsive to noxious stimulation, it follows that at least some of the *c-fos* projection neurons are nociceptive projection neurons. Our results provide important evidence supporting the hypothesis that by monitoring the expression of *c-fos* in response to peripheral noxious stimulation one is able to monitor the spatial distribution of neurons that contribute to the rostral transmission of nociceptive messages.

OPIATE MODULATION OF THE EXPRESSION OF *C-FOS* IN THE RAT SPINAL CORD

In a subsequent series of studies we examined the effect of opiate analgesics on the expression of *c-fos* in the spinal cord. We felt that this approach would offer a valuable way to further validate the nociceptive-specific nature of the *c-fos* pattern produced by noxious stimulation. We could also study the locus of action of narcotics and evaluate whether spinal and brainstem injection of the drug have comparable effects on the noxious stimulus-evoked expression of *c-fos*. For example, there is evidence for both spinal and supraspinal sites of morphine action (Basbaum and Fields, 1984). When injected directly onto the cord (epidurally or intrathecally), a potent analgesia is produced (Yaksh, 1981; Yaksh and Rudy, 1977). This is presumed to result either from a presynaptic inhibition of small-diameter primary afferents (Jessel and Iversen, 1977) or by direct postsynaptic inhibition of spinal nociceptive neurons, including some at the origin of ascending spinal pathways (Willcockson *et al*, 1984). The latter hypothesis is substantiated not only by the anatomical presence of opiate receptor binding in the dorsal horn (LaMotte *et al*, 1976) and the demonstration of immunoreactive opioid peptides associated with projection neurons (Ruda, 1982), but also by electrophysiological studies in which iontophoresis of morphine or enkephalin have been shown to inhibit the firing of spinal nociceptive neurons (Zieglgänsberger and Bayerl, 1976).

The mechanism of action of supraspinal morphine is more complicated and more controversial. Injection of opiates into the region of the PAG clearly evokes a profound analgesia (Pert and Yaksh, 1974; Lewis and Gebhart, 1977). Most studies suggest that the basis of this analgesia is an activation of a descending control system that inhibits the firing of the spinal nociceptors, resulting in no rostrad transmission of the afferent nociceptive input (Basbaum and Fields, 1978, 1984). The hypothesis that supraspinal injection of morphine increases descending control has, however, been questioned. Most importantly, LeBars and colleagues (1983 and this volume) have argued that morphine, when administered supraspinally, decreases descending control. In support of their hypothesis, they recorded from nociresponsive spinal neurons and found that intracerebroventricular or intracerebral injection of morphine increases, if anything, the discharge of spinal neurons to C-afferent inputs (Dickenson and LeBars, 1987). They proposed that the analgesia produced by supraspinal administration of morphine results from a decreased descending control, one which is necessary for the activation of a pain recognition system.

This hypothesis is very difficult to assess electrophysiologically. Since one cannot be certain of the blood levels after a single injection of morphine, one can generally only record from one or at most two cells per experiment. It is impossible to control for blood level changes after repeated injections of morphine. The fact that different laboratories perform their studies with different anesthetics complicates the comparison of data in different studies; it is also probable that the different laboratories have recorded from different cell groups. Brought down to its simplest form, the question can be phrased as follows. Is there a target at which morphine injection produces profound analgesia, without blocking the firing of spinal cord nociceptive neurons, or is the latter a prerequisite? By analyzing the noxious stimulus evoked expression of *c-fos* in rats made analgesic by systemic or intracerebroventricular administration of morphine, we can directly test the LeBars hypothesis. Importantly, the effect of the narcotic on large numbers of neurons can be assessed. Moreover, since the studies can be performed in the awake animal, one can be certain the drug is having an analgesic effect in the particular pain test which is being studied. We can also perform dose response curves to correlate the analgesia with the inhibition of the expression of *c-fos*; that is extremely difficult, if not impossible to do at the single cell level. Obviously, all of the caveats that bear on the significance of finding a cell which expresses *c-fos* must be considered in interpreting the results from such studies. Our preliminary data, however, suggest that this approach will indeed offer new insights into the differential mechanisms of action of narcotics administered at different CNS targets.

Our initial studies were directed at the effect of systemic administration of morphine (Presley *et al*, 1988a). Since we needed a relatively short duration noxious stimulus (one whose effect could be blocked by a single injection of narcotic), we returned to the formalin test for these studies. Rats were injected with different doses of morphine, one half hour before the formalin was injected into the plantar surface of the hindpaw. This time point was chosen so that the rats would receive the formalin at a time when morphine would be exerting its analgesic effect. The dose range chosen was 1 to 10mg/kg; sc. The rats were perfused two hours after the injection of the formalin. Since there is a delay in gene transcription and translation of the message, the immunohistochemical picture seen with *c-fos* is presumed to reflect the state of the *c-fos* activity about one-half hour before the animal is killed. Thus, we are probably evaluating the effect of the narcotic two hours after its injection and one and one-half hours after the noxious stimulus was administered. Behavioral evaluation confirmed that there was analgesia at all doses, but only at higher doses were the animals analgesic for the duration of the test.

Several conclusions were drawn from these initial studies. First, one can observe a dose dependent relationship for the effect of morphine on the behavior of the rats and this correlates with the numbers and distribution of neurons which express *c-fos* in response to the formalin injection. Second, we found that the effect of morphine on *c-fos* expression was most apparent in the ventral half of the spinal cord. For example, 2.5mg/kg sc, produced significant analgesia and decreased the expression of *c-fos* in laminae VII and VIII; there was only a small decrease in the numbers of cells in the superficial dorsal horn. Thus, one can apparently have relatively strong analgesia without complete suppression of the noxious stimulus-evoked expression of *c-fos* in the dorsal horn. As the dose of morphine was increased, there was progressively greater suppression of the neurons located superficially. At 10mg/kg there was almost complete suppression of the expression of *c-fos* in the spinal cord (Figure 3 and compare with control in Figure 2). Importantly, the suppression produced by this dose of morphine was completely reversed by the opiate antagonist naloxone.

These data indicate that there is a correlation between the potency of the analgesia produced by systemic injection of morphine and suppression of the expression of *c-fos* in the spinal cord. How this came about is, of course, unclear. It could have resulted from a direct inhibitory effect of the drug at the level of the spinal cord, or it could have resulted from binding of the drug at a supraspinal site, with subsequent activation of a descending inhibitory system. It should be pointed out that we never found signs of activation of *c-fos* in response to narcotic injection alone (*i.e.* in the absence of noxious stimulation), whether systemic or supraspinal. Since there is evidence that narcotics can, presumably via disinhibitory circuits, increase the discharge of neurons in the superficial dorsal horn (Fitzgerald and Woolf, 1980), this is an important observation. It indicates that immunocytochemically detectable levels of *c-fos* expression may not be found in all neurons whose activity level is increased. The particular stimulus that increased the discharge of the cell may be critical.

In order to assess the effect of supraspinally administered morphine on descending controls and to test the LeBars hypothesis described above, we have recently begun studies of the effect of intracerebroventricular injection of narcotics on the noxious stimulus-evoked expression of *c-fos* in the spinal cord. Cannulae were implanted into the third ventricle, just rostral to the level of the periaqueductal gray, at least two days before the study was performed. Importantly, we determined that the surgical procedure itself did not lead to the expression of *c-fos*; labelled cells were only seen in areas associated with the formalin-injected paw. The experiments involved injection of different doses of morphine five minutes before the formalin was injected into one hindpaw. The shorter time between injection of the morphine and the formalin was chosen because the maximal effect of icv morphine occurs earlier than after s.c. injection. Control animals received an injection of an equal volume of saline. As before, the rats were perfused two hours after injection of the formalin.

Our preliminary results from these studies demonstrated that intracerebroventricular injection of morphine produces analgesia in the formalin test and also reduces the expression of *c-fos* in the spinal cord. The reduction was found in all regions of the lumbar gray matter, including the superficial dorsal horn. With the small number of animals so far tested it is difficult to quantitate the amount of the suppression or to compare the amount of suppression with that seen after systemic injection of the drug. We also cannot tell whether there was a differential effect on the expression of *c-fos* in cells of the superficial dorsal horn *vs.* those located ventrally. These preliminary data do, however, suggest that morphine indeed activates an inhibitory control system when injected supraspinally. An important question to be addressed concerns the relative contribution of supraspinal and spinal sites to the analgesic action of different systemic doses of morphine. Quantitative studies of the changes in *c-fos* expression will hopefully provide answers to those questions.

GABAERGIC MODULATION OF THE EXPRESSION OF *C-FOS* IN THE RAT SPINAL CORD

In another series of studies we examined the effects exerted by the GABA analogue baclofen, the prototypic GABA B receptor agonist, on the noxious stimulus evoked-expression of *c-fos* in the rat spinal cord. Although its mechanism of action is not known, there is evidence for an antinociceptive action of baclofen in animals (Levy and Proudfit, 1977, 1979; Proudfit and Levy, 1978; Wilson and Yaksh, 1978). There is considerable GABA B binding on C-fiber primary afferents and thus a presynaptic blockade of impulse traffic is conceivable (Bowery *et al*, 1980; Price *et al*, 1984, 1987). In fact, baclofen binding sites are concentrated in the superficial dorsal horn; it was thus of particular interest to evaluate the differential effects of baclofen on the expression of *c-fos* immunoreactivity in superficial and deeper neurons of the spinal gray. We found that systemic administration of baclofen, at doses which did not produce significant flaccidity (5.0 and 7.5mg/kg), not only generated significant analgesia in the formalin test but also significantly reduced the numbers of cells which expressed *c-fos*. The reduction in cells was found in all laminae of the cord. These results corroborate other anatomical, physiological and pharmacological studies concerning the antinociceptive action of baclofen. We are presently examining the effects of administering baclofen at different sites to see if we can determine the target at which systemic administration of baclofen exerts its effect on the expression of *c-fos* in the spinal cord. We are also examining the effects of combining baclofen with subanalgesic doses of narcotics.

CONCLUSION

In conclusion these studies strongly support the original conclusions of Hunt *et al* (1987) that by monitoring *c-fos* expression in the spinal cord it is possible to assess the functionally determined patterns of activity that are produced by noxious peripheral stimulation. Our results emphasize that different patterns of activity are generated by different types of peripheral noxious stimuli. There are important rostro-caudal differences in the spread of activity. Of particular interest was the very widespread activity in marginal neurons produced by noxious visceral stimulation. Our results further emphasize that noxious stimuli generate a very complex mix of activity in dorsal and ventral horn neurons. Some of the latter may be particularly relevant to pain that is more prolonged. Anesthetic effects are particularly noticeable on the expression of *c-fos* in ventrally located neurons. Finally, our preliminary studies indicate how this approach can be used to analyze the mechanisms through which analgesics act in the freely moving animal.

ACKNOWLEDGEMENTS

We thank Dr. Jan Tuttleman for providing some of the antisera and for providing valuable insights into their application. This work was supported by PHS grants NS14627, NS21445 and AM32634. D. Menétrey was supported by the Centre National de la Recherche Scientifique, France, and by a fellowship from NATO.

REFERENCES

ABRAM, S.E. AND KOSTREVA, D.R. (1986) Spinal cord metabolic response to noxious radiant heat stimulation of the cat hind footpad. *Brain Research* **385**, 143-147.

BASBAUM, A.I. AND FIELDS H.L. (1978) Endogenous pain control mechanisms: Review and hypothesis. *Annals of Neurology* **4**, 451-462.

BASBAUM, A.I. AND FIELDS H.L. (1984) Endogenous pain controls systems: Brainstem spinal pathways and endorphin circuitry. *Annual Review of Neuroscience* **7**, 309-338.

BASBAUM, A.I. AND MENÉTREY, D. (1987) Wheat germ agglutinin-apoHRP gold: a new retrograde tracer for light- and electron-microscopic single- and double-label studies. *Journal of Comparative Neurology* **261**, 306-318.

BESSON, J.M. AND CHAOUCH, A. (1987) Peripheral and spinal mechanisms of nociception. *Physiological Reviews* **67**, 67-186.

BOWERY, N.G., HILL, D.R., HUDSON, A.L., DOBLE, A., MIDDLEMISS, D.N., SHAW, J.S. AND TURNBULL, M.J. (1980) (-) Baclofen decreases neurotransmitter release in the mammalian CNS by an action at a novel GABA receptor. *Nature* **283**, 92-94.

BROMBERG, M.B AND FETZ E.E. (1977) Responses of single units in cervical spinal cord of alert monkeys. *Experimental Neurology* **55**,469-482.

CERVERO, F. AND TATTERSALL, J.E.H. (1987) Somatic and visceral inputs to the thoracic spinal cord of the cat: Marginal zone (lamina I) of the dorsal horn. *Journal of Physiology* **388**, 383-395.

CERVERO, F. AND WOLSTENCROFT J.H.(1984) A positive feedback loop between spinal cord nociceptive pathways and antinociceptive areas of the cat's brain stem. *Pain*, **20**,125-138.

CIRIELLO, J, ROHLICEK, C.V., POULSEN, R.S. AND R.S. POLOSA, R.S. (1982) Deoxyglucose uptake in the rat thoracolumbar cord during activation of aortic baroreceptor afferent fibers. *Brain Research* **231**, 240-245.

CODERRE, T. AND WALL P.D. (1987) Ankle joint urate arthritis in rats: an alternative animal model of arthritis to that produced by Freund's adjuvant. *Pain* **28**, 379-393.

COLLINS, J.G. (1987) A descriptive study of spinal dorsal horn neurons in the physiologically intact, awake, drug free cat. *Brain Research* **416**, 34-42.

DEVOR, M. AND CLAMAN, D. (1980) Mapping and plasticity of acid phosphatase afferents in the rat dorsal horn. *Brain Research* **190**, 17-28.

DICKENSON, A.H. AND LEBARS, D. (1987) Supraspinal morphine and descending inhibitory action on the dorsal horn of the rat. *Journal of Physiology* **384**, 81-107.

DRAGUNOW, M. AND ROBERTSON, H.A. (1988) Localization and induction of *c-fos* protein-like immunoreactive material in the nuclei of adult mammalian neurons. *Brain Research* **440**, 252-260.

DUBUISSON, D. AND DENNIS, S.G. (1977) The formalin test: a quantitative study of the analgesic effects of morphine, meperidine, and brainstem stimulation in rats and cats. *Pain*, **4**,161-174.

DUNCAN, G.H., BUSHNELL, C.M., BATES, R. AND DUBNER, R. (1987) Task related responses of monkey medullary dorsal horn neurons. *Journal of Neurophysiology* **57**, 289-310.

FITZGERALD, M., AND WOOLF, C.J. (1980) The stereospecific effect of naloxone on rat dorsal horn neurones: Inhibition in superficial laminae and excitation in deeper laminae. *Pain* **9**, 293-306.

GIESLER, G.J. Jr., MENÉTREY, D. AND BASBAUM, A.I. (1979) Differential origins of spinothalamic tract projections to medial and lateral thalamus in the rat. *Journal of Comparative Neurology* **184**, 107-126.

GIESLER, G.J. Jr., YEZIERSKI, R.P., GERHART, K.D. AND WILLIS, W.D. (1981) Spinothalamic tract neurons that project to medial and/or lateral thalamic nuclei: Evidence for a physiologically novel population of spinal cord neurons. *Journal of Neurophysiology* **46**, 1285-1308.

GLAZER, E.J. AND BASBAUM, A.I. (1983) Opioid neurons and pain modulation: An ultrastructural analysis of enkephalin in cat superficial dorsal horn. *Neuroscience* **10**, 357-376.

GREENBERG, M.E. AND ZIFF, E.B. (1984) Stimulation of 3T3 cells induces transcription of the *c-fos* proto-oncogene. *Nature*. **311**, 433-438.

GREENBERG, M.E., ZIFF, E.B. AND GREENE, L.A. (1986) Stimulation of neuronal acetylcholine receptors induces rapid gene transcription. *Science* **234**, 80-83.

GREENBERG, M.E., GREENE, L.A. AND ZIFF, E.B. (1985) Nerve growth factor and epidermal growth factor induce rapid transient changes in proto-oncogene transcription in PC12 Cells. *Journal of Biological Chemistry* **260**, 14101-14110.

HSU, S., RAINE, L. AND FANGER, H. (1981) A comparative study of the antiperoxidase method and an avidin-biotin complex method for studying polypeptide hormones with radioimmunoassay antibodies. *American Journal of Clinical Pathology* **75**, 734-738.

HUNT, S.P., PINI, A. AND EVAN, G. (1987) Induction of *c-fos*-like protein in spinal cord neurons following sensory stimulation. *Nature* **328**, 632-634.

JANSCO, G. AND MAGGI , C.A. (1987) Distribution of capsaicin-sensitive urinary bladder afferents in the rat spinal cord. *Brain. Research* **418**, 371-376.

JESSEL, T.M. AND IVERSEN, L.L. (1977) Opiate analgesics inhibit substance P release from rat trigeminal nucleus. *Nature* **268**, 549-551.

JULIANO, S.L., BERNARD, J.-F., PESCHANSKI, M. AND BESSON, J.-M. (1987) Altered metabolic activity patterns in arthritic rats evoked by somatic stimulation. In: *Thalamus and Pain*, Eds. Besson, J.-M., Guilbaud, G. and Peschanski, M. Excerpta Medica, Amsterdam, N.Y., 155-170.

KRUIJER, W., SCHUBERT, D. AND VERMA, I.M. (1985) Induction of the proto-oncogene fos by nerve growth factor. *Proceedings of the National Academy of Science (USA)* **82**, 7330-7334.

KRUIJER, W., COOPER, J.A., HUNTER, T. AND VERMA, I.M. (1984) Platelet-derived growth factor induces rapid but transient expression of the *c-fos* gene and protein. *Nature* **312**, 711-720

LaMotte, C., PERT, C.B. AND SNYDER, S.H. (1976) Opiate receptor binding in primate spinal cord. Distribution and changes after dorsal root section. *Brain Research* **112**, 407-412.

LeBars, D., DICKENSON, A.H. AND BESSON, J.M. (1983) Opiate analgesia and descending control systems. *Advances in Pain Research and Therapy* **5**, 341.

LEVY, R.A. AND PROUDFIT, H.K. (1977) The analgesic action of baclofen [β-(4-chlorophenyl] gamma-aminobutyric acid. *Journal of Pharmacology and Experimental Therapeutics* **202**, 437-445.

LEVY, R.A. AND PROUDFIT, H.K. (1979) Analgesia produced by microinjection of baclofen and morphine at brain stem sites. *European Journal of Pharmacology* **57**, 43-55.

LEWIS, V.A. AND GEBHART, G.F. (1977) Evaluation of the periaqueductal gray as a morphine-specific locus of action and examination of morphine-induced and stimulation-produced analgesia at coincident PAG loci. *Brain Research* **124**, 283-303.

MENÉTREY, D. (1985) Retrograde tracing of neural pathways with a protein-gold complex. I. Light microscopic detection after silver intensification. *Histochemistry* **83**, 391-395.

MENÉTREY, D. (1987) Spinal nociceptive neurons at the origin of long ascending pathways in the rat: Electrophysiological, anatomical and immunohistochemical approaches. In: *Thalamus and Pain*, Eds. Besson, J.-M., Guilbaud, G. and Peschanski, M. Excerpta Medica, Amsterdam, N.Y., 21-34.

MENÉTREY, D. AND BASBAUM, A.I. (1987) Spinal and trigeminal projections to the nucleus of the solitary tract: A possible substrate for somatovisceral and viscerovisceral reflex activation. *Journal of Comparative Neurology* **255**, 439-450.

MENÉTREY, D., DE POMMERY, J. AND BESSON, J.M. (1984a) Electrophysiological characteristics of lumbar spinal cord neurone backfired from the lateral reticular nucleus in the rat. *Journal of Neurophysiology* **52**, 595-611.

MENÉTREY, D., DE POMMERY, J. AND ROUDIER, F. (1984b) Properties of deep spinothalamic tract cells in the rat, with special reference to ventromedial zone of lumbar dorsal horn. *Journal of Neurophysiology* **52**, 612-624.

MENÉTREY, D., ROUDIER, F. AND BESSON, J.M. (1983) Spinal neurones reaching the lateral reticular nucleus as studied in the rat by retrograde transport of horseradish peroxidase. *Journal of Comparative Neurology* **220**, 439-452.

MOLANDER, C. AND GRANT, G. (1985) Cutaneous projections from the rat hindlimb foot to the substantia gelatinosa of the spinal cord studied by transganglionic transport of WGA-HRP conjugate. *Journal of Comparative Neurology* **237**, 476-484.

MORGAN, J.I., COHEN, D.R., HEMPSTEAD, J.L. AND CURRAN, T. (1987) Mapping patterns of *c-fos* expression in the central nervous system after seizure. *Science* **237**, 192-196.

NESS, T.J. AND GEBHART, G.F. (1987) Characterization of neuronal responses to noxious visceral and somatic stimuli in the medial lumbosacral spinal cord of the rat. *Journal of Neurophysiology* **57**, 1867-1892.

OTSUKI, T., NAKAHAMA, H., NIIZUMA, H. AND SUZUKI, J. (1986) Evaluation of the analgesic effects of capsaicin using a new rat model for tonic pain. *Brain Research* **365**, 235-240.

PERT, A.AND YAKSH, T.L. (1974) Sites of morphine induced analgesia in the primate brain: relation to pain pathways. *Brain Research* **80**, 135-140.

PRESLEY, R., MENÉTREY, D., LEVINE, J.D. AND BASBAUM, A.I. (1988a) Morphine suppresses the noxious stimulation-evoked expression of the *c-fos* proto-oncogene product in spinal neurons. *Neurosci. Absts.* **18**, in press.

PRESLEY, R., MENÉTREY, D., LEVINE, J.D. AND BASBAUM, A.I. (1988b) Pentobarbital anesthesia suppresses expression of *c-fos* oncogene in rat spinal cord neurons. *Anesthesia and Analgesia.* (abstract) in press.

PRICE, G.W., KELLY, J.S. AND BOWERY, N.G. (1987): The location of $GABA_b$-receptor binding sites in mammalian spinal cord. *Synapse*, **1**, 530-538.

PRICE, G.W., WILKIN, G.P., TURNBULL, M.J. AND BOWERY, N.G. (1984): Are baclofen-sensitive $GABA_b$ receptors present on primary afferent terminals of the spinal cord? *Nature*, **307**, 71-74.

PROUDFIT, H.K. AND LEVY, R. (1978) Delimitation of neuronal substrates necessary for the analgesic action of baclofen and morphine. *European Journal of Pharmacology* **17**, 159-166.

RUDA, M.A., IADAROLA, M.J., COHEN, L.V. AND YOUNG, W.S., III (1988) *In situ* hybridization histochemistry and immunocytochemistry reveal an increase in spinal dynorphin biosynthesis in a rat model of peripheral inflammation and hyperalgesia. *Proceedings of the National Academy of Science (USA)* **85**, 622-626.

RUDA, M.A. (1982) Opiates and pain pathways: Demonstration of enkephalin synapses on dorsal horn projection neurons. *Science* **215**, 1523-1524,

SOKOLOFF, L., REIVICH, M., KENNEDY, C., DES ROSIERS, M.H., PATLAK, C.S., PETTIGREW, K.D., SAKURADA, O. AND SHINOHARA, M. (1977) The [^{14}C] deoxyglucose method for the measurement of local cerebral glucose utilization: Theory, procedure, and normal values in the conscious and anesthetized albino rat. *Journal of Neurochemistry* **28**, 897-916.

SORKIN, L.S., MORROW, T.J. AND CASEY, K.L. (1988) Physiological identification of afferent fibers and postsynaptic sensory neurons in the spinal cord of the intact, awake cat. *Experimental Neurology* **99**, 412-427.

SWETT, J.E. AND WOOLF, C.J. (1985) The somatotopic organization of primary afferent terminals in the superficial laminae of the dorsal horn of the rat spinal cord. *Journal of Comparative Neurology* **231**, 66-77.

TABER, R.I., GREENHOUSE, D.D., RENDELL, J.K. AND IRWIN, S. (1969) Agonist and antagonist interactions of opioids on acetic acid-induced abdominal stretching in mice. *Journal Pharmacology and Experimental Therapeutics* **169**, 29-38.

WILLCOCKSON, W.S., CHUNG, J.M., HORI, Y., LEE, K.H. AND WILLIS, W.D. (1984) Effects of iontophoretically released peptides on primate spinothalamic tract cells. *Journal of Neuroscience* **4**, 741-750.

WILSON, P.R. AND YAKSH, T.L. (1978): Baclofen is antinociceptive in the spinal intrathecal space of animals. *European Journal of Pharmacology* **51**, 323-330.

WONG-RILEY, M.T.T. AND KAGEYAMA, G.H. (1986) Localization of cytochrome oxidase in the mammalian spinal cord and dorsal root ganglia with quantitative analysis of ventral horn cells in monkeys. *Journal of Comparative Neurology* **245**, 41-61.

WOOLF, C.J. (1983): Evidence for a central component of post-injury pain hypersensitivity. *Nature* **306**, 686-688.

YAKSH, T.L. (1981) Spinal opiate analgesia. Characteristics and principles of action. *Pain* **11**, 293-346.

YAKSH, T.L. AND RUDY, T.A. (1977) Studies on the direct spinal action of narcotics in the production of analgesia in the rat. *Journal of Pharmacology and Experimental Therapeutics* **202**, 411-428.

ZIEGLGANSBERGER, W. AND BAYERL, H. (1976) The mechanisms of inhibition of neuronal activity by opiates in the spinal cord of the cat. *Brain Research* **115**, 111-128.

IN SITU HYBRIDIZATION HISTOCHEMICAL AND IMMUNOCYTOCHEMICAL ANALYSIS OF OPIOID GENE PRODUCTS IN A RAT MODEL OF PERIPHERAL INFLAMMATION

M.A. Ruda, L. Cohen, S. Shiosaka, O. Takahashi, B. Allen, E. Humphrey and M.J. Iadarola

Neurobiology and Anesthesiology Branch, National Institute of Dental Research
National Institutes of Health, Bethesda, Maryland 20892, USA

Three genes which encode families of opioid peptides have been described. They are 1: preproopiomelanocortin (POMC), 2: preproenkephalin (PPE), and 3: preprodynorphin (PPD) (Fig. 1). The peptide products of each of these opioidgenes have been identified in the spinal cord dorsal horn. Enkephalin-like immunoreactive (ENK-LI) cell bodies which likely originate from PPE (although the enkephalin sequence is present in each of the three opioid genes) have been observed in many laminae of the spinal cord (Miller and Seybold, 1987; Cruz and Basbaum, 1985; Bennett et al, 1982; Sumal et al, 1982; Conrath-Verrier et al, 1983; Hökfelt et al, 1977; Aronin et al, 1981; Glazer and Basbaum, 1981; Hunt et al, 1981; Merchenthaler et al, 1986; Ruda et al, 1986). Both the ENK-LI cell bodies and axons are concentrated in superficial dorsal horn laminae I and II, in deep dorsal horn laminae V and VI, and in the area around the central canal. Most enkephalin-like immunoreactivity in the dorsal horn likely originates from intrinsic dorsal horn neurons, while a few ENK-LI fibers may descend from the brainstem (Hökfelt et al, 1979) or originate in dorsal root ganglion neurons (Senba et al, 1982; Kawatani et al, 1984). The location of the PPD product, dynorphin (Goldstein et al 1979; Civelli et al 1985), has also been examined immunocytochemically in the spinal cord. Dynorphin-like immunoreactive (DYN-LI) neurons and axons are concentrated in laminae I, II, V, and VI, and in the area around the central canal (Sasek et al 1984; Cruz and Basbaum 1985; Miller and Seybold 1987). Similar to ENK-LI axons, DYN-LI axons in the dorsal horn arise predominantly from intrinsic neurons while a small number may be of primary afferent origin (Botticelli et al, 1981; Kawatani et al, 1984; Basbaum et al, 1986). No neuronal cell bodies containing POMC gene products have been found in the spinal cord although a few, scattered, varicose, POMC peptide immunoreactive axons have been observed in the dorsal horn (Tsou et al, 1986).

In order to investigate the role of opioids in spinal dorsal horn modulation of nociceptive inputs, we have examined opioid peptide gene expression in a model of peripheral inflammation and hyperalgesia. Using *in situ* hybridization histochemistry (ISHH) and immunocytochemistry (IC), mRNA and peptide alterations can be assessed at the level of individual neuronal cell bodies.

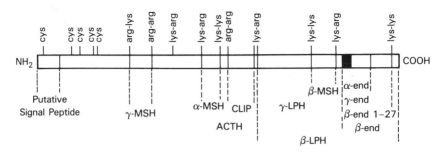

Pre-pro-opiomelanocortin

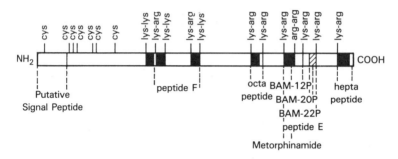

Pre-pro-enkephalin

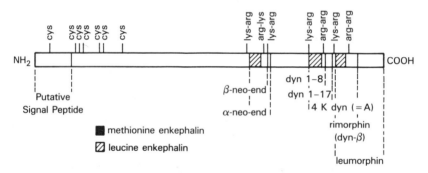

Pre-pro-dynorphin

FIGURE 1: Schematic representation of the structure of bovine preproopiomelanocortin (A), bovine preproenkephalin (B), and porcine preprodynorphin (C).

The methods used in these studies have been described in detail previously (Ruda *et al*; 1988). Briefly, inflammation of one hindpaw of rats was induced by intraplantar injection of a 1:1 emulsion of saline and complete Freund's adjuvant (CFA) (Iadarola *et al*, 1988). During the peak period of edema and hyperalgesia, animals used for IC were injected intrathecally with colchicine (day 2) and perfused with 4% paraformaldehyde (day 4). Animals for ISHH were killed by decapitation at 4 days of inflammation and their lumbar spinal cord frozen rapidly. These experiments were reviewed and approved by the NIDR Animal Care and Use Committee and conform to the guidelines of the International Association for the Study of Pain (Zimmermann *et al*, 1983).

ISHH employed 48 base oligodeoxyribonucleotide probes complementary to bases 862-909 of the PPD mRNA sequence or bases 454-501 of the PPE mRNA sequence.

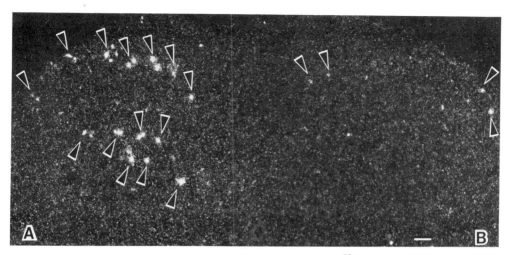

FIGURE 2: Autoradiogram of *in situ* hybridization using a [^{35}S] labelled oligomer to preprodynorphin (PPD). More neurons with a greater silver grain density (arrows) are visible on the side ipsilateral to the inflammation (A) as compared to the contralateral side of the same tissue section (B). Darkfield optics. Scale bar represents 100μm.

The probes were purified, labelled with ^{35}S-labelled deoxyadenosine [a-thio] triphosphate, hybridized to tissue sections and localized using autoradiographic techniques as previously described (Young *et al*, 1986).

IC employed standard PAP methodology (Ruda *et al*, 1984). The dynorphin antisera was raised in rabbits against dynorphin A-(1-8) conjugated to succinylated hemocyanin (Iadarola *et al*, 1986). Two different enkephalin antisera were used: a rabbit anti-leucine enkephalin (Immuno Nuclear) and a mouse monoclonal anti-enkephalin (Cuello *et al*, 1984) (Sera-lab).

PREPRODYNORPHIN MRNA AND DYNORPHIN A-(1-8) PEPTIDE

An increase in both PPD mRNA and dynorphin peptide was observed in the lumbosacral enlargement of the spinal cord of CFA-treated rats on the side ipsilateral to the inflammation at 4 days (Figs.2A and B; 3A and B). Neurons exhibiting the increase were concentrated in the medial portion of superficial laminae I and II and in laminae V and VI (Ruda *et al*, 1988). The superficial distribution corresponds to the somatotopic location within laminae I and II of nociceptive afferents innervating the inflamed limb. The dynorphin neurons in laminae III and IV did not exhibit an appreciable increase in the level of mRNA or peptide as compared to controls. The PPD mRNA increase was apparent from the increased density of silver grains overlying neuronal cell bodies (Fig. 2). Dynorphin A-(1-8) peptide increase was determined from the increased number of visible DYN-LI neuronal cell bodies using IC (Fig. 3A and B). An almost 3-fold increase in the number of labelled cells visible in the dorsal horn of the side ipsilateral to the inflammation was observed with both ISHH and IC labelling.

Some differences were apparent when ISHH and IC labelled neurons were compared. More labelled neurons exhibited above-threshold labelling using the ISHH method as compared to the IC method, suggesting a greater sensitivity for changes in mRNA using ISHH. Neurons in laminae I and II were more densely labelled than those in laminae V and VI using ISHH. With IC, individual labelling was comparable across laminae although the laminae V and VI neurons were more prominently stained or perhaps more noticeable because of the lesser terminal labelling in these laminae as

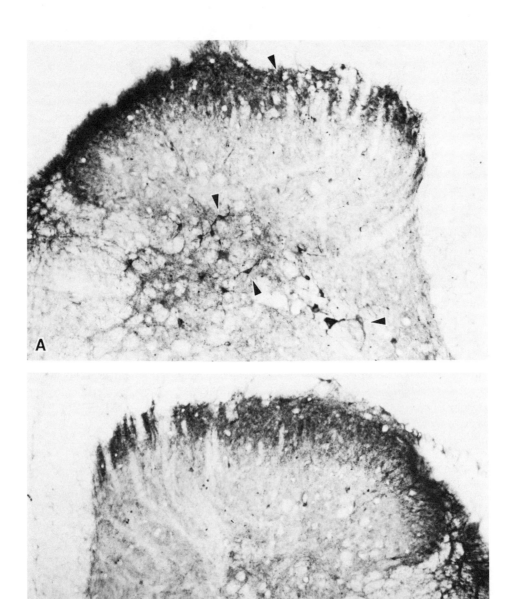

FIGURE 3: Immunocytochemical demonstration of dynorphin A-(1-8) and leucine-enkephalin in two neighboring sections of the lumbar spinal cord of the same animal with Freund's adjuvant-induced inflammation of the left hindpaw. Numerous stained cells (arrows indicate a few of the cells) are visible on the side ipsilateral to the inflammation (A,C) while few are seen on the contralateral side (B,D). Neurons in laminae V and VI are labelled particularly prominently. Scale represents 100μm.

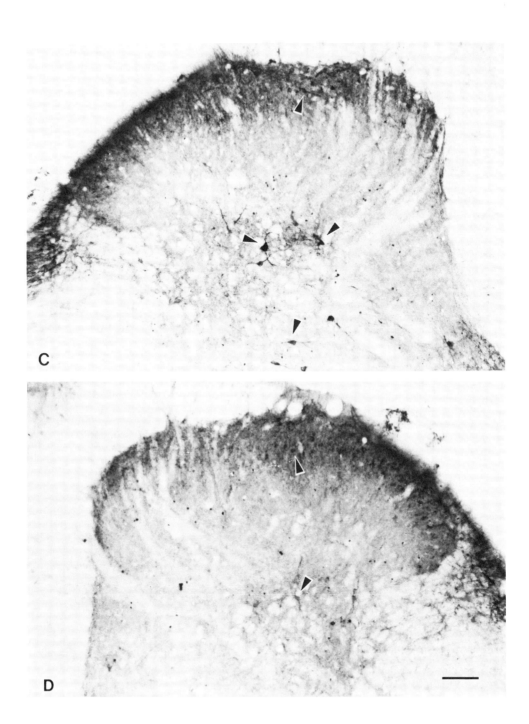

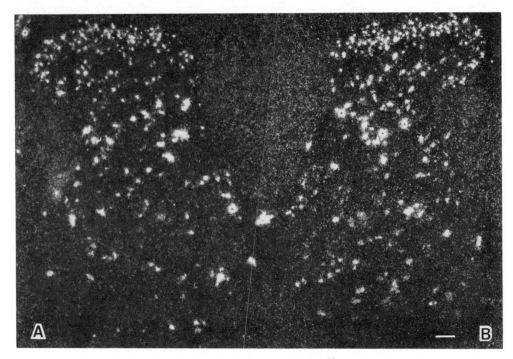

FIGURE 4: *In situ* hybridization histochemistry using a [^{35}S] oligonucleotide probe to preproenkephalin (PPE). Illustration shows left and right sides of a lumbar spinal cord section from an animal in which the left hindpaw had been injected with a saline-complete Freund's adjuvant emulsion. The distribution of labelled cells throughout all laminae of the spinal cord is illustrated using darkfield optics (A,B). In the dorsal horn, at higher magnification with bright-field optics, silver grains overlying labelled cells appear as black clusters (C,D; next page). The density of cell labelling is typically greater over neurons in laminae V and VI than over neurons in the superficial dorsal horn laminae. Density of cell labelling is similar ipsilateral (C) and contralateral (D) to the inflammation. Unlabelled cells are visualized with a neutral red counterstain. Scale represents 100μm.

compared to the superficial dorsal horn. Cell counts of labelled neurons using ISHH demonstrated a preponderance of neurons in laminae I and II as compared to laminae V-VI on both the ipsilateral (66% *vs* 29%) and contralateral (69% *vs* 12%) sides (Ruda *et al*, 1988). In contrast, the number of visible immunolabelled neurons was comparable in laminae I-II and V-VI, on the ipsilateral (41% *vs* 51%) and contralateral (33% *vs* 45%) sides (Ruda *et al*, 1988).

PREPROENKEPHALIN MRNA AND ENKEPHALIN PEPTIDE

Immunocytochemical staining of lumbar spinal cord sections for enkephalinlike immunoreactivity demonstrated an increased intensity of neuronal cell body staining on the side ipsilateral to the inflammation (Fig. 3C and D). Both enkephalin antisera exhibited a similar staining pattern, suggesting that they were recognizing the same neurons. The neurons exhibiting the increased staining intensity were concentrated in laminae I, II, V, and VI. Their distribution was similar although not identical to that of the DYN-LI neurons. There was some suggestion that there were perhaps fewer ENK-LI cells in laminae V-VI and more ENK-LI cells in laminae I-II exhibiting an increased peptide content as compared to DYN-LI labelled cells. The morphological types of ENK-LI cells were similar to that of the DYN-LI cells. In the transverse plane, laminae I and II ENK-LI neurons were typically small and ovoid, with a thin rim of cytoplasm

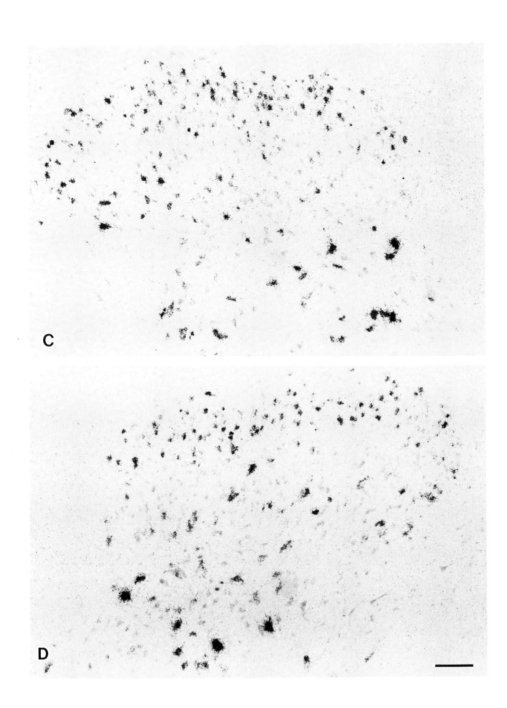

surrounding the nucleus. In laminae V and VI, ENK-LI neurons exhibited a variety of shapes including multipolar, triangular and bipolar. The intensity of the PAP reaction product was variable among the stained neurons.

In situ hybridization histochemistry using an oligonucleotide probe to PPE labelled cells in all laminae of the rat lumbosacral spinal cord, including an occasional cell in the motoneuronal cell groups (Fig. 5). The distribution of the labelled cells agrees with a previous study which used a cDNA probe to PPE (Harlan *et al*, 1987). No consistent differences in cell labelling could be discerned between spinal cord sections from untreated control animals and either the ipsilateral or contralateral sides of sections from animals with an inflamed hindpaw (compare Figs. 4 and 5). Although the density of silver grains overlying neurons in each lamina was variable, neurons in lamina V typically exhibited the greatest silver grain density. The greatest number of labelled cells was found in the superficial dorsal horn, in laminae I and II.

The distribution of labelled neurons was radically different using the PPE oligomer probe as compared to the PPD oligomer probe. Neurons exhibiting PPE mRNA were observed in more spinal cord laminae than those labelled for PPD mRNA. The density of cell labelling for PPE mRNA was typically greater than that for PPD mRNA. It is also interesting that at 4 days we could not detect an increase in PPE mRNA in any subpopulation of labelled neurons while at that time a large increase in PPD mRNA was observed.

Dorsal root ganglion neurons on the inflamed and control sides were examined for expression of PPE mRNA (Fig. 6). Only a few neurons in each ganglia were labelled

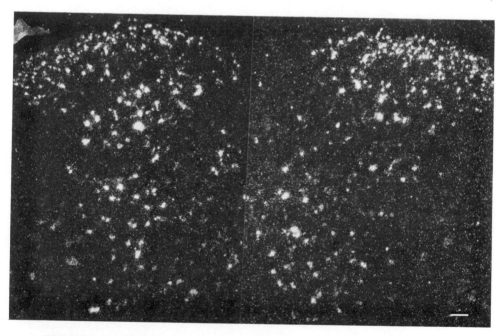

FIGURE 5: Darkfield photomicrographs of the lumbar spinal cord of a control rat. The tissue section has been hybridized with an [^{35}S] labelled oligonucleotide probe to preproenkephalin (PPE). The labelled cells are visualized autoradiographically with the clumps of silver grains, indicating labelled neurons, appearing bright white under darkfield optics. Labelled cells are observed in essentially all spinal cord laminae but are found infrequently in the motoneuronal cell groups, laminae VIII and IX. Scale bar represents 100μm.

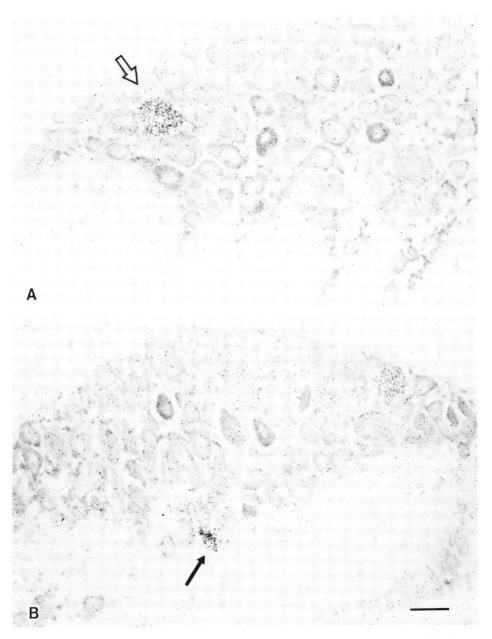

FIGURE 6: Sections from two different lumbosacral dorsal root ganglia (A,B) hybridized with an [^{35}S] oligonucleotide probe for preproenkephalin (PPE). Of the many ganglion cells visible in the neutral red counterstained sections, only three (arrows) are labelled. Both small (filled arrow) and large (open arrow) cells are labelled with a variable density of silver grains. Scale bar represents 50μm.

with the PPE probe. They included both small and large cell bodies with a variable intensity of cell staining. No appreciable differences were observed between the dorsal root ganglia ipsilateral or contralateral to the inflamed hindpaw.

These studies demonstrate that during peripheral inflammation and hyperalgesia there is a dramatic increase in PPD mRNA and dynorphin peptide. These results are in agreement with biochemical experiments of the spinal dorsal horn using this same model of inflammatory pain. RNA blot analysis of poly (A)+ RNA demonstrated a marked elevation of PPD mRNA; and RIA analysis showed a corresponding increase in dynorphin A-(1-8) peptide (Iadarola *et al*, 1988). Similar increases in dynorphin peptide and mRNA have been noted in a chronic polyarthritis model in the rat (Millan *et al*, 1986; Höllt *et al*, 1987).

In contrast, it is difficult to detect an increase in PPE mRNA in any subpopulation of dorsal horn neurons using ISHH in the same animal model. However, enkephalin-like immunoreactivity did appear to be elevated in subpopulations of dorsal horn neurons similar in laminar location to those exhibiting the dynorphin increase. RNA blot analysis with a probe for PPE in the same animal model exhibited only a slight increase in PPE mRNA (Iadarola *et al*, 1988). This small total increase would be difficult to detect with ISHH anatomical localization if it occurred as a small change in a large number of neurons. Although enkephalin peptide levels have not been examined using RIA, Iadarola and colleagues (1986, 1988) have measured the PPE derived peptide enkephalin-met^5-arg^6-gly^7-leu^8 (MERGL) and observed no significant change during the time course of the inflammation. A number of interpretations are possible to explain the differences in the enkephalin data. It is possible that at the concentration of dynorphin peptide in the up-regulated neurons, the antibodies to enkephalin are cross-reacting with the shared tetrapeptide (Tyr-Gly-Gly-Phe) in the pro-dynorphin peptide. Alternatively, since the enkephalin sequence is also encoded in the PPD gene, some enkephalin may be produced by post-translational processing of the PPD gene during inflammation. This enkephalin increase might be detected immunocytochemically but would not be related to an increased expression of the PPE gene. Further study is needed to address these issues.

It is clear from these studies that the two intrinsic spinal opioid systems, PPE and PPD, are acting differentially in a model of peripheral inflammation and hyperalgesia. The up-regulation of dynorphin mRNA and peptide content as determined using anatomical and biochemical methods suggest an important role for dynorphin systems in the CNS response to nociceptive inputs at the spinal level.

ACKNOWLEDGEMENTS

We would like to thank Dr. W.S. Young III for providing us with the synthetic probe to preprodynorphin mRNA and Drs R. Dubner, G. Bennett and R. Traub for their careful reading of this manuscript.

REFERENCES

ARONIN, N., DiFIGLIA, M., LIOTTA, A.S. AND MARTIN, J.B. (1981). Ultrastructural localization and biochemical features of immunoreactive leuenkephalin in monkey dorsal horn. *Journal of Neuroscience* **1**, 561-577.

BASBAUM, A.I., CRUZ, L. AND WEBER, E. (1986). Immunoreactive dynorphin B in sacral primary afferent fibers of the cat. *Journal of Neuroscience* **6**, 127-133.

BENNETT, G.J., RUDA, M.A., GOBEL, S. AND DUBNER, R. (1982). Enkephalin immunoreactive stalked cells and lamina IIb islet cells in cat substantia gelatinosa. *Brain Research* **240**, 162-166.

BOTTICELLI, L.H., COX, B.M. AND GOLDSTEIN, A. (1981). Immunoreactive dynorphin in mammalian spinal cord and dorsal root ganglia. *Proceedings of the National Academy of Science USA* **78**, 7783-7786.

CIVELLI, O., DOUGLASS, J., GOLDSTEIN, A. AND HERBERT, E. (1985). Sequence and expression of the rat prodynorphin gene. *Proceedings of the National Academy of*

Science USA **82**, 4291-4295.

CONRATH-VERRIER, M., DIETL, M., ARLUISON, M., CESSELIN, F., BOURGOIN, S. AND HAMMON, M. (1983). Localization of Met-enkephalin-like immunoreactivity within pain-related nuclei of cervical spinal cord, brainstem and midbrain in the cat. *Brain Research Bulletin* **11**, 587-604.

CRUZ, L. AND BASBAUM, A.I.(1985). Multiple opioid peptides and the modulation of pain: immunohistochemical analysis of dynorphin and enkephalin in the trigeminal nucleus caudalis and spinal cord of the cat. *Journal of Comparative Neurology* **240**, 331-348.

CUELLO, A.C., MILSTEIN, C., COUTURE, R., WRIGHT, B., PRIESTLEY, J.V. AND JARVIS, J. (1984). Characterization and immunocytochemical application of monoclonal antibodies against enkephalins. *Journal of Histochemistry and Cytochemistry* **32**, 947-957.

GLAZER, E.J. AND BASBAUM, A.I. (1981). Immunohistochemical localization of leucine-enkephalin in the spinal cord of the cat: Enkephalin-containing marginal neurons and pain modulation. *Journal of Comparative Neurology* **196**, 377-389.

GOLDSTEIN, A., TACHIBANA, S., LOWNEY, L.I., HUNKAPILLAR, M. AND HOOD, L. (1979). Dynorphin-(1-13), an extraordinarily potent opioid peptide. *Proceedings of the National Academy Science USA* **76**, 6666-6670.

HARLAN, R.E., SHIVERS, B.D., ROMANO, G.J., HOWELLS, R.D. AND PFAFF, D.W. (1987). Localization of preproenkephalin mRNA in the rat brain and spinal cord by *in situ* hybridization. *Journal of Comparative Neurology* **258**, 159-184.

HÖKFELT, T., ELDE, R., JOHANSSON, O., TERENIUS, L. AND STEIN, L. (1977). The distribution of enkephalin-immunoreactive cell bodies in the rat central nervous system. *Neuroscience Letters* **5**, 25-31.

HÖKFELT, T., TERENIUS, L., KUYPERS, H.G.J.M. AND DANN, O. (1979). Evidence for enkephalin immunoreactive neurons in the medulla oblongata projecting to the spinal cord *Neuroscience Letters* **14**, 55-60.

HÖLLT, V., HAARMANN, I., MILLAN, M.J. AND HERZ, A. (1987). Prodynorphin gene expression is enhanced in the spinal cord of chronic arthritic rats. *Neuroscience Letters* **73**, 90-94.

HUNT, S.P., KELLY, J.S., EMSON, P.C., KIMMEL, J.R., MILLER, R.J. AND WU, J.Y. (1981). An immunohistochemical study of neuronal populations containing neuropeptides or gamma-aminobutyrate within the superficial layers of the rat dorsal horn. *Neuroscience* **6**, 1883-1898.

IADAROLA, M.J., SHIN, C., McNAMARA, J.O. AND YANG, H.-Y.T. (1986). Changes in dynorphin, enkephalin and cholecystokinin content of hippocampus and substantia nigra after amygdaloid kindling. *Brain Research* **365**, 185-191.

IADAROLA, M.J., DOUGLASS, J., CIVELLI, O. AND NARANJO, J.R. (1986). Increased spinal cord dynorphin mRNA during peripheral inflammation. In *Progress in Opioid Research*, (NIDA Research Monograph 75), ed. Holaday, J.W., Law, P.-Y. and Herz, A., pp. 406-409. Washington, D.C.: U.S. Government Printing Office.

IADAROLA, M.J., DOUGLASS, J., CIVELLI, O. AND NARANJO, J.R. (1988). Differential activation of spinal cord dynorphin and enkephalin neurons during hyperalgesia: evidence using cDNA hybridization. *Brain Research* **455**, 205-212.

KAWATANI, M., NAGEL, J., HOUSTON, M.B., ESKAY, R., LOWE, I.P. AND deGROAT, W.C. (1984). Identification of leucine-enkephalin and other neuropeptides in pelvic and pudendal afferent pathways to the spinal cord of the cat. *Society for Neuroscience Abstracts* **10**, 589.

MERCHENTHALER, I., MADERDRUT, J.L., ALTSCHULER, R.A. AND PETRUSZ, P. (1986). Immunocytochemical localization of proenkephalin-derived peptides in the central nervous system of the rat. *Neuroscience* **17**, 325-348.

MILLAN, M.J., MILLAN, M.H., CZLONKOWSKI, A., PILCHER, C.W.T., HERZ, A. AND COLPAERT, F.C. (1986). A model of chronic pain in the rat: response of multiple opioid systems to adjuvant induced arthritis. *Journal of Neuroscience* **6**, 899-906.

MILLER, K.E. AND SEYBOLD, V.S. (1987). Comparison of met-enkephalin-, dynorphin A-, and neurotensin-immunoreactive neurons in the cat and rat spinal cords: I. lumbar cord. *Journal of Comparative Neurology* **255**, 293-304.

RUDA, M.A., BENNETT, G.J. AND DUBNER, R. (1986). Neurochemistry and neural circuitry in the dorsal horn. *Progress in Brain Research* **66**, 219-268.

RUDA, M.A., COFFIELD, J. AND DUBNER, R. (1984). Demonstration of postsynaptic opioid modulation of thalamic projection neurons by the combined techniques of retrograde horseradish peroxidase and enkephalin immunocytochemistry. *Journal of Neuroscience* **4**, 2117-2132.

RUDA, M.A., IADAROLA, M.J., COHEN, L.V. AND YOUNG, S.W. III. (1988). *In situ* hybridization histochemistry and immunocytochemistry reveal an increase in spinal dynorphin biosynthesis in a rat model of peripheral inflammation and hyperalgesia. *Proceeding of the National Academy of Science USA* **85**, 622-626.

SASEK, C.A., SEYBOLD, V.S. AND ELDE, R.P. (1984). The immunohistochemical localization of nine peptides in the sacral parasympathetic nucleus and the dorsal gray commissure in rat spinal cord. *Neuroscience* **12**, 855-874.

SENBA, E., SHIOSAKA, S., HARA, Y., INAGAKI, S., SAKANAKA, M., TAKATSUKI, K., KAWAI, Y. AND TOHYAMA, M. (1982). Ontogeny of the peptidergic system in the rat spinal cord: immunohistochemical analysis. *Journal of Comparative Neurology* **208**, 54-66.

SUMAL, K.K., PICKEL, V.M., MILLER, R.J. AND REIS, D.J. (1982). Enkephalin-containing neurons in substantia gelatinosa of spinal trigeminal complex: ultrastructure and synaptic interaction with primary sensory afferents. *Brain Research* **248**, 223-236.

TSOU, K., KHACHATURIAN, H., AKIL, H. AND WATSON, S.J. (1986). Immunocytochemical localization of pro-opiomelanocortin-derived peptides in the adult rat spinal cord. *Brain Research* **378**, 28-35.

YOUNG, S.W. III, BONNER, T.I. AND BRANN, M.R. (1986). Mesencephalic dopamine neurons regulate the expression of neuropeptide mRNAs in the rat forebrain. *Proceedings of the National Academy of Science USA* **83**, 9827-9831.

ZIMMERMANN, M. (1983). Ethical guide-lines for investigation of experimental pain in conscious animals. *Pain* **16**, 109-110.

IN VITRO STUDIES ON NEURONES OF THE SUPERFICIAL DORSAL HORN IN SLICES OF 9-16 DAY OLD RAT SPINAL CORD

C.A.Allerton, P.R.Boden and R.G.Hill*

Parke-Davis Research Unit, Addenbrookes Hospital Site, Hills Road
Cambridge CB2 2QB, U.K.

It is generally accepted that neurones in the substantia gelatinosa Rolandi (SG) play a critical role in the modulation of sensory inputs, especially those associated with the perception of pain. Their response to these inputs is, however, dependent upon their passive membrane properties and the way in which these properties are modulated by neurotransmitter substances. A knowledge of such factors is therefore important in the understanding of the functioning of the SG. One method of investigation is provided by *in vitro* slice preparations of spinal cord. These have been used previously to record from SG (Yoshimura and North, 1983; Schneider and Perl, 1985) but the electrophysiology of this region has not been well defined. We have established a spinal cord slice preparation modified from that of Randic and co-workers (Murase *et al*, 1982) and have used this to investigate some electrophysiological and pharmacological properties of SG neurones.

Transverse slices were cut from the spinal cord of 9-16 day old Wistar rats. The animal was anaesthetized with ether and cooled until its breathing was shallow. A dorsal laminectomy was performed to expose the lumbar and lower thoracic spinal cord, the dorsal roots cut and a 1-1.5cm length of cord excised. The dura was stripped and the cord cut into 400 μm transverse sections on a Vibratome. Slices were incubated in artificial cerebrospinal fluid (ACSF) for at least one hour.

A slice was then transferred to a recording chamber where it was completely submerged in ACSF which was pre-heated to 36°C and which flowed through the bath at a rate of 3ml/minute. The recording electrode was placed into the slice under visual control using a micromanipulator and a bipolar stimulating electrode was placed onto the dorsal root entry zone in a similar manner. Conventional intracellular recording was performed using 3M KCl filled glass microelectrodes with D.C. tip resistances of 40-100 MΩ . Neurones which we considered to be located in SG had a mean resting membrane potential (RMP) of 70±4 mV (n=6) and an apparent input resistance of 226±69 MΩ (n=6). This contrasted with the mean RMP of 67±1 mV (n=73) and mean input resistance of 83±4 MΩ (n=73) obtained for deeper dorsal horn neurones. The RMPs of the two neuronal populations were comparable but neurones in SG had a significantly

---

* Present Address: Smith, Kline and French Research Ltd, The Frythe, Welwyn, Herts AL6 9AR. U.K.

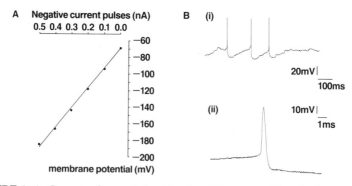

A   Negative current pulses (nA)
     0.5 0.4 0.3 0.2 0.1 0.0

membrane potential (mV)

B   (i)

20mV|
         100ms

     (ii)

10mV|
         1ms

FIGURE 1: A. Current-voltage relationship of an SG neurone. The abscissa shows the amplitude of the injected current pulses while the ordinate shows the potential to which the membrane was displaced. RMP was -69 mV and apparent input resistance of 243 MΩ , given by the gradient of the graph. B.(i) Series of action potentials fired spontaneously by an SG neurone from its RMP of -65 mV. (ii) One of these action potentials on a faster time scale.

higher input resistance than those located in the deeper laminae (Student's t-test, $p < 0.05$). The form of the current-voltage relationship was established by injecting saturating hyperpolarizing current pulses into the neurone through the recording electrode and measuring the resulting voltage displacement. Depolarizing pulses could not be injected into neurones without eliciting action potentials. Over the current range studied all SG neurones were found to have linear current-voltage relationships with no evidence of membrane rectification (Figure 1A).

At their RMP all SG neurones displayed a high level of spontaneous activity, both excitatory post-synaptic potentials (epsps) and action potentials. Action potentials overshot zero potential and were followed by after-hyperpolarizations which were less than 100 ms in duration (Figure 1B). Spontaneous epsps could be up to 30 mV in amplitude and many had more than one component. Computer analysis of these epsps showed that the decay phase was best fitted by a double (rather than a single) exponential and that their amplitude distribution followed that predicted by the Poisson equation. With the membrane potential held well negative to its firing threshold, epsps could be evoked in SG neurones by electrical stimulation of the dorsal root entry zone. Again, the decay phase was best fitted by a double exponential although the amplitude distribution approximated to a narrow normal distribution (Figure 2).

The actions of drugs on SG neurones were studied by superfusion on to the slice. The mu-selective opioid [D-Ala[2], MePhe[4], Gly-ol[5]] enkephalin had effects on 80% of SG neurones producing a hyperpolarization associated with a reduction in apparent input resistance and/or a reduction in spontaneous activity. The kappa-selective opioid U69,593 reduced spontaneous activity in 60% of SG neurones but had no membrane effects.

The use of a spinal cord slice preparation allows stable intracellular recordings from SG neurones to be made for many hours. Intracellular staining with HRP (Light et al, 1979) has shown that the cell bodies of SG neurones are the smallest in the spinal cord and this makes them probably the most difficult to investigate electrophysiologically. Intracellular recording from SG neurones in vivo is possible but there are many technical difficulties associated with such work. The slice offers greater stability of recording with the advantages that no anaesthetic is present and peripheral effects of drugs are eliminated. Disadvantages lie in its lack of natural inputs and in the transverse slice, the absence of ascending and descending pathways. SG neurones in this preparation have comparable RMPs but higher apparent input resistances than neurones in deeper laminae, correlating with their morphology (Light *et al*, 1979). These parameters are in agreement with those found in other preparations (Yoshimura and North, 1983). The high level of spontaneous activity is consistent with that found both in *in vitro* adult rat spinal cord preparations (Yoshimura and North, 1983) and in the *in vivo* situation (Cervero *et al*, 1979). This indicates a lack of tonic descending inhibition on to SG neurones *in vivo* as has been reported previously (Cervero *et al*, 1979).

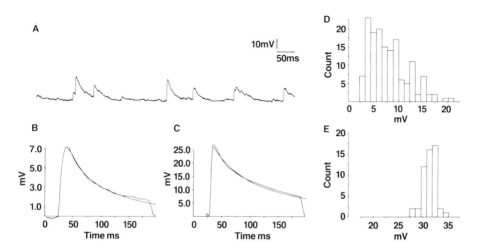

FIGURE 2: A: Series of spontaneous epsps seen in an SG neurone at its RMP of -75 mV. The average of 120 of these is shown in B and the decay phase was fitted by a double exponential. C: Average of 52 epsps evoked in another neurone held at -80 mV (RMP -64 mV). Again, the decay phase was fitted by a double exponential. D, E: Population histograms for the spontaneous and evoked epsps shown in B and C respectively. The abscissa shows the peak amplitude in mV while the ordinate represents the number of counts per bin. Epsps were analyzed using SAQ-5 (J. Dempster, University of Strathclyde).

The synaptic activation of SG neurones has been studied using both spontaneous and electrically evoked epsps. Spontaneous epsps have the expected Poisson distribution as the probability of quantal release is small and events are independent. They may be the result of spontaneously active dorsal root terminals or dorsal horn neurones. When the dorsal roots are stimulated electrically, the probability of quantal release is large so the distribution becomes normal in shape. The narrowness of this distribution implies consistent recruitment of the same fibre population by the electrical stimulus.

SG neurones have been studied pharmacologically by superfusion of drugs on to the preparation. To date, the actions of mu- and kappa-opioids have been examined and have been found to act as previously described in deeper dorsal horn (Allerton *et al*, 1987). There was, however, a greater probability of finding SG neurones responsive to opioids. This is consistent with autoradiographic data demonstrating a greater abundance of binding sites in superficial dorsal horn (Morris and Herz, 1987).

REFERENCES

ALLERTON, C.A., BODEN, P.R.AND HILL, R.G.(1987).Actions of mu- and kappa-opioids on deep dorsal horn neurones in rat transverse spinal cord slice *in vitro*. *Journal of Physiology* **396**, 153P.

CERVERO, F., MOLONY, V. AND IGGO, A.(1979).Supraspinal linkage of substantia gelatinosa neurones:effects of descending impulses.*Brain Research* **175**, 351-355.

LIGHT, A.R., TREVINO, D.L. AND PERL, E.R.(1979).Morphological features of functionally defined neurones in the marginal zone and substantia gelatinosa of the spinal dorsal horn *Journal of Comparative Neurology* **186**, 151-172.

MORRIS, B.J. AND HERZ, A.(1987).Distinct distribution of opioid receptor types in rat lumbar spinal cord. *Naunyn-Schmiedeberg's Archives Pharmacology* **336**, 240-243.

MURASE, K., NEDELJKOV, V. AND RANDIC, M.(1982).The actions of neuropeptides on dorsal horn neurones in the rat spinal cord slice preparation: an intracellular study. *Brain Research* **234**, 170-176.

SCHNEIDER, S.P. AND PERL, E.R.(1985).Selective excitation of neurons in the mammalian spinal dorsal horn by aspartate and glutamate *in vitro*: correlation with location and excitatory input. *Brain Research* **360**, 339-343.

YOSHIMURA, M. AND NORTH, R.A.(1983).Substantia gelatinosa neurones hyperpolarized *in vitro* by enkephalin. *Nature* **305**, 529-530.

OPIOID AND SEROTONERGIC EFFECTS ON LAMINA I AND DEEPER DORSAL HORN NEURONES

P. J. Hope, N. El-Yassir, S. M. Fleetwood-Walker and R. Mitchell*

Department of Preclinical Veterinary Sciences and *MRC Brain Metabolism Unit
University of Edinburgh, Edinburgh EH9 1QH, U.K.

INTRODUCTION

It has been suggested that lamina I cells may play a pre-eminent role in nociception and may therefore be subject to specific modulation from descending and segmental systems. Serotonin is one of the transmitters thought to be involved in descending control of nociception (see LeBars, 1988, for a recent review). The major part of the serotonergic input to the dorsal horn originates from the nucleus raphe magnus (NRM) and adjacent reticular formation (Bowker et al, 1982). The spinal cord, however, appears to contain more than one type of 5-HT receptor (Mitchell and Riley, 1985) suggesting complex 5-HT actions. The presence of three opioid receptor subtypes and a number of endogenous opioid peptides within the dorsal horn, also suggests a complex role for opioids in the processing of somatosensory information. The analgesic actions of μ, δ and κ agonists, administered intrathecally in behavioural studies, support this proposal (Schmauss and Yaksh, 1984). This study investigated the sites of action of opioid and 5-HT receptor subtypes on nociceptive transmission, in restricted laminae within the dorsal horn of the rat.

METHODS

Extracellular recordings were made from neurones characterised as multireceptive (responding to innocuous brush and noxious pinch and/or radiant heat) or nocispecific (responding only to noxious stimuli) neurones. Recording sites were determined histologically, following pontamine sky blue ejection. A variety of opioid and serotonin agonists and antagonists were applied ionophoretically in the vicinity of lamina I neurones which were often antidromically identified as projecting to the parabrachial area of the brainstem (spinomesencephalic tract cells). In some experiments, concentric bipolar electrodes were placed in the region of NRM and the effect of stimulation (0.4 ms width, 5-300 μA, 33-100 Hz) were assessed on dorsal horn neurones located mainly in laminae III-V.

RESULTS AND DISCUSSION

Actions of 5-HT and NRM Stimulation

The effect of 5-HT and its agonists on responses of lamina I cells to cutaneous stimulation are summarised in Table I. Ionophoretically applied 5-HT caused both selective and non-selective inhibitory effects on lamina I cells. The selective inhibitory effect of 5-HT on the nociceptive input was mimicked by RU 24969, which indicates that the selective antinociceptive effect of 5-HT may be mediated through a $5-HT_{1B}$ type receptor. The non selective inhibitory effect on all evoked responses however, appears to be mediated through a $5-HT_{1A}$ type receptor, since it was mimicked by 8-OH-DPAT, a highly selective 1A receptor agonist. Our previous results (El-Yassir et al, 1988), suggest a similar influence of different 5-HT receptor subtypes on sensory processing in laminae III-V.

TABLE I

Effects of 5-HT and 5-HT receptor agonists on dorsal horn lamina I neurones. The nociceptive response (to noxious pinch and/or heat) was judged to be selectively inhibited by a particular compound when this response was significantly reduced whilst responses to DLH and/or brush were not significantly affected (Student's t test on pooled data). Non-selective effects represented significant alterations of different evoked responses from control values.

Compound	Selective inhibition of the nociceptive responses	Non-selective inhibition of all evoked responses tested	No effect	Total Nº of cells
5-HT	5	2	2	9
8-OH-DPAT (a $5-HT_{1A}$ receptor agonist)	-	6	-	6
RU 24969 (a $5-HT_{1B}$ receptor agonist)	5	-	-	5

When the NRM was electrically stimulated the predominant effect was a selective inhibition of the nociceptive responses (14/20 cells, including one lamina I multireceptive cell). Some cells (6/20, including a nocispecific lamina l cell), however, displayed non selective inhibition of all evoked responses tested. Both these effects were reversed by the $5-HT_1$ antagonist cyanopindolol in 6/6 cases while ketanserin, a selective $5-HT_2$ receptor antagonist was ineffective in 4/4 cases. Neither antagonist on its own, altered evoked activity. The selective antinociceptive action of the $5-HT_{1B}$ receptor agonist suggests that the relevant receptors may be located specifically around the nociceptive input to the cell either presynaptically, or in a restricted area on the postsynaptic dendritic tree. The blanket inhibitory effect of the $5-HT_{1A}$ receptor agonist, on the other hand, suggests that the relevant receptors are located on or near the soma. In vivo, these receptors may play a role in inducing Diffuse Noxious Inhibitory Controls. The serotonergic supply to the different 5-HT receptor types may descend from anatomically discrete regions in the NRM and adjacent reticular formation, which may in turn be differentially activated.

The μ agonist DAGO, consistently inhibited nociceptive responses of both nocispecific and multireceptive cells (12/12), whilst DLH-evoked activity in both types of lamina I cells and brush-evoked responses of multireceptive cells were unaffected. The action of DAGO was reversed by naloxone. In a previous study (Fleetwood-Walker *et al*, 1988), we demonstrated that a selective antinociceptive influence of μ agonists was also exerted on deeper dorsal horn neurones via the substantia gelatinosa (lamina II). Therefore, μ agonists exert a widespread influence throughout the dorsal horn. In contrast, the δ agonist (DPDPE) had no influence on deeper neurons when ionophoresed in lamina II (Fleetwood-Walker *et al*, 1988), while in this study it was found to inhibit selectively the nociceptive responses of multireceptive lamina I neurons. This effect was reversed by the δ antagonist, ICI 174864. On nocispecific neurones, DPDPE had a variety of effects, causing non-selective inhibition of both DLH-evoked and nociceptive responses (7/15 cells), selective anti-nociception (5/15 cells) or no effect (3/15 cells). The predominantly non selective effect of DPDPE suggests a direct action on a population of nocispecific lamina I neurones. Receptor autoradiographic data support our evidence that δ actions would be restricted to lamina I and not deeper laminae 6. Kappa agonists (DYNO A 1-13 and U50488H) failed to exert any effect in the superficial dorsal horn, in accord with the finding of J.-M. Besson (reported in this meeting) that κ-receptors are located mainly in deeper dorsal horn laminae.

In conclusion, our present and previous results (El-Yassir *et al*, 1988; Fleetwood-Walker *et al*, 1988) suggest a differential role for two 5-HT_1 receptor subtypes, but not the 5-HT_2 receptor type in mediating the effect of 5-HT descending from NRM on both lamina I and deeper dorsal horn neurones. Like 5-HT, μ sites seem to modulate nociceptive transmission in both superficial and deeper dorsal horn laminae. In contrast δ and κ agonist actions seem to have a specific laminar distribution. Delta sites appear to be specifically responsible for modulating nociceptive transmission in lamina I. Kappa sites, on the other hand, seem to play a role only in deeper dorsal horn laminae.

REFERENCES

BOWKER, R. M., WESTLUND, K. N., SULLIVAN, M. C. AND COULTER, J. D. (1982). Organization of descending serotonergic projections to the spinal cord. In *Descending Pathways to the Spinal Cord*. H. G. Kuypers and G. F. Martin (Eds). *Progress in Brain Research*, Vol. **57**, pp. 239-265. Elsevier: Amsterdam.

EL-YASSIR, N., FLEETWOOD-WALKER, S. M. AND MITCHELL, R. (1988). Heterogeneous effects of serotonin in the dorsal horn of rat: the involvement of 5-HT, receptor subtypes. *Brain Research*, in press.

FLEETWOOD-WALKER, S. M, HOPE, P. J., MITCHELL, R., EL-YASSIR, N. and MOLONY, V. (1988). The influence of opioid receptor subtypes on the processing of nociceptive inputs in the spinal dorsal horn of the cat. *Brain Research*, **451**, 213-226.

LEBARS, D. (1988). Serotonin and Pain. In *Neuronal Serotonin*, N. N. Osborne and M. Hamon (Eds) pp. 171-229. John Wiley and Sons Ltd. Chichester.

MITCHELL, R. AND RILEY, S. (1985). Characterization of receptors for 5-hydroxytryptamine in spinal cord. *Biochemical Society Transactions*, **13**, 955.

MORRIS, B. J. AND HERZ, A. (1987). Distinct distribution of opioidreceptor types in rat lumbar cord. Naunyn *Schmiedeberg's Archives of Pharmacology*, **336**, 240-243.

SCHMAUSS, C. AND YAKSH, T. L. (1984). *In vivo* studies on spinal opiate receptor systems mediating antinociception. II. Pharmacological profiles suggesting a differential association of Mu, Delta and Kappa receptors with visceral chemical and cutaneous thermal stimuli in the rat. *Journal of Pharmacology and Experimental Therapeutics*, **228**, 1-12.

DISCUSSION ON SECTION V

Rapporteur: S. P. Hunt

MRC Molecular Neurobiology Unit, University of Cambridge Medical School
Hills Road, Cambridge CB2 2QH, U.K.

The session on Neurotransmitters and Peptides in the superficial dorsal horn was introduced by P.M. Headley who emphasised the problems inherent in many of the experimental approaches used and the lack of correlation between results obtained with different techniques. He pointed out that many peptidergic neurons could also be releasing fast acting transmitters such as glutamate and that this may explain the presence of the large dense core vesicles mixed with a small clear vesicle population within primary afferent endings. Reference to the peripheral role of substance P and calcitonin gene related polypeptide (CGRP) in the response to injury and maintaining the periphery was often made during the session.

E.R. Perl discussed the possible role of glutamate and ATP as primary afferent neurotransmitters. Using a hamster horizontal slice preparation, glutamate was found not to be a universal excitant of neurons. Less than fifty per cent of neurons excited by dorsal root volleys were excited by exogenous application of glutamate. It was also impossible to tell whether glutamate application was mimicking the action of neurotransmitter released from primary afferents or the results of polysynaptic activation. Immunohistochemical investigation with anti-glutamate antibodies revealed a mixed population of dorsal root ganglion cells of large and small diameter. At the electron-microscopic level, using gold labelling techniques, some *central* terminals were labelled within the substantia gelatinosa. Gold particles could however be seen over the non-vesicular cytoplasmic compartment. The role of glutamate as a primary afferent neurotransmitter clearly remains controversial.

A. Duggan presented results from the use of an antibody coated microprobe, detecting the release of either substance P or somatostatin. Somewhat surprisingly, he found that substantial release of substance P occurred only with temperatures of 52° C applied for greater than 15 minutes. It was suggested that there may be two populations of small diameter sensory fibres, one of which contains peptide but which only responds with central release of neurotransmitter following peripheral injury. This brought to mind both the *nocifensor* concept of Lewis and the proposal that peptide and non-peptide containing small diameter fibres formed parallel channels by which sensory information could reach the dorsal horn. Duggan also suggested that there was a significant release of peptide from the pial membranes, perhaps because of a collateral sensory innervation to this structure. He displayed considerable scepticism over the possibility that any transmitter candidate released by the spinal cord could be measured by intrathecal perfusion, although this view was contested. Unlike substance P, there was a measurable basal release of somatostatin and this increased following thermal but not mechanical stimulation. It was suggested that release was from intrinsic cord neurons and that basal release levels reflected local damage by the electrode.

A. Basbaum continued the analysis of signal transduction from periphery to central projection neurons with his analysis of the rapid induction of the c-fos proto-oncogene within dorsal and ventral horn neurons following noxious peripheral stimulation. The c-fos protein was entirely nuclear and the distribution of labelled neurons was dependent upon the peripheral site of stimulation. Joint, visceral and muscle stimulation produced a distribution of positive cells predominantly in lamina I (largely avoiding lamina II) and in deeper regions of the spinal cord including laminae V, X and VII-VIII. Cutaneous stimulation labelled predominantly lamina II, the substantia gelatinosa, and lamina I. Using double labelling techniques, he reported that approximately 40% of lamina I neurons were projection cells but that in deeper layers the majority of c-fos positive cells were interneurons. Pretreatment with opioid drugs substantially reduced the number of c-fos positive cells seen following peripheral formalin injection. However, the observation that there was a preferential loss of deeper c-fos positive neurons may have been due to an overall drop in the intensity of the stimulus. Cell counts would be needed to substantiate a differential failure of labelling in deep versus superficial spinal cord laminae. Some evidence was also produced to indicate that total behavioural analgesia did not prevent the appearance of c-fos positive neurons in superficial cord laminae following peripheral stimulation.

During the discussion the significance of the c-fos positive population of neurons was questioned and the presence of other relevant but unlabelled populations proposed. This was not denied by the speaker, but the close correlation between c-fos positive cells and the later appearance of other gene products such as dynorphin in cells of the same laminae of the spinal cord was thought to be too great to be coincidental. The c-fos protein is thought to play a role in the control of gene transcription.

M. A. Ruda presented evidence to show that dynorphin gene regulation was substantially affected 3-5 days following plantar injection of Freund's adjuvant - the basis for a peripheral model of inflammation. In contrast, using a combination of in situ hybridization to detect message and immunocytochemistry to identify protein, the changes in enkephalin message and peptide were more modest. Dynorphin positive neurons were found throughout layers I and V, precisely within those areas where c-fos immunoreactivity was seen at much earlier time points: it was reported that c-fos mRNA could be identified thirty minutes after the injection of adjuvant. There was an approximately 800% increase in dynorphin mRNA over control values while enkephalin levels increased only by 50-60%.

The significance of this observation was questioned and the observation that dorsal rhizotomy has similar effects discussed. The idea that injury itself was the necessary stimulus was considered but a general consensus was not reached.

SECTION VI

SUPERFICIAL DORSAL HORN CHANGES FOLLOWING PERIPHERAL INJURY

INTRODUCTION TO SECTION VI

Patrick D. Wall

Cerebral Functions Research Group, Department of Anatomy, University College London
London WC1E 6BT, U.K.

Fifty years ago, awful battles were fought in the country where this meeting took place. Two poets who died at that time write of the wider meanings of pain:

Where in the fields by Huesca the full moon
Throws shadows clear as daylight, soon
The innocence of this quiet plain
Will fade in sweat and blood, in pain
As our decisive hold is lost or won.
All round, the barren hills of Aragón
Announce our testing has begun.

John Cornford

¡Oh blanco muro de España!
¡Oh negro toro de pena!

(Oh white wall of Spain!
Oh black bull of pain!)

Federico García Lorca
(translated by Allen Josephs)

In the following four chapters, four new factors are introduced and analysed in which peripheral injury disturbs the function of the spinal cord. Each is different but we need a way in which they can be considered together. Furthermore we need a scheme by which to analyse the causal factors which are responsible for the abnormal cord activity. This is particularly important since the intent of the work is to be able to understand and treat disease states and we need a scheme for comparison of experimental models with diseases. It would be fatuous to propose a single cause and every reason to expect multiple interacting mechanisms. It is highly unlikely that a particular pain has a purely peripheral or a purely central origin. Peripheral mechanisms are not incompatible with central mechanisms. For that reason, the phrase *nociceptive pain* may be inappropriate in its implication that only the periphery need be considered. However it is the scientists' and clinicians' duty to identify the major components in any particular condition. In order to do that there are good tactical and practical reasons to start in the periphery and to move centrally. The reason is that the periphery is more open to analysis and therapy. The analytic scheme I would propose is summarised as follows.

PAIN FOLLOWING PERIPHERAL INJURY MAY BE CAUSED BY:

(1) Factors which remain entirely peripheral.

    A. Presence of an abnormal ongoing afferent barrage.
    B. Absence of a normal ongoing afferent barrage.
    C. Sensitization and desensitization to normally effective stimuli.
    D. Appearance of responses to novel stimuli.

(2) Changes in dorsal root ganglion cells induced by:

    A. Nerve impulses.
    B. Transport mechanisms.

(3) Changes in afferents central terminals induced by:

    A. Nerve impulses.
    B. Transport mechanisms.

(4) Postsynaptic changes in the spinal cord induced by:

    A. Peripheral nerve impulses.
    B. Transport mechanisms in peripheral afferents.
    C. Changed descending controls.

(1) FACTORS WHICH REMAIN ENTIRELY PERIPHERAL

A. Presence of an abnormal ongoing barrage. This is the most classical and straightforward hypothesis (Willis, 1985 for review). The proposal would be that central cells remain stable, line-labelled, hard wired and dedicated to a single function while the cause of the central abnormality resides in the abnormal afferent barrage. Tissue damage directly excites nerve endings and the secondary effects of neurogenic and cellular inflammation add to the excitation. When peripheral nerve itself is damaged, the damaged nerve membrane becomes spontaneously active and therefore adds new ectopic impulses to the afferent signals (Devor, 1989; Wall and Gutnick, 1974a and b). The experimental test of the importance of this factor is to match the properties of the afferent barrage with the properties of the central responses. There is often a good match of the two with brief stimuli under anaesthesia but it often breaks down in circumstances where either prolonged stimuli are tested or in clinical situations (Adriaensen *et al*, 1984; Campbell *et al*, 1988; Woolf, 1984).

B. Absence of the normal afferent barrage. This factor is often neglected. Its most dramatic manifestation is the appearance of a phantom sensation immediately after local anaesthetic block of afferents (Bromage and Melzack, 1974). Some single units in cord (Devor and Wall, 1981a and b; Hylden *et al*, 1987), dorsal column nuclei (Dostrovsky *et al*, 1976), midbrain (Mooney *et al*, 1987), thalamus (Nakahama *et al*, 1966; Wall and Egger, 1971) and cortex (Merzenich *et al*, 1985) have been shown to change receptive fields after peripheral block or section. In human disease and in some animal models such as the one described here by Bennett, differential block of some components might be a crucial factor.

C. Sensitization and desensitization. After stimulation, peripheral endings change their sensitivities for long periods (Campbell *et al*, 1989, for review). There is good evidence for this, particularly in Aδ nociceptive afferents which decrease their thresholds after brief noxious stimuli. While this would seem an obvious explanation of

408

primary hyperaesthesia after injury, one should share the extreme caution of the major contributors to the field. They often report a mismatch between the sensitised afferent responses and the sensitised central responses (Campbell *et al*, 1989 for review). We have here an example of the possibility of simultaneous peripheral and central change in which neither factor alone explains the overall phenomenon. One must also warn that the disappearance of pain with local anaesthesia does not prove that the causative factors are entirely peripheral. It could be that in addition to an injury-induced abnormal barrage, there has been a sensitization of central structures which overreact to normal afferent impulses carried by unchanged afferents. Peripheral local anaesthesia in that situation will block both the abnormal barrage and the normal input which arrives on abnormally sensitive central cells.

D. Appearance of responses to novel stimuli. Damaged nerves and nerve endings are excited by sympathetic nerve impulses (Roberts and Elardo, 1985; Wall and Gutnick, 1974a and b; Devor, 1989, for review). While attention has rightly concentrated on the novel alpha excitatory effect of noradrenaline, one should not forget that other possibly excitatory chemicals are released primarily and secondarily by sympathetic efferent action and by injury (Levine *et al*, 1985).

(2) CHANGES IN DORSAL ROOT GANGLIA

A. Induced by nerve impulses. Once injury has occurred in the periphery a cascade of changes sweep centrally in addition to the nerve impulses continuously generated in the periphery. No location should be neglected without experimental examination to confirm that peripheral injury does or does not induce changes in that location. For example, in work to be published by Devor and Wall, it will be shown that substantial excitatory cross talk can develop between myelinated axon's cells in the dorsal root ganglion.

B. Induced by transport mechanisms. Peripheral axotomy but not section of the dorsal roots induces marked changes in the chemistry of dorsal root ganglion cells (Jessell and Dodd, 1989, for review). Like cut peripheral axons, the cells become highly mechanosensitive, spontaneously active and sensitive to norepinephrine (Wall and Devor, 1983). This means that the spinal cord receives an abnormal chemical input and nerve impulse input originating not only from the region of injury but also from the dorsal root ganglia. It is commonly proposed that these changes occur since the cells are cut off from their supply of nerve growth factor, NGF (Fitzgerald *et al*, 1985). This is supported by showing a prevention of the changes by providing a substitute supply of NGF. However one should be cautious that there may be chemicals other than NGF which play a role. The change in the dorsal root ganglia can be so severe that some die thereby converting a peripheral nerve lesion into a central lesion as the central terminals of spinal afferents degenerate (Ygge and Aldskogius, 1984). While most work has concentrated on the effect of nerve lesions, it should not be forgotten that the chemical content of C fibres depends on their target tissue. The chemistry of afferents changes following cross anastomosis of peripheral nerves (McMahon and Gibson, 1987). It is therefore possible that the chemistry of dorsal root ganglia may change in the presence of pathological peripheral tissue even if the nerves are intact.

(3) CHANGES IN AFFERENT CENTRAL TERMINALS

A. Induced by nerve impulses. The arrival of sensory impulses in the spinal cord triggers central mechanisms which feed back onto the afferent terminals of the fibres which have carried the afferent volley and onto their passive neighbours (Lloyd, 1949).

This feedback changes the transynaptic effectiveness of subsequent arriving impulses as in presynaptic inhibition (Eccles, 1964).

It is an obvious suggestion, as yet untested experimentally, that there could be a central equivalent of the peripheral axon reflex. In the periphery, action potentials in C fibres release compounds which alter blood flow, plasma extravasation and nerve sensitivity. Central C fibre terminals contain the same chemicals as peripheral terminals and their release could have the same effect on blood vessels and on nerve fibres in the spinal cord as occurs in the periphery.

B. Induced by transport mechanisms. The chemical changes which take place in the dorsal root ganglia are necessarily reflected in the central terminals since the ganglion cells are the source of many of the chemicals located in the terminals (Fitzgerald, 1989 for review). We do not know precisely the functional role of any of the chemicals which exist in sensory terminals and which are known to be released on excitation. It is reasonable to expect that their release will have slow and fast effects on the physiology and morphology of postsynaptic cells (Jessell and Dodd, 1989, for review).

If peripheral nerve lesions occur in the neonate, there is a serious failure of development of the central terminals of the cut axons and a compensatory expansion of the terminal arborizations of intact neighbours (Fitzgerald and Vrbova, 1985). There is no clear evidence that such obvious sprouting occurs in adults as discussed in the chapter by Snow.

(4) POSTSYNAPTIC CHANGES IN THE SPINAL CORD

A. Induced by nerve impulses. During injury and surgery and particularly if nerves are sectioned, there are brief periods of intense high frequency injury discharge (Wall *et al*, 1974). These short bursts of maximal high frequency firing may have special central effects as discussed in the chapter by Bennett *et al*. Whatever may be the special effects of these intense bombardments, Woolf's chapter shows that much less dramatic increases of afferent barrage trigger long latency long duration changes of excitability which are sustained by an intrinsic spinal cord mechanism. The chapters by Basbaum *et al* and by Hunt *et al* show that injury-induced afferent barrages also evoke central chemical and metabolic alterations with a somewhat longer latency and duration than those discussed by Woolf. The new central chemistry described by Besson and by Bennett has a sufficiently long latency in its appearance that it could be either impulse triggered or the consequence of transport changes or both.

The analysis of these prolonged central changes triggered by the arrival of nerve impulses will have important practical consequences. For example, it had been assumed in the past that the reason patients were in postoperative pain was that they were reacting moment by moment to the nociceptive input generated from the damaged tissue created by the surgery. Now we must consider the possibility that the massive barrage generated during the surgery had left the spinal cord in a prolonged hyperexcitable state. Tests for this new hypothesis are now in progress and consist of examining the prolonged postoperative effect of adequate brief block of the input during surgery and of adequate preoperative narcotic medication (McQuay *et al*, 1988; Bach *et al*, 1988). The results suggest that it may be possible to prevent postoperative pain as well as to treat it when it occurs.

B. Induced by transported chemicals. It is reasonable to propose that the changes observed in spinal cord with a latency of many days after peripheral nerve lesions are caused by changes in transported chemicals. Prolonged block of afferent and efferent fibres with tetrodotoxin (Wall *et al*, 1982) does not produce the same changes as occur after peripheral injury, as are described in the chapter by Dubner *et al*. However, we know that sectioned peripheral nerve generates an abnormal afferent barrage as well as changing the chemistry of afferents. It is possible that both of these abnormalities contribute to the central changes; and this needs experimental investigation. This is particularly true in such conditions as induced polyarthritis where the relative roles of afferent barrage, changed transport and systemic disease need unravelling.

Peripheral nerve lesions provoke central anatomical, chemical and physiological changes (Mendell, 1984). The physiological changes include changes of inhibitions, receptive field size and modality. The unmyelinated afferents appear to be particularly important in transferring the signal from periphery to centre (Wall *et al*, 1982). Many of the central changes can be prevented by supplying the cut end of the nerve with a supply of Nerve Growth Factor (Fitzgerald *et al*, 1985). This suggests that a cause of the central change is the failure of delivery of a substance normally present. However it would be premature to propose that NGF is the only chemical messenger involved in the central chemical detection of peripheral injury.

C. Induced by descending controls. Since messages arriving at the spinal cord by way of nerve impulses and of chemical transport are in turn relayed to the brain stem, thalamus and hypothalamus, we must expect the possibility that changes observed in the spinal cord are in fact produced by changes of descending controls (Yaksh, 1986, for review). Most of the studies on these feedback systems, in common with most work on responses of dorsal horn cells, have examined the brief effect of brief stimuli. We now know that there may be very prolonged periods of response even after brief stimuli (Woolf, 1984; Wall and Woolf, 1984). Chronic responses are not necessarily a tonic repetition of acute responses. Most work on descending controls has emphasised their inhibitory effect. Therefore one might expect a homeostatic negative feed-back onto the spinal cord tending to reduce evoked over-activity. However, in pathology, these negative feedbacks might fail or even be replaced by excitatory tonic controls.

This brief scheme provides a series of steps on which one may seek the location and nature of the phenomena.

REFERENCES

ADRIAENSEN, H., GYBELS, J., HANDWERKER, H.O. AND VAN HEES, J. (1984) Nociceptor discharge and sensations due to prolonged noxious mechanical stimulation, a paradox. *Human Neurobiology* 3, 53-58.

BACH, S., NORENG, M.F. AND TJELLDEN, N.V. (1988) Phantom limb pain in amputees during the first 12 months following limb amputation after preoperative lumbar epidural blockade. *Pain* 33, 297-302.

BROMAGE, P.R. AND MELZACK, R. (1974) Phantom limbs and the body schema. *Canadian Anaesthesiology Society Journal* 21, 267274.

CAMPBELL, S.N., RAJA, R.H., COHEN, D.C., MANNING, A.A., KHAN, A.A. AND MEYER, R.A. (1989) Peripheral neural mechanisms of nociception. Chapter 1, in *The Textbook of Pain*, Eds. P.D. Wall and R. Melzack, Churchill Livingstone, London.

CAMPBELL, J.N., RAJA, S.N., MEYER, R.A. AND MACKINNON, S.E. (1988) Myelinated afferents signal the hyperalgesia associated with nerve injury. *Pain*, 32, 89-94.

DEVOR, M. (1989) The pathophysiology of damaged peripheral nerve. Chapter 3, In, *The Textbook of Pain*, second edition, Eds. P.D. Wall and R. Melzack, Churchill Livingstone, London.

DEVOR, M. AND WALL, P.D. (1981a) The effect of peripheral nerve injury on receptive fields of cells in the cat spinal cord. *Journal of Comparative Neurology*, **199**, 277-291.

DEVOR, M. AND WALL, P.D. (1981b) Plasticity in the spinal cord sensory map following peripheral nerve injury in rats. *Journal of Neuroscience*, **1**, 679-684.

DOSTROVSKY, J., MILLAR, J. AND WALL, P.D. (1976) The immediate shift of afferent drive of dorsal column nucleus cells following deafferentation, A comparison of acute and chronic deafferentation in gracile nucleus and spinal cord. *Experimental Neurology* **52**, 480-495.

ECCLES, J.C. (1964) Presynaptic inhibition in the spinal cord. In, *Progress in Brain Research* vol. **12**, *Physiology of Spinal Neurons,* Ed. J.C. Eccles and J.P. Schade, Elsevier, Amsterdam.

FITZGERALD, M. (1989) The course and termination of primary afferent fibres. Chapter **2** in, *The Textbook of Pain*, 2nd edition, Eds. P.D. Wall and R. Melzack, Churchill Livingstone, London.

FITZGERALD, M. AND VRBOVA, G. (1985) FRAP plasticity afferent terminal fields and of dorsal horn terminal growth in the neonatal rat. *Journal of Comparative Neurology*, **240**, 414422.

FITZGERALD, M., WALL, P.D., GOEDERT, M. AND EMSON, P.C. (1985) Nerve growth factor counteracts the neurophysiological and neurochemical effects of chronic sciatic nerve injury. *Brain Research*, **332**, 131-141.

HYLDEN, J.L.K., NAHIN, R.L. AND DUBNER, R. (1987) Altered responses of nociceptive cat lamina I spinal dorsal horn neurons after chronic sciatic neuroma formation. *Brain Research*, **411**, 341-350.

JESSELL, T.M. AND DODD, J. (1989) Functional chemistry of primary afferent neurons. Chapter **2**, in *The Textbook of Pain*, 2nd editions, Eds. P.D. Wall and R. Melzack, Churchill Livingstone, London.

LEVINE, J.D., GOODING, J., DONATONI, P., BORDON, L. AND GRETZL, E.J. (1985) The role of polymorphonuclear leukocytes in hyperalgesia. *Journal of Neuroscience*, **5**, 3025-3029.

LLOYD, D.P.C. AND MCINTYRE, A.K. (1949) On the origin of dorsal root potentials. *Journal of General Physiology,* **32**, 409443.

MCMAHON, S.B. AND GIBSON, S. (1987) Peptide expression is altered when afferent nerves reinnervate inappropriate tissue. *Neuroscience Letters*, **73**, 9-15.

MCQUAY, H.J., CARROLL, D. AND MOORE, R.A. (1988) Postoperative orthopaedic pain. *Pain* **33**, 291-296.

MENDELL, L.M. (1984) Modifiability of spinal synapses. *Physiological Reviews* **64**, 260-324.

MERZENICH, M.M., NELSON, R.J., KAAS, J.H., STRYKER, M.P., JENKINS, W.M., ZOOK, J.M., CYANDER, M.S. AND SCHOPPMANN, A. (1985) Variability in hand surface representations in areas 3b + I in adult owl and squirrel monkeys. *Journal of Comparative Neurology* **258**, 281-297.

MOONEY, R.D., NIKOLETSEAS, K. AND RHOADES, R.W. (1987) Transection of the infraorbital nerve in newborn hamsters alters the somatosensory but not the visual representation in the superior colliculus. *Journal of Comparative Neurology*, **266**, 1.

NAKAHAMA, H., NISHIOKA, S. AND OTSUKA, T. (1966) Excitation and inhibition in ventrobasal thalamic neurons before and after cutaneous input deprivation. *Progress in Brain Research*, **21**, 180-185.

ROBERTS, W.J. AND ELARDO, S.M. (1985) Sympathetic activation of A-δ nociceptors.

Somatosensory Research, **3**, 33-44.

WALL, P.D. AND DEVOR, M. (1983) Sensory afferent impulses from dorsal root ganglia as well as from the periphery in normal and nerve injured rats. *Pain*, **17**, 321-339.

WALL, P.D. AND EGGER, M.D. (1971) Formation of new connections in adult rat brains after partial deafferentation. *Nature* **232**, 542-545.

WALL, P.D., FITZGERALD, M. AND WOOLF, C.J. (1982) Effects of capsaicin on receptive fields and on inhibitions in the rat spinal cord. *Experimental Neurology*, **78**, 425-436.

WALL, P.D. AND GUTNICK, M. (1974a) Ongoing activity in peripheral nerves, II. The physiology and pharmacology of impulses originating in a neuroma. *Experimental Neurology*, **38**, 580-593.

WALL, P.D. AND GUTNICK, M. (1974b) Properties of afferent nerve impulses originating from a neuroma. *Nature*, **248**, 740743.

WALL, P.D., MILLS,R., FITZGERALD, M. AND GIBSON, S.J. (1982) Chronic blockade of sciatic nerve transmission by tetrodotoxin does not produce central changes in the dorsal horn of the spinal cord of the rat. *Neuroscience Letters*, **30**, 315-320.

WALL, P.D., WAXMAN, S. AND BASBAUM, A.I. (1974) Ongoing activity in peripheral nerve, III. Injury discharge. *Experimental Neurology*, **45**, 576-589.

WALL, P.D. AND WOOLF, C.J. (1984) Muscle but not cutaneous Cafferent input produces prolonged increases in the excitability of the flexion reflex in the rat. *Journal of Physiology*, **356**, 443-458.

WILLIS, W.D. (1985) *The Pain System*. Karger, Basel.

WOOLF, C.J. (1984) Long term alteration in the excitability of the flexion reflex produced by peripheral tissue injury in the chronic decerebrate rat. *Pain*, **18**, 325-343.

YAKSH, T.L. (1986) Editor, *Spinal afferent processing*, Plenum, New York.

YGGE, J. AND ALDSKOGIUS, H. (1984) Intercostal nerve transection and its effect on the dorsal root ganglion. *Experimental Brain Research*, **55**, 402-408.

OPIOID RECEPTORS IN THE DORSAL HORN OF INTACT AND DEAFFERENTED RATS: AUTORADIOGRAPHIC AND ELECTROPHYSIOLOGICAL STUDIES

J. M. Besson[1,2], M. C. Lombard[1,2], J. M. Zajac[3], D. Besse[1,2], M. Peschanski[1] and B. P. Roques[3]

Unité de Recherche de Neurophysiologie Pharmacologique (I.N.S.E.R.M., U.161)[1] and Laboratoire de Physiopharmacologie de la Douleur, Ecole Pratique des Hautes Etudes[2], 2 rue d'Alésia, 74014 Paris; Unité de Recherche de Pharmacochimie Moléculaire (I.N.S.E.R.M., U.266 and C.N.R.S. UA 498)[3], 4 avenue de l'Observatoire 75006 Paris, France

The direct depressive effect of opioids on the transmission of nociceptive processing at the spinal level is well documented (see refs in Le Bars and Besson, 1981; Duggan and North, 1984; Yaksh and Noueihed, 1985; Zieglgänsberger, 1986; Besson and Chaouch, 1987). Both pre- and postsynaptic mechanisms have been proposed as an explanation of the depressive effects of opioids on the activity of nociceptive dorsal horn neurons. Despite the lack of morphological evidence for a direct presynaptic control by enkephalinergic axo-axonic synapses, there is evidence for a presynaptic action of opioid substances (Fields *et al*, 1980; Jessell and Iversen, 1977; Lamotte *et al*, 1976; MacDonald and Nelson, 1978; Mudge *et al*, 1979; Sastry, 1979). In addition both electrophysiological (Barker *et al*, 1978; Zieglgänsberger and Tulloch, 1979; Yoshimura and North, 1983) and immunocytochemical (Aronin *et al*, 1981; Hunt *et al*, 1980; Ruda, 1982; Ruda *et al*, 1984) investigations support postsynaptic sites of action of opioids.

Both mechanisms seem to play a major role in the action of opioids since there is a reduction of 40-50% in the levels of opioid receptors in the superficial dorsal horn after dorsal rhizotomy (Lamotte *et al*, 1976; Ninkovic *et al*, 1981) and at least 50% of lumbar spinothalamic cells receive enkephalinergic terminals (Ruda *et al*, 1984).

The first part of this paper is devoted to the characterization of the various types of opioid receptors encountered in the superficial layers of the dorsal horn of the spinal cord using highly selective tritiated ligands and autoradiography. The presence of μ, δ and κ binding sites in this area were determined following various combinations of dorsal root rhizotomies in order to evaluate quantitatively the percentage of presynaptic and postsynaptic receptors. In addition, the density of endopeptidase 24.11 (enkephalinase) was measured after lesions, using [^{3}H]-HACBO-Gly as a selective marker (Waksman *et al*, 1986).

The second part of this paper is an attempt to gauge, with electrophysiological techniques, the relative importance of pre-and postsynaptic effects of morphine on the transmission of nociceptive information in the dorsal horn. To this end the effects of morphine were compared on dorsal horn neurons in deafferented and *intact* spinal rats.

415

TABLE I

Modifications of opioid receptors after rhizotomy, peripheral nerve lesion and
neonatal treatment with capsaicin

Authors	Species	Lesions (unilateral)	Delay	Ligands	Methods	Modifications
LaMotte et al, 1976	Monkey	C2-C8	2-4 weeks	[^{3}H] Naloxone	binding	↓ laminae I-III
Ninkovic et al, 1981	Rat (Wis.)	C4-C6	1 week	[^{3}H] Etorphine (μ δ)	RAG	↓ 40% laminae I-IIo
Ninkovic et al, 1982	Monkey	C3-C6	8 days	[^{3}H] Etorphine (μ δ)	RAG	↓ 43% laminae I-II
Daval et al, 1987	Rat (S-D)	C4-C6	1 week	[^{3}H] DAGO (μ)	RAG	↓ 43% laminae I-II
Jessell et al, 1979	Rat	L5-L6	3-4 weeks	[^{3}H] Diprenorphine	binding	↓ 47%
	Rat	Sciatic	1-57 days	[^{3}H] Diprenorphine		small decrease after 28 days
Fields et al, 1980	Rat (S-D)	Sciatic	1 month	[^{3}H] Morphine (μ)	binding	↓ dorsal roots L5-L6 μ 34% δ 51%
				[^{3}H] DADLE (δ)		
Gamse et al, 1979	Rat	Capsaicin (50mg/kg neonate)	5 months	[^{3}H] Diprenorphine	binding	↓ 37% laminae I-III
Nagy et al, 1980	Rat (Wis.)	Capsaicin (50mg/kg neonate)	3 months	[^{3}H] Naloxone	binding	↓ 38% (dorsal horn)
Daval et al, 1987	Rat (S-D)	Capsaicin (50mg/kg neonate)	3 months	[^{3}H] DAGO (μ) [^{3}H] DSTLE (δ)	RAG	↓ 31% μ ↓ 36% δ laminae I-II

OPIOID RECEPTORS AND SUPERFICIAL DORSAL HORN

Various techniques have demonstrated the presence of opioid receptors in the superficial laminae of the dorsal horn (see refs. in Wamsley, 1983). There are many binding sites in the substantia gelatinosa. This area has been demonstrated to be critical in the action of morphine and enkephalins in iontophoretic studies (Duggan et al, 1977; Morton et al, 1987). These results are also in keeping with reports showing that the superficial layers of the dorsal horn are rich in enkephalin containing terminals and interneurones (Hökfelt et al, 1977).

It is likely that each of the three main types of opioid receptors are located within the superficial dorsal horn; numerous studies, using receptor autoradiography, visualized μ (Pert et al, 1975, 1976; Atweh and Kuhar, 1977; Pearson et al, 1980; Ninkovic et al, 1982; Wamsley et al, 1982), δ (Goodman et al, 1980), κ (Slater and Patel, 1983; Gouarderes et al, 1985), μ, δ and enkephalinase (Waksman et al, 1986) and μ, δ and κ (Morris and Herz, 1987) binding sites in the superficial layers of the dorsal horn.

As shown in Table I, a reduction of 40-50% in the levels of opioid receptors in the superficial dorsal horn occurs after dorsal root rhizotomy; a decrease in opioid receptor binding has also been observed after peripheral nerve transection and after capsaicin treatment of neonatal rats. Overall, these studies suggest that some receptors are situated on thin primary afferent terminals. Further evidence for opiate binding sites on primary afferent fibers was provided by the demonstration of opiate binding in dorsal root ganglia (Young et al, 1980; Ninkovic et al, 1982), and dorsal roots (Fields et al, 1980). Interestingly, a high level of opioid binding was found in the neuritic outgrowth from dorsal root ganglia (Hiller et al, 1978) in foetal mouse dorsal root ganglia and spinal cord tissue cultures.

The effects induced by either surgical or chemical lesions (Table I) are difficult to interpret:

- a large number of binding studies were performed on membrane preparations of spinal cord. In such preparations, it is impossible to localise the site of the reduced binding.
- most of the ligands used are not selective. For example, the so-called δ agonist DADLE displays a high cross-reactivity for μ sites (Zajac et al, 1983). Diprenorphine and etorphine interact with various types of receptors and their use in conjunction with cold-blockers does not allow a clear distinction between each type of receptor (Delay-Goyet et al, 1987).
- finally after surgical lesions, studies have not been performed after short and long survival periods. Such studies could assess the possible involvement of transynaptic degeneration which occurs in the dorsal horn 3 weeks after rhizotomy (see refs in Csillik and Knyihar-Csillik, 1986).

To examine the effects of lesions on opioid binding in the superficial dorsal horn, we have used highly selective μ, δ and κ ligands and quantitative autoradiography. These studies were performed in normal rats and in animals that underwent various dorsal root rhizotomies.

Additionally, in order to evaluate whether opioid receptors and enkephalin degrading enzymes are similarly affected by these experimental conditions, we also labelled, in the same animals, neutral endopeptidase (NEP, enkephalinase). To label NEP we used [^{3}H]-HACBO-Gly, a specific ligand developed in our laboratory (Waksman et al, 1986).

Experimental procedures

Male Sprague-Dawley albino rats were sacrificed by decapitation and their cervical spinal cords were rapidly removed. The whole piece was frozen in isopentane (-40°C). Frontal sections (10-15 μm thick) were cut on a cryostat (-20°C), thaw-mounted onto gelatine-control slides and kept at -80°C. Three sets of adjacent sections were prepared for incubation with one of the four ligands.

The sections were brought back to room temperature, then incubated in 50mM Tris-HCl buffer (pH 7.4) at 25°C for 60 min with one of four ligands. [^{3}H]-DAGO (Tyr-D-Ala-Gly-(Me)Phe-Gly-ol) (1.59 TBq/mmol, CEN Saclay) was used at a final concentration of 3nM to label μ sites. [^{3}H]-DTLET (Tyr-D-Thr-Gly-Phe-Leu-Thr) (2.1 TBq/mmol, CEN Saclay) was used at a final concentration of 3nM to label δ sites Ethylketocyclazocine, [^{3}H]-EKC (1TBq/mmol, NEN) was used at a final concentration of 10 nM, in the presence of 100 nM of cold DAGO and 100 nM of cold DTLET, to label κ sites. For these three ligands, the non-specific binding was evaluated in the same conditions in the presence of 10μM levorphanol (Hoffman-La Roche). [^{3}H]-HACBO-Gly (N-(2RS)-3-hydroxyamino-carboxyl-2-benzyl-1-oxopropyl-glycine) (1.1 TBq/mmol, CEN Saclay) was used at a concentration of 3 nm. In this case, the non-specific binding was assessed in the presence of 10μM thiorphan.

At the end of the incubation the sections were washed twice in ice-cold buffer for 10 min, rinsed in the cold water and air-dried. Labelled sections were closely apposed to tritium sensitive film (LKB) and exposed for 14-17 weeks at 4°C. The autoradiograms were revealed in Kodak D19b.

Spinal cord sections were Nissl-stained using cresyl violet for histological determination of anatomical boundaries. The averaged optical density values were converted to binding density values by reference to tritium standards (Amersham).

417

Autoradiography of opioid receptors and neutral endopeptidase in the superficial dorsal horn of normal rats

With each of the 4 types of ligand a high density of labelling was observed in the superficial layers of the dorsal horn (lamina I and, mainly, lamina II; *substantia gelatinosa*). The grain density fell sharply in lamina III, where it did not differ significantly from that observed in the white matter. For all ligands, microscopic examination revealed no obvious difference between the grain density in the superficial layers at different rostro-caudal levels of the cord, including the spinal trigeminal subnucleus caudalis. Quantitative analyses were performed in the two superficial layers of the dorsal horn at cervical levels.

Assuming that the K_D values of the ligands are similar to those found in rat brain (Waksman *et al*, 1987), the percentages of μ, δ and κ receptors were, respectively, $71\pm3\%$, $22\pm3\%$ and $7\pm2\%$. Such an evaluation can be performed since DAGO and DTLET exhibited a very low affinity ($K_I < 10,000$ nM) for κ sites. Furthermore, under the experimental conditions used for autoradiography, the cross-reactivity of [^{3}H]-DTLET with μ sites remained negligible (Zajac and Roques, 1989).

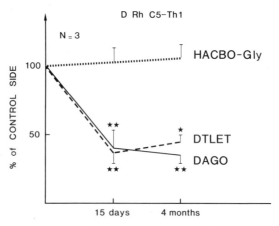

FIGURE 1: Effects of dorsal root rhizotomy (C5-Th1) on binding of [^{3}H]-DAGO, [^{3}H]-DTLET and [^{3}H]-HACBO-Gly in the superficial layers of the dorsal horn. Binding densities were analyzed in C7 segment 15 days and 4 months after rhizotomy. The results are expressed as percentage of the binding density of the control side (*P<0.02; **<0.01).

The density of κ receptors was relatively low and contrasts with previous reports showing a high density of κ binding sites in the dorsal horn (Slater and Patel, 1983; Gouarderes *et al*, 1985; Traynor and Wood, 1987; Czlonkowski *et al*, 1983). Unfortunately, in these studies the labelling of κ sites was performed by using non-specific tritiated ligands (etorphine, bremazocine) in the presence of high concentration of μ and δ blockers. We have seen in the same experimental conditions that the quantity of κ sites measured with [^{3}H]- etorphine was greater than that evaluated with [^{3}H]- EKC (Delay-Goyet *et al*, 1987). In these experiments we demonstrated that [^{3}H]- etorphine still binds to a number of μ and δ sites in the presence of high concentrations of μ and δ ligands. This finding suggests that previous studies overestimated the number of κ sites. Our interpretation agrees well with that of Mack *et al* (1984) who reported low quantities of κ sites measured with [^{3}H]-EKC. Thus, from our present experiments, it appears that the rat spinal cord contains few κ receptors.

Effects induced by dorsal root rhizotomies

Surgical procedures were performed on Sprague-Dawley rats using ketamine as general and xylocaine as local anesthetics. Due to the low concentration of [³H]-EKC binding sites, rhizotomy was used only in studies of μ and δ binding sites and of endopeptidase 24.11.

Extensive rhizotomy C5-Th1

Using a dissecting microscope, a dorsal hemilaminectomy of vertebrae C4 to Th1 was made on the right side and the five corresponding dorsal roots C5 to Th1 (inclusive) were sectioned intradurally proximal to the ganglia, through small individual openings of the dura matter. Care was taken not to damage the blood vessels running along the dorsal roots. The surgical wound was washed with saline and the muscles and skin were sutured, layer by layer.

In comparison to the intact side, there was a marked decrease of μ and δ binding sites at all the levels of the deafferented cord. This finding is similar to previous reports (Table I). The decrease was the greatest ($\simeq$60-70% for both μ and δ binding sites) in C7. This level corresponds to the middle of the deafferented area. At Th1, the decrease was approximately 25%. It is interesting that the same amount of decrease was observed 15 days and four months (Fig. 1) after the rhizotomy. This finding suggests first that the transsynaptic degeneration which occurs 3 weeks after rhizotomy does not eliminate a significant additional number of opioid binding sites, and second that degenerating dorsal horn neurons bear a small proportion of postsynaptically located opioid receptors.

C-fibres within Lissauer's tract do not project more than 3 segments (see refs in Fitzgerald, 1984). Thus, after extensive deafferentation, it was likely that C7 segment, the center of the lesion, did not receive any fine afferent input. This conclusion is supported by the fact that even larger rhizotomies (C4-Th2) did not induce additional decreases in opioid binding sites. Thus, it is reasonable to conclude that the 60% decrease in both [³H]-DAGO and [³H]-DTLET labelling is related to the loss of presynaptic binding sites localized on primary afferent fibers. The remaining binding sites (40% of binding in intact animals) probably reflect the existence of a significant population of postsynaptic binding sites. The existence of postsynaptic opioid binding sites is supported by the observation of numerous spinothalamic neurones receiving direct enkephalinergic projections in the superficial layers of the dorsal horn (Ruda, 1982; Ruda *et al*, 1984). In addition, it must be pointed out that both μ and δ receptors decreased in the same proportion, indicating that pre- and postsynaptic components have similar ratios of receptors.

In sharp contrast with the results obtained with μ and δ opioid sites, the density of endopeptidase 24.11 labelled by [³H]- HACBO-GLY was not altered by rhizotomies (Fig. 1). This finding indicates that this enkephalin degrading enzyme is not associated with primary afferent fibers. In contrast, presynaptic localization of NEP in the pallidum and substantia nigra (Waksman *et al*, 1987) has been observed previously.

Rhizotomy C4-Th2 leaving C7 intact

As previously mentioned, C fibers passing in Lissauer's tract do not project more than 3 segments. With such a lesion, we were able to examine the opioid receptors on a single root.

This is shown for μ receptors in Fig. 2 where there is a dramatic decrease of binding on both sides of the peak that corresponds to C7 segment. In the area of the spared root the percentages of each of the three types of receptors were similar to those measured in intact animals. Our preliminary results indicate that the binding in C7 segment is less than that found in C7 intact animals. The difference in binding levels in C7 (approximately 20%) is probably due to the removal of primary afferent inputs from dorsal roots surrounding C7.

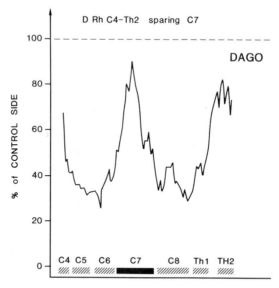

FIGURE 2: μ binding sites in the superficial layers of the dorsal horn in a rat that underwent dorsal rhizotomy from C4-Th2 but sparing C7. Labelling was performed with [^{3}H]-DAGO 8 days after the lesion. The curve represents a moving average of 5 successive values, each measured every 150 μm.

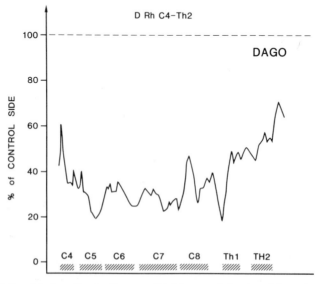

FIGURE 3: μ binding sites in the superficial layers of the dorsal horn in a rat that underwent a dorsal rhizotomy from C4-Th2. Same measurements as for Fig. 2. The spinal cord is longer in this case because the rat was 3 weeks older than in Fig. 2.

The possibility of innervation from nearby dorsal roots is also suggested by findings illustrated in Fig. 3 which shows the effects produced by a large rhizotomy that included C7. In this case there is a consistent decrease in each deafferented segment. Near the limit of the lesion in C4 and Th2, binding levels were higher than those measured within the 5 segments in the center of the lesion.

THE RELATIVE IMPORTANCE OF PRE- AND POSTSYNAPTIC EFFECTS OF MORPHINE ON THE TRANSMISSION OF NOCICEPTIVE MESSAGES IN THE DORSAL HORN OF SPINAL RAT

We wished to evaluate semi-quantitatively the postsynaptic effects of morphine. We therefore studied the effects of morphine on the increased spontaneous activity of dorsal horn neurons induced by a large chronic dorsal rhizotomy (C5-Th1) in the spinal rat.

Experiments were carried out between 11 and 41 days following the surgery. As already mentioned (see section I), it seems highly probable that segment C7 was totally deafferented. This conclusion was supported by the finding that the neurones recorded in C7 could never be activated by ipsilateral stimulation. Contralateral stimulation was also ineffective although short lasting inhibitions could be produced by contralateral mechanical stimulation.

The impossibility of characterizing the neurones on a functional basis could give rise to problems in the analysis of the results. We used spinal animals in order to avoid interactions of morphine with descending systems. The combination of spinalization and deafferentation precludes any characterization of the neurones using conventional physiological techniques. We have therefore attempted to classify the cells by pharmacological means. Many electrophysiological studies have clearly shown that the depressive effect of morphine is selectively exerted on dorsal horn neurones responding to noxious stimuli rather than on cells responding exclusively to non noxious stimuli (see refs in Le Bars and Besson, 1981; Duggan and North, 1984). Using either 2 mg/kg of morphine or 2 then 4 mg/kg I.V., we presume that cells that were depressed by the opiate may be nociceptive neurones. Obviously this is somewhat arbitrary but it does not prejudice our conclusions as to a post-synaptic action of morphine since with the doses of 2 plus 4 mg/kg, nearly two-thirds of the cells had their activity depressed by morphine (Fig. 4).

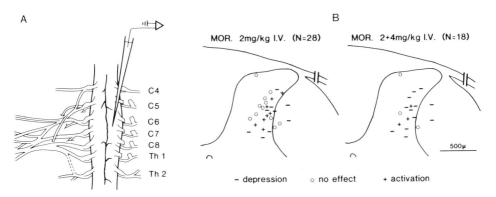

FIGURE 4: Left: Drawing showing the extent of rhizotomy and the level of the recording tracks (C7); Right: location of the recorded units that received either 2 or 2 + 4 mg/kg I.V. of morphine.

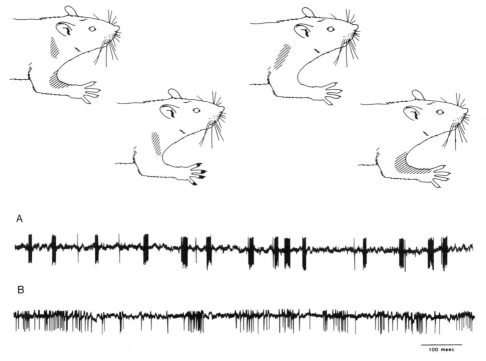

FIGURE 5: Top: examples of the location and extent of the scratching behavior induced by the C5-Th1 dorsal rhizotomy. Bottom: two examples (A and B) of spontaneous neuronal hyperactivity recorded in the dorsal horn of deafferented rats.

Effects of morphine on the spontaneous activity of dorsal horn neurons in the deafferented rat

Most of the rats developed scratching behaviour after the dorsal rhizotomy. As shown in Fig. 5, the scratching wounds were situated in partially afferented areas adjacent to the deafferented zone but sometimes spread to the totally insensitive zone.

As previously described (Lombard and Larabi, 1983) dorsal horn neurons in deafferented rats have a relatively high level of background activity (Fig. 5) which generally consists of spontaneous bursting activity and/or long lasting discharges.

Total population (Fig. 4)

The mean frequency of the control spontaneous firing rate for the 28 neurons studied was 26.01 ± 4.46 impulses per second. Morphine (2 mg/kg I.V.) did not produce a significant change in the spontaneous firing rate while for the 18 neurons which received an additional dose of 4 mg/kg I.V. (total dose 6 mg/kg), given 10 to 20 minutes after the initial injection, the activity was decreased to $68.86 \pm 9.78\%$ of the control values ($P < 0.001$). The maximum depressive effect of morphine was present 5 minutes after injection.

Morphine-sensitive depressed cells

In this group we included all 14 neurons influenced either by 2 mg (2 neurons) or 2 + 4 mg/kg of morphine (12 neurons). The depressive effects of morphine were dose

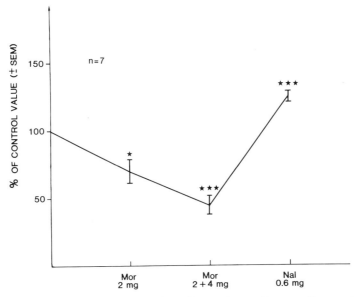

FIGURE 6: Dose-dependent depressive effects of morphine on the spontaneous hyperactivity of seven morphine sensitive depressed cells.

dependent and the mean firing rate was decreased to 76.48±8.39% (P < 0.001) of the control values respectively for 2 and 2 + 4 mg/kg of morphine. In all cases (9 neurons) these effects were clearly reversed by naloxone (0.6 mg/kg I.V.). In addition, 10 minutes after the administration of the opiate antagonist the level of spontaneous activity was significantly greater than the activity recorded before morphine. Fig. 6 illustrates the action of morphine on 7 neurons tested with the two doses of morphine and naloxone.

In order to evaluate the relative roles of pre- and postsynaptic mechanisms in the inhibitory effects of morphine, we have compared these findings with those induced in non-deafferented animals. We have chosen the arthritic rat since dorsal horn neurones have a marked *spontaneous* activity (Menétrey and Besson, 1982) compared to the low levels or complete lack found in normal rats.

Effects of morphine on the spontaneous *activity of dorsal horn neurones in the arthritic rat*

All neurons recorded were characterized as nociceptive non-specific neurones. Each neuron had an input from C fibers. Their mean firing level (35.72±6.62 Hz, n = 13) was similar to that found in deafferented neurons that were inhibited by morphine (28.10±5.78Hz n = 14).

In arthritic rats, morphine 2 mg/kg I.V. strongly depressed the firing of all neurons tested. The firing rate was reduced to 46.03±7.47% (P < 0.001) of the control value. The effects of morphine were reversed by naloxone. It must be emphasized that after naloxone the spontaneous firing rate was markedly increased over the levels recorded before morphine (mean firing: 200.7±29.40% of the control value; P < 0.001). This dose of 2 mg/kg of morphine was twice as effective in the arthritic rat (a 53.97±7.47% decrease of activity) as compared to the deafferented animal (23.52±8.39%), a highly significant difference (P < 0.001) (Fig. 7).

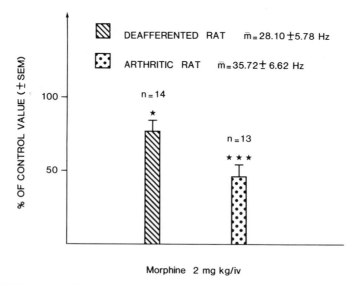

FIGURE 7: Comparison of the effect of 2 mg/kg of morphine on the spontaneous activity of dorsal horn neurons in deafferented and arthritic rats.

DISCUSSION

This study demonstrates a dose-dependent depressive effect of morphine on the hyperactivity of deafferented dorsal horn neuron receptors. This study is the first to demonstrate a post-synaptic effect of morphine following its systemic administration. We have also demonstrated in this study that about 40% of the total number of opioid binding sites are located postsynaptically.

The results from this physiological model using the deafferented animal agree with those from electrophysiological, immunohistochemical and behavioural approaches. As discussed by Willcockson et al (1986) electrophysiological studies have provided several possible postsynaptic actions of morphine. These include an inhibitory or blocking action on receptor-activated sodium channels (Barker et al, 1978, 1980; Zieglgänsberger and Bayerl, 1976; Zieglgänsberger and Tulloch, 1979), an increased potassium conductance (Yoshimura and North, 1983) and an increased chloride conductance (Barker et al, 1980). From immunohistochemical studies it has been clearly established that some lamina I and V dorsal horn neurons at the origin of the spinothalamic tract are directly contacted by enkephalin terminals (Ruda, 1982; Ruda et al, 1984). These connections are considerable in number since 67% of spinothalamic tract neurones in the monkey cervical cord have these terminals (Ruda, 1984). Finally, it has been shown in freely moving mice that intrathecal morphine can suppress the behavioural syndrome (biting and scratching) elicited by intrathecal administration of SP (Hylden and Wilcox, 1983) or excitatory aminoacids (Aanonsen and Wilcox, 1987). This latter result is in good agreement with the fact that iontophoretic morphine depresses the excitatory responses induced by glutamate on primate spinothalamic neurons (Willcockson et al, 1986). Our experiments with systemic morphine in deafferented rats further support a postsynaptic site of action.

From the comparison of the results obtained in deafferented and arthritic rats, it appears that the removal of presynaptic receptors diminishes by about half the depressive effects of morphine on the spontaneous activity of dorsal horn neurons. It is interesting that the spontaneous activity in the arthritic rat results mainly from a sensitization of peripheral fibres (see discussion in Menétrey and Besson, 1982; Guilbaud *et al*, 1985). These experiments are the first attempts to define physiologically the relative involvement of pre- and postsynaptic mechanisms in the spinal action of morphine. Although speculative, our data suggest that both mechanisms are of similar importance.

These results can also explain why morphine is more effective in combating pain originating in nociceptors than it is for pain arising from deafferentation. In fact, despite the paucity of clinical studies, morphine has a reputation for minimal effects on this latter type of pain (Tasker, 1984). This is supported by a recent study of Arner and Meyerson (1988) assessing the responsiveness of different types of chronic pain (including deafferentation) to intravenous opioids in a placebo controlled double-blind randomized trial. Theoretically these results are somewhat surprising since even though the spinal action seems reduced in the deafferented rat, it is difficult to exclude direct supraspinal actions of morphine on areas rich in opioid receptors. Obviously there is a need for future clinical investigations to answer this question clearly.

REFERENCES

AANONSEN, L. M., WILCOX, G. L., (1987) Nociceptive action of excitatory aminoacids in the mouse: effects of spinally administered opioids, phencyclidine and sigma agonists. *J.Pharmacol. Exp. Ther.*, **243** 9-19.

ARNER, S. AND MEYERSON, B. A., (1988). Lack of analgesic effect of opioids on neuropathic and idiopathic forms of pain. *Pain*, **33**, 11-23.

ARONIN, N., DIFIGLIA, M., LIOTTA, A. S., AND MARTIN, J. S. (1981). Ultrastructural localization and biochemical features of immunoreactive leu-enkephalin in monkey dorsal horn. *J. Neurosci.* **1**, 561-577.

ATWEH, S. F. AND KUHAR, M. J. (1977). Autoradiographic localization of opiate receptors in rat brain. I. Spinal cord and lower medulla. *Brain Res.*, **124**, 53-67.

BARKER, J. L., GRUOL, D. L., HUANG, M., MACDONALD, J. F., AND SMITH, T. G. (1980). Peptide receptor functions on cultured spinal neurons. In *Neural Peptides and Neuronal Communications.* E. Costa and M. Trabucchi, eds., pp. 409-423, Raven Press, New York.

BARKER, J. L., SMITH, T. G. AND NEALE, J. H. (1978). Multiple membrane actions of enkephalin revealed using cultured spinal neurons. *Brain Res.*, 154-158.

BESSON, J. M. AND CHAOUCH, A. (1987). Peripheral and spinal mechanisms of nociception. *Physiol. Rev.*, **67**, 67-185.

CSILLIK, B. AND KNYIHAR-CSILLIK, E. (1986). *The Protean Gate.* Akademiai Kiado, Budapest.

CZLONKOWSKI, A., COSTA, T., PRZEWLOCKI, R., PASI, A. AND HERZ, A. (1983). Opiate receptor binding sites in human spinal cord. *Brain Res.* **267**, 392-296.

DAVAL, G., VERGE, D. AND BASBAUM, A. I., BOURGOIN, S. AND HAMON, M. (1987). Autoradiographic evidence of serotonin binding sites on primary afferent fibres in the dorsal horn of the rat spinal cord. *Neurosci. Lett.*, **83**, 71-76.

DELAY-GOYET, P., ROQUES, B. P. AND ZAJAC, J. M. (1987). Differences of binding characteristics of non-selective opiates towards μ and δ receptors types. *Life Sci.*,**441**, 723-731.

DUGGAN, A. W., HALL, J. W. AND HEADLEY, P. M. (1977). Suppression of transmission of nociceptive impulses by morphine: selective effects of morphine administered in the region of the substantia gelatinosa. *Brit. J. Pharmacol.*, **61**, 65-

76.

DUGGAN, A. W. AND NORTH, R. A. (1984). Electrophysiology of opioids, *Pharmacol. Rev.*, **35**, 219-281.

FIELDS, H. L., EMSON, P. C., LEIGH, B. K., GILBERT, R. F.T. AND IVERSEN, L. L. (1980). Multiple opiate receptor sites on primary afferent fibres. *Nature*, **284**, 351-353.

FITZGERALD, M. (1984). The course and termination of primary afferent fibers. In *Textbook of Pain*. Edited by P. D. Wall and R. Melzack, Churchill Linvingstone, pp. 34-48.

GAMSE, R., HOLZER, P. AND LEMBECK, F. (1979). Indirect evidence for presynaptic location of opiate receptors on chemosensitive primary sensory neurones. *Naunyn-Schmiedeberg's Arch. Pharmacol.*, **308**, 281-285.

GOODMAN, R. R., SNYDER, S. H., KUHAR, S. H. AND YOUNG, W. S. III (1980). Differentiation of d and μ opiate receptor localization by light microscopic autoradiography, *Proc. Natl. Acad. Sci. U.S.A.*, **77**, 6239-6243.

GOUARDERES, C., CROS, J. AND QUIRION, R. (1985). Autoradiographic localization of μ, δ and κ opioid receptor binding sites in rat and guinea pig spinal cord. *Neuropeptides*, **6**, 331-342.

GUILBAUD, G., IGGO, A. AND TEGNER, R. (1985). Sensory receptors in ankle joint capsules of normal and arthritic rats. *Exp. Brain Res.*, **58**, 29-40.

HILLER, J. M., SIMON, E. J., CRAIN, S. M. AND PETERSEN, E. R. (1978). Opiate receptors in cultures of fetal mouse dorsal root ganglia (DRG) and spinal cord: Predominance.in DRG neurites. *Brain Res.*, **145**, 396-400.

HÖKFELT, T., LJUNGDAHL, A.,TERENIUS, L., ELDE, R. AND NILSSON, G. (1977). Immunohistochemical analysis of peptide pathways possibly related to pain and analgesia: enkephalin and substance P. *Proc. Nat. Acad. Sci. U. S.A.*, **74**, 3081-3085.

HUNT, S. P., KELLY, J. S. AND EMSON, P. C. (1980). The electron microscopic localization of methionine enkephalin within the superficial layers (I and II) of the spinal cord. *Neuroscience* **5**, 1871-1890.

HYLDEN, J. L. K. AND WILCOX, G. L. (1983). Pharmacological characterization of substance P-induced nociception in mice: modulation by opioid and noradrenergic agonists at the spinal level. *J. Pharmacol. Exp. Ther.*, **226**, 398-404.

JESSELL, T. M. AND IVERSEN, L. L. (1977). Opiate analgesics inhibit substance P release from rat trigeminal nucleus. *Nature*, **268**, 549-551.

JESSELL, T., TSUNOO, A., KANAZAWA, I. AND OTSUKA, K. (1979). Substance P: Depletion in the dorsal horn of rat spinal cord after section of the peripheral processes of primary sensory neurons. *Brain Res.*, **168**, 247-259.

LAMOTTE, C., PERT, C. B. AND SNYDER, S. H. (1976). Opiate receptor binding in primate spinal cord; Distribution and changes after dorsal root section. *Brain Res.*, **112**, 407-412.

LE BARS, D. AND BESSON, J. M. (1981). The spinal site of action of morphine in pain relief: from basic research to clinical applications. *Trends in Pharmacol. Sciences* **2**, 323-325.

LOMBARD, M. C. AND LARABI, Y. (1983). Electrophysiological study of cervical dorsal horn cells in partially deafferented rat. In *Advances in pain Research and therapy*, vol.5 , edited by J. J. Bonica *et al*, Raven Press, New York, pp. 147-153.

MACDONALD, R. L. AND NELSON, P. G. (1978). Specific opiate-induced depression of transmitter release from dorsal root ganglion cells in culture. *Science*, **199**,1449-

11451.

MACK, K. J. KILLIAN, A. AND NEYHENMEYER, J. A. (1984). Comparison of μ, δ and κ opiate binding sited in rat brain and spinal cord. *Life Sci.*, **34**, 281-285.

MÉNÉTREY, D. AND BESSON, J. M. (1982). Electrophysiological characteristics of dorsal horn cells in rats with cutaneous inflammation resulting from chronic arthritis. *Pain*, **13**, 343-364.

MORRIS, B. J. AND HERZ, A. (1987). Distinct distribution of opioid receptor types in rat lumbar spinal cord. *Naumyn-Schmiedeberg's Arch. Pharmacol.*, **336**, 240-243.

MORTON, C. R., ZHAO, Z.Q. AND DUGGAN, A. (1987). Kelatorphan potentiates the effect of (Met) enkephalin in the substantia gelatinosa of the cat spinal cord. *Eur. J. Pharmacol.*, **140**, 195-201.

MUDGE, A. W., LEEMAN, S. E. AND FISCHBACH, G. D. (1979). Enkephalin inhibits release of substance P from sensory neurons in culture and decreases action potential duration. *Proc. Natl. Acad. Sci. U.S.A.*, **76**, 526-530.

NAGY, J. I., VINCENT, S. R., STAINES, W. M., FIBIGER, H. C., REISINE, T. D. AND YAMAMURA, H. I. (1980). Neurotoxic action of capsaicin on spinal substance P neurons. *Brain Res.*, **186**, 435-444.

NINKOVIC, M., HUNT, S. P. AND GLEAVE, J. R. W. (1982). Localization of opiate and histamine H1-receptors in the primate sensory ganglia and spinal cord. *Brain Research*, **241**, 197-206.

NINKOVIC, M., HUNT, S. P. AND KELLY, J. S. (1981). Effect of dorsal rhizotomy on autoradiographic distribution of opiate and neurotensin receptors and neurotensin-like immunoreactivity within the rat spinal cord. *Brain Res.*, **230**, 111-119.

PEARSON, J., BRANDEIS, L., SIMON, E. AND HILLER, J. (1980). Radioautography of binding of tritiated diprenorphine to opiate receptors in the rat. *Life Sciences* **26**, 1047-1052.

PERT, C. B., KUHAR, M. J. AND SNYDER, S. H. (1975). Autoradiographic localization of the opiate receptor in rat brain. *Life Sci.*, **16**, 1849-1854.

PERT, C. B. KUHAR, M. J. AND SNYDER, S. H. (1976). Opiate receptor: Autoradiographic localization in rat brain. *Proc. Natl. Acad. Sci. U.S.A.*, **73**, 3729-3733.

RUDA, M. A. (1982). Opiates and pain pathways: demonstration of enkephalin synapses on dorsal horn projection neurones, *Science*, **215**, 1523-1525.

RUDA, M. A., COFFIELD, J. AND DUBNER, R. (1984). Demonstration of postsynaptic opioid modulation of thalamic projection neurons by the combined techniques of retrograde horseradish peroxidase and enkephalin immunohistochemistry, *J. Neurosci.*, **4**, 2117-2132.

SASTRY, B. R. (1979). Presynaptic effects of morphine and methionine-enkephalin in feline spinal cord. *Neuropharmacology*, **18**, 367-375.

SLATER, P. AND PATEL, S. (1983). Autoradiographic localization of opiate κ receptors in the rat spinal cord. *Eur. J. Pharmacol.*, **92**, 159-160.

TASKER, R. R. (1984). Deafferentation. In *Textbook of Pain*. Edited by P. D. Wall and R. Melzack, Churchill Linvingstone, pp. 119-132.

TRAYNOR, J. R. AND WOOD, M. S. (1987). Distribution of opioid binding sites in spinal cord. *Neuropeptides*, **10**, 313-320.

WAKSMAN, G., HAMEL, E., DELAY-GOYET, P. AND ROQUES, B. P. (1987). Neutral endopeptidase 24.11, μ and δ opioid receptors after selective brain lesions: an autoradiographic study. *Brain Res.*, **436**, 205-216.

WAKSMAN, G., HAMEL, E., FOURNIE-ZALUSKI, M. C. AND ROQUES, B. P. (1986). Autoradiographic comparison of the distribution of the neutral endopeptidase *enkephalinase* and of μ and δ opioid receptors in rat brain. *Proc. Natl. Acad. Sci. (USA)*, **86**, 1523-1527.

WAMSLEY, J. K. (1983) Opioid receptors: autoradiography. *Physiol. Rev.* **35**, 69-83

WAMSLEY, J. K., ZARBIN, M. A., YOUNG, W. S. AND MUHAR, M. J. (1982). Distribution of opiate receptors in the monkey brain: an autoradiographic study. *Neurosci.*, **7**, 595-613.

WILLCOCKSON, W. S., KIM, J., SHIN, H. K., CHUNG, J. M. AND WILLIS, W. D. (1986). Actions of opioids on primate spinothalamic tract neurones. *J. Neurosci.*, **6**, 2509-2520.

YAKSH, T. L. AND NOUEIED, R. (1985). The physiology and pharmacology of spinal opiates. *Ann. Rev. Pharmacol. Toxicol.*, **25**, 433-462.

YOUNG, W. S. III, WAMSLEY, J. K., ZARBIN, M. A. AND KUHAR, M. J. (1980). Opioid receptors undergo axonal flow. *Science*, **210**, 76-77.

YOSHIMURA, M. AND NORTH, R. A. (1983). Substantia gelatinosa neurones hyperpolarized in vitro by enkephalin. *Nature*, **305**, 529-530.

ZAJAC, J. M., GACEL, J., PETIT, F., DODEY, P., ROSSIGNOL, P. AND ROQUES, B. P. (1983). Deltakephalin, TYR-D-THR-GLY-PHE-LEU-THR: A new highly potent and fully specific agonist for opiate-receptors. *Biochem. Biophys. Res. Comm.*, **11**, 390-397.

ZAJAC, J. M. AND ROQUES, B. P. (1989). Properties required for reversible and irreversible radiolabelled probes for selective characterization of brain receptors and peptidase by autoradiography. In *Brain imaging: Techniques and Applications,* Eds. Shariff, N. A. and Lewis, M. E., Ellis Horwood Ltd.

ZIEGLGANSBERGER, W. (1986). Central control of nociception. In: *Handbook of Physiology, The nervous system* **IV**. V. B. Mountcastle, F. E. Bloom, S. R. Geiger (eds.), Williams and Wilkins, Baltimore.

ZIEGLGANSBERGER, W. AND BAYERL, H. (1976). The mechanism of inhibition of neuronal activity by opiates in the spinal cord of the cat. *Brain Res.*, **115**, 111-128.

ZIEGLGANSBERGER, W. AND TULLOCH, I. F. (1979). The effects of methionine- and leucine-enkephalin on spinal neurones of the cat. *Brain Res.*, **167**, 53-64.

NEURONAL PLASTICITY IN THE SUPERFICIAL DORSAL HORN FOLLOWING PERIPHERAL TISSUE INFLAMMATION AND NERVE INJURY

R. Dubner, J.L.K. Hylden, R.L. Nahin and R.J. Traub

Neurobiology and Anesthesiology Branch, National Institute of Dental Research, National Institutes of Health, Bethesda MD 20892, U.S.A.

INTRODUCTION

Inflammation and hyperalgesia are common components of many acute and chronic pain conditions including postsurgical acute pain, cancer pain and arthritis. Pathological changes in peripheral nerve produced by trauma, metabolic disorders or viral infections sometimes result in painful neuropathies characterized by spontaneous pain, hyperalgesia and allodynia. Experimental studies in which the effects of peripheral tissue inflammation are compared with the effects of nerve injury on neuronal responsiveness in the peripheral and central nervous systems should provide insights into our understanding of the pathophysiology associated with these acute and chronic pain conditions.

Numerous animal studies in the last two decades have examined the electrophysiological responses of spinal and medullary dorsal horn neurons to noxious stimulation (Dubner and Bennett, 1983). Neurons that respond exclusively to noxious stimuli (nociceptive-specific, NS) and those that respond to innocuous stimuli, but maximally to noxious stimuli (wide-dynamic-range, WDR), are found in the superficial and deep layers of the dorsal horn. Subpopulations of these neurons send major projections to the thalamus, the midbrain and the medulla. Both NS and WDR neurons receive input from peripheral nociceptive afferents (Dubner and Bennett, 1983). Several laboratories have examined changes in the responsiveness of cutaneous peripheral nociceptive afferents following inflammation and tissue damage or after nerve injury (Dubner and Bennett, 1983; Devor, 1984; Raja et al, 1984; LaMotte et al, 1982). Unmyelinated and myelinated cutaneous nociceptive afferents exhibit increases in spontaneous activity and greater sensitivity to innocuous and noxious stimuli following inflammation. These peripheral nervous system changes are thought to account, at least in part, for the hyperalgesia and spontaneous pain associated with cutaneous inflammation. In addition, peripheral nerve injury leads to neuroma formation and primary afferents that exhibit spontaneous activity, increased mechanosensitivity and responsiveness to sympathetic efferent activity. Such changes may explain some of the pain associated with various neuropathies. Few studies have examined the responses of dorsal horn nociceptive neurons following cutaneous tissue inflammation (Menétrey and Besson, 1982; Calvino *et al*, 1987). Some investigators have produced experimental neuromas but have focused their attention on cells in the dorsal horn that respond to innocuous stimuli (Devor and Wall, 1981; Lisney, 1983; Pubols, 1984; Brown *et al*, 1984) rather than examining the effects of nerve transection on the responses of dorsal horn nociceptive neurons.

It is important to determine whether the changes in the peripheral nervous system associated with cutaneous tissue or nerve injury are reflected in the activity of different

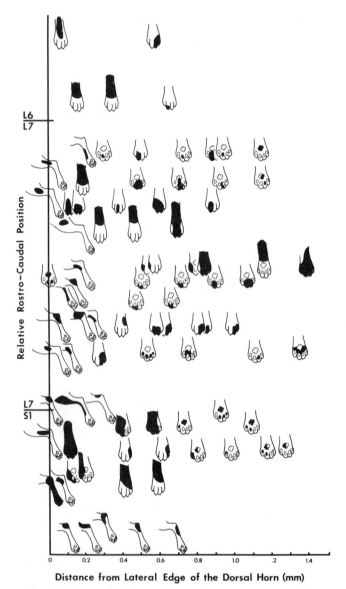

Distance from Lateral Edge of the Dorsal Horn (mm)

FIGURE 1: Receptive fields of lamina I neurons recorded from control cats. The borders of spinal segment L7 are indicated on the ordinate which represents the lateral boundary of the dorsal horn. The medial boundary of the dorsal horn (right side of the figure) was located 1.0 to 1.4 mm from the lateral edge depending on the rostrocaudal position. The sketches of the receptive fields are placed according to the mediolateral and rostrocaudal positions from which they were recorded. Each row of sketches gives the results of a series of electrode penetrations in a single animal. Data from several cats are combined (n=4). From Hylden *et al* (1987).

subpopulations of dorsal horn neurons and whether there are alterations in dorsal horn activity that cannot be explained by these peripheral neural changes. We chose to examine the effects of cutaneous inflammation and nerve injury on an identified nociceptive cell population found in rat, cat and monkey. Dorsal horn lamina I consists of many neurons that respond exclusively or maximally to noxious stimuli and project via the dorsolateral funiculus to the thalamus, midbrain and bulbar reticular formation (Hylden *et al*, this volume). The lamina I component of the spinothalamic and spinomesencephalic tracts in rat and cat is almost exclusively represented by NS neurons. Lamina I neurons in these tracts were identified in the present study by antidromic stimulation of their axons at C2 spinal cord levels and by electrical stimulation of the sciatic nerve. We have examined the response properties of this nociceptive subpopulation in two models of injury (Hylden *et al*, 1987, 1989). First, we induced neuroma formation in the cat by tightly ligating and transecting the common sciatic nerve. The nerve was cut distal to the ligation and drawn into a polyethylene tube to promote neuroma formation (Aguayo *et al*, 1973). Electrophysiological data were obtained from 12 animals with 20 to 82 day-old neuromata. An additional 8 control animals were studied, three of them following acute section of the sciatic nerve. Second, we studied the properties of these same neurons in the rat spinal dorsal horn 4 hours to five days following the injection of complete Freund's adjuvant (CFA) into the plantar surface of the hindpaw. CFA results in edema and hyperalgesia of the limb that peaks in 4-6 hours and persists for more than five days (Iadarola *et al*, 1988). Although there is deep tissue inflammation accompanying the injection of CFA, we have concentrated on the cutaneous inflammation as assessed behaviorally and the reflection of these cutaneous changes in the defined subpopulation of lamina I neurons. We also examined the receptive field properties of cutaneous primary afferent nociceptive afferents following adjuvant-induced inflammation. In addition, there are changes in dynorphin gene expression and dynorphin peptide content localized to the ipsilateral lumbar dorsal horn during the same time period (Iadarola *et al*, 1988; Ruda *et al*, 1988).

ALTERED RESPONSIVENESS IN THE CAT FOLLOWING NEUROMA FORMATION

A total of 95 neurons in the superficial dorsal horn were studied in intact control animals (n=5). Seventy-five percent were classified as NS and 24 percent as WDR neurons. All neurons were activated by electrical stimulation of the sciatic nerve at latencies consistent with input from A-δ and C fibers. Receptive fields were generally small and most commonly located on one or more toes or toe pads (Fig. 1). Few receptive fields (6 of 95) included some aspect of the leg proximal to the ankle. Figure 1 illustrates the somatotopic organization of the receptive fields. Cells with receptive fields on the toes occupied the medial two-thirds of lamina I and comprised the majority of sciatic nerve-innervated cells. Cells with receptive fields on the foot or ankle, or both, were located more laterally. Cells with receptive fields on the upper leg and thigh were recorded only in the one or two most lateral electrode penetrations within 0.2 mm of the lateral edge of the dorsal horn.

Acute transection of the sciatic nerve in three animals resulted in an almost complete lack of receptive fields for lamina I neurons. Only 2 of 54 cells activated by sciatic nerve stimulation proximal to the transection had receptive fields. These two cells responded to stimulation of the lateral thigh and were located on the lateral edge of the dorsal horn. Those cells located in the medial three-fourths of the dorsal horn that normally receive input from the toes and feet were not activated by peripheral

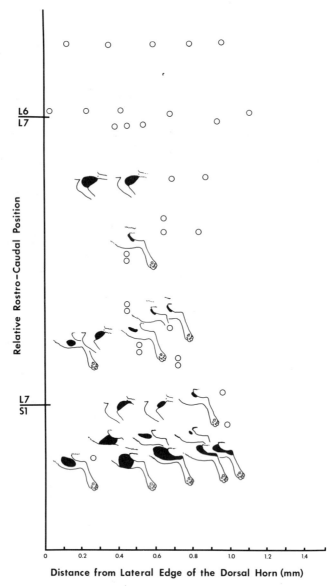

FIGURE 2: Receptive fields of lamina I neurons from cats with chronic transections of the ipsilateral sciatic nerve. Same boundaries of the figure as in Fig. 1. Open circles indicate the position of cells with no apparent receptive field. Data from several cats with chronic nerve section 2 or more months earlier (n=4). From Hylden et al(1987).

stimuli and were identified only by their response to sciatic nerve stimulation or by antidromic stimulation.

Seventy five cells located in lamina I of the dorsal horn, ipsilateral to sciatic transection performed 20-82 days previously, had very different responses. First, two-thirds had no receptive fields and could only be identified by their response to electrical stimulation of the sciatic nerve proximal to the ligation or by antidromic stimulation. The remaining cells (24 of 75) could be activated by cutaneous stimulation and were mainly classified as NS (60%) or WDR (24%) neurons. All the responding cells had

432

receptive fields proximal to the ankle. Their responses were usually atypical in that they were difficult to reproduce with repeated stimulation, exhibited bursting responses followed by silent periods or had shifting receptive fields. Only two cells responded to pressure on the neuroma itself. Two of ten cats had a higher than average number of lamina I cells with ongoing spontaneous activity. The mediolateral distribution of cells recorded from 4 cats with chronic (2 months) neuromata is shown in Fig. 2. Cells with proximal receptive fields were not concentrated at the lateral edge of the dorsal horn, but were observed medially, as well. All the sampling methods were the same; fewer total cells were recorded in the neuroma animals than in the intact control animals. Therefore, statistics were performed on the proportion of cells with proximal receptive fields at each mediolateral position. The mediolateral distribution of cells with proximal receptive fields in animals with chronic sciatic transection was significantly different from that of intact control animals (Chi square, $p < 0.01$). Figure 3 shows the incidence of proximal receptive fields in control, acute and chronic nerve section animals. The mean percentage of cells with proximal receptive fields in 12 animals with chronic sciatic section was significantly greater than that observed in intact controls ($p < 0.05$, t-test).

These data indicate that the somatotopic organization of the superficial dorsal horn changes after chronic peripheral deafferentation. Our conclusions are drawn from three lines of evidence: 1) the frequency of lamina I neurons with proximal receptive fields increases following chronic deafferentation; 2) the mediolateral distribution of cells with proximal receptive fields shifts medially following these lesions; and 3) many neurons exhibit irregular physiological responses as compared to intact control cats. These findings support those of others (Devor and Wall, 1981; Lisney, 1983; Snow and Wilson, 1985) who reported similar changes in the deeper layers of the dorsal horn in low threshold mechanoreceptive as well as some nociceptive neurons.

We were disappointed not to find any changes in the excitability of the lamina I neurons that might account for the hyperalgesia and allodynia found in human painful peripheral neuropathies. Only two cells responded to pressure on the neuroma and only two of ten animals with chronic neuromata exhibited an increase in ongoing spontaneous activity, suggesting that activity from the neuromata may not be reflected in the responses of lamina I neurons. In addition, these two cats did not exhibit any behaviors that might indicate they were in pain. In fact, sciatic nerve ligation did not produce any signs of hyperalgesia or allodynia in any of the cats. In contrast, experimental nerve lesions in which there is only partial disruption of peripheral nerve fibers do produce behavioral hyperalgesia and allodynia in rats and may prove to be more useful models for examining central nervous system changes associated with pain (Bennett and Xie, 1988; Bennett et al, this volume).

ALTERED RESPONSIVENESS IN THE CAT FOLLOWING ADJUVANT-INDUCED INFLAMMATION

Complete Freund's adjuvant (CFA) injected into the hindpaw of a rat produces an intense inflammation, characterized by erythema, edema and hyperalgesia, which lasts for several days (Iadarola et al, 1988). The inflammation is limited to the injected paw and the animals exhibit normal grooming and locomotor behavior except for guarding of the inflamed paw. This model of inflammation was approved by the Institute Animal Care and Use Committee and the experiments conform to the guidelines proposed by the International Association for the Study of Pain (Zimmermann, 1983). The time course of the edema and hyperalgesia associated with the inflammation was assessed by measuring the paw diameter with calipers and by assessing the withdrawal latency to a radiant heat stimulus presented through the glass floor of a chamber to which the rats had been acclimated (Hargreaves *et al*, 1988). Typically, paw diameter increased by 40% within 6 hours after CFA injection and remained elevated for more than 5 days. The animals' paw withdrawal latency to the radiant heat stimulus decreased from a preinjection baseline of 9-10 sec to 2-3 sec within 6 hours after CFA treatment. This change in latency corresponds to a decrease in withdrawal threshold; the temperature at which the animals withdraw their paws is reduced from 45°C to 39°C (Hargreaves *et al*, 1988). Paw withdrawal latencies were still reduced at 24 hours (about 3 sec) but began to approach control values by 5 days (6-7 sec). We concentrated on the characterization of neuronal responses to cutaneous stimulation since one of our major behavioral measures, hyperalgesia, was in response to heating of the skin.

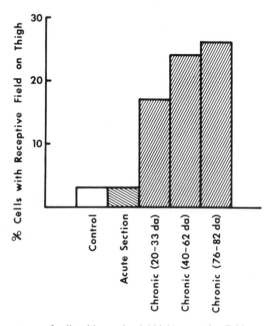

FIGURE 3: Percentage of cells with proximal (thigh) receptive fields recorded in control (n=5) animals and after acute (n=3) or chronic nerve transection (n=4 in each of 3 time periods). No effort was made to correct for mediolateral position of cells. The number of neurons per column ranges from 15 to 95. From Hylden *et al*(1987).

Twenty-nine neurons identified as lamina I projection neurons by antidromic stimulation were studied in control rats. They were classified as NS (93%) or WDR (7%). All neurons were activated by electrical stimulation of the sciatic nerve at latencies consistent with primary afferent input from A-δ and C fibers. Receptive fields were located on one or more toes on the dorsal, ventral or lateral surfaces of the paw (Fig. 4A). Spontaneous activity was recorded in a few cells, but was never more than 1-2 Hz. Noxious heat thresholds ranged from 43-50°C with a mean of 47°C (n=19). Mechanical thresholds measured with von Frey filaments averaged 5.4 grams force (54 mN). Thirty-seven lamina I projection neurons were studied in rats that received injections of CFA 5 days earlier. Almost all were NS neurons (98%) and had thermal and mechanical thresholds similar to NS neurons encountered in control rats. However, they often had more complex receptive fields than those observed in control rats

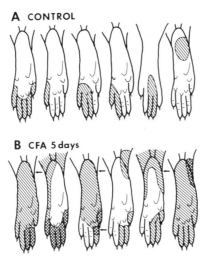

A CONTROL

B CFA 5 days

FIGURE 4: Some examples of receptive fields of lamina I projection neurons recorded in control rats (A) and 5 days after injection of CFA (B). Lamina I neurons in rats with inflamed hindpaws tended to have larger receptive fields, often including the entire surface of the foot. In addition, many of these cells had complex receptive field patterns including areas of differing sensitivity (different shading in sketches), discontinuous receptive fields or responses to joint movement (arrows). From Hylden *et al* (1988).

(Fig.4B). About 50% of the neurons had one or more of the following: discontinuous fields, fields with areas of differing sensitivity to mechanical stimulation measured with von Frey filaments, or they responded to joint movement as well as to cutaneous input. In addition, the receptive fields from the inflamed paws were 2.4 times larger than the receptive fields on control hindpaws (Fig. 4B, 5) as demonstrated by thermal and electrical in addition to mechanical stimulation. Control rats mostly had small receptive fields whereas cells in 5 day CFA-treated rats varied in size with some including the entire surface of the hindpaw (Fig. 5). There was also a significant increase in the number of cells exhibiting spontaneous activity as compared to control animals (87% *vs* 24%, $p < 0.05$, Chi square). Noxious mechanical and thermal thresholds throughout the new receptive field were unchanged as compared with control animals.

We studied the properties of 25 lamina I projection neurons from 4 to 8.5 hours after CFA injection into the hindpaw. All were classified as NS neurons. The response properties of neurons encountered early in this time period (< 6 hours, n=9) were essentially the same as those in control animals. In the period from 6-8.5 hours (n=16), the response properties resembled lamina I cells studied in the 5 day CFA-injected rats. The percentage of cells exhibiting spontaneous activity was significantly increased over controls (87% *vs* 24%, $p < 0.05$, Chi square) and there was an expansion of receptive field size (Fig. 5) in comparison to control animals ($p < 0.05$, ANOVA/Dunnett's). Although mechanical thresholds were unchanged, noxious heat thresholds were significantly decreased as compared to controls (mean of 44°C versus 47°C; $p < 0.05$, ANOVA/Dunnett's).

Figure 6 illustrates the receptive fields of two lamina I neurons that were observed for two hours beginning approximately 5 hours after CFA injection. The receptive fields first included some of the toes plus an adjacent area of the plantar surface of the foot. Within 30 min, both receptive fields had expanded to include more of the ventral surface of the foot as well as the heel and ankle area. The receptive field of one of the

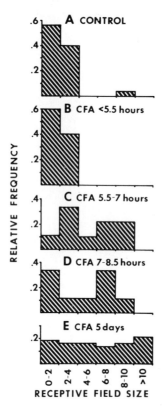

FIGURE 5: The distribution of receptive field size of lamina I projection neurons in control rats (A) and at the indicated times after the injection of CFA into the ipsilateral hindpaw. Receptive field size was normalized to account for the size of the hindpaw in different animals; the area of the ventral surface of the paw was set equal to 10. Relative frequency indicates the fraction of the total number of cells in each histogram bin. The total number of cells in each bin were : A: 27 cells; B, C, D: 8 cells; F: 38 cells. ANOVA across the time periods indicated in B-D showed a significant main effect of time on receptive field size (p < 0.05). From Hylden *et al* (1988).

cells continued to expand (Fig. 6A) until almost the entire surface area of the foot was included. Von Frey thresholds did not appear to change during this time period. Noxious heat thresholds were not determined.

In preliminary experiments, we have investigated the response properties of A-δ and C primary cutaneous nociceptive afferents following inflammation by recording activity from the dorsal root ganglion approximately 24 hours after CFA injection into the hindpaw. We have found no evidence of enlarged receptive fields of either A-δ or C nociceptive cutaneous afferents recorded from rats with inflamed paws. Receptive fields were single 1-3 mm spots in both control and CFA rats. Mechanical thresholds were similar in both groups and comparable to those of dorsal horn lamina I neurons. Noxious heat thresholds were not determined. Previous studies have revealed that C nociceptive cutaneous afferents exhibit sensitization to heat stimuli following inflammation (Kocher *et al*, 1987). We suspect that further study of primary C nociceptive afferents in the present model would reveal similar effects.

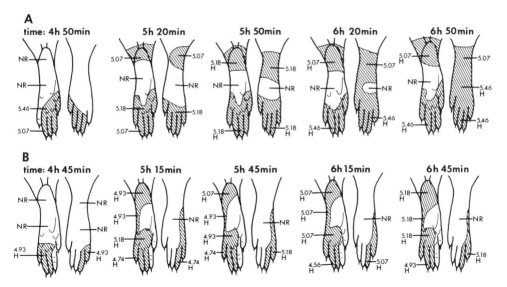

FIGURE 6: The receptive field properties of two lamina I projection neurons were monitored for a 2 hour period approximately 5 to 7 hours after CFA injection. Each pair of sketches represents a dorsal and ventral view of the injected hindpaw and the apparent receptive field at that time. Mechanical thresholds were determined with von Frey filaments and the force in log units (10 times the force in mg) is indicated near the shaded regions. Response to heat was determined using a radiant heat lamp which heated an area of skin less than 5 mm in diameter. H indicates a response to heat. NR indicates no response to mechanical stimulation. From Hylden et al (1988).

These findings in rats indicate that CFA-induced behavioral hyperalgesia and edema correlate with changes in the activity of lamina I dorsal horn neurons. The expansion of receptive fields, the increase in spontaneous activity, and the increased sensitivity to thermal stimuli occurred in parallel with the peak effects on hyperalgesia and edema which occurred within 6 hours of CFA treatment. The responses of dorsal horn lamina I neurons in polyarthritic rats also exhibit increases in spontaneous activity and atypical responses (Ménétrey and Besson, 1982). However, these authors found lowered thresholds to mechanical stimulation of edematous tissue and higher thresholds to radiant heat. This is in contrast to our own findings of lowered thresholds to heat and no change in mechanical sensitivity in the zone of inflammation. We found no evidence that NS neurons had lowered mechanical thresholds nor did we find an increased incidence of WDR projection neurons in lamina I following inflammation. The different models used and the different assessment methods employed in the two studies may account for these variant findings. A more recent study in polyarthritic rats from the same laboratory has focused on the responses of neurons in laminae IV-VI (Calvino et al, 1987). In addition to confirming the findings of Ménétrey and Besson (1982), an expansion of the classical excitatory receptive fields of these neurons was noted, similar to our findings in lamina I following CFA-induced inflammation. Our preliminary findings in the inflammation model suggest that the expansion of receptive fields of lamina I neurons cannot be explained by alterations in the receptive field size of primary nociceptive afferents. In addition, we found no evidence of increased mechanical sensitivity of primary nociceptive afferents following inflammation, similar to previous reports (Reeh et al, 1986; Kocher et al, 1987). In contrast, inflammation induced by carrageenan or mustard oil has been shown to produce increases in spontaneous activity and heat sensitivity of C nociceptive afferents in the rat hindlimb (Reeh *et al*, 1986; Kocher *et al*, 1987) and sensitization of peripheral nociceptors may account at least in part for similar increases in responsivity of lamina I neurons in the CFA-induced inflammation model.

DISCUSSION AND CONCLUSIONS

One of the major findings in these studies was that both sciatic nerve transection and CFA-induced inflammation produce an expansion of the receptive field zones of lamina I neurons. We asked the question whether this expansion of receptive fields can be accounted for entirely by peripheral mechanisms or whether changes central to the peripheral receptor or peripheral nerve are necessary to explain the findings. In neither instance is the expansion explained by changes in the receptive fields of primary afferents. Following chronic sciatic nerve transection, approximately 25% of lamina I neurons activated by sciatic nerve electrical stimulation exhibited receptive fields that suggested an activation of these neurons by input from the saphenous or posterior cutaneous nerve territories on the proximal limb. There is no evidence for such a major redistribution of neighboring peripheral nerve terminals in the sciatic cutaneous territory following sciatic nerve crush, nor is there evidence for a redistribution of central terminals of peripheral nerves following sciatic nerve section (Devor and Claman, 1980; Seltzer and Devor, 1984). Therefore, the receptive field changes following chronic sciatic nerve transection are possibly explained by functional reorganization in the dorsal horn.

There are a number of changes occurring at the peripheral site of cutaneous inflammation that might account for the expansion of receptive fields of lamina I neurons. First, changes in the tissue environment of nociceptors, produced by the edema, could result in an increase in their responsiveness to mechanical stimuli located at a distance from the actual borders of the receptive field. We ruled out this possibility by recording from peripheral nociceptors and demonstrating no change in the size of their receptive fields in CFA-injected rats as compared to control rats. We also ruled out this mechanism by showing that the enlarged receptive fields were sensitive to electrical and thermal stimuli. Second, peripheral sensitization following inflammation (Kocher *et al*, 1987) results in an increase in spontaneous activity and an enhanced response to suprathreshold thermal stimuli. The resulting increase in evoked neuronal barrage produced by thermal stimuli could provide sufficient input at previously ineffective synapses (see below) to activate the lamina I neurons. We ruled out this possibility by activating the neurons with electrical stimuli at similar thresholds throughout the expanded receptive field (Hylden *et al*, 1989). Such stimuli presented outside the small receptive fields found in normal rats were ineffective. Such evidence also rules out the possibility that the enlarged receptive fields can be explained by the sensitization of previously silent and unresponsive afferents (Schaible and Schmidt, 1988). However, the increase in spontaneous activity of many nociceptors providing input to a lamina I neuron following inflammation could produce sufficient membrane depolarization to result in activation by electrical stimuli at previously ineffective synapses. We did find an increase in spontaneous activity of lamina I neurons after CFA injection as compared to controls. We ruled out this third possible explanation based on peripheral receptor changes by anesthetizing most of the receptive field of some neurons leaving only a part of the *expanded* portion of the field intact (Hylden *et al*, 1989). Under this condition, the lamina I projection neurons could still be activated by electrical stimulation with little or no change in threshold. On the basis of the above experimental manipulations, we conclude that the expansion of receptive fields of lamina I neurons following cutaneous inflammation cannot be explained by alterations in peripheral receptor mechanisms, and may involve central mechanisms.

It should be noted that the sciatic nerve transection model results in a reduction in peripheral input to the dorsal horn. We found that few cats with chronic neuromata had an increase in spontaneous activity as compared to control cats, suggesting that spontaneous activity from neuromata was of little consequence, if present at all (Jänig, 1988). In contrast, previous studies indicate that inflammation produces an increase in the nociceptive barrage entering the dorsal horn due to the increased activation of nociceptors (Reeh et al, 1986; Kocher et al, 1987). Can the same mechanisms account for the changes in size of receptive fields in both models? The expansion of receptive fields in the inflammation model occurs too rapidly to be explained by central sprouting of afferent terminals. Although such a mechanism is possible following chronic sciatic nerve transection, there is no evidence that it occurs (Rodin et al, 1983; Rodin and Kruger, 1984; Seltzer and Devor, 1984). The most likely explanations involve either an increase in synaptic efficacy of excitatory inputs or a release of inhibitory inputs resulting in a net increase in excitation in the dorsal horn. Slow and long-term depolarizations in dorsal horn neurons produced by neuropeptides such as substance P (Urban and Randic, 1984) and calcitonin gene-related peptide (Ryu et al, 1988) provide a reasonable mechanism in the inflammation model since these neuropeptides are found in nociceptive afferents and are released during noxious stimulation (Oku et al, 1987). Weak, ineffective, excitatory inputs on distal dendrites and excitatory inputs under presynaptic or postsynaptic inhibitory control would be facilitated during slow depolarization of lamina I nociceptive neurons. Subliminal inputs would reach threshold for excitation resulting in expansion of the apparent receptive field of a dorsal horn neuron. Such an unmasking of previously existing synapses has been produced by electrical stimulation of ineffective inputs (Merrill and Wall, 1972; Mendell et al, 1978; Pubols et al, 1986), punctate burns to the skin (McMahon and Wall, 1984), repetitive electrical stimulation (Cook et al, 1987) and cold block (Dostrovsky et al, 1976).

An increase in excitatory drive produced by slow depolarization is an unlikely explanation for the expansion of receptive fields found after sciatic nerve transection. In this condition, there is a loss of excitatory input and a depletion of primary afferent neuropeptides (Wall et al, 1981). A release of inhibition provides a more likely explanation for the expansion of receptive fields after sciatic nerve transection. The blocking of inhibitory transmitters by picrotoxin or strychnine results in an expansion of receptive fields after acute sciatic denervation (Yokota and Nishikawa, 1979; Saade et al, 1985; Markus and Pomeranz, 1987). Peripheral deafferentation leads to a reduction in the amplitude of the dorsal root potential and primary afferent depolarization (Wall and Devor, 1981) and a reduction in the mechanism of surround inhibition which influences the responses of WDR neurons (Yokota and Nishikawa, 1979). A loss of inhibitory inputs to NS neurons in lamina I could also lead to an expansion of receptive fields. The appearance of proximal limb fields in lamina I NS neurons after sciatic transection may represent such an expansion in the absence of the normal innervation of the sciatic territory (a *doughnut* receptive field as compared to a fully expanded field found following inflammation).

What role do expanded receptive fields play in the appearance of hyperalgesia associated with inflammation and partial deafferentation? Dubner et al (1987) have proposed that WDR neurons are a critical neuronal population in the mechanism of *tic douloureux*. Minor deafferentation in the trigeminal system may lead to an expansion of the low-threshold portions of the receptive fields of WDR neurons so that the temporal and spatial profile of neural activity now mimics that ordinarily produced by noxious stimulation. Thus, a punctate tactile stimulus will be perceived as a sharp, localized, pin-prick or electric shock-like sensation. A similar mechanism may account for the allodynia produced by mild tactile stimulation in cases of partial deafferentation associated with painful neuropathies following traumatic injury (Campbell *et al*, 1988). In both *tic douloureux* and some painful neuropathies, the pain is produced by activation of myelinated low-threshold mechanoreceptive afferents which normally activate WDR neurons. An expansion of these fields and the accompanying loss of inhibitory inputs would produce an increased excitation of these WDR neurons. The finding that there is no increased sensitivity to noxious heat in these painful neuropathies or in *tic douloureux* (Dubner *et al*, 1987) suggests that NS neurons may not play an important role in the hyperalgesia and allodynia associated with these conditions. However, NS neurons may play a role in the hyperalgesia associated with inflammation. The expansion of receptive fields accompanying inflammation may provide an additional mechanism besides primary afferent sensitization to account for the appearance of hyperalgesia. The expanded receptive fields will lead to a greater number of NS or WDR neurons activated by a stimulus. The increase in discharge frequency may ultimately be perceived as more intense pain. A strange paradox in our inflammation model is the absence of increased sensitivity to mechanical stimulation. This parallels the absence of mechanical sensitization of primary nociceptive afferents. The increase in effective input convergence on NS and WDR neurons produced by expanded receptive fields could account for the behavioral hyperalgesia produced by mechanical stimulation in models of inflammation (Millan *et al*, 1986; Hargreaves *et al*, 1988).

REFERENCES

AGUAYO, A.J., PEYRONNARD, J.M. AND BRAY, G.M. (1973). A quantitative ultrastructural study of regeneration from isolated proximal stumps of transected unmyelinated nerves. *Journal of Experimental Neurology* **32**, 256-270.

BENNETT, G.J. AND XIE, Y.-K. (1988). A peripheral mononeuropathy in rat that produces disorders of pain sensation like those seen in man. *Pain* **33**, 87107.

BROWN, A.G., FYFFE, R.E.W., NOBLE, R. AND ROWE, M.J. (1984). Effects of hindlimb nerve section on lumbosacral dorsal horn neurones in the cat. *Journal of Physiology* **354**, 375-394.

CALVINO, B., VILLANUEVA, L. AND LEBARS, D. (1987). Dorsal horn (convergent) neurones in the intact anaesthetized arthritic rat. I. Segmental excitatory influences. *Pain* **28**, 81-98.

CAMPBELL, J.N., RAJA, S.N., MEYER, R.A. AND MACKINNON, S.E. (1988). Myelinated afferents signal the hyperalgesia associated with nerve injury. *Pain* **32**, 89-94.

COOK, A.J., WOOLF, C.J., WALL, P.D. AND MCMAHON, S.B. (1987). Dynamic receptive field plasticity in rat spinal cord dorsal horn following C-primary afferent input. *Nature* **325**, 151-153.

DEVOR, M. (1984). The pathophysiology and anatomy of damaged nerve. In *Textbook of Pain*, eds. WALL, P.D. and MELZACK, M., pp. 49-64. Edinburgh: Churchill Livingstone.

DEVOR, M. AND CLAMAN, D. (1980). Mapping and plasticity of acid phosphatase afferents in the rat dorsal horn. *Brain Research* **190**, 17-28.

DEVOR, M. AND WALL, P.D. (1981). Plasticity in the spinal cord sensory map following peripheral nerve injury in rats. *Journal of Neuroscience* **1**, 679684.

DOSTROVSKY, J.O., MILLAR, J. AND WALL, P.D. (1976). The immediate shift of afferent drive of dorsal column nucleus cells following deafferentation: a comparison of acute and chronic deafferentation in gracile nucleus and spinal cord. *Experimental Neurology* **52**, 480-495.

DUBNER, R., AND BENNETT, G.J. (1983). Spinal and trigeminal mechanisms of nociception. *Annual Review Neuroscience* **6**, 381-418.

DUBNER, R., SHARAV, Y., GRACELY, G.H. AND PRICE, D.D. (1987). Idiopathic trigeminal neuralgia: sensory features and pain mechanisms. *Pain* **31**, 23-33.

HARGREAVES, K., DUBNER, R., BROWN, F., FLORES, C. AND JORIS, J. (1988). A new and sensitive method for measuring thermal nociception in cutaneous hyperalgesia. *Pain* **32**, 77-88.

HYLDEN, J.L.K., NAHIN, R.L. AND DUBNER, R. (1987). Altered responses of nociceptive cat lamina I spinal dorsal horn neurons after chronic sciatic neuroma formation. *Brain Research* **411**, 341-350.

HYLDEN, J.L.K., NAHIN, R.L., TRAUB, R.J. AND DUBNER, R. (1989). Physiological characterization of spinal lamina I projection neurons in rats with unilateral adjuvant-induced inflammation. (submitted)

IADAROLA, M.J., DOUGLASS, J., CIVELLI, O. AND NARANJO, J.R. (1988). Differential activation of spinal cord dynorphin and enkephalin neurons during hyperalgesia: evidence using cDNA hybridization. *Brain Research*, In press.

JANIG, W. (1988). Pathophysiology of nerve following mechanical injury. In *Proceedings of the Fifth World Congress on Pain*, eds. DUBNER, R., GEBHART, G.F. and BOND, M.R., pp. 89-108. Amsterdam: Elsevier.

KOCHER, L., ANTON, F., REEH, P.W. AND HANDWERKER, H.O. (1987). The effect of carrageenan-induced inflammation on the sensitivity of unmyelinated skin nociceptors in the rat. *Pain* **29**, 363-373.

LAMOTTE, R.H., THALHAMMER, J.G., TORBJÖRK, H.E. AND ROBINSON, C.J. (1982). Peripheral neural mechanisms of cutaneous hyperalgesia following mild injury by heat. *Journal of Neuroscience* **2**, 765-781.

LISNEY, S.J.W. (1983). Changes in the somatotopic organization of the cat lumbar spinal cord following peripheral nerve transection and regeneration. *Brain Research* **259**, 31-39.

MARKUS, H. AND POMERANZ, B. (1987). Saphenous has weak ineffective synapses in sciatic territory of rat spinal cord: electrical stimulation of the saphenous or application of drugs reveal these somatotopically inappropriate synapses. *Brain Research* **416**, 315-321.

MCMAHON, S.B. AND WALL, P.D. (1984). Receptive fields of rat lamina I projection cells move to incorporate a nearby region of injury. *Pain* **19**, 235-247.

MENDELL, L.M., SASSOON, E.M. AND WALL, P.D. (1978). Properties of synaptic linkage from long ranging afferents onto dorsal horn neurons in normal and deafferented cats. *Journal of Physiology* **285**, 299-310.

MENÉTREY, D. AND BESSON, J.M. (1982). Electrophysiological characteristics of dorsal horn cells in rats with cutaneous inflammation resulting from chronic arthritis. *Pain* **13**, 343-364.

MERRILL, E.G. AND WALL, P.D. (1972). Factors forming the edge of a receptive field: the presence of relatively ineffective afferent terminals. *Journal of Physiology* **226**, 825-846.

MILLAN, M.J., MILLAN, M.H., CZLONKOWSKI, A., HÖLLT, V., PILCHER, C.W.T., HERZ,

A. AND COLPAERT, F.C. (1986). A model of chronic pain in the rat: Response of multiple opioid systems to adjuvant-induced arthritis. *Journal of Neuroscience* 6, 899-906.

OKU, R., SATOH, M., AND TAKAGI, H. (1987). Release of substance P from the spinal dorsal horn is enhanced in polyarthritic rats. *Neuroscience Letters* 74, 315-319.

PUBOLS, L.M. (1984). The boundary of proximal hindlimb representation in the dorsal horn following peripheral nerve lesions in cats: a reevaluation of plasticity in the somatotopic map. *Somatosensory Research* 2, 19-32.

PUBOLS, L.M., FOGLESONG, M.E. AND VAHLE-HINZ, C. (1986). Electrical stimulation reveals relatively ineffective sural nerve projections to dorsal horn neurons in the cat. *Brain Research* 371, 109-122.

RAJA, S.N., CAMPBELL, J. AND MEYER, R. (1984). Evidence for different mechanisms of primary and secondary hyperalgesia following heat injury to the glabrous skin. *Brain* 107, 1179-1188.

REEH, P.W., KOCHER, L. AND JUNG, S. (1986). Does neurogenic inflammation alter the sensitivity of unmyelinated nociceptors in the rat? *Brain Research* 384, 42-50.

RODIN, E.B. AND KRUGER, L. (1984). Absence of intraspinal sprouting in dorsal root axons caudal to a partial spinal hemisection: a horseradish peroxidase transport study. *Somatosensory Research* 2, 171-192.

RODIN, E.B., SAMPOGNA, S.L. AND KRUGER, L. (1983). An examination of intraspinal sprouting in dorsal root axons with the tracer horseradish peroxidase. *Journal of Comparative Neurology* 215, 187-198.

RUDA, M.A., IADAROLA, M.J., COHEN, L.V. AND YOUNG III, W.S. (1988). *In situ* hybridization histochemistry and immunocytochemistry reveal an increase in spinal dynorphin biosynthesis in a rat model of peripheral inflammation and hyperalgesia. *Proceedings National Academy of Science USA* 85, 622-626.

RYU, P.D., GERBER, G., MURASE, K. AND RANDIC, M. (1988). Actions of calcitonin gene-related peptide on rat spinal dorsal horn neurons. *Brain Research* 441, 357-361.

SAADE, N., JABBUR, S.J. AND WALL, P.D. (1985). Effects of 4-amino-pyridine, GABA and bicuculline on cutaneous receptive fields of cat dorsal horn neurons. *Brain Research* 344, 356-359.

SCHAIBLE, H.-G. AND SCHMIDT, R.G. (1988). Direct observation of the sensitization of articular afferents during an experimental arthritis. In *Proceedings of the Fifth World Congress on Pain*, eds. DUBNER, R., GEBHART, G.F. and BOND, M.R., pp. 44-50. Amsterdam: Elsevier.

SELTZER, Z. AND DEVOR, M. (1984). Effect of nerve section on the spinal distribution of neighboring nerves. *Brain Research* 306, 31-37.

SNOW, P.J. AND WILSON, P. (1985). Plasticity of somatosensory maps in the adult mammalian spinal cord. *Society Neuroscience Abstract* 11, 965.

URBAN, L. AND RANDIC, M. (1984). Slow excitatory transmission in rat dorsal horn: possible mediation by peptides. *Brain Research* 290, 336-341.

WALL, P.D. AND DEVOR, M. (1981). The effect of peripheral nerve injury on dorsal root potentials and on transmission of afferent signals into the spinal cord. *Brain Research* 209, 95-111.

WALL, P.D., FITZGERALD, M. AND GIBSON, S.J. (1981). The response of rat spinal cord cells to unmyelinated afferents after peripheral nerve section and after changes in substance P levels. *Neuroscience* 6, 2205-2215.

YOKOTA, T. AND NISHIKAWA, Y. (1979). Action of picrotoxin upon trigeminal subnucleus caudalis neurons in the monkey. *Brain Research* 171, 369-373.

ZIMMERMAN, M. (1983). Ethical guidelines for investigations of experimental pain in conscious animals. *Pain* 16, 109110.

AFFERENT INDUCED ALTERATIONS OF RECEPTIVE FIELD PROPERTIES

Clifford J. Woolf

Cerebral Functions Research Group, Department of Anatomy and
Developmental Biology, University College London, Gower Street
London WC1E 6BT, U.K.

INTRODUCTION

The connections between neurones in the nervous system are elaborate,complex and highly ordered. This order is achieved by genetic and epigenetic influences operating on neuronal differentiation, proliferation and migration during development together with the surface and cell-mediated factors that control the accurate guidance of axons to their targets (Easter *et al*, 1985). A key issue in contemporary neurobiology is the extent to which the ordered synaptic connections that exist in the adult are modifiable. If modifiability does occur a further question arises whether it represents part of the normal operation of the system or whether it is a pathological response to grossly abnormal circumstances. In this chapter I will present evidence that suggests that a modifiability of the properties of dorsal horn neurones in response to afferent input is an integral component of their functional repertoire and that in particular it contributes to the pathophysiology of acute pain. A major role of unmyelinated primary afferents will be seen from this analysis to be the modification of the excitability of dorsal horn neurones over prolonged periods in addition to their role in providing information by fast transmitter mechanisms on the onset, duration, location, intensity and quality of those peripheral stimuli that activate these fibres.

Classical neurophysiology has until recently been dominated by the view that information is conducted along axons as impulses lasting a few milliseconds and that the transfer of information from one neurone to another is via mechanisms that produce perturbations in excitability that only last for a few tens of milliseconds at most. The properties of any given circuit in the nervous system, if this view were true, would simply be the result then of the spatial organization of the neurones that make up the circuit, the sign of the synaptic inputs and the non-linear spatial and temporal integrating properties of the postsynaptic membrane. The reason why this model of neural networks is unsatisfactory is because it is based on the assumption that synaptic efficacy is temporally static. New models of nerve networks need to incorporate the recent findings that have demonstrated slow postsynaptic potentials, voltage dependent blockade of receptors, voltage dependent dendritic currents, prolonged afterpotentials, second messenger mediated changes in membrane properties, transmitter generated alterations in protein phosphorylation and gene expression. All of these factors can

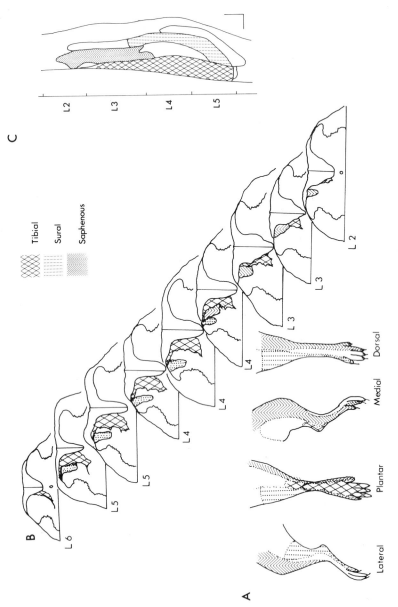

FIGURE 1: A: Outlines of the hindlimb of the rat showing lateral, plantar, medial and dorsal views of the skin surface. The peripheral fields of the tibial, sural and saphenous nerves are illustrated. B: A series of transverse sections of the lumbar dorsal horn of the rat for the L6 to the L2 segments illustrating the relative locations of the central terminal fields of the three nerves established by transganglionic HRP transport (Woolf and Fitzgerald, 1986). C: A plan view of the dorsal horn of the lumbar spinal cord through lamina 2 showing the central terminal fields of the three nerves. The straight lines on the left represents the midline, the next line to the right is the medial border of the dorsal horn while the line on the extreme right is the lateral border of the dorsal horn. Scale bars, vertical 1mm, horizontal 0.2mm (Adapted from Swett and Woolf, 1985).

independently or together result in situations in which the response evoked by a particular synaptic input to a neurone may change over a period of hundreds of milliseconds to days as a result of previous inputs from the same or other synapses. The consequence of the modifiability of synaptic transmission is that it ensures that functional changes, either adaptive or maladaptive, can occur dynamically in the central nervous system in response to changes in the environment. These changes may be short lasting, as the effects of C-afferent fibre input on motor and dorsal horn neurones have been shown to be (Woolf, 1983; Wall and Woolf, 1984; Cervero *et al*, 1984; Cook *et al*, 1987) or permanent, as for the changes that underlie long term memory (Byrne, 1987) and possibly chronic pain. In order to appreciate the functional plasticity of neurones in the spinal cord it is essential first to attempt to understand the basic anatomical and functional elements in the spinal cord that contribute to the organization of the receptive fields of the neurones.

FACTORS CONTRIBUTING TO THE RECEPTIVE FIELD PROPERTIES OF DORSAL HORN NEURONES

Primary Afferent Neurones: Peripheral Terminals

Order in the organization of the nervous system is particularly well demonstrated by the structure and function of primary afferent neurones. Primary afferent neurones are characterized by functional specificity (Burgess and Perl, 1973). The transduction mechanisms of the different classes of afferents have finely tuned sensitivities and are therefore able to extract information concerning specific aspects of peripheral stimuli with little overlap with the sensitivities of other classes of afferents. Cutaneous mechanosensitive afferents for example may be uniquely sensitive to movement of a hair, indentation of a touch dome, vibration, or intense potentially damaging stimuli. Threshold, rate of adaptation and size of peripheral receptive field are important properties of these afferents individually (Lynn and Carpenter, 1982), but collectively the density of innervation and the polyneuronal innervation of structures such as hair follicles are also important, as are regional differences in both skin thickness and the distribution of the different types of skin appendages such as hair (Millard and Woolf 1988). The functional specificity of primary afferents is not fixed. The threshold and response characteristics of nociceptors have, for example, been repeated shown to alter following the application of tissue damaging stimuli in the vicinity of their receptive fields with both peripheral sensitization and desensitization occurring (LaMotte, 1984).

The release of chemicals from damaged tissue, from inflammatory cells or as a result of the antidromic activation of afferent terminals may all participate in this phenomenon. Peripheral sensitization although clearly important cannot however be used to explain all the sensory disorders that result from peripheral injury, particularly mechanical hypersensitivity and secondary hyperalgesia (spread of tenderness beyond the site of the injury) (Raja *et al*,1984; Woolf, 1985).

Primary Afferent Neurones: Central Terminals

In the rat, the skin of the hindlimb is innervated by several cutaneous or mixed nerves: the sural, lateral sural, tibial, superficial peroneal, lateral femoral cutaneous, posterior cutaneous and saphenous nerves. Each nerve has its own peripheral territory or nerve field with little overlap between adjacent fields (Swett and Woolf, 1985) (Fig. 1A). The transganglionic transport of either wheatgerm agglutin conjugated horseradish peroxidase (WGA-HRP) (Swett and Woolf, 1985; Molander and Grant, 1985) or free HRP (Woolf and Fitzgerald, 1986) can be used to map the central terminal fields of these nerves (Fig. 1B). The WGA-HRP labels C-afferents most effectively resulting in maximum reaction product in lamina 2 while free HRP has a time-dependent transport in different afferents, first labelling lamina 1, then 2, and finally laminae 3 to 5 (Woolf and Fitzgerald, 1986).

The central terminal fields of each nerve, whether labelled with WGA-HRP or free HRP, have a specific spatial location in the mediolateral and rostrocaudal planes of the lumbar dorsal horn with very little overlap between adjacent fields (Swett and Woolf, 1985). The spatial arrangement is somatotopically organized, including the splitting of representation, so that the contiguous borders of nerve fields in the periphery are maintained centrally. Plan views of the dorsal horn illustrate this clearly (Fig. 1C). Intracellular recordings from single functionally identified primary afferents followed by the ionophoresis of HRP permit the morphology and the spatial distribution of the collaterals arbors of individual afferents to be visualized (Light and Perl, 1979, Brown, 1981; Woolf, 1987c) and this data can then be used for an analysis of their topographical arrangements. The mediolateral location of the collaterals of a single hair follicle afferent are, for example, aligned in a narrow longitudinal sheet the position of which reflects the location of peripheral receptive field of the afferent (Fitzgerald et al, 1988). The distribution of the central terminals of individual afferents within the nerve fields are not, however, arranged so that they generate a point to point representation of the surface of the skin (Fitzgerald et al, 1988).

Because of the limited size of the central terminal fields of individual nerves relative to the size of the central terminals of individual afferents, hair follicle afferents with receptive fields in the sural peripheral field will, for example, have overlapping central terminals in the sural central terminal field even though their peripheral receptive fields do not overlap. Therefore while there is a topographical order in the representation of the skin surface, accurate localization of a peripheral stimulus cannot be predicted solely by identifying the central terminal field of the afferents that are activated by the stimulus. In order to encode in the spinal cord the accurate location of a peripheral stimulus, both presynaptic factors, such as the synaptic density and spatial organization of afferents activated by a peripheral stimulus and postsynaptic factors such as the patterns of mono and polysynaptic excitation and inhibition evoked in response to the stimulus, must be involved.

Although lamina 2 is somatotopically organized in terms of nerve fields (Swett and Woolf, 1985), there is little information on the somatotopic organization of individual A-δ and C afferent terminals (Light and Perl, 1979; Sugiura et al, 1986).

Second Order Neurones

The presynaptic neuropil provides a framework for the generation of the cutaneous receptive field properties of dorsal horn neurones. The laminar location of the afferents is a reflection of their class and function; A-β in laminae 3 to 5; A-δ in 1 and 5 and C predominantly in 1 and 2 (Light and Perl, 1979; Brown, 1981; Sugiura et al,1986; Woolf, 1987). The mediolateral and rostrocaudal spatial distribution is a reflection of peripheral receptive field location.

In assessing the way in which information concerning peripheral stimuli is transferred to dorsal horn neurones it is necessary to examine three factors: 1) the nature of the synaptic contact between primary afferents and second order neurones, 2) the spatial distribution of the dendrites of second order dorsal horn neurones relative to the spatial distribution of primary afferents and 3) polysynaptic interactions between primary afferents and dorsal horn neurones.

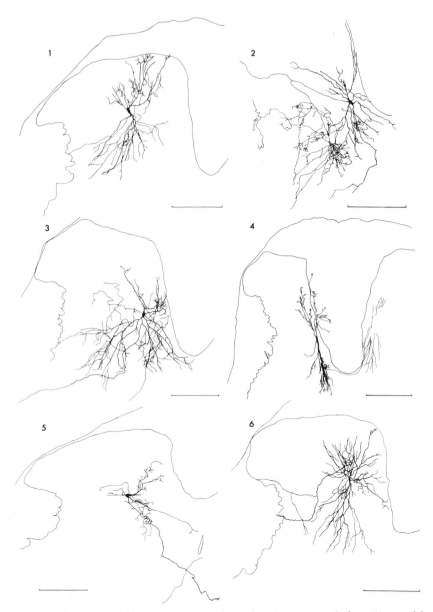

FIGURE 2: Camera lucida reconstructions of 6 lamina V neurons made from 50μm serial transverse sections of the 4th segment of the lumbar spinal cord. Cell 1: No axon or axon collaterals could be identified (reconstructed from 12 sections). Cell 2: An axon arising from the cell body and generating a dense ventrolateral network of collaterals can be seen (9 sections). Cell 3: The axon from this cell arises from a dendrite and projects to the ipsilateral ventrolateral quadrant (12 sections). Cell 4: Note the contralateral axonal collaterals (12 sections). Cell 5: The axon of this neuron projected rostrally in the contralateral ventral quadrant (11 sections). Cell 6: This neuron gave off an axon to the ipsilateral dorsolateral funiculus (see Fig. 11) (13 sections). Scale bars 250μm. (Reproduced with permission from Woolf and King, 1987).

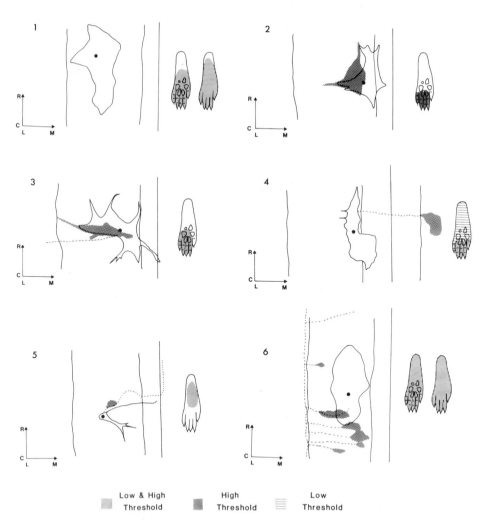

FIGURE 3: Plan views made from serial sections of 6 lamina V neurons. The diagrams are numbered so that no. 1 represents cell 1 in Fig. 2 etc. For each diagram the vertical solid line on the left represents the lateral border of the dorsal horn, the next vertical line to the right represents the medial dorsal horn and the straight line on the extreme right, the midline. The dot represents the cell body, the continuous line connects the maximal medio-lateral extent of the dendrites from each section so as to represent schematically the dendritic envelope. The dotted line represents the axons and the shaded area the distribution of the axonal collaterals. No. 4 shows the medial edge of the contralateral dorsal horn as well as that from the ipsilateral one. The scale in the mediolateral and rostrocaudal plane is 200μm (R - rostral, C - caudal, L - lateral, M - medial). The location, size and response properties of the cutaneous receptive field of each neuron is illustrated next to the appropriate plan diagram with the appropriate key below. (Reproduced with permission from Woolf and King, 1967)

Quantitative analysis of primary afferent synaptic transmission has at present been largely confined to the connections between Ia afferents and motoneurones (Jahr and Yoshioka, 1986) where a fast excitatory transmitter acting on amino acid receptors of the kainate and quisqualate class has been demonstrated. The only similar study on dorsal horn neurones was performed on co-cultures of dorsal root ganglion cells and unidentified spinal neurones and also supported a role for fast excitatory transmitters of the glutamate class (Jessell and Jahr, 1986). Glutamate is present in primary afferent neurones (Battaglia *et al*, 1986) and glutamate receptors are present in the dorsal horn (Monoghan and Cotman, 1985). Glutamate has both powerful direct (TTX resistant) and indirect (TTX sensitive) excitatory actions on dorsal horn neurones both in the superficial (Schneider and Perl, 1985) and in the deep dorsal horn (King *et al*, 1988b) suggesting that this or a related amino acid may be responsible for fast transmission between primary afferents and second order cells. There is accumulating evidence however that both the N-methyl-D-aspartate excitatory amino acid receptor and peptides such as substance P may contribute to postsynaptic changes that last for considerably greater periods than the quisqualate/kainate receptor activation that appears to mediate fast excitatory post synaptic potentials (see later).

If second order dorsal horn neurones were functionally dominated by monosynaptic primary afferent inputs then, with the assumption that segmental and descending inhibitory influences were weaker than the monosynaptic ones, it would be expected that given the order in the presynaptic arrangement of primary afferents and their capacity to excite the cells by fast transmitter systems, the location, threshold and modality of the peripheral receptive fields of dorsal horn neurones would be determined by the extent and location of their dendrites relative to the central terminals of primary afferent fibres. Do neurones with large receptive fields have a greater dendritic spread than those with small receptive fields? Are the dendrites of nociceptive specific cells restricted to laminae 1 and 2? Do wide dynamic range neurones have dendrites that span the superficial and deep laminae of the dorsal horn?

The technique of intracellular recording with HRP injection permits these issues to be addressed. The results of such studies have demonstrated the following: 1) There is no clear relationship between the presence of C-fibre inputs to dorsal horn neurones (which may be mono- and poly-synaptic in origin) and the spread of their dendrites to laminae 1 and 2 (Ritz and Greeenspan, 1985; Woolf and King, 1987). 2) The modality and submodality responsiveness of dorsal horn neurones and their dorsoventral dendritic spread are not tightly correlated (Light *et al*, 1979; Woolf and Fitzgerald, 1983; Bennett *et al*, 1984; Renehan *et al*,1986; Woolf and King, 1987). 3) There is no relationship between the mediolateral spread of dendrites of deep dorsal horn neurones and the area of their cutaneous receptive fields (Ritz and Greenspan, 1985; Egger *et al*, 1986; Woolf and King, 1987).

The results of one such study on neurones in the deep dorsal horn of the rat are shown in Figs. 2 and 3 (Woolf and King, 1987). All neurones were wide dynamic range or multireceptive neurones with both A and C fibre inputs. Fig. 2 shows the diversity of the morphology of these cells with similar receptive field properties; while all cells had a clear C-fibre input only one had extensive dendrites in lamina 2. Plan views of these same neurones are illustrated in Fig. 3 together with diagrams of their receptive fields. It is apparent from this diagram that dendritic spread and receptive field size are not correlated in any simple way.

The conclusion from this and the other studies is that polysynaptic input dominates over monosynaptic input in shaping the receptive fields of dorsal horn neurones. Clearly many neurones do receive monosynaptic inputs from primary afferents but they also receive inputs indirectly via interneurones and many of them transfer this convergent input onto other neurones in the dorsal horn. Cutting dorsal roots which results in the degeneration of all primary afferent terminals, results in the loss only of a minority of synapses on dorsal horn neurons (A. Light, personal communication).

MODIFIABILITY OF RECEPTIVE FIELD PROPERTIES

The complexity of the somatosensory nervous system is such that in stepping from primary afferents, which are characterized by functional and morphological specialization, to second order dorsal horn neurones, specialization, when viewed from the perspective of individual neurones, is apparently lost. Although cells with a selective sensitivity to highly specific stimuli are present (Chung et al, 1986) the vast majority of neurones are dominated by convergent inputs from low and high threshold mechano-, thermo- or chemo-sensitive primary afferents from skin, deep tissue or viscera (see Willis and Coggeshall, 1978).

The cutaneous receptive fields of dorsal horn neurones while somatotopically organized (Wall, 1960; Applebaum et al, 1975; Brown et al, 1983; Woolf and Fitzgerald, 1986) do not have the same degree of high spatial order that primary afferents have nor is there any apparent columnar organization of receptive fields of cells lying in superficial and deep laminae (Woolf and Fitzgerald, 1986).

Assessment and classification of the cutaneous receptive fields of neurones in the dorsal horn have largely been based on the assumption that the receptive field properties of these neurones are fixed and unchangeable. Variation in receptive field properties has however been observed both spontaneously (Dubuisson et al, 1979;

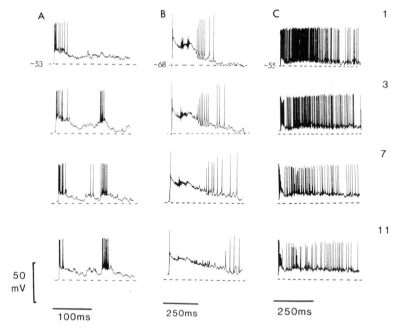

FIGURE 4: The change in the postsynaptic potentials, membrane potential and amplitude of action potentials produced in lamina V neurones recorded in the deep dorsal horn of decerebrate spinal rats by repeated stimulation of the sciatic nerve at C fibre strength (1Hz). A: shows *wind-up* with each successive stimulus increasing the amplitude of the long latency C-fibre evoked PSP. B: shows a neurone for which each stimulus produces a longer lasting PSP; sitting on the progressively more depolarized membrane potential this results in a greater inactivation of the action potentials. C: shows a neurone with which the repeated stimulation produced incremental depolarization of the membrane resulting eventually in inactivation of action potentials. The dotted lines represent the resting membrane potential before the C-fibre stimulation. (Adapted from Woolf and King, 1987).

Woolf and Fitzgerald, 1983), in response to descending influences (Wall, 1967; MacMahon and Wall, 1988) pharmacological agents (Zieglgänsberger and Puil, 1973; Saade *et al*, 1985) and more recently as a result of afferent input (McMahon and Wall, 1984; Cervero *et al*, 1984; Cook *et al*, 1987, Ferrington *et al*, 1987; Schaible *et al*, 1987).

Primary Afferent Input and the Modifiability of the Receptive Fields of Dorsal Horn Neurones

One of the first indications that afferent input could alter the response properties of spinal neurones for prolonged periods emerged from studies on flexor α-motoneurones. In the decerebrate spinal rat these neurones are characterized by lack of spontaneous activity and discrete high threshold cutaneous receptive fields, stimulation within which evokes a phasic discharge of the motoneurones (Woolf and Swett, 1984; Cook and Woolf, 1985). Peripheral tissue injury results in the development of a background discharge in these motoneurones, a reduction in the threshold of their receptive fields and a change in the pattern of the reflex from phasic to tonic (Woolf, 1983, 1984; Woolf and McMahon, 1985). These post-injury hypersensitivity changes, which resemble post-injury pain hypersensitivity states in man (Woolf,1987a), can be duplicated by brief (20s) low frequency (1Hz) trains of electrical stimuli to peripheral nerves provided that the stimulus intensity is sufficient to activate C-afferents (Wall and Woolf, 1984; Woolf and Wall, 1986).

Different C afferents have, moreover, different central effects depending on the tissue they innervate, muscle afferents have more prolonged actions than cutaneous afferents (Woolf and Wall, 1986). The sizes of the cutaneous receptive fields of flexor motoneurones expand following peripheral injury or brief C afferent conditioning stimuli. This includes in many cases the recruitment of novel contralateral inputs (Woolf, 1983). The injury induced alterations in the flexor motoneurones are not associated with prolonged alterations in the excitability of the motoneurones and are therefore likely to be the result of changes upstream from the motoneurones (Cook *et al*, 1986).

Brief afferent conditioning stimuli identical to those that change the flexion reflex have been shown to induce prolonged changes in the receptive field properties of dorsal horn neurones including a population that projects to the brain (Fig. 4) (Cook *et al*, 1987). These changes which have a time course similar to the facilitation of the flexion reflex include both expansions in the size of receptive fields and a change in the types of stimuli that activate these cells. The neurone illustrated in Fig. 4, a lamina 1 projection cell, had, prior to a conditioning stimulus, a stable high threshold receptive field. Following a 20s, 1Hz stimulation of the nerve to the gastrocnemius soleus muscle three changes occurred to this neurone (see Fig. 4): 1) the size of its receptive field expanded, 2) the response to a standard pinch increased when measured in terms of number of action potentials generated and 3) the cell began to respond to low intensity stimuli. These changes, which were found in the majority of cells examined in this study in decerebrate spinal rats, indicate that a static classification of a neurones receptive field does not take into account its potential response repertoire. A *nociceptive specific* neurone in one context may, for example, begin to respond to low threshold afferent fibres in another. The failure to appreciate that the present response properties of a neurone are to some degree a reflection of the history of its past inputs may explain the lack of success in correlating the function of dorsal horn neurones with their structure. Expansions in receptive fields following brief C fibre inputs have been observed by other groups (Cervero *et al*, 1984).

Peripheral tissue injury, like afferent conditioning stimuli produces marked alterations in dorsal horn neurons that cannot be simply accounted for by peripheral sensitization (Ferington et al, 1987; Schaible et al, 1987) and these changes are reflected by changes in the receptive fields of neurones in the thalamus (Guilbaud et al, 1987). We have found, for example, that the application of mustard oil to the skin, a stimulus that predominantly or exclusively activates chemosensitive C-afferents (Woolf and Wall, 1986), produces a long lasting and substantial expansion in the receptive fields of dorsal horn neurones for periods greater than the afferent barrage generated by the conditioning input (Woolf et al, 1988).

This data on the modifiability of the receptive fields of dorsal horn neurones has two important implications. Firstly the concept that the functional organization of the dorsal horn is the product of a rigid hard wired set of neural networks must be wrong and secondly that the C-afferent fibre input can produce a central sensitization that is likely to contribute to the pathogenesis of pain (Woolf, 1987). The remainder of this chapter will be an attempt to address these issues by asking what are the possible mechanisms underlying this functional plasticity and what implications there are for our analysis of the way in which the spinal cord processes sensory information.

Factors Responsible for Synaptic Modifiability in the Spinal cord

Studies into the mechanisms of memory and learning have provided considerable information on how synaptic contacts between neurones can change in the adult central nervous system and have demonstrated that these changes may either be transient (short term memory) or permanent (long term memory). It is perhaps ironic that one of the most successful models of *memory* is the sensitization of the gill withdrawal reflex in Aplysia (Byrne, 1987) because this system may turn out to be a more appropriate model of hyperalgesia (Walters, 1987) than of learning. If conservation of the mechanisms underlying synaptic plasticity occurs during evolution, some of the changes that have been described so successfully for Aplysia may also be relevant for the mammalian spinal cord.

Two categories of synaptic plasticity are possible, homosynaptic plasticity where input in a given synapse results in a subsequent change in its efficacy, and heterosynaptic plasticity where input in one synapse may change the efficacy of another unactivated synapse. In both cases pre and postsynaptic mechanisms may be operational.

Presynaptic changes

Homosynaptic potentiation has been extensively studied for the Ia monosynaptic contact with motoneurones (Mendell, 1984), for long term potentiation (LTP) in the hippocampus (Bliss et al, 1986) and in Aplysia (Byrne, 1987). Repeated activation of an afferent can result both in increases and decreases in synaptic efficacy related to changes in the amount of transmitter released. Control of transmitter release may be localized to the axon terminal depending on calcium entry, suitable stores of transmitter, and transmitter release mechanisms, or it may be affected by anterograde transport from the cell body over a long time course, so that gene expression may be able to influence synaptic transmission. Autoreceptors and presynaptic axo-axonic and dendro-axonic contacts may be able to regulate synaptic efficacy over varying time periods but direct synaptic contact may not be necessary if modulators such as neuropeptides can act as local hormones spreading from the site of release for considerable distances. In Aplysia presynaptic changes are particularly important; they involve a 5-HT mediated increase in cAMP and protein phosphorylation which changes a potassium channel thereby producing facilitated transmitter release (Shuster *et al*,1985). These changes can be transient due to post-translational changes or may be persistent due to changes in gene expression (see Byrne, 1987). Presynaptic increases in glutamate release from the hippocampus have also been claimed to contribute to LTP (Bliss *et al*, 1986). Although most studies on presynaptic changes in synapses have looked at direct influences operating on the presynaptic terminal there is evidence that eicosanoid second messengers that are derived from arachidonic acid that are produced postsynaptically can diffuse across the postsynaptic membrane and the synaptic cleft to influence presynaptic elements (Greenberg *et al*, 1987). By this means, as well as the axo-axonic and dendro-axonic inputs from intervening interneurones, it is conceivable that heterosynaptic plasticity could be the result of presynaptic changes.

Postsynaptic Changes

The capacity for synaptic contacts to modify the postsynaptic membrane are enormous. This was originally regarded only to involve the release of transmitters that transiently opened receptor gated ion channels. More recently it has become appreciated both that slow postsynaptic currents can occur and that, operating via GTP binding proteins and second messengers, transmitters can indirectly modify receptor or ion channel properties, for example by phosphorylating them (Black *et al*, 1987).

Persistent Afferent Induced Postsynaptic Changes

That slow postsynaptic potentials may be an important element of the activity evoked by primary afferents on dorsal horn neurones has been shown by *in vitro* analysis of both spinal cord slices (Urban and Randic, 1984; Yoshimura and Jessell, 1987) and of the hemisected spinal cord (King *et al*, 1988a; Woolf *et al*, 1988). These changes appear not to be potassium mediated and are not evoked by low threshold afferents. In our studies in neonatal rat (12 day) hemisected spinal cord preparations, we have found that repeated stimulation of the dorsal root at 0.5Hz at a strength that recruits unmyelinated afferents produces both a progressive incremental depolarization during the train of stimuli and a sustained depolarization for some minutes after the cessation of the input (Woolf *et al*, 1988). This depolarization, in addition to augmenting the input from the conditioning dorsal root, also changes the input from an adjacent test root. No such changes occur when low threshold afferents are stimulated. Intracellular recordings from rat dorsal horn neurones *in vivo* show similar changes (Fig. 5) (Woolf and King, 1987). Not all dorsal horn neurones show this build up of a depolarization when C-fibres are repetitively stimulated. Some neurones show no change, others exhibit only an increase in their long latency C-fibre evoked postsynaptic potentials (Fig. 5A) resulting in *wind-up* (Mendell, 1966); others do again show a long lasting depolarization (tens of seconds) (Fig. 5, B and C) which is sufficient in some cells to inactivate the action potential (Woolf and King, 1987). Similar to the results obtained *in vitro*, A-β or A-δ afferents stimulated at low frequencies (1-10Hz) do not produce any depolarizations equivalent to those generated by C fibres (Woolf and King, 1987).

C-fibre stimulation can be demonstrated then to have three actions on dorsal horn neurones: 1) it produces a fast transmitter mediated excitatory input on those cells on which the C-fibres make a direct monosynaptic contact; 2) it has the capacity, when the afferents are stimulated repeatedly, to produce progressive response increments (windup) and this is associated in some cells with a substantial, prolonged depolarization (Fig. 5); and 3) brief C-fibre inputs can produce prolonged alterations in

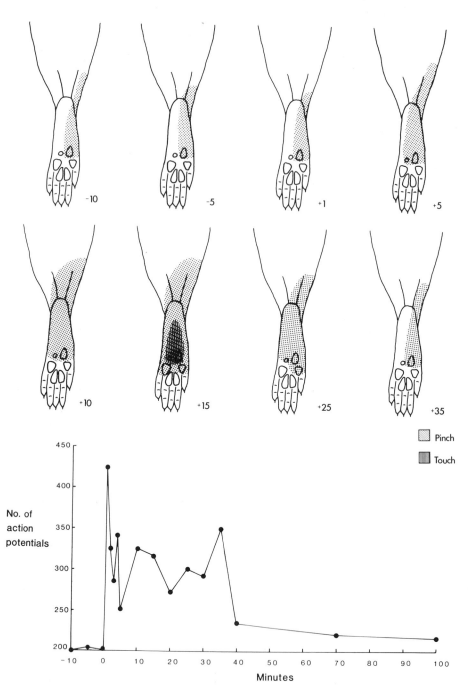

FIGURE 5: A: Expansion of the pinch receptive field of a dorsal horn neuron recorded extracellularly in the rat following a C-fibre strength conditioning stimulus at time 0 to the gastrocnemius-soleus nerve (1Hz, 20s). Note that 15 min after the conditioning stimulus the neuron begins to respond to a low intensity mechanical stimulus (touch). B: Changes in the total number of action potentials in a neuron evoked by a standard pinch applied for 3s to the medial edge of the foot following the gastrocnemius soleus conditioning stimulus at time 0. (Reproduced with permission from Cook *et al*, 1987).

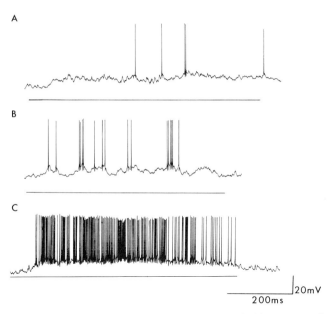

FIGURE 6: Intracellular recordings of the supra and subthreshold responses of a neurone in lamina 5 of the fourth lumbar segment of the rat spinal cord to a standard pinch applied to different regions of the skin. A: The responses elicited by stimulating the dorsum of the foot proximal to toe 5. B: responses elicited by stimulating the plantar skin above toe 2, C: the response evoked by a pinch to the plantar surface of toe 5. The solid lines beneath each trace represent the onset and duration of the stimulus. Note from top to bottom the larger depolarization and the greater number of action potentials evoked.

receptive field properties (Fig. 4) that outlast the period both of the stimulus and of the depolarization. What is not clear yet is the relationship between the mechanisms responsible for these different actions although, based on evidence from a variety of sources, the following scheme is possible.

PROPOSED MECHANISM OF C FIBER INDUCED PLASTICITY OF DORSAL HORN NEURONES

C-fibres may have two different transmitter systems, a fast excitatory amino acid system coexisting in the same neurones with neuropeptides such as substance P or calcitonin gene related peptides *etc*. (Battaglia *et al*, 1986). The excitatory amino acid transmitter, acting via quisqualate/kainate receptors will produce a short lasting inward current, generating a monosynaptic fast epsp. Co-release of peptides will produce further inward currents with a longer latency and a longer duration as a result of acting on calcium and sodium channels and by decreasing potassium outward currents (Nowak and MacDonald, 1982; Murase *et al*, 1986). The depolarization produced by these two sources could result in the removal of the voltage-dependent magnesium block of NMDA channels (Mayer *et al*, 1984). This could result in further depolarization by augmenting the net inward current. Additional calcium could enter the cells via the open NMDA channel (MacDermott *et al*, 1986). The NMDA antagonist APV (5-aminophosphovaleric acid) has the capacity both to reduce glutamate depolarization on dorsal horn neurones (King *et al*, 1988b) and to reduce windup (Davies and Lodge, 1987). In the hippocampus APV blocks LTP (Herron *et al*, 1986). Prolonged depolarization evoked in dorsal horn neurones is likely therefore to be a combination of peptide mediated actions and of amino acid actions on NMDA receptors. Depolarization of a neurone as a result of either a transmitter or a neuromodulator action will, as a result of the recruitment of voltage dependent channels in dendrites and the soma change the prepotentials, the action potential width, and the amplitude and duration of the after potentials; in this way it will alter the firing pattern of the cell (Llinas, 1984; Mayer, 1985; Murase and Randic, 1983). How can these changes which extend the actions of a transmitter input from milliseconds to tens of seconds produce changes that last for minutes or hours. The key to this must be a change in intracellular calcium and/or other second messengers. The depolarization may itself increase calcium entry into the cell either by opening voltage dependent calcium channels or by removing the magnesium blockade of NMDA receptors. In the hippocampus for example, depolarization combined with selective afferent input is sufficient to induce LTP (Wigstrom et al, 1986). Alternatively the changes in second messengers may be independent of the depolarization and may instead be produced by a receptor mediated increase in cyclic AMP, cyclic GMP. IP3 etc. Substance P and glutamate have recently been shown to regulate intracellular Ca^{2+} levels in dorsal horn cells (Womack et al, 1988). An example of the actions of afferent inputs on second messengers/Ca^{2+} in the dorsal horn is the increase in the activity of glycogen phosphorylase in the dorsal horn that occurs in response to C-afferent fibre stimulation and that can be abolished by APV (Woolf, 1987b). We are currently using in vitro spinal cord preparations to study whether this proposed scheme for the production of plasticity by C afferents is correct.

Studies in Aplysia (Shuster et al, 1985) have shown how second messenger systems via protein kinases and altered gene expression can modify excitability for prolonged periods. A particularly interesting recent finding that C-afferent inputs to the spinal cord can also alter gene expression (Hunt et al, 1987) provides a mechanism for producing truly long lasting changes in response properties following brief afferent inputs.

The importance of C-afferent induced alterations in the dorsal horn and of the site and nature of the molecular mechanisms is not purely academic. If post-injury pain hypersensitivity states in man are produced by mechanisms similar to those that occur in animals, then means either of interrupting the development of or of reversing the prolonged facilitations, open the prospect of introducing new classes of analgesic drugs.

HOW ARE CHANGES IN DORSAL HORN EXCITABILITY TRANSLATED INTO CHANGES IN RECEPTIVE FIELD PROPERTIES?

The tip of the iceberg

The spatial organization of primary afferent and second order neurones and their pattern of mono and polysynaptic interactions as discussed earlier in the chapter provide the basis for the ordering of the receptive field properties of dorsal horn neurones. Perturbation in the excitability of the spinal cord by activation of C afferents can however alter these receptive field properties. How does this actually occur. The most reasonable explanation is that second order dorsal horn neurones have two different excitatory receptive field zones which are potentially interchangeable depending on changes in their excitability. The first is a firing zone, stimulation within which elicits a discharge of action potentials by means of a combination of suprathreshold mono and polysynaptic excitatory inputs. It is this firing zone which has been studied in most extracellular analyses of the dorsal horn. The second zone is the subliminal fringe. Stimulation of this part of the receptive field elicits a distinct but subthreshold input to the neurones (Brown and Fyffe,1981; Brown *et al*, 1987; Woolf and King 1988) which can only be analysed by intracellular recording (see Fig. 6). In this example a neurone in lamina 5 of the lumbar spinal cord of a decerebrate-spinal rat is shown to respond differently to identical mechanical stimuli applied to three different areas of skin on the hindpaw. In Fig. 6C the response elicited by pinching toe 5 is seen to be a substantial depolarization with a high frequency action potential discharge. This part of the skin is in the neurone's firing zone. Stimulation of the plantar skin above toe 2 elicits the response shown in Fig. 6B. Again a depolarization is elicited but it is of smaller amplitude and elicits fewer action potentials. When the dorsal surface of the foot is stimulated (Fig. 6A) a depolarization consisting of compound excitatory post synaptic potentials is generated with few or no action potentials. This is an example of the subliminal zone of the cutaneous receptive field. The size of this zone varies from neurone to neurone but is present in a majority of dorsal horn neurones we have examined so far. Using intracellular recordings to define the receptive fields of dorsal horn neurones (firing and subliminal zones) we have found that we can produce an expansion in the size of the receptive field by activating C-fibres (Woolf and King, 1988). This expansion involves an increase in the firing zone both to incorporate the subliminal zone and usually to extend beyond it. In other words increasing the excitability of the dorsal horn results in receptive fields (defined as the firing zone) expanding into a new part of the subliminal zone of the cell that was not identifiable before the conditioning stimulus. There are two explanations for this. The first is that the subthreshold inputs activated by stimulating these regions of skin in the control situation are so small relative to the spontaneous fluctuations in membrane potential that they cannot be recognized but when a conditioning stimulus is delivered their synaptic efficacy increases to a point at which action potentials can be generated. Secondly because polysynaptic inputs dominate over monosynaptic inputs in driving the cells, and when the excitability of many converging cells is increased by an afferent conditioning stimulus, there will be not only direct effects on the cell one is recording from but also increases in polysynaptic inputs from other cells whose receptive fields have expanded. Given that different interneurones are likely to have different strengths of synaptic inputs onto any neurone and that most of these will be subthreshold in control situations, the possibility exists for substantial changes in the properties of any neurone in the affected network, both by direct means and by the indirect transfer of changes in other neurones. We cannot investigate the properties of the dorsal horn by examining the properties of single neurones alone. A similar conclusion has recently been made for the nervous system in general: *the real basis for overall functional responses is the dynamic interaction of specific individual components arranged in repertoires of neuronal groups or populations with different mapped reentrant structures rather than fixed assignment of function to anatomically distinct regions* (Edelman, 1987). Neurones may not operate solely by acting as selective sensors of particular inputs predetermined by fixed anatomical connections. Instead there is tremendous capacity for dynamic plasticity by altering the software. The evidence presented in this review points to C-afferent fibres, either directly or indirectly via the cells on which they terminate in the superficial dorsal horn, having the capacity to produce prolonged changes in most of the neurons of the dorsal horn. Because C fibre inputs are associated in man with prolonged pain, with diminished sensory thresholds and with the spread of sensitivity, such a C-fibre mediated central sensitization may represent a key feature of the pathogenesis of acute pain. Speculation and analysis of the function of the superficial laminae of the dorsal horn has until now been dominated by the view that the cells in this region are primarily concerned with the control of sensory input into the spinal cord by producing inhibition. We now have data indicating that this region of the spinal cord has in addition a role in controlling excitability by producing excitation.

REFERENCES

APPLEBAUM, A.E., BEALL, J.E., FOREMAN, R.D. AND WILLIS, W.D. (1975) Organization and receptive fields of primate spinothalamic tract neurons. *Journal of Neurophysiology*, **38**, 572-586.

BATTAGLIA, G., RUSTIONI, A., ALTSCHULER, R.A. AND PETRUSZ, P. (1986) Glutamate immunoreactive neurons in the dorsal root ganglia contain Substance P. *Society for Neuroscience Abstracts*, **12**, 333.

BENNETT, G.J., NISHIKAWA, N., LU, G-U., HOFFERT, M.J. AND DUBNER, R.(1984) The morphology of dorsal column postsynaptic spinomedullary neurons in the cat. *Journal of Comparative Neurology*, **224**, 568-578.

BLACK, I.B., ADLER, J.E., DREYFUS, C.F., FRIEDMAN, W.F., LaGAMMA,E.F. AND ROACH, A.H. (1987) Biochemistry of information storage in the nervous system. *Science*, **236**, 1263-1268.

BLISS, T.V.P., DOUGLAS, R.M., ERRINGTON, M.L. AND LYNCH, M.A. (1986) Correlation between long term potentiation and release of endogenous amino acids from dentate gyrus of anaesthetised cats. *Journal of Physiology*, **377**, 391-408.

BROWN, A.G. (1981) *Organization in the spinal cord: the anatomy and physiology of indentified neurones.* Springer-Verlag, Berlin.

BROWN, A.G., BROWN, P.B., FYFFE, R.E.W. AND PUBOLS, L.M. (1983) Receptive field organization and response properties of spinal neurones with axons ascending the dorsal columns in the cat. *Journal of Physiology*, **337**, 575-588.

BROWN, A.G. AND FYFFE, R.E.W. (1981). Form and function of dorsal horn neurones with axons ascending the dorsal columns in the cat. *Journal of Physiology*, **321**, 31-47.

BROWN, A.G., KOERBER, H.R. AND NOBLE, R. (1987) An intracellular study of spinocervical tract cell responses to natural stimuli and single hair afferent fibres in cats. *Journal of Physiology*, **382**, 331-354.

BURGESS, P.R. AND PERL, E.R. (1973) Cutaneous mechanoreceptors and nociceptors. In: *Handbook of sensoy physiology, somatosensory system*, vol. **2**, edited by A. Iggo, Springer, Heidelberg, pp. 29-78.

BYRNE, J.H. (1987) Cellular analysis of associative learning. *Physiological Reviews*, **67**, 329-439.

CERVERO, F., SCHOUENBORG, J., SJÖLUND, B.H. AND WADDELL, P.J. (1984) Cutaneous inputs on dorsal horn neurones in adult rats treated at birth with capsaicin. *Brain Research*, **300**, 45-57.

CHUNG, J.M., SURMEIER, D.J, LEE, K.H., SORKIN, L.S., HONDA, C.N., TSANG, Y., AND WILLIS, W.D. (1986) Classification of primate spinothalamic and somatosensory thalamic neurones based on cluster analysis. *Journal of Neurophysiology*, **56**, 308-327.

COOK, A.J. AND WOOLF, C.J. (1985) Cutaneous receptive field and morphological properties of hamstring flexor α-motoneurone in the rat. *Journal of Physiology*, **364**, 249-263.

COOK, A.J., WOOLF, C.J., AND WALL., P.D. (1986) Prolonged C-fibre mediated facilitation of the flexion reflex is not due to changes in afferent terminal or motoneurone excitability. *Neuroscience Letter*, **70**, 91-96.

COOK, A.J., WOOLF, C.J., WALL, P.D. AND MCMAHON, S.B. (1987) Dynamic receptive field plasticity in rat spinal dorsal horn following C-primary afferent input. *Nature*, **325**, 151-153.

DAVIES, S.N. AND LODGE, D. (1987) Evidence for involvement of N-methylaspartate receptors in wind-up of Class 2 neurones in the rat. *Brain Research*, **424**, 402-406

DUBUISSON, D., FITZGERALD, M. AND WALL, P.D. (1979) Ameboid receptive fields of cells in laminae 1, 2, and 3. *Brain Research*, **177**, 376-378.

EASTER, S.S., PURVES, D., RAKIC, P. AND SPITZER, N.C. (1985) The changing view of neural specificity. *Science*, **230**, 507-511.

EDELMAN, G.M. (1987) *Neural Darwinism: The Theory of Neuronal Group Selection.* Basic Books, New York, p.371.

EGGER, M.D., FREEMAN, N.C.G., JACQUIN, M., PROSHANSKY, E. AND SEMBA, K. (1986) Dorsal horn cells in the cat responding to stimulation of the plantar cushion. *Brain Research*, **383**, 68-83.

FERRINGTON, D.G., SORKIN, L.S. AND WILLIS, W.D. (1987) Responses of spinothalamic tract cells in the superficial dorsal horn of the primate lumbar spinal cord. *Journal of Physiology*, **388**, 681703.

FITZGERALD, M., SHORTLAND, P. AND WOOLF, C.J. (1988) The somatotopic arrangement of single hair follicle afferent terminals in the dorsal horn of the rat lumbar spinal cord. *Journal of Physiology*, **398**, 32P.

GREENBERG, S.M., CASTELLUCCI, V.F., BAYLEY, H. AND SCHWARTZ, J.H. (1987) A molecular mechanism for long term sensitization in Aplysia. *Nature*, **329**, 62-65.

GUILBAUD, G., BENOIST, J.M., NEIL, A., KAYSER, V. AND GAUTRON, M. (1987) Neuronal response thresholds to and encoding of thermal stimuli during carrageenin-hyperalgesic inflammation in the ventrobasal thalamus of the rat. *Experimental Brain Research*, **66**, 421-431.

HERRON, C.E., LESTER, R.A., COAN, E.J. AND COLLINRIDGE, G.L. (1986) Frequency-dependent involvement of NMDA-receptors in the hippocampus: a novel synaptic mechanism. *Nature*, **322**, 365-268.

HUNT, S.P., PINI, A. AND EVAN, G. (1987) Induction of C-fos-like protein in spinal cord neurones following sensory stimulation. *Nature*, **328**, 632-634.

JAHR, C.E. AND YOSHIOKA, K. (1986) Ia afferent excitation of motoneurones in the *in vitro* newborn and spinal cord is selectively antagonized by kynurenate. *Journal of Physiology*, **370**, 515530.

JESSELL, T.M. AND JAHR, C.E. (1986) Synaptic interactions between dorsal root ganglia and dorsal horn neurones in cell culture: amino acids, nucleotides and peptides as possible fast and slow excitatory transmitters. In, *Fast and Slow Chemical Signalling in the Nervous System*, ed. L.L. Iversen and E. Goodman, Oxford University Press, Oxford.

KING, A.E., THOMPSON, S.W.N., URBAN, L. AND WOOLF, C.J. (1988a) The responses recorded *in vitro* of deep dorsal horn neurones to direct and orthodromic stimulation in the young rat spinal cord. *Neuroscience*, **27**, 231-242.

KING, A.E., THOMPSON, S.W.N., URBAN, L. AND WOOLF, C.J. (1988b) An intracellular analysis of amino acid induced excitation of deep dorsal horn neurones in the rat spinal cord slice. *Neuroscience Letters*, **89**,286-292.

LAMOTTE, R.H. (1984) Can sensitization of nociceptors account for hyperalgesia after skin injury? *Human Neurobiology*, **3**, 47-52.

LIGHT, A.R. AND PERL, E.R. (1979) Spinal termination of functionally identified primary afferent neurons with slowly conducting myelinated fibres. *Journal of Comparative Neurology*, **186**, 133-150.

LIGHT, A.R, TREVINO, D.L. AND PERL, E.R. (1979) Morphological features of functionally defined neurons in the marginal zone and substantia gelatinosa of the spinal dorsal horn. *Journal of Comparative Neurology*, **186**, 151-172.

LLINAS, R. (1984) Comparative electrobioloy of mammalian central neurons. In: *Brain Slices*, Ed. R. Dingledine, Plenum Press, New York, pp. 7-24.

LYNN, B. AND CARPENTER, S.E. (1982) Primary afferent units from the hairy skin of the rat hind limb. *Brain Research*, **238**, 29-43.

MAYER, M.L. (1985) A chloride activated chloride current generates the after-depolarization of rat sensory neurons in culture. *Journal of Physiology*, **364**, 217-239.

MAYER, M.L., WESTBROOK, G. AND LAND GUTHRIE, P.B. (1984) Voltage-dependent lock by Mg^{2+} of NMDA responses in spinal cord neurones. *Nature*, **309**, 261-263.

MACDERMOTT, A.B., MAYER, M.L., WESTBROOK, G.L., SMITH, D.J. AND BARKER, J.L. (1986) NMDA-receptor activation increases cytoplasmic calcium concentrations in cultured spinal cord neurones. *Nature*, **321**, 519521.

MCMAHON, S.B. AND WALL, P.D. (1984) Receptive fields of lamina 1 projection cells move to incorporate a nearby region of injury. *Pain* **19**, 235-247.

MCMAHON, S.B. AND WALL, P.D. (1988) Descending excitation and inhibition of spinal lamina 1 projection neurones in the rat. *Journal of Physiology*, **396**, 59P.

MENDELL, L.M. (1966) Physiological properties of unmyelinated fibre projections to the spinal cord. *Experimental Neurology*, **16**, 316-332.

MENDELL, L.M. (1984) Modifiability of spinal synapses. *Physiological Reviews*, **64**, 260-324.

MILLARD, C.L. AND WOOLF, C.J. (1988) The sensory innervation of the hairs of the rat hindlimb; a light microscopic analysis. *Journal of Comparative Neurology* (in press).

MOLANDER, C. AND GRANT, G. (1985) Cutaneous projection from the hindlimb foot to the substantia gelatinosa studied by transganglionic transport of WGA-HRP. *Journal of Comparative Neurology*, **237**, 476484.

MOLANDER, C., XU, Q. AND GRANT, G. (1984) The cytoarchitectonic organization of the spinal cord in the rat. I. The lower thoracic and lumbosacral spinal cord. *Journal of Comparative Neurology*, **230**, 133-141.

MONOGHAN, D.T. AND COTMAN, C.W. (1985) Distribution of N-methylaspartate sensitive C-[^{3}H] glutamate binding sites in rat brain. *Journal of Neuroscience*, **5**, 2909-2919.

MURASE, K. AND RANDIC, M. (1983) Electrophysiological properties of rat spinal dorsal horn neurones *in vitro*; calcium dependent action potentials. *Journal of Physiology*, **334**, 141-153.

MURASE, K. AND RANDIC, M. (1984) Actions of substance P on rat spinal dorsal horn neurones. *Journal of Physiology*, **346**, 203-217.

MURASE, K., RYU, P.D. AND RANDIC, M. (1986) Substance P augments a persistent slow inward calcium sensitive current in voltage clamped spinal dorsal horn neurones of the rat. *Brain Research*, **265**, 369376.

NOWAK, L.M. AND MACDONALD, R.L. (1982) Substance P: ionic basis for depolarizing responses of mouse spinal cord neurons in cell culture. *Journal of Neuroscience*, **2**, 1119-1128.

RAJA, S., CAMPBELL, J.N. AND MEYER, R.A. (1984) Evidence for different mechanisms of primary and secondary hyperalgesia following heat injury to the glabrous skin. *Brain* , **107**, 1179-1188.

RENEHAN, W.E., JACQUIN, M.F., MOONEY, R.D. AND RHOADES, R.W. (1986) Structure-function relationships in rat medullary and cervical dorsal horns. II. Medullary dorsal horn cells. *Journal of Neurophysiology*, **55**, 1187-1201.

RITZ, L.A. AND GREENSPAN, J.D. (1985) Morphological features of lamina V neurons receiving nociceptive input in cat sacrocaudal spinal cord. *Journal of Comparative Neurology*, **238**, 440-452.

SAADE, N., JABBUR, S.J. AND WALL, P.D. (1985) Effects of 4-aminopyridine and bicuculline on cutaneous receptive fields of cat dorsal horn cells. *Brain Research*, **344**, 356-359.

SCHAIBLE, H.G., SCHMIDT, R.F. AND WILLIS, W.D. (1987) Enhancement of the responses of ascending tract cells in the cat spinal cord by acute inflammation of the knee joint. *Experimental Brain Research*, **66**, 489-499.

SCHNEIDER, S.P. AND PERL, E.R. (1985) Selective excitation of neurones in the mammalian spinal dorsal horn by aspartate and glutamate *in vitro*: correlation with location and excitatory input. *Brain Research*, **360**, 339-343.

SHUSTER, M.J., COMARDO, J.S., SIEGELBAUM, S.A. AND KANDEL, E.R. (1985) Cyclic AMP-dependent protein kinase closes serotonin sensitive K^+ channels of Aplysia sensory neurons in cell free membrane preparations. *Nature*, **313**, 392-395.

SUGIURA, Y., LEE, C.L. AND PERL, E.R. (1986) Central projections of identified, unmyelinated (C) afferent fibres innervating mammalian skin. *Science*, **234**, 358-361.

SWETT, J. AND WOOLF, C.J. (1985) The somatotopic organization of primary afferent terminals in the superficial laminae of the dorsal horn of the rat spinal cord. *Journal of Comparative Neurology*, **231**, 66-77.

URBAN, L. AND RANDIC, M. (1984) Slow excitatory transmission in rat dorsal horn: possible mediation by peptides. *Brain Research*, **290**, 336-341.

WALL, P.D. (1960) Cord cells responding to touch, damage and temperature of the skin. *Journal of Neurophysiology*, **23**, 197-210.

WALL, P.D. (1967) The laminar organization of dorsal horn and effects of descending impulses. *Journal of Physiology*, **188**, 403-423.

WALL, P.D. AND WOOLF, C.J. (1984) Muscle but not cutaneous C-afferent input produced prolonged increases in the excitability of the flexion reflex in the rat. *Journal of Physiology*, **356**, 443-458.

WALTERS, E.T. (1987) Site specific sensitization of defensive reflexes in *Aplysia: A simple model of long-term hyperalgesia*. Journal of Neuroscience, **7**, 400-407.

WIGSTROM, H.B., GUSTAFSSON, B., HUANG, Y.Y. AND ABRAHAM, W.G. (1986) Hippocampal long lasting potentiation is induced by pairing single afferent volleys with intracellularly injected depolarized current pulses. *Acta Physiological Scandanavica*, **126**, 317-319.

WILLIS, W.D. AND COGGESHALL, R.E. (1978) *Sensory mechanisms of the spinal cord.* John Wiley, New York.

WOMACK, M.D., MACDERMOTT, A.B. AND JESSELL, T.M. (1988) Sensory transmitters regulate intracellular calcium in dorsal horn neurones. *Nature* **334**, 351-353.

WOOLF, C.J. (1983) Evidence for a central component of postinjury pain hypersensitivity. *Nature*, **308**, 686-688.

WOOLF, C.J. (1984) Long term alterations in the excitability of the flexion reflex produced by peripheral tissue injury in the chronic decerebrate rat. *Pain*, **18**, 325-343.

WOOLF, C.J. (1985) Central and peripheral components of the hyperalgesia that follows peripheral tissue injury. In, *Development, Organization and Processing*, Eds. M. Rowe and W.D. Willis, Alan Liss, New York, pp. 317-323.

WOOLF, C.J. (1987a) Physiological, inflammatory and neuropathic pain. *Advances and Technical Standards in Neurosurgery*, **15**, 39-62.

WOOLF, C.J. (1987b) Excitatory amino acids increase glycogen phosphorylase activity in the rat spinal cord. *Neuroscience Letters*, **73**, 209-214.

WOOLF, C.J. (1987c) The central termination f cutaneous mechanoreceptive afferents in the rat lumbar spinal cord. *Journal of Comparative Neurology*, **261**, 105-119.

WOOLF, C.J. AND FITZGERALD, M. (1983) The properties of neurones recorded in the superficial dorsal horn of the rat spinal cord. *Journal of Comparative Neurology*, **221**, 313-328.

WOOLF, C.J. AND FITZGERALD, M. (1986) The somatotopic organization of cutaneous afferent terminals and dorsal horn neuronal receptive fields in the superficial and deep laminae of the rat lumbar dorsal horn. *Journal of Comparative Neurology*, **221**, 517-531.

WOOLF, C.J. AND KING A.E. (1987) Physiology and morphology of multireceptive neurons with C-afferent fibre inputs in the deep dorsal horn of the rat lumbar spinal cord. *Journal of Neurophysiology*, **58**, 105-119.

WOOLF, C.J. AND KING A.E. (1988). Subliminal fringes and the plasticity of dorsal horn neuron's receptive field properties. *Society for Neuroscience Abstracts* **14**.

WOOLF, C.J. AND MCMAHON, S.B. (1985) Injury-induced plasticity of the flexor reflex in chronic decerebrate rats. *Neuroscience*, **16**, 395404.

WOOLF, C.J. AND SWETT, J.E. (1984) The cutaneous contribution to the hamstring flexor reflex in the rat: an electrophysiological and anatomical study. *Brain Research*, **303**, 299-312.

WOOLF, C.J., THOMPSON, S.W.N. AND KING, A.E. (1988) Prolonged primary afferent induced alterations in dorsal horn neurones, an intracellular analysis *in vivo* and *in vitro*. *Journal of Physiology (Paris)*, in press.

WOOLF, C.J. AND WALL, P.D. (1986) The relative effectiveness of C primary afferent fibres of different origins in evoking a prolonged facilitation of the flexor reflex in the rat. *Journal of Neuroscience*, **6**, 1433-1443.

YOSHIMURA, M. AND JESSELL, T.M. (1987) Membranes properties and afferent evoked synaptic responses of substantia gelatinosa neurones in rat spinal cord slices. *Society for Neuroscience Abstracts*, **13**, 1389.

ZIEGLGANSBERGER, W. AND PUIL, E.A. (1973) Actions of glutamic acid on spinal neurones. *Experimental Brain Research*, **17**, 35-49.

NEUROCHEMICAL AND ANATOMICAL CHANGES IN THE DORSAL HORN OF RATS WITH AN EXPERIMENTAL PAINFUL PERIPHERAL NEUROPATHY

Gary J. Bennett, Keith C. Kajander, Yoshinori Sahara,
Michael J. Iadarola and *Tomosada Sugimoto

Neurobiology and Anesthesiology Branch, National Institute of Dental Research,
National Institutes of Health, Bethesda, MD, USA and *Second Department of Oral
Anatomy, Osaka University, Faculty of Dentistry, Osaka, Japan

INTRODUCTION

Many of the neuropathic pain states that occur when human somatosensory nerves are damaged by disease or trauma are thought to involve pathological changes within the spinal segments innervated by the affected nerve. Investigations in animals that have had a peripheral nerve transected or crushed have revealed several neurochemical changes within the spinal cord that may be of pathophysiological significance. Both transection and crush injuries cause a complete peripheral denervation, but their behavioral consequences differ (Wall *et al*, 1979a). Rats with a transection have a marked tendency to attack the denervated region (autotomy); animals with a crush injury display autotomy infrequently and when present it is mild. It has been hypothesized that autotomy is an animal's response to a neuropathic pain state (Wall *et al*,1979a,b; Rodin and Kruger, 1984; Coderre *et al*, 1986).

Complete peripheral denervation is a special case of nerve damage that does not produce all of the abnormal pain sensations that occur with neuropathies that spare at least some afferent fibers' normal connections with the periphery. An animal model of this latter condition has been described recently in which unilateral nerve damage is produced by tying loosely constrictive ligatures around the sciatic nerve of a rat (Bennett and Xie, 1988). The constrictions evoke intraneural edema that causes the nerve to strangulate beneath the ligatures. The behavior of these animals indicates that the nerve damage produces hyperalgesia, allodynia, and spontaneous pain that begin in about two days and lasts for 2-3 months. We describe here the preliminary results of our investigation of some of the neurochemical and neuroanatomical changes that occur within the spinal dorsal horn of animals with this painful peripheral neuropathy.

METHODS

Animals and tissue

Adult male rats of the Sprague-Dawley strain were anesthetized with sodium pentobarbital and had loosely constrictive ligatures placed around one sciatic nerve at mid-thigh level as described in detail elsewhere (Bennett and Xie, 1988). Spinal cords, and in some cases dorsal root ganglia, were collected at various times after nerve injury. For immunocytochemistry and enzyme histochemistry, the animals were deeply anesthetized and perfused transcardially with saline until exsanguinated and were then fixed with 4% paraformaldehyde. The spinal segments that receive the majority of the sciatic nerve input (L3-L5) were identified, cryoprotected with sucrose, and sectioned in the transverse or sagittal plane. Some cases (see Results) were pretreated with colchicine. This was accomplished, under general anesthesia, with an intrathecal cannula introduced through a slit in the atlanto-occipital membrane and threaded caudally to the level of the thoraco-lumbar junction. The cannula was removed after the injection of 10 μl of a 1% colchicine solution in saline. The animals were sacrificed 24h later.

For radioimmunoassay, the animals were deeply anesthetized and guillotined. A transverse cut was made through the sacrum, a 19g needle was inserted into the vertebral canal, and saline was injected forcibly until the spinal cord was ejected from the cervical transection. On an ice-cold glass plate, the region of the lumbar enlargement corresponding approximately to segments L3-L5 was isolated, divided at the midline, and separated into dorsal and ventral horn samples (quadrants) by a cut at the level of the central canal. The samples were immediately frozen on dry ice and were stored at -70°C until assayed.

For the demonstration of trans-synaptic effects on intrinsic spinal neurons, deeply anesthetized animals were perfused transcardially with saline followed by fixative (1% paraformaldehyde, 1% glutaraldehyde, and 0.05 mM $CaCl_2$ in 0.12 M phosphate buffer). A 1.5 mm thick block from the L4-L5 junction was osmicated, dehydrated, and embedded in plastic. Transverse 1 mm sections were stained with toluidine blue. Additional details of the tissue preparation and the criteria for the identification of trans-synaptically altered neurons (*dark neurons*) are given elsewhere (Sugimoto *et al*, 1984, 1985, 1987a,b).

Histochemistry and immunocytochemistry

Fluoride-resistant acid phosphatase (FRAP) was demonstrated in freefloating sections using Gomori's method and 0.1 mM NaF. Substance P (SP), calcitonin gene-related peptide (CGRP), and dynorphin (DYN) immunoreactivities were demonstrated in free-floating sections using the peroxidase-antiperoxidase method and diaminobenzidine as the chromogen according to a protocol given elsewhere (Ruda *et al*, 1982). Antisera for SP and CGRP were obtained commercially (Immunonuclear and Peninsula Labs, respectively). The antiserum for DYN was raised in rabbits inoculated with dynorphin A-(1-8) conjugated to succinylated hemocyanin; its characteristics are described elsewhere (Iadarola *et al*, 1986). The staining obtained with the SP and CGRP antisera is completely eliminated when the working dilution of the antisera is preadsorbed with the immunizing peptide. Preadsorption of the DYN antisera with 10^{-6} M dynorphin A-(1-8) completely eliminated all staining. However, preadsorption with met-enkephalin-[Arg^6,Gly^7,Leu^8] also completely blocked staining, but at a 10-fold greater concentration (10^{-5} M). Leu- and metenkephalin did not eliminate staining at a concentration of 10^{-3} M.

Radioimmunoassay

The radioimmunoassay procedure has been described in detail elsewhere (Iadarola *et al*, 1985, 1986). Assays employed ^{125}I-DYN A-(1-8), ^{125}I[Tyr^0]-CGRP-(28-37), and ^{125}I-[Tyr^8]-SP as tracers. The properties and specificities of the DYN antisera (Iadarola *et al*, 1986) and SP antisera (Pang and Vasko, 1986) are given elsewhere. Briefly, the DYN antisera does not cross-react with leu- enkephalin, met-enkephalin-[Arg^6,Gly^7,Leu^8], DYN A-(1-6), DYN A-(1-7), or alpha-neo-endorphin. There is approximately 3% cross-reactivity with DYN A-(1-9) and 0.05% cross-reactivity with DYN A-(113) and DYN A1(1-17). The SP antiserum has less than 0.01% cross-reactivity with eleodoisin, physalaemin and similar peptides and about 0.1% cross-reactivity with Arg-vasopressin and angiotensin II. The CGRP antisera was raised in rabbit (Iadarola and Flores, unpublished). It is C-terminally directed and has full cross-reactivity for CGRP-(1-37) and [Tyr^0]-CGRP-(28-37). No cross-reactivity has been detected for cholecystokinin, neuropeptide Y and FMRFamide-like peptides.

RESULTS

Fluoride-resistant acid phosphatase

The normal staining pattern for FRAP consists of a dense band that covers about the middle third of the thickness of the substantia gelatinosa (Fig. 1, top row). Five days after nerve injury 3 of 4 cases had distinctly pale patches in this band in the sciatic nerve territory ipsilateral to the nerve damage. At 10 and 20 days after the injury every case (n=9) had a complete, or very nearly complete, depletion of FRAP activity throughout the sciatic nerve territory in the ipsilateral substantia gelatinosa (Fig. 1). The location of this depletion is exactly the same as that which follows sciatic nerve transection (Devor and Claman, 1980). There was also a prominent decrease in the number of FRAP cells in ganglia L4-L5; most rat sciatic afferents originate from these two ganglia (Devor *et al*, 1985). The depletion was partly recovered after 3-5 months (n=6). Contralateral FRAP activity was normal at all times.

Substance P and calcitonin gene-related peptide

The immunocytochemical changes seen for these two peptides were very similar but slightly more clear-cut in the case of CGRP. We suspected that several of the 8 cases examined had a small decrease in staining density for these peptides on the side of the nerve damage at 5 and 10 days after injury, but the changes were small. Twenty days after injury, however, every case (n=9) had unmistakeable changes in both peptides on the nervedamaged side. The dense band of SP and CGRP staining that covers laminae I-IIa was markedly, but not totally, depleted throughout the sciatic nerve territory (Fig. 1, 2nd and 3rd rows). Dorsoventrally oriented SP and CGRP fibers traverse laminae III-IV and these were also partly depleted. For both peptides, immunoreactive varicose fibers form dense, discontinuous plexi in the lateral, reticulated part of lamina V. These plexi were severely depleted. No changes were seen in the SP and CGRP staining that occurs in the region around the central canal. The L4 and L5 dorsal root ganglia had obvious reductions in the number of small cells with SP and CGRP immunoreactivity. Some of the large cells in the ganglia show a coarsely granular CGRP stain; these cells were not clearly affected. By 3-5 months after the injury the staining patterns for SP and CGRP had returned to near normal. SP and CGRP staining contralateral to the nerve damage appeared to be normal at all times.

Radioimmunoassays confirmed and extended the immunocytochemical observations. Relative to the control side, the SP content of the dorsal horn on the side of the nerve damage was significantly depleted by 15-21% at both 10 and 20 days (p < 0.01; paired t test). Similarly, CGRP in the dorsal horn of the nerve-damaged side was significantly depleted (16-19%) at 10 and 20 days (p < 0.05).

Dynorphin

Our initial immunocytochemical observations on DYN changes were in animals with 20 day old injuries. These animals appeared to have a small increase in DYN immunoreactivity on the side of the nerve damage. Close inspection showed that the increase was accompanied by the appearance of faintly stained cell bodies. In order to accentuate any possible increase in cell body DYN content, we made all of our subsequent observations on animals that had received an intrathecal injection of colchicine (100 mg) 24 h before sacrifice. To date, only the 10 (n=4) and 20 (n=6) day postinjury times have been examined. At both of these times every case has had a dramatic increase in the number of DYN-positive cells on the nerve-damaged side and many of these cells were stained more intensely than the cells on the contralateral side (Fig 1, bottom row). The increase in the frequency and staining intensity was seen in DYN neurons in laminae V-VI. Laminae I-II also contain DYN-positive cells but the heavy immunoreactivity in this region has so far prevented us from determining whether there is any change.

Radioimmunoassay of tissue from animals (not colchicinized) 10 and 20 days postinjury confirmed the DYN increase. The dorsal horn's DYN content was increased significantly by 192-366% (p < 0.01).

Dark neurons

The creation of a chronic neuroma of the inferior alveolar nerve or the production of repeated bursts of injury discharges in the nerve result in the appearance of dark neurons in the superficial dorsal horn when the nerve injury is combined with subconvulsive doses of a strychnine. Neither the nerve injury nor the strychnine produces dark neurons by themselves (Sugimoto et al, 1984, 1985, 1987a,b). In 1 mm toluidine blue-stained sections, the affected neurons have increased cytoplasmic and nucleoplasmic staining density (hence *dark neurons*) and several other distinctive abnormalities are noted with the electron microscope (Sugimoto et al, 1984). It is not known whether these abnormalities are indicative of a disuse atrophy or of an irreversible degeneration.

We have detected dark neurons in the superficial laminae of the dorsal horn of rats (n=5) within 8 days of the onset of the painful peripheral neuropathy described here and without administration of any convulsant drug. The altered appearance of these cells is the same as that seen in previous studies (Sugimoto et al, 1984, 1985, 1987a,b). The average incidence of dark neurons in sections from the spinal cords of intact animals is very low (0-3 per section). Rats with the neuropathy had a 3-5 fold increase in the incidence of dark neurons that was bilateral but was significantly greater ipsilateral to the nerve damage. Most of the dark neurons were small and in laminae I-III. The incidence of dark neurons in sections from the cervical enlargement of these same animals was not elevated.

DISCUSSION

The intraspinal depletion of FRAP, SP, and CGRP can be attributed to the disappearance of these substances from the terminals of primary afferent neurons

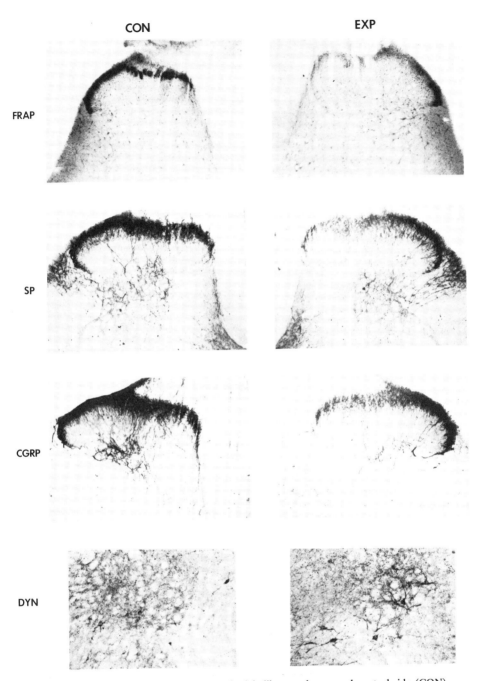

CON   **EXP**

FRAP

SP

CGRP

DYN

FIGURE 1: All rows: Each pair shows the labelling on the normal control side (CON) and on the nerve-damaged experimental side (EXP) from the same section. FRAP: Note the activity remaining in the lateral-most part of the dorsal horn on the nerve-damaged side. This region corresponds to the territory of the posterior cutaneous nerve of the thigh, which was not damaged by the ligation injury. The size of this unaffected nerve territory varies slightly with the rostrocaudal level of the section. SP: Note the decrease in the fibers that descend through laminae II-IV. CGRP: The decrease in the immunoreactivity in lamina V is especially clear in material stained for this peptide. DYN: Immunoreactive spinal neurons in the lateral, reticulated part of lamina V on both sides of the same section. Colchicine was administered intrathecally 24 h before sacrifice.

whose axons travel in the damaged sciatic nerve. The primary afferent origin of the FRAP and CGRP is certain. FRAP is contained only in small-diameter primary afferent neurons with unmyelinated axons (reviewed by Ruda et al, 1986). Intraspinal CGRP is found only in primary afferent terminals and in motoneurons (Gibson et al, 1984). The CGRP-positive varicose fiber systems in laminae I–V are clearly of primary afferent origin. The identification of the origin of the SP that is depleted cannot be unequivocal because of the large number of SP-positive profiles originating from both intrinsic spinal neurons and from descending axons (see Ruda et al, 1986). However, three observations indicate that at least the majority of the depleted SP is from primary afferent terminals: (1) There was a decrease in the number of SP-positive primary afferent somata in the appropriate ganglia, (2) the pattern of the depletion matched the distribution of the sciatic nerve terminals in laminae I–II, and (3) a large majority of SP-containing primary afferents also contain CGRP and the patterns of depletion for SP and CGRP were nearly identical.

The depletion of these three substances reveals the intraspinal terminal distributions of at least two, and perhaps three, different subsets of small-diameter primary afferents. One of these subsets contains FRAP. Only a tiny percentage of the FRAP-containing primary afferent neurons have co-existent SP or CGRP (see Ruda et al, 1986) and the location of their terminal field in the middle of the substantia gelatinosa is unlike that of any other primary afferent marker. The SP and CGRP depletions show the terminal distributions of one or perhaps two subsets of primary afferents. A large majority of SP-containing primary afferent neurons contain co-existent CGRP (Gibson et al, 1984). This must account for the great similarity in their patterns of depletion. However, only a minority of the CGRP-containing cells have co-existent SP (Gibson et al, 1984) and it is thus possible that the pattern of CGRP depletion also indicates the terminal distribution of a subset of CGRP-containing afferents that do not have co-existent SP. However, we were unable to see any difference between the patterns of depletion for CGRP and SP.

It is of interest to note that the CGRP- and SP-containing terminal plexi in the lateral, reticulated part of lamina V were obviously depleted. Myelinated nociceptors are known to terminate in this region (Light and Perl, 1979) and it has been suggested that unmyelinated nociceptors might do likewise (see Ruda et al, 1986 and Sugiura in this volume). It is also of interest that myelinated nociceptors are known to terminate in the central canal region (Light and Perl, 1979) and the neuropeptide staining in this region suggests the possibility of unmyelinated input (see Ruda et al, 1986 and Sugiura in this volume). Nerve damage did not seem to cause any depletion of SP and CGRP staining in the region around the central canal.

Why are these substances depleted? The most obvious possibility is that the nerve injury causes the death of many small-diameter primary afferent neurons, but this is not so. In our preliminary EM observations (Y. Sahara and G.J. Bennett, unpublished) we have not detected any sign of degeneration in the nerve proximal to the injury. Moreover, even a complete sciatic transection kills only a few cells (Devor et al, 1985). Even if it is granted that there is little mortality, one might still suppose that the injury has so debilitated the cells that they are incapable of manufacturing much of anything. But this is not so. Sciatic nerve section, for example, leads to a greatly increased synthesis of vasoactive intestinal polypeptide (McGregor et al, 1984; Shehab and Atkinson, 1984, 1986). It seems most probable that the injury evokes a profound change in gene expression leading to a de novo synthesis of substances needed for repair.

Evidence for such a change has been seen in axotomized cells in the superior cervical ganglion (Hall *et al*, 1978).

There is a pronounced difference between the SP depletion that follows a sciatic nerve transection and that which follows a crush injury. The transection effect is marked and is apparent within a few days. Crush also results in a complete interruption of all the axons in the nerve, but the SP depletion that it produces is small (or absent), is of delayed onset, and recovers quickly (Barbut *et al*, 1981; McGregor *et al*, 1984). The depletion of SP (and CGRP) caused by the injury described here is very similar in terms of both magnitude and time-course to the depletion produced by a transection, although it is important to recall that the injury produced by our ligation method does not cause a complete denervation. Gorio and his colleagues (1986) have recently presented evidence indicating that the critical difference between transection and crush is that the former exposes the injured axons to the extraneural *milieu* while the latter does not. They showed that a transection-like SP depletion occurs after a crush if the nerve is cut below the crush. The results presented here are difficult to reconcile with this hypothesis. The ligation injury clearly produces a depletion of SP like that produced by a transection, but the ligation injury is less likely to breach the neural sheath than the crush injury.

The injuries produced by transection, crush and the ligation method all evoke a total depletion of FRAP. This result appears to be in marked contrast to the differential effect of transection or ligation *vs* crush on primary afferent SP and CGRP levels; it suggests that there might be several mechanisms underlying injury-evoked changes in primary afferent neurochemistry.

The experimental painful neuropathy evoked a dramatic increase in the DYN content of intrinsic spinal neurons. A very similar effect has been observed in Freund's adjuvant-induced polyarthritis (Millan *et al*, 1985) and in a model of inflammation and hyperalgesia produced by injecting one of a rat's hindpaws with an inflammatory agent (Iadarola *et al*, 1986, 1988a,b; Ruda *et al*, 1988). The immunocytochemical evidence for the DYN increase seen in the inflammation model has been substantiated by demonstrations of an increase in the mRNA that codes for DYN (Iadarola *et al*, 1986, 1988a,b; Ruda *et al*, 1988). The experimental neuropathy, the inflammation model, and the polyarthritis all create pain states that can persist for days or months. It is thus possible that the increased DYN synthesis reflects the activation of an intrinsic anti-nociceptive system in the dorsal horn.

The preliminary observations reported here indicate that there is an increase in the incidence of dark neurons in animals with the painful peripheral neuropathy. Dark neurons have been shown to appear after neuroma formation and repetitive injury discharge. It has been hypothesized that in these situations the trans-synaptic effect is due to excessive primary afferent activity producing damaging levels of postsynaptic depolarization, perhaps like that which underlies excitatory amino acid neurotoxicity (Sugimoto *et al*, 1984, 1987a). Our preliminary electrophysiological analysis of primary afferent activity (Kajander and Bennett, 1988) suggests that excessive primary afferent input may also be of significance in the appearance of dark neurons in animals with the experimental peripheral neuropathy. The physiological consequences of the appearance of dark neurons are unknown. However, because most of the affected neurons are small laminae II-III cells, it is possible that inhibitory local circuit neurons are preferentially disabled after nerve injury. The resulting disinhibition may account for at least some aspects of the abnormal pain sensations.

REFERENCES

BARBUT, D., POLAK, J.M. AND WALL, P.D. (1981). Substance P in spinal cord dorsal horn decreases following peripheral nerve injury. *Brain Research* **205**, 289-298.

BENNETT, G.J. AND XIE, Y.-K. (1988). A peripheral mononeuropathy in rat that produces disorders of pain sensation like those seen in man. *Pain* **33**, 87-107.

CODERRE, T.J., GRIMES, R.W. AND MELZACK, R. (1986). Deafferentation and chronic pain in animals: an evaluation of evidence suggesting autotomy is related to pain. *Pain* **26**, 61-84.

DEVOR, M. AND CLAMAN, D. (1980). Mapping and plasticity of acid phosphatase afferents in the rat dorsal horn. *Brain Research* **190**, 17-28.

DEVOR, M., GOVRIN-LIPPMANN, R., FRANK, I. AND RABER, P. (1985). Proliferation of primary sensory neurons in adult rat dorsal root ganglion and the kinetics of retrograde cell loss after sciatic nerve section. *Somatosensory Research* **3**, 139-167.

GIBSON, S.J., POLAK, J.M., BLOOM, S.R., SABATE, I.M., MULDERRY, P.M., GHATEL, M.A., McGREGOR, G.P., MORRISON, J.F.B., KELLY, J.S. EVANS, R.M. AND ROSENFELD, M.G. (1984). Calcitonin gene-related peptide immunoreactivity in the spinal cord of man and of eight other species. *Journal of Neuroscience* **4**, 3101-3111.

GORIO, A., SCHIAVINATO, A., PANOZZO, C., GROPPETTI, A., DiGIULIO, A.M. AND MANTEGAZZA, P. (1986). On the causes regulating the loss of peptides in the spinal cord following sciatic nerve lesions. *Society for Neuroscience Abstracts* **12**, 377.

HALL, M.E., WILSON, D.L. AND STONE, G.C. (1978). Changes in protein metabolism following axonotomy: a two-dimensional analysis. *Journal of Neurobiology* **9**, 353-366.

IADAROLA, M.J., BRADY, L.S., DRAISCI, G. AND DUBNER, R. (1988a). Enhancement of dynorphin gene expression in spinal cord following experimental inflammation: stimulus specificity, behavioral parameters and opioid receptor binding. *Pain*, **35**, 313-326.

IADAROLA, M.J., DOUGLASS, J., CIVELLI, O. AND NARANJO, J.R. (1986). Increased spinal cord dynorphin mRNA during peripheral inflammation. In *Progress in Opioid Research, (NIDA Research Monograph 75)*, ed. Holaday, J.W., Law, P.-Y. and Herz, A., pp. 406409. Washington, D.C.: U.S. Government Printing Office.

IADAROLA, M.J., DOUGLASS, J., CIVELLI, O. AND NARANJO, J.R. (1988b). Differential activation of spinal cord dynorphin and enkephalin neurons during hyperalgesia: evidence using cDNA hybridization. *Brain Research*, **455**, 205-212.

IADAROLA, M.J., PANULA, P., MAJANE, E.A. AND YANG, H.Y.-T. (1985). The opiod octapeptide met[5]-enkephalin-Arg[6]-Gly[7]-Leu[8]: characterization and distribution in rat spinal cord. *Brain Research* **330**, 127-134.

IADAROLA, M.J., SHIN, C., McNAMARA, J.O. AND YANG, H.-Y.T. (1986). Changes in dynorphin, enkephalin and cholecystokinin content of hippocampus and substantia nigra after amygdala kindling. *Brain Research* **365**, 185-191.

KAJANDER, K.C. AND BENNETT, G.J. (1988). Analysis of the activity of primary afferent neurons in a model of neuropathic pain in the rat. *Society for Neuroscience Abstracts* **14**, in press.

LIGHT, A.R. AND PERL, E.R. (1979). Spinal termination of functionally identified primary afferent neurons with slowly conducting myelinated fibers. *Journal of Comparative Neurology* **186**, 133-150.

MCGREGOR, G.P., GIBSON, S.J., SABATE, I.M., BLANK, M.A., CHRISTOFIDES, N.D., WALL, P.D., POLAK, J.M. AND BLOOM, S.R. (1984). Effect of peripheral nerve section and nerve crush on spinal cord neuropeptides in the rat; increased VIP and PHI in the dorsal horn. *Neuroscience* **13**, 207-216.

MILLAN, M.J., MILLAN, M.H., PILCHER, C.W.T., CZLONKOWSKI, A., HERZ, A. AND COLPAERT, F.C. (1985). Spinal cord dynorphin may modulate nociception via a kappa opioid receptor in chronic arthritic rats. *Brain Research* **340**, 156-159.

PANG, I.-H. AND VASKO, M.R. (1986). Morphine and norepinephrine but not 5-hydroxytryptamine and γ-aminobutyric acid inhibit the potassium-stimulated release of substance P from rat spinal cord slices. *Brain Research* **376**, 268-279.

RODIN, B.E. AND KRUGER, L. (1984). Deafferentation in animals as a model for the study of pain: an alternative hypothesis. *Brain Research Reviews* **7**, 213-228.

RUDA, M.A., BENNETT, G.J. AND DUBNER, R. (1986). Neurochemistry and neural circuitry in the dorsal horn. In: *Progress in Brain Research*, Vol.66, ed. Emson, P.C., Rossor, M.N. and Tohyama, M., pp 219-268. Amsterdam: Elsevier.

RUDA, M.A., COFFIELD, J. AND STEINBUSCH, H.W.M. (1982). Immunocytochemical analysis of serotonergic axons in laminae I and II of the lumbar spinal cord of the cat. *Journal of Neuroscience* **2**, 1660-1671.

RUDA, M.A., IADAROLA, M.J., COHEN, L.V. AND YOUNG, W.S. (1988). *In situ* hybridization histochemistry and immunocytochemistry reveal an increase in spinal dynorphin biosynthesis in a rat model of peripheral inflammation and hyperalgesia. *Proceedings of the National Academy of Sciences (U.S.A.)* **85**, 622-626.

SHEHAB, S.A.S. AND ATKINSON, M.E. (1984). Sciatic nerve section has variable effects on primary afferent neuropeptides. *Journal of Anatomy* **139**, 725.

SHEHAB, S.A.S. AND ATKINSON, M.E. (1986). Vasoactive intestinal polypeptide (VIP) increases in the spinal cord after peripheral axotomy of the sciatic nerve originates from primary afferent neurons. *Brain Research* **372**, 37-44.

SUGIMOTO, T., TAKEMURA, M., OKUBO, J. AND SAKAI, A. (1984). Subconvulsive dose of strychnine enhances the transneuronal effect of peripheral sensory nerve transection. *Brain Research* **323**, 320325.

SUGIMOTO, T., TAKEMURA, M., OKUBO, J. AND SAKAI, A. (1985). Strychnine and L-allylglycine but not bicuculline and picrotoxin induce transsynaptic degeneration following transection of the inferior alveolar nerve in adult rats. *Brain Research* **341**, 393-398.

SUGIMOTO, T., TAKEMURA, M., SAKAI, A. AND ISHIMARU, M. (1987a). Rapid transneuronal destruction following peripheral nerve transection in the medullary dorsal horn is enhanced by strychnine, picrotoxin and bicuculline. *Pain* **30**, 385-393.

SUGIMOTO, T., TAKEMURA, M., SAKAI, A. AND ISHIMURA, M. (1987b). Strychnine-enhanced transsynaptic destruction of medullary dorsal horn neurons following transection of the trigeminal nerve in adult rats including evidence of involvement of the bony environment on the transection neuroma in the peripheral mechanism. *Archives of Oral Biology* **32**, 623-629.

WALL, P.D., DEVOR, M., INBAL, R., SCADDING, J.W., SCHONFELD, D., SELTZER, Z. AND TOMKIEWICZ, M.M. (1979a). Autotomy following peripheral nerve lesions: experimental anaesthesia dolorosa. *Pain* **7**, 103-113.

WALL, PD., SCADDING, J.W. AND TOMKIEWICZ, M.M. (1979b). The production and prevention of experimental anaesthesia dolorosa. *Pain* **6**, 175182.

A COMPARISON OF THE RECEPTIVE FIELD PLASTICITY OF NOCIRECEPTIVE AND MULTIRECEPTIVE DORSAL HORN NEURONES FOLLOWING NOXIOUS MECHANICAL STIMULATION

Jennifer Laird and Fernando Cervero

Department of Physiology, University of Bristol, Medical School, University Walk
Bristol BS8 1TD, U.K.

INTRODUCTION

We have previously shown that the ability of both Multireceptive (Class 2) and Nocireceptive (Class 3) dorsal horn neurones to encode the intensity of noxious mechanical stimuli is altered after a series of noxious pinches applied to their receptive field (RF) (Cervero et al, 1988). Further, the RF size of some dorsal horn neurones is known to increase following a brief period of electrical stimulation at C-fibre intensity (Cervero et al, 1984; Cook et al, 1987). We have now investigated the effect of a series of 2 minute noxious pinches upon the excitatory RF and mechanical threshold of Class 3 cells, predominantly recorded in the superficial dorsal horn. However, since only very small changes in RF size were observed in this population the responses of a sample of Class 2 neurones were also examined and the results included in this study to provide a comparison under the same experimental conditions.

METHODS

Single-unit recordings were made using glass micropipettes in the sacral dorsal horn of barbiturate-anaesthetised rats (60 mg.kg^{-1} i.p. induction; 10 mg.kg^{-1} i.v. maintenance). Blood pressure, end-tidal CO_2 and body temperature were monitored and kept within normal physiological limits. Neurones were classified on the basis of their response to innocuous stimuli (brush, touch) and to noxious stimuli (pin-prick, pinch, press). The RF area was then carefully mapped and marked on the skin of the tail. Mechanical thresholds were determined using von Frey hairs.

A series of 2 minute pinches of constant intensity (8 N) were applied by a feedback controlled device to the centre of the RF at intervals ranging from 10 to 30 min. Changes in the area of the RF and in mechanical thresholds were monitored during and after the test series. For the purposes of comparison only the high threshold RFs of Class 2 neurones will be considered in this report although these cells also had distinct low threshold RFs. The response of the neurones to each of the 2 minute pinches was also recorded and analysed. Only one cell per animal was usually tested with a series of tail pinches.

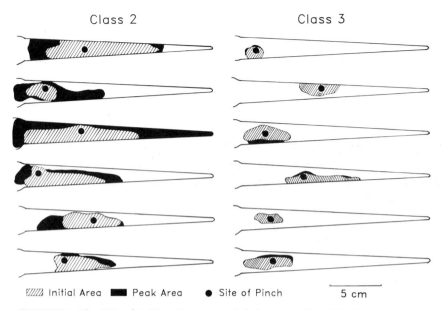

Class 2   Class 3

▨▨ Initial Area   ■ Peak Area   ● Site of Pinch   5 cm

FIGURE 1: The RFs of 6 Class 2 neurones (left-hand panel) and 6 Class 3 neurones (right-hand panel) are shown, drawn on a standard diagram of the rat's tail. The hatched area indicates the size of the RF when it was initially mapped before the application of any noxious stimuli. The solid area indicates the size of the RF at the point of maximum increase observed during the course of the test series.

The position of the recording electrode was marked and the section of spinal cord processed histologically in order to determine the location of the neurone in the dorsal horn.

RESULTS

Sixteen Class 3 neurones were tested. Of these 3 had an Aδ fibre input only (Class 3a) and the remaining 13 had both Aδ and C fibre input (Class 3b). No distinction between these two sub-groups of cells has been made in describing these results. All but one of the 16 neurones were located in the superficial dorsal horn. Ten Class 2 neurones were tested all of which had both A and C fibre input. One of the 10 cells was recorded in lamina I and the rest were recorded in the deep dorsal horn mainly in or around lamina V.

Class 3 neurones

RF properties before noxious pinch: The mean initial size of RFs for the Class 3 cells was 331.6 mm^2 (S.E. = 49.6). RF position on the tail did not appear to be related to either the input properties of the neurone or its recording site in the dorsal horn. The mechanical thresholds of the Class 3 cells before the first press ranged between 40 and 180 mN, though only 2/16 had thresholds below 80 mN.

RF changes after noxious stimuli: Five neurones showed no detectable changes in RF size. The remainder showed increases restricted to the immediate vicinity (within 2 cm) of the noxious pinch (Fig. 1). In 2/16 cells these changes developed only after more than one pinch and increased gradually with several pinches in 7/16 to reach the maximum observed value. The increases were short-lived after the initial pinch stimuli (5-15 min) but recovery was much slower or absent after 4 or 5 successive pinches. The mean increase for the population was 38.3 mm^2 (S.E. = 11.95) (Fig. 2).

Mechanical thresholds: The mechanical thresholds of 7/16 neurones dropped after the stimulus series and the thresholds of the remaining cells were constant or varied without a trend. More than one pinch was required before changes were seen in 50% of cells and thresholds below 40 mN were not observed until after more than three noxious pinches. No threshold below 20 mN was ever observed.

Response to the 2 minute pinch: All neurones responded for the whole duration of the initial 8 N pinch. In general, an initial phasic burst lasting 10-20 s was seen followed by steady tonic firing for the rest of the stimulus period. These responses to the pinch stimuli were analysed to obtain some indication of the excitability of the cells. None of the components analysed revealed any overall trends although some cells responded less well after several pinches and one Class 3 cell produced only an initial phasic burst to the 3rd, 4th or 5th pinches suggesting a decrease in excitability.

Class 2 neurones

RF properties before noxious pinch: Class 2 neurones had larger RFs as a group (mean=896.7 mm^2; S.E.=174.5) than the Class 3 cells although the two groups overlapped to some extent. All of the Class 2 neurones had mechanical thresholds below 22 mN when initially measured.

RF changes after noxious stimuli: All of the neurones showed large increases in their high threshold RF area immediately after the first pinch in the series, and 5/10 showed further increases on subsequent pinch stimuli (Fig. 1). Some degree of recovery was seen in 5 cells but it developed with a slower time course (> 20 min) than the recovery observed in the Class 3 cells. A complete return to the originally mapped RF boundaries was never seen. The mean increase for the population was 642.3 mm^2 (S.E.=175.8) (Fig. 2).

Mechanical thresholds: No change in mechanical threshold was seen in 4/10 cells. The thresholds of the remaining cells dropped after the pinch stimuli.

Response to the 2 minute pinch: All neurones responded for the whole duration of all of the 8 N pinches. The general form was similar to that of the Class 3 cells, that is an initial phasic burst, followed by tonic firing. Likewise, none of the components of the response that were analysed revealed any overall trends although some cells had decreased responses after several pinches.

CONCLUSIONS

These results show that prolonged mechanical stimulation of the cutaneous RF of Class 3 dorsal horn cells produces small or no changes in RF size. In contrast Class 2 neurones show large changes in response to a pinch stimulus under the same experimental conditions. Similar increases in RF size of dorsal horn cells have previously been reported in response to electrical stimulation of peripheral nerves at C-fibre intensity (Cervero *et al*, 1984, Cook *et al*, 1987) and to thermal injury (McMahon and Wall 1983).

The differences seen in our study between the two groups of cells do not appear to be related to the location of the neurones within the dorsal horn. Although the majority of the Class 3 cells were recorded in the superficial dorsal horn, the one Class 3 cell recorded in lamina VI behaved in the same manner as the other Class 3 neurones. Similarly, though most of the Class 2 cells were recorded in or close to lamina V those recorded in the superficial dorsal horn responded in the same way as the rest of the Class 2 group.

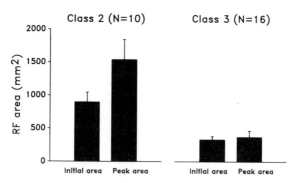

FIGURE 2: Bar graphs showing the mean RF area before noxious stimuli and at the point of maximum increase during the test series for the sample of Class 2 neurones (left-hand panel) and the sample of Class 3 neurones (right-hand panel). The error bars denote the standard error of the mean.

Changes in the RF size of a dorsal horn neurone may be a consequence of sensitisation of the primary afferents providing the input to that cell. High threshold mechanoreceptors (HTM) connected to Aδ fibres are known to be particularly sensitive to lateral stretch. Reeh and colleagues (1987), using the same stimulating device and rat tail preparation as the ones described here, demonstrated that the RF of an Aδ HTM could increase up to 2 cm adjacent to the site of a noxious pinch. It is therefore possible that the small increases in RF size observed in our sample of Class 3 cells were entirely due to peripheral changes without the need for a central component. The Class 2 neurones, however, exhibited increases considerably larger than the 2 cm observed in the primary afferents and therefore a central mechanism must be involved.

The differences between the two groups of dorsal horn neurones in their response to prolonged noxious mechanical stimulation suggest that the Class 3 cells are more resistant to change or are more hard-wired than the Class 2 cells. However, this difference may only exist in the responses during the first few hours after injury, rather than in the chronic or abnormal state. It has been reported (see Dubner et al, this volume) that no changes in RF size of Class 3 lamina I neurones are observed for the first 6 hours after subcutaneous injection of Freund's adjuvant but marked increases occur thereafter.

REFERENCES

CERVERO F., HANDWERKER H.O. AND LAIRD J.M.A. (1988). Prolonged noxious mechanical stimulation of the rat's tail: responses and encoding properties of dorsal horn neurones. *Journal of Physiology* **404**, 419-436.

CERVERO F., SCHOUENBORG J., SJÖLUND B.H. AND WADDELL P.J. (1984). Cutaneous inputs to dorsal horn neurones in adult rats treated at birth with capsaicin. *Brain Research* **301**, 47-57.

COOK A.J., WOOLF C.J., WALL P.D. AND MCMAHON S.B. (1987). Dynamic receptive field plasticity in rat spinal cord dorsal horn following C-primary afferent input. *Nature* **325**, 151-153.

MCMAHON S. AND WALL P.D. (1983). The receptive fields of rat lamina I projection neurones move to incorporate a nearby region of injury. *Pain* **19**, 235-247.

REEH P.W., BAYER J., KOCHER L. AND HANDWERKER H.O. (1987). Sensitisation of nociceptive cutaneous nerve fibres from the rat's tail by noxious mechanical stimulation. *Experimental Brain Research* **65**, 505-512.

DISCUSSION ON SECTION VI

Rapporteur: M. Devor

Neurobehavior Unit, Dept. Zoology Life Sciences Institute, Hebrew University
Jerusalem 91904, Israel

Among our motives in studying the superficial layers of the dorsal horn is the dream of understanding, and eventually controlling, chronic intractable pains that sometimes accompany peripheral injury. It is clear that changes in transduction and conduction in peripheral nerves and their receptor endings play an important role, and these must not be ignored. However, there are also changes in central signal processing. Session VI dealt with such changes.

The nature of the problem was brought home by Bennett in his presentation of a novel animal model of neuropathic pain. Within 2 days of partial constriction of the sciatic nerve, and persisting for about 2 months, Bennett's rats maintained a protective posture and showed exaggerated responses to cutaneous thermal, and perhaps also mechanical, stimuli on the foot. Fortunately, the discomfort was moderate (the rats were active, gained weight, groomed, and interacted socially), laying to rest serious ethical objections. Analysis of peripheral and central pathophysiology induced by the lesion has only just begun.

SPINAL CORD PATHOPHYSIOLOGY

A forecast of the types of central changes that might, in time, emerge appeared in the presentations of Besson, Dubner and Woolf, who investigated other forms of peripheral injury and irritation. Besson emphasized the role of intrinsic and descending circuits in controlling the modality convergence of wide dynamic range (*multireceptive*) neurons. Using rat models of deafferentation and of experimental rheumatoid arthritis, results were described which suggested the possible involvement of endogenous opioids in mediating segmental control over noxious inputs. Such injuries bring about substantial depletion of opioid receptors in the upper layers of the dorsal horn, with different receptor subtypes reacting differently. Besson suggested that loss of opioid inhibition resulting from receptor depletion may contribute to elevated spontaneous discharge in dorsal horn neurons and to elevated excitability as expressed in changes in neuronal responsiveness to peripheral stimuli. A lively discussion surrounded the relative importance of μ, δ and κ-opioid receptors in segmental control, particularly in light of new evidence of injury-induced upregulation of spinal dynorphin, an endogenous κ ligand (see chapter by Ruda).

There was general agreement among the speakers that peripheral noxious stimulation, including inflammation and electrical stimulation of afferent C-fibers, can cause expansion of receptive fields (RFs) of nociceptive specific and/or of wide dynamic range neurons (also see Cervero *et al*, 1984, and Laird and Cervero, this volume). Wall and Woolf added that for some neurons, at least, brief periods of noxious input can recruit additional afferent types, changing what originally appeared to be nociceptive selective neurons into ones with a wide dynamic range (*eg.* Cook *et al*, 1987). Headley and Giesler raised the natural question of how cells with nociceptive input could ever appear to have stable sensitivity and boundaries in routine testing. Merely mapping the RF ought instantly to change it in a Heisenbergian nightmare! The consensus reply was that below some threshold level of intensity and frequency of noxious stimulation RFs are relatively stable; above that level RFs of at least some classes of neurons can be altered.

Surprisingly, the *opposite* of exaggerated afferent input also expands RFs! Dubner, describing recent experiments in cats, showed that nerve section induces lamina I spinomesencephalic neurons to expand their area of input, replacing the RF lost as a result of the nerve section by a novel one proximally up the leg (Hylden *et al*, 1987). This reiterates a finding that had previously been made for cells in deeper laminae of the dorsal horn (Devor and Wall, 1978; Dostrovsky *et al*, 1982; Lisney, 1983; Markus *et al*, 1984; Wilson, 1987).

TRIGGERS

How is it possible that excess stimulation and nerve division both produce RF expansion? This paradox was anticipated by Wall in the 2x2 matrix of questions he posed in his introductory remarks. Is the peripheral signal that triggers central changes carried by electrical impulses or by substances transported in the axoplasmic freight? And whichever, is it a positive signal (excess activity or substances generated as a result of injury), or a negative one (reduced activity or block of normal trophic support)? Although a complete picture cannot yet be assembled, many of the pieces of the puzzle are in hand. For example, there can be little doubt that the signal for rapid (seconds to minutes) RF changes, such as those reported by Woolf, are carried centripetally by action potentials. The changes themselves, however, might be induced by neuromodulatory substances transported from the sensory cell body and released centrally upon the arrival of action potentials. Modulatory effects of this sort are well known in invertebrate preparations (*eg* Kaczmarek and Levitan, 1987).

The persistent expanded RFs in peripheral inflammation models may reflect altered trophic interactions, or alternatively, continued release of neuromodulatory substances driven by persistent nociceptor input. Possible sources of such persistent noxious input were questioned in light of Dubner's failure in preliminary studies to find sensitisation of cutaneous nociceptive afferents in his peripheral inflammation model. Iggo and Perl pointed to joints and deep tissue as likely sources; receptor sensitisation in these tissues is well documented. Woolf made a similar point when he emphasized the particularly striking changes in cutaneous RFs following electrical stimulation of muscle, as opposed to cutaneous nerves.

Persistent expanded RFs following division of peripheral nerves is more difficult to account for. Two facts, however, must be kept in mind. First, nerve section does not necessarily mean afferent silence. Both the emerging nerve-end neuroma, and axotomized sensory neurons in the dorsal root ganglia, provide sustained abnormal afferent impulse traffic. Indeed, chronic nerve block without injury does not induce RF expansion (Wall *et al*, 1982). Second, as pointed out by Bennett in this session, and many other speakers earlier, peripheral injury down- and up-regulates numerous spinal modulatory substances, both ones transported centrally and ones synthesized centrally. RF plasticity in response to chronic noxious input and to nerve injury might, therefore, turn out to have a common basis.

MECHANISM

Whatever triggers it, the mechanism underlying respecification of RF modality and spatial convergence in the dorsal horn is becoming increasingly clear. In his early seminal papers on RF plasticity, Wall layed out two alternative hypotheses. One was that RFs change upon the creation of new anatomical connections. The second was that such changes reflect the strengthening of pre-existing, but latent, synaptic inputs. Although sprouting appeared a viable alternative in the past, Basbaum reminded us of the consistent failure of attempts to obtain positive evidence of sufficiently long-distance sprouting (*eg* Seltzer and Devor, 1984). In contrast, evidence favoring the second hypothesis has continued to accumulate.

Wall's use in this context of the terms *silent* and *relatively ineffective* synapses has inspired visions of all manner of peculiar physiological entities. Thus, at this meeting, there was talk of afferent fibers that end blindly in terminals devoid of synaptic vesicles and release machinery. I do not doubt the possibility of such structures nor that they would be ineffective synaptically. However, emphasis on the bizarre obscures the essence of the idea. There is nothing unconventional about the *relatively ineffective* synapses hypothesized. Indeed, *most* CNS synapses are *relatively ineffective*. This point was made elegantly by Woolf in his intracellular records of neurons caught in the very process of modality and somatotopic respecification. Subthreshold synaptic potentials filled the baseline of his records, but only EPSPs from afferents within the RF were large enough to reach spike threshold. Upon intense noxious peripheral stimulation, the membrane potential of the neuron began slowly to move in the direction of depolarization. As a result, EPSPs previously ineffective at driving the neuron began to reach threshold and the RF (defined by spikes) expanded.

There are many perfectly conventional pre- and postsynaptic mechanisms capable of changing the relative effectiveness of initially subliminal synaptic inputs, as well as abundant anatomical substrates for them. Advanced analysis of this problem will no doubt converge on the biophysical and biochemical processes that have been the bread-and-butter of other branches of neurophysiology for some years now. To quote Woolf, at least some of us will certainly have to give up being *in-vitro* virgins.

ON THE RELATION OF *RELATIVELY INEFFECTIVE* SYNAPSES TO NEUROPATHIC PAIN

Imagine a group of spinal projection neurons whose activity normally signals pain to a conscious brain. If the effectiveness of subliminal low threshold afferent input increased, then weak stimuli would come to evoke pain (Fig. 1A). Experiments reported by Dubner (Hylden *et al*, 1987) examined effects of peripheral deafferentation on neurons with primarily nociceptive input. They found that following section of the nerves that served the RF, the newly emerging proximal RFs did not have low threshold input. Of course, the animals had not shown behavioral signs of pain in response to weak proximal stimulation (allodynia), and so novel low-threshold RFs should perhaps not have been expected for this particular cell type. The general approach is clever, though, and may yet pay off in models of allodynia such as that presented by Bennett.

From the aforementioned, it is obvious how altered modality convergence could yield neuropathic pain (Fig. 1A). But why should RF expansion in the *absence* of modality change be relevant to this problem? Dubner discussed a possible answer (Hayes *et al*, 1979; Dubner *et al*, 1987; see also Devor, 1984). Consider the same population of pain signalling spinal neurons. Before RF expansion, a particular noxious stimulus at one spot will activate a particular number of neurons (call this number n). Let us now imagine that RF expansion triples the amount of RF overlap. The same noxious stimulus will now activate 3n neurons (Fig. 1B). The increased ascending signal could well yield augmented pain sensation even though there has been no change in the modality convergence of RFs of individual cells.

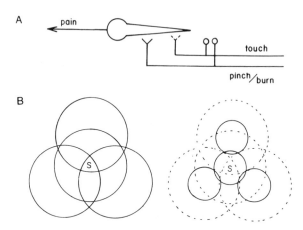

FIGURE 1: Two ideas on how changes in spinal signal processing following peripheral injury could yield neuropathic pain. The first (A) is based on changed modality convergence; the second (B) is based on changed spatial convergence. (A) This spinal neuron, whose activity signals pain, has *relatively ineffective* input from low threshold afferents (touch fiber, dashed synaptic terminal). Strengthening of this latent input yields pain on weak peripheral stimulation (allodynia). (B) Solid circles in the right-hand sketch represent receptive fields (RFs) of spinal neurons whose activity evokes pain. Noxious stimulation at S normally activates only the cell with the central RF. After RF expansion (left hand sketch), the same stimulus falls within the RF of all four neurons yielding an augmented ascending volley and more pain (hyperalgesia).

It was stressed by many of the speakers that not all neurons are alike. As expressed by L. Pubols, *each is an individual upon which anecdotes can be spun.* Nonetheless, few would doubt that organizing principles exist and should be sought. It seems reasonable that the relatively isodendritic neurons of the spinal core (Ramon-Moliner and Nauta, 1966), whose dendrites span many layers of afferent type segregation (dorsoventrally) and range widely across somatotopic fields (mediolaterally and rostrocaudally), should have greater potential for RF plasticity than the relatively idiodendritic neurons of the upper layers. However, RF modality and spatial properties are modifiable in neurons in all laminae. Indeed, according to P. Hope, even spinocervical tract neurons, those we thought would prove to be the most rigid of all, can be demonstrated to expand their RF upon stimulation with certain tachykinins (also see Zieglgänsberger and Herz, 1971). To a greater or lesser extent, it is likely that all classes of spinal sensory neurons have some potential for plasticity in the modality and/or spatial domains.

ACKNOWLEDGEMENT

Supported by NATO and by the United States-Israel Binational Science Foundation.

REFERENCES

CERVERO, F., SCHOUENBORG, J., SJÖLUND, B.H. AND WADDELL, P.J. (1984) Cutaneous inputs to dorsal horn neurones in adult rats treated at birth with capsaicin. *Brain Research* **301**, 47-57.

COOK, A.J., WOOLF, C.J., WALL, P.D. AND MCMAHON, S.B. (1987) Dynamic receptive field plasticity in rat spinal cord dorsal horn following C-primary afferent input. *Nature* **325**, 151-153.

DEVOR, M. (1984) Pain and "state"-induced analgesia: an introduction. In: M.D. Tricklebank and G. Curzon (eds.) *Stress-Induced Analgesia* Wiley, New York pp.1-18.

DEVOR, M. AND WALL,P.D. (1978) Reorganization of spinal cord sensory map after peripheral nerve injury. *Nature* **275**, 75-76.

DOSTROVSKY, J.O., BALL, G.J., HU, J.W. AND SESSLE, B.J. (1982) Functional changes associated with partial tooth pulp removal in neurons of the trigeminal spinal tract nucleus, and their clinical implications. In: R.G. Hill and B. Matthews (Eds.) *Anatomical, Physiological and Pharmacological Aspects of Trigeminal Pain*, Elsevier, Amsterdam.

DUBNER, R., SHARAV, Y., GRACELY, R.H. AND PRICE, D.D. (1987) Idiopathic trigeminal neuralgia: sensory features and pain mechanisms. *Pain* **31**, 23-33.

HAYES, R.L., PRICE, D.D. AND DUBNER, R. (1979) Behavioral and physiological studies of sensory coding and modulation of trigeminal nociceptive input. In: *Advances in Pain Research and Therapy* Vol. 3 J.J.Bonica, J. Liebeskind and D. Albe-Fessard (Eds.) Raven Press, N.Y. pp. 219-243.

HYLDEN, J.L.K., NAHIN, R.L. AND DUBNER, R. (1987) Altered responses of nociceptive cat lamina I spinal dorsal horn neurons after chronic sciatic neuroma formation. *Brain Research* **411**, 341350.

KACZMAREK, L.K. AND LEVITAN, I.B. (1987) *Neuromodulation: the Biochemical Control of Neuronal Excitability* Oxford Univ. Press, N.Y.

LISNEY, S.J.W. (1983) Changes in the somatotopic organization of the cat lumbar spinal cord following peripheral nerve transection and regeneration. *Brain Research* **259**, 31-39.

MARKUS, H., POMERANZ, B., KRUSHELNYCKY, D. (1984) Spread of saphenous projection map in spinal cord and hypersensitivity of the foot after chronic sciatic denervation in adult rat. *Brain Research* **296**, 27-39.

RAMON-MOLINER, E. AND NAUTA, W.J.H. (1966) The iso-dendritic core of the brainstem. *Journal of Comparative Neurology* **126**, 311-335.

SELTZER, Z. AND DEVOR, M. (1984) Effect of nerve section on the spinal distribution of neighboring nerves. *Brain Research* **306**, 3137.

WALL, P.D., MILLS,R., FITZGERALD, M. AND GIBSON, S.J. (1982) Chronic blockade of sciatic nerve transmission by tetrodotoxin does not produce central changes in the spinal cord of the rat. *Neuroscience Letters* **30**, 315-320.

WILSON, P. (1987) Absence of mediolateral reorganization of dorsal horn somatotopy after peripheral deafferentation in the cat. *Experimental Neurology* **95**, 432-447.

ZIEGLGANSBERGER, W. AND HERZ, A. (1971). Changes of cutaneous receptive fields of spino-cervical-tract neurones and other dorsal horn neurones by microelectrophoretically administered amino acids. *Experimental Brain Research* **13**, 111-126.

SECTION VII

EFFECTS OF TECHNICAL APPROACHES ON CURRENT OPINIONS ABOUT THE SUPERFICIAL DORSAL HORN

INTRODUCTION TO SECTION VII

Ronald Dubner

Neurobiology and Anesthesiology Branch, National Institute of Dental Research
National Institutes of Health, Bethesda MD 20892, U.S.A.

The remarkable achievements in our understanding of the organization of the dorsal horn are mainly a consequence of technical advances over the last two decades. New behavioral methods have provided information on the sensory discriminative capacities of nociceptive neurons including those in the dorsal horn. The refinement of single unit recording techniques has led to definitive studies of the nociceptive properties of neurons in the superficial dorsal horn. The utilization of horseradish peroxidase histochemistry has resulted in new observations on the morphology of cell types and on the origin and destination of projection neurons in the dorsal horn. Immunological and pharmacological methodology including radioimmunoassays, immunocytochemistry and microiontophoresis have increased our knowledge of the neurochemical mediators involved in dorsal horn function. Electron microscopy has provided insights into structural organization. Biochemical studies have revealed an array of receptor-mediated second messenger systems that influence dorsal horn activity. Finally, recent advances in molecular biology indicate that changes in gene expression in the dorsal horn are associated with peripheral tissue damage and nerve injury.

In the face of such exciting new findings, we sometimes lose sight of the possible limitations of our technical approaches. Our interpretations of results are often influenced by preconceived notions of how the system might function. In order to increase our objectivity in drawing conclusions from our data, we need to take into account the applicability of the techniques we employ. I would like to discuss the limitations of some of the methods we use by focusing on the present controversy regarding the role of different classes of dorsal horn nociceptive neurons in sensory discrimination. The term sensory discrimination refers to the ability to identify the features of environmental stimuli such as their quality, intensity, location and duration. Noxious stimuli elicit simple reflexes as well as complex escape and avoidance behaviors related to their aversive or unpleasant character. Thus, the experience of pain is multidimensional, and it may be inappropriate to consider all neurons that respond to noxious stimulation as part of sensory discriminative pathways. Multiple lines of evidence are often necessary to establish the functional role of different nociceptive neurons.

The terminology we use to describe different classes of nociceptive neurons must indeed be confusing to the naive reader. Neurons that respond to hair movement or light touch but maximally to intense forms of mechanical stimulation such as pinch or pinprick are referred to as wide-dynamic-range (WDR), multireceptive, convergent, class II or class III, depending on the author of the paper. Neurons that respond almost exclusively to noxious stimulation are called nociceptive-specific (NS), high-threshold, nocireceptive, class II or class III. My personal preference is to refer to them as WDR and NS neurons and I will use that terminology to be consistent with my own previous publications.

On the basis of their exclusive response to noxious or near-noxious stimuli, NS neurons have been assumed to play a role in the detection and discrimination of intense forms of mechanical, thermal and chemical stimuli (Perl, 1971; Cervero *et al*, 1976). The presumed *non-selective* response of WDR neurons to a range of stimuli has led investigators to question their role in sensory discriminative processes (Perl, 1984). Such concerns about the sensory capacities of WDR neurons have some validity when one considers the limitations of the techniques we employ in studying nociceptive neurons. A major problem is the types of stimuli used in determining the sensory encoding capacities of a neuron. Most investigators categorize the neurons based on mechanical or electrical stimulation, and neither is definitive. In classifying a neuron as WDR or NS, it is difficult to rule out that intense mechanical stimulation is merely activating low-threshold mechanoreceptive afferents at higher discharge rates, resulting in a low-threshold mechanoreceptive dorsal horn neuron being mislabelled. Similarly, classifying a WDR neuron based on electrical stimulation of A-β and C afferents is inconclusive since both non-nociceptive and nociceptive afferents conduct impulses in these ranges. In contrast, noxious thermal stimuli are definitive in establishing that a neuron responds in the noxious range, since such stimuli activate only nociceptive myelinated and unmyelinated afferents (Price and Dubner, 1977). Therefore, the classification of a WDR neuron is most adequately established when mechanical, electrical and noxious thermal stimuli are employed. It is important to determine that single-hair displacement or gentle stroking of the skin with forces that do not activate nociceptive afferents is sufficient to produce a response in WDR neurons (Price *et al*, 1979).

The classification of a neuron as WDR or NS does not necessarily lead to the conclusion that the neuron encodes stimulus feature information in the noxious range. A combination of different lines of evidence are necessary to infer a role in sensory discrimination (Price and Dubner, 1977). An important criterion is the ability of the neuron to exhibit graded responses to systematic alterations in stimulus intensity. The most useful stimulus for such an analysis is noxious heat (Dubner, 1985). Few studies employ such parametric analyses. In fact, most studies use only one stimulus level to determine whether a response to noxious stimulation is present. The use of only one point on a stimulus-response curve does not establish the sensory encoding capacity of a neuron and is fraught with error especially when the purpose of the study is to examine the effect of different manipulations on the neuronal responsiveness. If the stimulus is either very intense or very weak, and the response is not on the sensitive portion of the stimulus-response curve, manipulations that are thought to increase or decrease responsiveness will have little or no effect.

Another important criterion in establishing the role of a nociceptive neuron in sensory discrimination is its location and the destination of its axon. It is not useful to discuss the wide dynamic range properties of motoneurons or spinocerebellar neurons in terms of their sensory-discriminative capacities. However, a dorsal horn neuron which can be antidromically activated from the ventrobasal thalamus would have anatomical connections consistent with a role in pain sensation.

The destinations of the axons of dorsal horn neurons are multiple. Dorsal horn neurons are components of spinothalamic, spinomesencephalic, spinocervical, dorsal column postsynaptic and spinomedullary pathways (Hylden *et al*, this volume; Willis, 1985). The use of techniques that determine the projection sites of dorsal horn neurons is critical in the interpretation of the functional role of subpopulations. Yet, a minority of physiological and pharmacological studies employ antidromic techniques to determine the projections of dorsal horn neurons. This is in spite of the knowledge that such methodology can lead to the elegant demonstration of new nociceptive pathways (Burstein *et al*, 1987).

A further problem with our methods of classifying dorsal horn neurons relates to the behavioral state of the animals. Most experiments are performed on anesthetized, decerebrate or spinalized animals. There is considerable evidence that supraspinal descending mechanisms suppress the responses of dorsal horn neurons to noxious stimuli (Willis, 1982). Therefore, sensitivity to noxious stimuli is enhanced in the spinalized animal. WDR neurons appear to be more common in such preparations than in decerebrate animals (Willis, 1982). Anesthetics such as barbiturates have been shown to suppress the activity of WDR neurons. Paradoxically, Collins (this volume) has found many cat dorsal horn WDR neurons in anesthetized animals as compared to very few in awake animals. This is in contrast to the high percentage of WDR neurons observed in the awake monkey medullary dorsal horn (Hoffman *et al*, 1981; Dubner *et al*, 1988). There are a number of possible explanations for this discrepancy including species differences, dorsal horn segment differences and the methods of searching for neurons. However, there also are major differences in neuronal responsiveness in untrained versus trained animals. Dubner *et al* (1988) used monkeys trained to detect noxious heat stimuli and these animals accepted noxious heat stimuli throughout their threshold to tolerance range. They received 100-300 trials of noxious heat per day for months and correctly detected stimuli at better than 90% levels. In contrast, Collins (this volume) utilized untrained cats that reflexly withdrew from stimuli that approached noxious levels. The predominance of low-threshold neurons in the Collins study may be due to the cats avoiding noxious stimuli by escaping innocuous ones. This would result in few of the neurons being exposed to noxious stimuli and possibly explain the predominance of low-threshold neurons in the study.

The correlation of behavior in trained monkeys with neuronal activity provides the most conclusive data on the sensory discriminative capacities of dorsal horn WDR and NS neurons (Dubner *et al*, 1988). With such methods, it can be established that neuronal responses to graded noxious stimuli covary with the perceived intensity of such stimuli. The findings from such studies argue for the importance of WDR neurons in sensory discrimination. WDR neurons exhibit greater heat sensitivity in comparison to NS neurons. The ability of monkeys to perform successfully in thermal detection tasks, determined from threshold responses and detection speeds, is dependent on the activity of WDR neurons. The neuronal discharge of NS neurons alone cannot provide the minimal information necessary to account for the monkeys' ability to detect increases in noxious heat intensity in the 44° to 47°C range. The similar detection speeds in monkeys and humans, and the high correlation of detection speed with the perceived intensity of these same noxious heat stimuli in human subjects, support the conclusion that WDR neurons participate in neural coding mechanisms leading to the perception of pain.

The role of NS neurons in sensory discrimination is less clear. NS neurons may provide sensory discriminative information in response to temperatures of 47°C or greater. They also may provide signals related to the motivational and affective components of the pain experience. Many NS neurons originate from lamina I of the rat, cat and monkey and project to the midbrain periaqueductal gray and cuneiform nuclei which have extensive efferent connections with hypothalamic and limbic structures (see Hylden *et al*, this volume). Therefore, activation of NS neurons may evoke complex emotional reactions related to pain sensations. Furthermore, the midbrain periaqueductal gray is the site of origin of descending pathways which project to the medulla and the spinal cord (Willis, 1982) and which modulate the output of dorsal horn nociceptive neurons. NS lamina I neurons may be a component of the afferent loop that activates these descending systems (Hylden *et al*, this volume).

In conclusion, our interpretation of the function of dorsal horn nociceptive neurons and their role in the extraction of features of environmental stimuli is often dependent on the techniques we employ to study their properties. Although major advances have been made in our understanding of dorsal horn organization, we need to pay more attention to the limitations of the techniques used and how they influence our findings.

REFERENCES

BURSTEIN, R., CLIFFER, K.D. AND GIESLER, Jr., G.J. (1987). Direct somatosensory projections from the spinal cord to the hypothalamus and telencephalon. *Journal of Neuroscience* **7**, 4159-4164.

CERVERO, F., IGGO, A. AND OGAWA, H. (1976). Nociceptor-driven dorsal horn neurones in the lumbar spinal cord of the cat. *Pain* **2**, 5-24.

DUBNER, R. (1985). Specialization in nociceptive pathways; sensory-discrimination, sensory modulation and neuronal connectivity. In *Advances in Pain Research and Therapy,* eds. FIELDS, H.L., DUBNER, R. and CERVERO, F., pp.111-137. New York: Raven Press.

DUBNER, R., CHUDLER, E.H. AND KENSHALO, Jr., D.R. (1988). Specialized pathways that subserve pain sensation. In *Bio-warning System in the Brain*, eds. TAKAGI, H., OOMURA, Y., ITO, M. and OTSUKA, M., pp. 41-53. Tokyo: University Tokyo Press.

HOFFMAN, D.S., DUBNER, R., HAYES, R.L. AND MEDLIN, T.P. (1981). Neuronal activity in medullary dorsal horn of awake monkeys trained in a thermal discrimination task. I. Responses to innocuous and noxious thermal stimuli. *Journal of Neurophysiology* **46**, 409-427.

PERL, E.R. (1971). Is pain a specific sensation?. *J. Psychiat. Res.* **8**, 273-287.

PERL, E.R. (1984). Why are selectively responsive and multireceptive neurons both present in somatosensory pathways?. In *Somatosensory Mechanisms*, eds. von EULER, C., FRANZEN, O., LINDBLOM, U. and OTTOSON, D., pp. 141-161. New York: Plenum Press.

PRICE, D.D. AND DUBNER, R. (1977). Neurons that subserve the sensory-discriminative aspects of pain. *Pain* **3**, 307-338.

PRICE, D.D., HAYASHI, H., DUBNER, R. AND RUDA, M.A. (1979). Functional relationships between neurons of marginal and substantia gelatinosa layers of primate dorsal horn. *Journal of Neurophysiology* **42**, 1590-1608.

WILLIS, W.D. (1982). Control of nociceptive transmission in the spinal cord. In *Progress in Sensory Physiology*, ed. OTTOSON, D., pp. 1-159. Heidelberg: Springer-Verlag.

WILLIS, JR., W.D. (1985). *The Pain System: The Neural Basis of Nociceptive Transmission in the Mammalian Nervous System*. In Pain and Headache, Vol. **8**, ed. GILDENBERG, P.L., pp. 1-331. Basel: Karger.

WHAT MODULATES TONIC MODULATION OF SPINAL DORSAL HORN NEURONS?

J.G. Collins

Departments of Anesthesiology and Pharmacology, Yale University
School of Medicine, 333 Cedar Street, New Haven, CT 06510 U.S.A.

INTRODUCTION

The purpose of this chapter is neither to answer the question raised by the title (we must assume that anything we do to the preparation may alter modulatory systems), nor to provide a review of spinal dorsal horn physiology and pharmacology, but rather to provide examples of the possible impact that changes in tonic modulatory systems may have upon our understanding of sensory processing in the spinal dorsal horn. As such this chapter will rely heavily upon data from our laboratory with citations of only the most poignant examples of other investigators work to support our contentions.

Each preparation imposes upon the nervous system its own set of uncontrollable variables. Our use of the intact, awake, drug-free preparation (to be referred to in this chapter as the intact preparation) allows us to avoid the effects of anesthesia, decerebration, spinal cord transection, and acute surgical preparation, all of which would be expected to have an influence on tonic modulatory systems in the central nervous system. The intact preparation, which is not without its own set of uncontrolled variables, has begun to provide insights into the degree of tonic modulation on some spinal dorsal horn neurons. It is our contention that acute preparations (a preparation in which anesthesia, decerebration and/or spinal cord transection as well as significant surgical trauma are present) with altered tonic modulatory influences are less likely to depict the entire response profile of neurons under study. Just as one frame of a motion picture does not provide the information necessary to understand the complete story, dependence on acute preparations may provide only a static image of a very dynamic process of sensory transmission within the spinal dorsal horn. It is hoped that this chapter will provide examples of the wide response profile that some dorsal horn neurons are capable of, and, at the very least, raise in the reader's mind renewed curiosity about the physiologic role that such neurons may play in spinal sensory processing.

EVIDENCE IN SUPPORT OF TONIC MODULATION

Many well-designed and executed studies have demonstrated the existence of supraspinal modulatory influences on spinal dorsal horn neurons. Wall (1967) reported on the effects of a reversible cold block of the spinal cord on spinal dorsal horn neurons;

he clearly demonstrated that descending systems can change the response profile of some neurons. In that study, when descending modulation was presumably disrupted by a reversible cold block of the spinal cord above the region from which neuronal activity was being recorded, neuronal response profiles were altered. Neurons in the lumbar dorsal horn that had only responded to low threshold stimuli and that had not increased their activity with increasing stimulus intensity responded, after cold block, with a greater firing frequency as the stimulus intensity increased. In the absence of the cold block the neurons could be classified as low threshold (LT). During cold block the same neurons could be classified as wide dynamic range (WDR) neurons. Other laboratories have reported similar effects (Brown, 1971; Handwerker et al, 1975).

Work conducted in intact, awake, drug-free monkeys has revealed additional types of changes that can occur in the response profile of medullary dorsal horn neurons. Hayes et al, (1981) demonstrated that by altering behavioral paradigms they could induce profound changes in the ability of some neurons to respond to peripheral stimulation. They reported on one neuron that was recorded in the medullary dorsal horn and that had receptive fields on both sides of the monkey's face. Activation of the neuron could be elicited when either receptive field was contacted by a 49°C stimulus: activation of the neuron, however, depended upon the behavioral relevance of the stimulus. Stimulation of one side of the face always caused activity. However, stimulation of the other side of the face with the same 49°C stimulus only raised neuronal activity above baseline if the stimulus was behaviorally relevant. These findings could be interpreted to mean that when the animal needed information about the thermal stimulus in order to perform the behavioral task it *allowed* normally ineffective receptive fields to influence the activity of the neuron under study.

The above are just two examples of a wealth of data that suggest the existence of some dorsal horn neurons with *silent synapses*. The synapses are silent in the sense that their ability to evoke action potentials in dorsal horn neurons appears to be inhibited under certain circumstance. Removal of the tonic inhibitory influences immediately results in a change in the afferent input that is capable of evoking action potentials. We will now present data from our own work that begins to define the degree to which the response profile of some dorsal horn neurons may be modified by changes in inhibition of *silent synapses*.

INTACT, AWAKE, DRUG-FREE MODEL

The technique used in our laboratory to study the physiology and pharmacology of spinal dorsal horn neurons in intact, awake, drug-free cats has been described elsewhere (Collins, 1985). Although not without its own problems, the technique makes it possible to study cord function in a preparation in which tonic modulatory systems are assumed to be capable of operating normally. Sterile implantation of a recording chamber over the lumbar enlargement and subsequent implantation of a chronic jugular vein catheter provide a preparation that, following several weeks of recovery from surgery, has a *window to the cord* through which multiple microelectrode penetrations may be made. As the animals sit quietly in a restraint box, an electrode may be manipulated until extracellular activity of a single dorsal horn neuron is discriminated from background activity. With each neuron serving as its own control, stimulus response functions are determined for brush, pinch and heat stimuli. Pinch is applied with forceps that are instrumented with strain gauges so that a record of the change in stimulus intensity is available for data analysis. Thermal stimulation, depending upon receptive field location, is applied with either a contact or radiant heat stimulator. Both pinch and heat are terminated when the animal begins to withdraw from the stimulus. We interpret the reflex movement of the animal as an indication that the stimulus is approaching the noxious range. Receptive field size is determined by lightly rubbing the skin from the center of the receptive field outward.

The animals have not been trained to use the stimuli in any behavioral paradigm and, with the exception of having been adapted to stimulus presentation, are naive to the protocol that is employed during data collection. Animals that have been trained to use the stimuli as part of a behavioral paradigm may have altered modulatory systems that act to maximize information input. Since we are interested in defining the role that tonic modulation has on spinal dorsal horn neurons we have chosen to use a system in which such biasing is, in our opinion, less likely to occur even though the absence of a behavioral paradigm associated with stimulus presentation can decrease the precision of stimulus control.

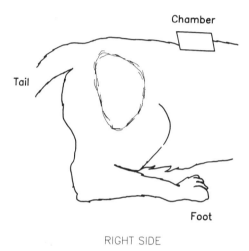

RIGHT SIDE

FIGURE 1: The limits of a single neuron's receptive field area that was sensitive to light rubbing of the skin. The receptive field was mapped four times over the two-hour period (solid line = control; dotted line = 30 min.; short dashed line = 60 min.; long dashed line = 120 min.). There was no significant change in the border of the receptive field during that time as is evident by the overlap of the lines.

We are able to record from neurons (typically laminae IV - VI) with receptive fields on the feet, legs, and hips of the animals (Collins, 1987). Since changes in receptive field size are of particular interest we prefer to study neurons with receptive fields on the hips where receptive field mapping is easier to accomplish. Mapping is done by lightly rubbing the skin to determine the outer limit of the area from which activation may be produced. The limits of that area are then marked with a water soluble, non-toxic paint.

We initially observed differences in neuronal responses between intact, awake, and intact, barbiturate-anesthetized animals; but because they were population studies we could not determine if the presence of the barbiturate was responsible for the changes. However, by using the intact preparation, in which each neuron is its own control we were able to evaluate drug effects on the response properties of individual neurons. In our early drug studies we used pentobarbital and obtained evidence for significant barbiturate-induced changes in the response properties of some spinal dorsal horn neurons (Collins and Ren, 1987). The most obvious change was that some neurons had their response to noxious stimuli unmasked following pentobarbital administration (20 mg/kg). Some cells also had their low threshold receptive field area changed in size by pentobarbital. We hypothesized that these changes were due to a non-specific barbiturate inhibition of descending inhibitory systems, not unlike that demonstrated in acute preparations with a reversible cold block of the spinal cord. We further hypothesized that serotonergic systems were likely to be involved in the process and thus began to examine the effects of systemic methysergide administration (0.05 to 2.0 mg/kg) on spinal dorsal horn neurons in the intact preparation. We will concentrate on three types of changes as examples of the impact of changing modulatory systems on our understanding of cord function.

TABLE I

Methysergide-induced, dose-dependent changes in receptive field area*

	Methysergide Dose (mg/kg)					
Control	0.05	0.10	0.25	0.5	1.35	2
100	107.2±11.2	125.5±23.7	136.3±16.9	155.1±23.5	137.6	189.8
(13)	(6)	(6)	(7)	(8)	(1)	(1)

*values are expressed as percent of control ± S.D.; numbers in parentheses indicate sample size.

INCREASED RECEPTIVE FIELD SIZE

As shown in Figure 1, the limits of a spinal dorsal horn neuron's receptive field from which light rubbing may cause activation tends to be constant over time. This is seen not only in control studies but also in neurons in which methysergide produces no change in the area of the receptive field from which low threshold stimulation can elicit activity. In the intact preparation many dorsal horn neurons appear to have receptive fields that are constant over time and that are not altered by systemic methysergide.

In contrast, Figure 2 demonstrates a typical methysergide induced increase in the area from which activation could be produced. This change has been observed to reverse spontaneously with time and as seen in Table I appears to be dose dependent. We have not been able, with systemic administration, to determine the maximum extent of the change since high doses of systemically administered methysergide produce agitation that limits recording. It is hoped that intrathecal administration will eliminate that problem.

We have attempted to determine if there is a directional selectivity associated with changes in receptive field area. When the data are pooled from all neurons in which receptive field changes occur, the change in area is equally distributed in all directions but an analysis of the direction of maximum increase indicates that the receptive fields tended to move the furthest in the distal direction.

UNMASKING OF RESPONSES TO HIGHER INTENSITY STIMULATION

Studies of spinal dorsal horn neurophysiology have resulted in the description of several *types* of neurons based upon their response profiles to a series of stimuli of increasing intensity. Low threshold neurons respond well to low intensity (non-noxious) stimuli but do not increase their response to higher intensities of stimulation. At the other end of the spectrum, high threshold neurons are only activated when their receptive fields are contacted by stimuli that are near or in the tissue damaging range. A third cell type that is driven by both non-noxious and noxious stimuli has been called, among other terms, a wide dynamic-range neuron. The impact of descending modulation on WDR neurons has been demonstrated in countless experiments. Typically, the noxiously evoked response of the WDR neurons has been shown to be significantly influenced by modulatory systems. In fact, that very aspect of WDR neuron activity, the ease with which inhibition of noxiously-evoked activity is produced, has been a major reason for the WDR neuron type being attributed such a prominent role in the spinal transmission of pain information.

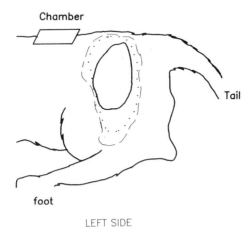

FIGURE 2: The limit of a single neuron's receptive field area that was sensitive to light rubbing of the skin was plotted before and after the systemic administration of methysergide. Methysergide increased this neuron's receptive field with the higher dose producing the greatest change from control (solid line=control, dotted line=0.25 mg/kg; dashed line=0.50 mg/kg). Areas were determined 15 minutes after each dose of drug was administered.

Following the development of the technique for recording from intact preparations we set out to study WDR neurons. We were, however, impeded by the very low number of such neurons that were encountered, in spite of the fact that much higher numbers of WDR neurons were encountered in the same animals when they were anesthetized with pentobarbital. It quickly became apparent that tonic inhibitory systems were active in the intact animal to block the response of many WDR neurons to higher intensities of stimulation. We have been able to demonstrate that the systemic administration of methysergide is capable of reducing the impact of those tonic inhibitory systems such that some of those spinal dorsal horn neurons that were considered to be LT neurons during control studies were reclassified as WDR neurons after methysergide administration.

Figure 3 demonstrates the change in a spinal dorsal horn neuron's response to thermal stimulation of its receptive field. During drug-free control studies the neuron was not activated by thermal stimulation in spite of the fact that the animal withdrew from the stimulus (47°C, 8 seconds). Following 0.25 mg/kg of systemically-administered methysergide, the cell responded briskly to the stimulus. Similar changes, as will be seen below, were also observed when noxious pinch stimuli were employed.

The change in activity seen in Figure 3 depicts a problem in interpretation that must be considered when classifying spinal dorsal horn neurons. In this instance a contact thermal stimulus was employed. Contact during control caused minimal activation but after methysergide administration contact of the stimulus with the skin elicited a rapidly-adapting response that was equal to that produced by the 47°C stimulus. The animal withdrew from the thermal stimulus but did not withdraw from initial contact with the skin. If thermal activation is signalled by increased activity in the neuron it is not obvious how the nervous system discriminates between the first and second burst of activity.

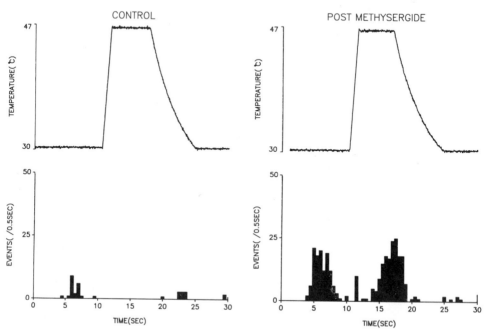

FIGURE 3: The effects of systemic methysergide administration on a dorsal horn neuron's response to thermal stimulation. The top traces are of the thermal stimulus that was applied with a contact probe which had a baseline temperature of 30°C. Control contact with the skin caused a small response that adapted rapidly. Heating the probe to 47°C caused no increase in neuronal activity above the level of spontaneous activity. In contrast after methysergide (0.15 mg/kg) contact caused a rapidly adapting response that was followed by activation of the neuron during the time that the probe was at 47°C. In both cases the animal withdrew near the end of the 8 second stimulus. This cell's response to pinch was also unmasked by methysergide.

MODIFIED STIMULUS RESPONSE FUNCTIONS

The use of a pinch stimulus produced by forceps that are instrumented with strain gauges has allowed us to observe an additional effect of methysergide on some spinal dorsal horn neurons. As indicated above, increased responses to both thermal and pinch stimuli were observed following methysergide administration. In some instances increased response to both stimuli were observed in the same cell. However, not only was the level of neuronal activity in response to a pinch stimulus increased but as shown in Figure 4 the change in firing frequency much more accurately reflected the change of stimulus intensity. Prior to methysergide administration the cell typically demonstrated an on- and off- response associated with initial contact with the skin and with removal of the forceps from the skin (this occurs when the animal begins to withdraw from the pinch). These responses were greater than any other evoked activity during the pinch. There was no correspondence between the magnitude of the stimulus and the evoked neuronal activity. Following methysergide administration some neurons had a completely different response profile. As we see in Figure 4, the maximum response is now seen at maximum pinch intensity and as the animal is withdrawing from the stimulus. Of equal interest, the neuronal activity now appears to contain information about the rate of change of the stimulus. This effect, as well as the enhanced activation by stimuli approaching the noxious range has been observed to recover spontaneously over a period of two hours. This spontaneous reversal suggests a drug dependent effect that briefly impedes tonic inhibitory systems.

WHAT, IF ANYTHING, DO THE CHANGES TELL US?

Data obtained from the pentobarbital and methysergide studies of more than 100 neurons reveals that approximately 25% of the cells displayed at least one of the above

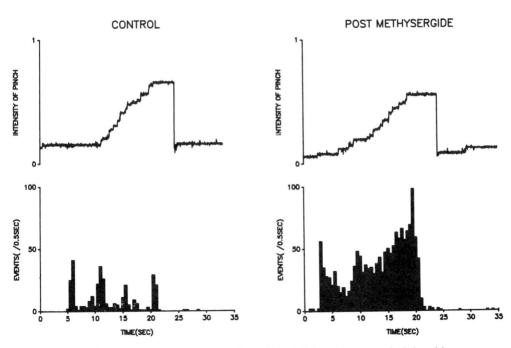

FIGURE 4: The effect of systemic methysergide administration on a spinal dorsal horn neuron's response to a pinch stimulus applied to the peripheral receptive field. Top: the output voltage from strain gauges mounted on the forceps with which the pinch was applied. The skin fold was initially placed in the forceps; the response to contact was allowed to adapt before the pressure was increased. Pinch was terminated when the animal withdrew reflexly. The output voltage was recorded on a ramp and hold display so that the start of the plateau near the end of the intensity plot represents the time when the stimulus was terminated. Prior to methysergide (0.15 mg/kg) the neuron gave an on- and off- response associated with contact and removal of the forceps. Following drug, the maximum response was seen at maximum pinch and the overall level of activity was greater throughout the duration of the pinch. Prior to drug there was no similarity between the slope of the pinch and the slope of the neuronal response. After drug there was a close correspondence between the two slopes.

changes following drug administration. For some neurons all these changes were evident. A discussion of the interpretation of the changes described above can be divided into two areas, the first of which relates to effects of technical approaches on current opinion about the superficial dorsal horn. The second concerns the physiologic role of neurons that have potential response properties that are tonically inhibited.

The impact of technical approaches on our understanding of spinal dorsal horn neurophysiology may be profound. Each technique will impose its own set of uncontrolled and unrecognized or perhaps unrecognizable variables. Our findings in the intact, awake, drug-free preparation as well as work by others using intact or acute preparations suggest that acute preparations are likely to freeze a neuron's response profile within a particular narrow limit that is determined by the impact of the preparation on the nervous system. The resultant static image of a potentially dynamic process may provide important information about sensory processing but it must not impede our willingness to see the potential of a much more dynamic system - a system that may, from moment to moment, depending upon the previous history of the organism, change its ability to process information about peripheral stimuli. If the preparation that we are currently using is physiologically intact (some would argue that is not the case) and is providing us with a correct, although limited, view of tonic modulation then our image of the WDR neuron as a static entity needs to be reevaluated. This is especially true in light of the role that WDR neurons have been assigned in the transmission of information about pain.

The role of the WDR neuron in sensory processing, especially its role in pain signalling, has been challenged. The two extreme points of the argument suggest that either activation of WDR neurons is a sufficient condition to produce pain in man (Mayer et al, 1975, Price and Mayer, 1975) or that, at best, WDR responses to painful stimuli may, under pathological conditions, be a source of abnormal somatosensory experience (Perl, 1984) I would like to propose for discussion a *middle of the ground* role for WDR neurons in pain processing.

It is clear that a tissue damaging stimulus causes changes in the way that the nervous system responds to subsequent stimulation, whether it be noxious or non-noxious. The hyperalgesic state that can be induced either by tissue damage or by the injection of various chemicals (*e.g.* capsaicin) is associated with an increased sensitivity not only to noxious stimuli but also to non-noxious stimuli. Part of this is clearly due to changes in the sensitivity of peripheral receptors but there is also evidence that changes in central mechanisms are involved (Hardy et al, 1950; Woolf 1983). We hypothesize that neurons of the type that are unmasked in the intact animal provide the neural basis by which the nervous system increases its detection of stimuli around an area of damage. The increased receptive field area for non-noxious stimuli could be associated with the region of secondary hyperalgesia. The unmasking of a response to higher intensity stimuli, in conjunction with the increased correspondence between stimulus intensity and neuronal activity, could be associated with the lowering of thresholds to painful stimulation.

The apparent dynamic range of these convertible neurons that are so greatly influenced by tonic inhibition may provide a system that is capable of opening new channels for information processing when appropriate stimuli impinge on peripheral receptive fields.

A final point that needs to be raised relates to aspects of an acute preparation that may influence modulatory systems. When discussing the effect of experimental methods on the responses evoked from a preparation we often concentrate on type and depth of anesthesia, and the presence or absence of decerebration or spinal cord transection because of their obvious impact on the nervous system. An area of additional concern should be the impact of the surgery itself. Price and Mayer (1975) have suggested that the surgical preparation of peripheral nerves increases spontaneous activity of dorsal horn neurons. The effect of distal noxious stimulation on spinal dorsal horn neurons has been well described (*e.g.*, Gerhardt *et al*, 1981). It is clear that spinal cord pharmacology is influenced by distal noxious stimulation (*e.g.* Yaksh *et al*, 1980). Although the exact impact of acute surgery is likely never to be understood, it is reasonable to assume that modulatory systems are influenced by that aspect of an acute preparation.

CONCLUSION

Some spinal dorsal horn neurons appear to have a capability to respond to high intensity stimuli that is normally inhibited by tonic modulatory systems. Technical approaches associated with acute preparations in which these neuron types have been studied may have significantly altered the influence of the tonic modulatory systems on their response profiles. As a result, our opinion about the superficial dorsal horn includes a view that is much more static than the processes themselves. There appear to be neurons in the dorsal horn with dynamic properties that may provide a means by which sensory processing may be significantly altered by the previous history of the organism.

In response to the question contained in the title of this chapter, it seems appropriate to propose that many of the technical approaches used in our study of dorsal horn physiology and pharmacology may influence tonic modulatory system. Since that may be the case it is important for us to continue to define the role of tonic modulation on dorsal horn sensory processing.

ACKNOWLEDGEMENTS

This work has been supported in part by NIH GM29065 and NS 23033. That support as well as collaboration by K. Ren, Y. Saito, H. Iwasaki, J. Tang and the excellent technical support and animal care by A. Kerman-Hinds and T. Morgan have made these projects possible.

REFERENCES

BROWN A.G. Effects of descending impulses on transmission through the spinocervical tract. *J. Physiol.* **219**: 103-125, 1971.

COLLINS J.G. A technique for chronic extracellular recording of neuronal activity in the dorsal horn of the lumbar spinal cord in drug-free, physiologically intact, cats. *J. Neurosci. Methods* **12**: 277-287, 1985.

COLLINS J.G. A descriptive study of spinal dorsal horn neurons in the physiologically intact, awake, drug-free cat. *Brain Research* **416**: 34-42, 1987

COLLINS J.G. AND REN, K. WDR response profiles of spinal dorsal horn neurons may be unmasked by barbiturate anesthesia. *Pain* **28**: 369-378, 1987.

GERHARDT K.D., YEZIERSKI R.P., GIESLER G.J. AND WILLIS W.D. Inhibitory receptive fields of primate spinothalamic tract cells. *J. Neurophysiol.* **46**: 1309-1325, 1981.

HANDWERKER H.O., IGGO A. AND ZIMMERMAN M. Segmental and supraspinal actions on dorsal horn neurons responding to noxious and non-noxious skin stimuli. *Pain* **1**: 147-165, 1975.

HARDY J.D., WOLFF H.G. AND GOODELL H. Experimental evidence on the nature of cutaneous hyperalgesia. *J. Clin. Invest* **29**: 115-140, 1950.

HAYES R.L., DUBNER R. AND HOFFMAN D.S. Neuronal activity in medullary dorsal horn of awake monkeys trained in a thermal discrimination task. II. Behavioral modulation of responses to thermal and mechanical stimuli. *J. Neurophysiol.* **46**: 428-445, 1981.

MAYER D.J., PRICE D.D. and BECKER D.P. Neurophysiological characterization of the anterolateral spinal cord neurons contributing to pain perception in man. *Pain* **1**: 51-58, 1975.

PERL E.R. Why are selectively responsive and multireceptive neurons both present in somatosensory pathways? In: *Somatosensory Mechanisms.* Wenner-Gren International Symposium Series Vol. 41, C. von Euler, O. Frazier, U. Lindbloom, and D. Ottoson eds. pp 141-161, 1984.

PRICE D.D. AND MAYER D.J. Neurophysiological characterization of the anterolateral quadrant neurons subserving pain in M. Mulatta. *Pain* **1**: 59-72, 1975.

WALL P.D. The laminar organization of the dorsal horn and effects of descending impulses. *J. Physiol.* **188**: 403-425, 1967.

WOOLF C.J. Evidence for a central component of post-injury pain hypersensitivity. *Nature* **306**: 686-688, 1983.

YAKSH T.L., JESSELL J.M., GANSE L., MUDGE A.W. AND LERMAN S.E. Intrathecal morphine inhibits substance P release from mammalian spinal cord *in vivo*. *Nature* **286**: 155-156, 1980.

ON THE INFLUENCE OF ANAESTHESIA, STIMULUS INTENSITY AND DRUG ACCESS IN PHARMACOLOGICAL TESTS OF SENSORY PROCESSING IN THE SUPERFICIAL DORSAL HORN

P. Max Headley, Chris G. Parsons, David C. West and Xiao-Wei Dong

Department of Physiology, School of Medical Sciences, University of Bristol
University Walk, Bristol BS8 1TD, U.K.

SUMMARY

Anaesthetic and analgesic agents have been tested, by intravenous administration in spinalized animals, for effects on somatosensory responses of single neurones in spinal lamina I. In these electrophysiological experiments on α-chloralose anaesthetized rats and decerebrate cats, the anaesthetic agents tested were α-chloralose, methohexitone, ketamine and the steroid mixture alphaxalone/alphadolone. The potencies of these agents in reducing nociceptive responses did not match their potencies as anaesthetics. Thus supplementary doses of α-chloralose, or full anaesthetic doses of ketamine, had only small effects on nociceptive responses whilst alphaxalone/alphadolone had marked effects at doses representing a small proportion of its accepted anaesthetic dose. In tests with opioids, both mu (morphine and fentanyl) and kappa ligands (U-50,488 and tifluadom) reduced neuronal responses to thermal and mechanical noxious stimuli in parallel, so long as the peripheral stimuli were adjusted such as to evoke similar frequency discharges in the cell under study. Relative to the mu agonists, the kappa opioids were much more potent than has been reported for topical spinal administration. These results are discussed with respect to the importance of the stimulus intensities used, the access of drugs from the site of administration to the site(s) of their action, and the anaesthetic agent(s) employed in electrophysiological studies.

INTRODUCTION

In recent years we have been performing pharmacological tests investigating the effects of opioid analgesics, anaesthetics and neurotransmitter agonists and antagonists on the somatosensory responses of neurones in several laminae of the spinal cord. We have become increasingly aware of technical aspects which limit the interpretation of experimental results and yet which are not always taken into account. This chapter will attempt to highlight some of these technical points.

METHODS

Fuller details of experimental methods are given in Headley et al (1987a).

Experiments were performed on anaesthetized rats and decerebrate cats, all of which were spinalised at mid-low thoracic levels so that systemic drugs could be tested for effects on spinal neurones in the absence of indirect effects due to their supraspinal actions. Rats were anaesthetised with α-chloralose (80-100mg/kg i.p. or 50mg/kg i.v.; 10mg/ml in saline), supplemented with halothane in oxygen during surgery. Cats were decerebrated at midcollicular level under steroid anaesthesia (alphaxalone and alphadolone, Saffan, Glaxovet). All animals had tracheal, carotid and jugular cannulae. Most animals received a single large dose of a short-lasting soluble corticosteroid (betamethasone, 1mg/kg i.v.) at the start of surgery. When blood loss during surgery was appreciable the appropriate volume of whole blood or plasma was given. Blood pressure was monitored throughout and experiments terminated if systolic pressure fell below 100mm Hg (other than when transient effects were induced by some of the test drugs). Fluid therapy was given in the form of plasma expander (Haemaccel, Hoechst) and isotonic saline at a total rate of approximately 80ml/kg/24hrs. All cats and most rats were paralysed with pancuronium and were ventilated (with oxygen) to maintain end tidal CO_2 close to 4%.

Peripheral stimuli were designed to mimic natural conditions as far as is practicable, whilst being controlled electronically for constancy of intensity, duration and repetition interval. There is always a compromise to be made between shorter repetition intervals which permit more accurate assessment of drug effects, and longer intervals which are less likely to result in damage to the peripheral receptive field. Our normal repetition interval was between 3 and 4 minutes. On those occasions when inflammation was evident the experiment was terminated. Stimuli used included noxious heat (via a contact thermode with feedback control), noxious mechanical pinch (intensity controlled by a regulated gas supply) and a range of innocuous stimuli involving deflection of hair, skin or joints at variable frequencies.

Single neurones were recorded extracellularly with glass micropipettes. These usually had three barrels which were filled with 3.5M NaCl in the recording barrel, quisqualate Na (5mM in 200 mM NaCl at pH 7.5) and pontamine sky blue (2% in 0.5M Na acetate). The amino acid was ejected as an aid to locating cells; the dye was ejected at selected recording sites for retrospective histology. In some experiments 7-barrel pipettes were used and were filled with selections of excitatory amino acids and their antagonists. Spike configuration was carefully monitored on a digital delay line to ensure that activity of only a single cell was processed. Neuronal firing rate, counts of spikes during stimulus-related epochs, and, as appropriate, thermode temperature and pinch force were plotted on a pen recorder. The spike counts were processed by a microcomputer to give on-line analysis of the effects of drugs on neuronal responses.

On the majority of cells two different stimuli were alternated in a regular cycle. At least three cycles of responses were used to calculate the control values on which the effects of i.v. drugs were based. Drug tests were considered technically acceptable only when reversal by at least 50% of the apparent drug effect was observed. We attempted to compare as many different drugs as possible on single cells tested under closely comparable conditions of physiological state and peripheral stimuli. The interval between such tests was based on the known half life of the drugs and/or our assessment of the half recovery time from drug effects (when the half life in plasma is known these values correspond closely). For this reason the selection of test anaesthetic agents and of receptor-selective opioids was made largely on the basis of their having experimentally convenient half lives.

Many analgesic and anaesthetic drugs affect blood pressure. Such changes were

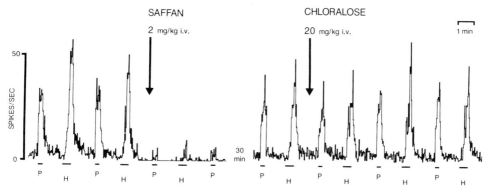

FIGURE 1: Comparison of the effects of sub-anaesthetic doses of the steroid anaesthetic mixture alphaxalone/alphadolone (Saffan) and of α-chloralose on nociceptive responses of a lamina I neurone in a rat. Trace of spike discharge rate (counted in 2 s epochs) against time. The cell was activated by alternating mechanical and thermal noxious stimuli (P: pinch toe 3 for 15 s; H: heat toes 4-5 (*ie* lateral toes) and lateral plantar foot, ramping from 37°C baseline to 48°C, for 30 s). Stimulus repetition cycle was 3 min 30 s. α-chloralose anaesthetized spinalized rat.

minimised firstly by making injections over 30 seconds or more and secondly by giving drugs in logarithmically cumulative doses. Tests were also performed with amyl nitrite (by inhalation) to mimic the hypotensive effects seen with some agents; in no case were drug effects mimicked by such induced hypotension.

RESULTS AND DISCUSSION

Of the cells recorded in this study, all but two could be activated by low threshold peripheral natural stimuli as well as by noxious stimuli. On most of these cells, however, the maximal firing rate that could be attained with the low intensity stimuli was much less than that attained during noxious stimuli. This contrasts with many multireceptive lamina propria neurones which respond at similarly high frequencies to both repetitive low and maintained high intensity stimuli.

A. Relative Potencies of Anaesthetic Agents

In common with many others we used α-chloralose as the anaesthetic of choice; in fact, however, there is relatively little information on the use of this anaesthetic in rats. Our tests on the effects of chloralose on nociceptive responses of lamina I neurones have been limited to testing supplementary doses in rats already lightly anaesthetised with this anaesthetic. Under these conditions doses which represent 40-100% of the full i.v. anaesthetic dose (which is 50-60mg/kg) had relatively weak effects on nociceptive responses of lamina I cells. An example is shown in Figure 1 which shows minimal effects of a 20mg/kg dose, even 10 minutes after the injection, which is the time when chloralose effects are likely to be maximal (eg Collins *et al*, 1983).

In contrast, doses of the steroid anaesthetic mixture alphaxalone/alphadolone affected nociceptive responses at doses appreciably below those accepted as the standard anaesthetic dose, which is given as 9mg/kg i.v. in cats (manufacturer's data sheet) and as 10-20mg/kg i.v. in rats (Green, 1982). In the example of Figure 1, a dose of 2mg/kg i.v. in a chloralose-anaesthetized rat caused a marked reduction of both thermal and mechanical nociceptive responses. Figure 2 illustrates another case, this time in a decerebrate cat, in which cumulative doses up to 4mg/kg i.v. caused a

501

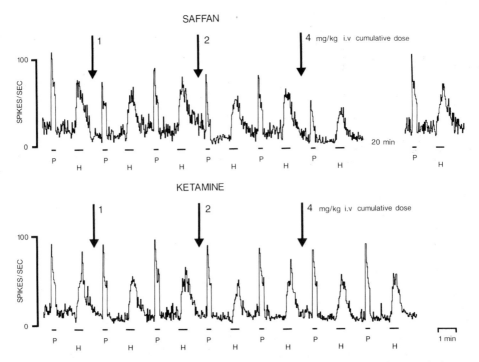

FIGURE 2: Comparison of the effects of sub-anaesthetic doses of the steroid anaesthetic mixture alphaxalone/alphadolone (Saffan) (upper trace) and of the dissociative anaesthetic ketamine (lower trace) on nociceptive responses of a lamina I neurone. The activating stimuli were noxious pinch (P) to toe 3 for 15 s and noxious heat (H) to toepad 2, ramped from 37°C to 48°C, for 30 s. Stimulus repetition interval 3 min. Decerebrate spinalized cat.

progressive and marked reduction of responses. In fact 4mg/kg of the steroid given i.v. will cause transient anaesthesia in cats when given as a rapid bolus (F Boissonade and B Matthews, personal communication and data presented at this meeting) but would probably not do so when given over several minutes as shown in Figure 2.

The spinal actions of the dissociative anaesthetic ketamine are of interest for several reasons. In man this agent is an effective analgesic for somatic pain even at sub-anaesthetic doses (see White et al, 1982). There are disputed claims that, following topical spinal administration, it has antinociceptive actions both in man (eg. Bion, 1984; but cf. eg. Rubin et al, 1983) and in rats (eg. Pekoe and Smith, 1982; cf. Tung and Yaksh, 1981; Brock-Utne et al, 1985). The veterinary literature, however, does not support ketamine as having potent analgesic actions in sub-primate species. Figure 2 illustrates that at sub-anaesthetic doses ketamine did not affect the nociceptive responses of a lamina I cell in a cat. In Figure 3 is shown a test with a full anaesthetic dose (24mg/kg in cats) but even at this dose the nociceptive responses were scarcely affected. In this series of experiments ketamine was tested on 2 cells responding to alternating noxious heat and noxious pinch stimuli. Responses to heat were as resistant to ketamine as were those to noxious pinch.

At sub-anaesthetic doses ketamine and related dissociative anaesthetics are, in all species tested to date, selective non-competitive antagonists of the actions of the excitatory amino acid N-methyl-D-aspartate (NMDA) (Anis et al, 1983; Lodge et al, 1983). These agents have the advantage over available competitive NMDA antagonists in that they readily penetrate the blood-brain barrier and can therefore be used systemically to test for NMDA receptor involvement in synaptic pathways. Figure 4 illustrates a test in which the stimulus cycle was of a noxious pinch and of the excitatory amino acid analogues NMDA and quisqualate, administered microelectrophoretically. The responses to NMDA were reduced early in the cumulative dose regime whilst responses to noxious pinch and quisqualate remained relatively unchanged. Lamina I neurones are thus like other dorsal horn neurones, but unlike motoneurones and some ventral horn interneurones, in that their nociceptive responses are resistant to ketamine (see Headley *et al*, 1987a). There is however evidence that NMDA antagonists do block the process of wind-up of responses of deeper dorsal horn neurones to electrical stimulation of primary afferents (Davies and Lodge, 1987; Dickenson and Sullivan, 1987).

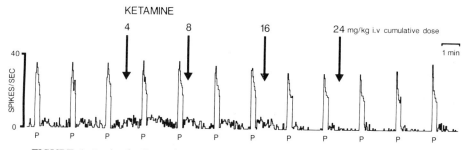

FIGURE 3: Lack of effect of a full anaesthetic dose of the dissociative anaesthetic ketamine on nociceptive responses of a lamina I neurone. Cell activated by noxious pinch stimuli (P: toe 4 for 15 s) repeated every 2 min. Decerebrate spinalized cat.

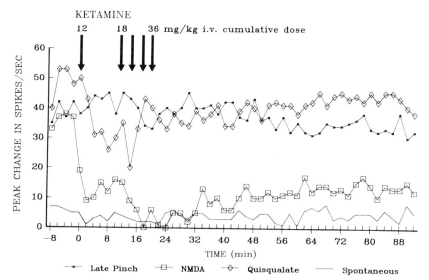

FIGURE 4: Ketamine reduces responses to the excitatory amino acid N-methyl-D-aspartate (NMDA) but not responses to the amino acid quisqualate or nociceptive responses of a lamina I neurone. Cell activated in a regular 2 min cycle by noxious pinch stimuli applied to toe 4 for 10 s (Late Pinch) and by microelectrophoretic administrations of NMDA (50nA) and quisqualate (50nA). The graph plots, for each stimulus, the increment of spike discharge frequency above the spontaneous rate. α-chloralose anaesthetized spinalized rat.

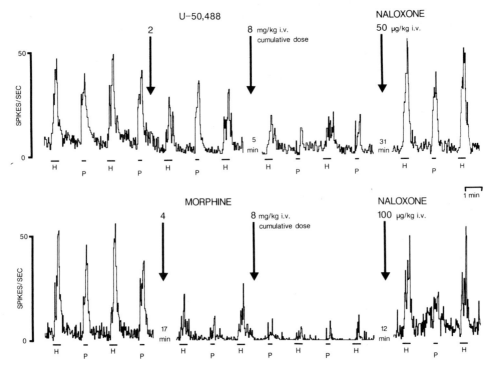

FIGURE 5: Comparison of the effects of the mu opioid fentanyl on nociceptive responses of a lamina I neurone. The opioid reduced thermal and mechanical nociceptive responses to varying degrees depending on the relative firing rates elicited by the two stimuli. Stimulus parameters: noxious heat (H) for 30 s, ramped from 37°C to 48.5°C on medial plantar foot (upper) or to 48°C on lateral plantar foot (lower); noxious pinch for 15 s to toe 4 (upper) or toe 3 (lower). Stimulus repetition cycle 3 min 30 s. α-chloralose anaesthetized spinalized rat.

The implication of this result is therefore that NMDA receptors do not mediate the synaptic responses investigated despite the fact that the neurones are sensitive to this amino acid. This highlights the danger of attributing a physiological function to the simple finding that cells are responsive to a putative neurotransmitter (or an analogue). Nonetheless such neuronal sensitivity (for example to substance P) has frequently been interpreted as evidence in favour of a function for the relevant agent.

We have also tested barbiturate anaesthetics on spinal neurones. Methohexitone is the drug of choice in that it has a short plasma half life, and in tests on reflex responses it had actions similar to those of pentobarbitone (Headley et al, 1987b). On lamina I cells it reduced nociceptive responses at doses of approximately half the induction dose (quoted as about 8mg/kg by Green, 1982). Such an effect is illustrated in Figure 7 (which should be viewed in relation to the discussion below).

On some cells low intensity peripheral stimuli were alternated with noxious stimuli. On this rather small sample of cells, none of the four anaesthetic agents tested showed any consistent selectivity between the two types of stimulus, although on some (but not all) of these cells the mu opioid fentanyl did reduce the nociceptive responses preferentially.

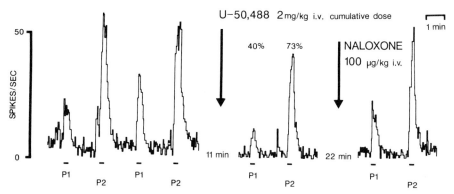

FIGURE 6: The kappa opioid U-50,488 showing apparent selectivity between responses to two different intensity pinch stimuli delivered alternately by the same pincher device. Note that the responses to the less intense stimulus were reduced to a greater extent; in terms of the number of spikes elicited by each stimulus the smaller response was reduced to 40% of control whereas the larger response was reduced to only 73% of control. Pinch stimuli delivered to toe 4 for 15 s; P2 was twice the force of P1. α-chloralose anaesthetized spinalized rat.

B. The Importance of Stimulus Intensity in Tests on Anaesthetics and Opioids

In our electrophysiological studies of mu and kappa opioid effects on nociceptive reflex responses we have obtained results markedly different to the majority of reflex tests based on behavioural measurements with intrathecally-administered opioids. Thus whilst in behavioural tests kappa agonists are generally described as being ineffective in thermal tests such as the tail flick and hotplate tests (for review see eg Yaksh and Noueihed, 1985), we have not observed such a difference in electrophysiological measures of reflex output (Headley *et al*, 1984, 1987c; Parsons *et al*, 1986; Parsons and Headley, 1988). The kappa agonists U-50,488 (Figure 8) and tifluadom (not illustrated) are similarly equieffective between thermal and mechanical nociceptive responses when tested on cells in lamina I. We have become increasingly convinced that two technical limitations of most behavioural tests account for the discrepancy between the behavioural and our electrophysiological results and, further, that an erroneous interpretation has been made of the relative spinal actions of mu and kappa agonists. One of these technical aspects concerns the adequate matching of stimulus intensity between thermal and non-thermal inputs. We have previously reported that when recording reflex responses of single motoneurones even quite small mismatches in firing rate can result in marked but false selectivity between responses (Parsons *et al*, 1986; Headley *et al*, 1987c). The same false selectivity can be seen with lamina I cells, though it appears to be rather less marked.

Mu agonists such as fentanyl are generally said to affect thermal and non-thermal responses equally. Figure 5 indicates that this can indeed be the case; but it also indicates that apparent selectivity between thermal and mechanical tests is observed whenever the peripheral stimuli are not matched such as to elicit similar firing rates on the cell under study. Thus in the top trace, where the stimuli were well matched, the responses were reduced fairly closely in parallel. On the same cell, when the responses were less well matched (lower trace), the same drug caused an apparent relatively selective reduction of the smaller response.

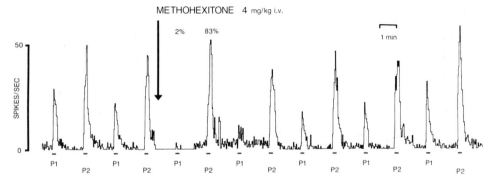

FIGURE 7: The barbiturate anaesthetic methohexitone, like the opioids, showed apparent selectivity for the smaller of the responses evoked by alternating pinch stimuli of different intensities. Same cell and same stimulus parameters as in Figure 6.

The same effect can be demonstrated more clearly when the same stimulus modality is alternated at different intensities. This was the case in the examples of Figures 6 and 7, in which one pincher device was used to exert different pressures to the same site. In these examples from two lamina I cells, both the selective kappa opioid U-50,488 and the barbiturate anaesthetic methohexitone showed similar propensities for reducing the smaller of the alternating pinch responses to a greater extent than the larger responses. This apparent selectivity by one drug between responses to the same stimulus modality indicates the problem of interpreting tests performed in behavioural studies where different modality stimuli are tested in different animals at different intensities and applied to different receptive fields.

A caveat with all experiments utilising a mechanical pinch stimulus concerns the possible contribution of slowly adapting mechanoreceptors to the evoked *nociceptive* responses. Whilst such activation seems likely, the contribution cannot be measured directly. However, the following four points, taken together, indicate that it is unlikely that such a contribution affects our interpretation significantly. Firstly the pinch stimuli used elicit clearly aversive responses in both man and rats. Secondly, in those tests in which noxious heat and pinch stimuli were alternated, both mu and kappa opioids, and the anaesthetics, affected the two types of responses to the same degree, so long as the stimuli were matched; this applied not only to the relatively small sample of lamina I neurones tested but also to all the lamina propria neurones and motoneurones we have studied, a sample of over 80 neurones. Thirdly since the opioids (to a greater extent than the anaesthetics) were selective in reducing mechanical as well as thermal nociceptive responses over mechanical nonnociceptive responses, the implication is that the responses to mechanical pinch are primarily nociceptive in content. Fourthly and most importantly, if, in those tests with alternating intensities of pinch, the smaller responses contained a relatively higher proportion of low threshold information, then it would be expected that these responses would be less, not more, affected by the opioids.

C. Access of Opioid Agonists to Spinal Sites of Action

Not only have we found that kappa opioid are equally effective between thermal and non-thermal nociceptive responses, but we find that the relative potencies of kappa and mu opioids in our tests are grossly different to those quoted in most behavioural tests; this is the case whether the administration in the latter is systemic or topical. With systemic administration in spinally intact animals it is not possible to distinguish spinally from supraspinally-mediated effects; and with topical administration there remains the complication that the lipophilicity of drugs profoundly affects the rate at which they are absorbed into the circulation and hence the degree to which they effectively penetrate the spinal grey. The relative effectiveness of mu agonists with very different lipophilicities was investigated by Durant and Yaksh (1986) and by Yaksh *et al* (1986). In their tests effective epidural doses of fentanyl could exceed the systemically effective dose whereas the effective dose of intrathecal morphine was two to three orders less than the systemically effective dose. Put another way, the relative potencies of fentanyl and morphine are around 500-1000:1 after i.v. administration to intact animals (Janssen *et al*, 1963) whereas they are only 2:1 following intrathecal administration (Yaksh *et al*, 1986). Kappa agonists with structures similar to U-50,488 are much more lipophilic than is morphine (Cheney *et al*, 1985) and have been observed to be redistributed from CNS tissue rapidly after local administration (Leighton *et al*, 1988). In spite of the above observations, the relative spinal potencies of topical morphine and U-50,488 are still generally taken as an indication of the relative effectiveness of spinal mu and kappa receptors.

In our tests with i.v. administration in spinalized animals, the relative potencies of fentanyl and morphine on reflex responses are 500-1000:1 (Parsons *et al*, 1986; Headley

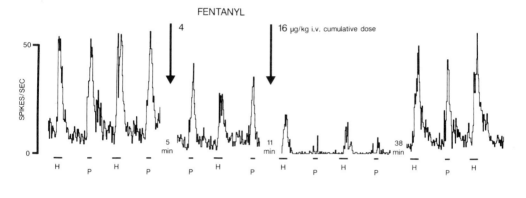

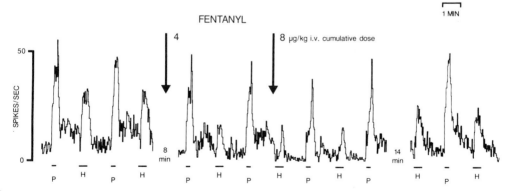

FIGURE 8: Comparison of the potencies of the mu opioid morphine and the kappa opioid U-50,488 on nociceptive responses of a lamina I neurone. The two agonists were similarly potent in this test and both reduced thermal and mechanical nociceptive responses in parallel. Heat stimulus (H) to lateral toes and plantar foot, ramped from 37°C to 48°C for total 30 s. Pinch stimulus (P) to toe 3 for 15 s. Stimulus cycle 3min 30 s. α-chloralose anaesthetized spinalized rat.

et al, 1987c). The same potency ratio applies to lamina I cells, as can be seen by comparing the effective doses on the cell illustrated in Figures 5 and 8.

With intravenous administration, the potency ratio for morphine:U-50,488 on reflex responses is approximately 1:1 in our electrophysiological studies (Headley *et al*, 1987c; Parsons and Headley, 1988) and similar potencies have been reported for spinally-intact rats in behavioural tests with mechanical (although not with thermal) noxious stimuli (eg Leighton *et al*, 1988). The same ratio applies in the lamina propria and also on the majority of lamina I neurones examined, as is shown by the tests illustrated in Figure 8. In contrast the potency ratios reported following topical administration are markedly different. With intrathecal administration in behavioural tests on thermally elicited reflexes the ratio is > 100:1 (Yaksh and Noueihed, 1985). In electrophysiological tests of dorsal horn neurones, and using topical administration, the relative potencies are evidently > 30:1 (Dickenson and Sullivan, 1986; Knox and Dickenson, 1987); and by microelectrophoretic administration U-50,488 is ineffective on lamina I neurones (Fleetwood-Walker *et al*, 1987; Hope *et al*, this meeting). The appropriate control in tests utilising local administration of kappa opioids is to perform parallel tests with a mu agonist of lipophilicity similar to the kappa agent; but this has not been performed. In the absence of such tests the lack of effect of locally administered kappa opioids cannot be interpreted as implying lack of physiologically or pharmacologically relevant kappa receptors. However, comparative microelectrophoretic studies between mu and kappa opioid peptides of similar structure and presumably with similar degrees of hydrophilicity, still indicate differences between kappa and mu ligands (Fleetwood-Walker *et al*, 1987), suggesting that lipophilicity is not the only factor involved in the discrepancies described above.

CONCLUSIONS

The results presented above indicate that the relative potencies of injectable anaesthetics in reducing nociceptive responses do not match their relative potencies as general anaesthetics, whether the measure is made on spinal motoneurones (Headley *et al*, 1987b) or on lamina I cells (see above). This has clear implications for the interpretation of electrophysiological data gathered from anaesthetized preparations. Our results are not yet sufficiently extensive to permit a re-evaluation of published data, but they do indicate that more specific consideration should be given to the choice of anaesthetic.

Our choice of α-chloralose as a base anaesthetic for these studies receives justification from the relative lack of effect of supplementary doses of this anaesthetic. There is an obvious requirement to test this agent in decerebrate rats in a manner akin to that performed in cats by Collins *et al* (1983) who found that chloralose did affect spinal neuronal responses to an appreciable degree. We have not yet performed such tests. Preliminary results in our laboratory do, however, suggest that αchloralose has similarly weak effects when tested on reflexes in rats anaesthetized with constant infusions of alphaxalone/alphadolone (N.A. Hartell, unpublished observations).

The question of matching the firing rates of responses to alternating stimuli has been addressed before in other situations. The point seems, however, not to be fully appreciated by most workers carrying out behavioural tests on analgesic agents (but see Hayes *et al*, 1987; MJ Millan, pers. comm.). The latency measurements generally given for tail flick tests are very much shorter than those obtaining in writhing or paw pressure tests, and the relative vigour of the motor response too indicates that motoneuronal discharge rates are likely to be very different between these tests. There have been few

508

behavioural tests in which different modality stimuli have been matched so as to evoke similar latency responses and even fewer in which the stimuli are administered sufficiently close together anatomically to evoke activity in a similar pool of central neurones; when this is done the selectivity of kappa opioids between thermal and non-thermal responses is greatly reduced (Millan MJ and Herz A, pers. comm.). Under these conditions, results in behavioural tests thus closely match our electrophysiological results.

The tests performed on the relative potencies of morphine and fentanyl, hydrophilic and lipophilic mu opioids respectively, indicate that the spinal receptor population responds to these agonists in the same proportion as do receptors activated in the intact animal (our potency ratios being similar to those for i.v. administration in behavioural tests; see Janssen et al, 1963). It is therefore clear that the very low potency ratio between these agents, as seen following topical spinal administration, is due to differential access to receptor sites rather than to any difference is receptor activation (see Durant and Yaksh, 1986; Yaksh et al, 1986). The potency difference between hydrophilic morphine and lipophilic kappa ligands following topical administration should *not* therefore be interpreted in terms of differential mu and kappa receptor numbers or efficacy in the spinal cord, unless further evidence for such a difference can be found. To the contrary, our finding that morphine and U-50,488 are equipotent following i.v. administration (see also Leighton et al, 1988) indicates that the accepted interpretation is incorrect. Other evidence regarding kappa functions in the rat spinal cord is similarly disparate. For instance in studies of opioid binding sites, some evidence implies that kappa binding sites are virtually non-existent in the spinal cord of the rat (eg Lahti et al, 1985) whereas other reports indicate kappa sites may be the predominant opioid sites (Traynor et al, 1982; Czlonkowski et al, 1983; Slater and Patel, 1983). In addition, the presence of dynorphin in lamina I (eg Ruda, this meeting) implies that kappa receptors are likely to be present in superficial laminae. Moreover, the fact remains that, in spinalized preparations, systemically-administered kappa ligands are effective at reducing nociceptive responses of spinal motoneurones, lamina propria neurones (Headley et al, 1984) and of lamina I neurones (see above) in the rat as well as in the cat.

In summary, we have found that three aspects of the interpretation of pharmacological and physiological data need to receive more emphasis than is usually given to them. The choice of anaesthetic, the intensity of somatosensory stimulus used and the access of drugs from the site of administration to the site of action all need detailed consideration; in the absence of such consideration, as is often the case, experimental data can only too easily be misinterpreted.

ACKNOWLEDGEMENTS

This work was supported by the Medical Research Council and by the Wellcome Trust.

REFERENCES

ANIS NA, BERRY SC, BURTON NR AND LODGE D (1983). The dissociative anaesthetics, ketamine and phencyclidine, selectively reduce excitation of central mammalian neurones by N-methyl-D-aspartate. *British Journal of Pharmacology* **79**: 565-575.

BION JF (1984). Intrathecal ketamine for war surgery. A preliminary study under field conditions. *Anesthesia* **39**: 1023-1028.

BROCK-UTNE JG, DOWNING JW, MANKOWITZ E AND RUBIN J (1985). Intrathecal ketamine in rats. *British Journal of Anaesthesia* **57**: 837.

CHENEY BV, SZMUSZKOVICZ J, LAHTI R AND ZICHI DA (1985). Factors affecting binding of trans-*N*-[2-(methyl-amino)cyclohexyl]benzamides at the primary morphine receptor. *Journal of Medicinal Chemistry* **28**: 1853-1864.

COLLINS JG, KAWAHARA M, HOMMA E AND KITAHATA LM (1983). α-chloralose suppression of neuronal activity. *Life Sciences* **32**: 2995-2999.

CZLONKOWSKI A, COSTA T, PRZEWLOCKI R, PASI A AND HERZ A (1983). Opiate receptor binding in human spinal cord. *Brain Research* **267**: 392-396.

DAVIES SN AND LODGE D (1987). Evidence for involvement of *N*-methylaspartate receptors in wind-up of class 2 neurones in the dorsal horn of the rat. *Brain Research* **424**: 402-406.

DICKENSON AH AND SULLIVAN AF (1986). Electrophysiological studies on the effects of intrathecal morphine on nociceptive neurones in the rat dorsal horn. *Pain* **24**: 211-222.

DICKENSON AH AND SULLIVAN AF (1987). Evidence for a role of the NMDA receptor in the frequency dependent potentiation of deep rat dorsal horn nociceptive neurones following C fibre stimulation. *Neuropharmacology* **26**: 1235-1238.

DURANT PAC AND YAKSH TL (1986). Epidural injections of bupivacaine, morphine, fentanyl, lofentanil, and DADL in chronically implanted rats: a pharmacologic and pathologic study. *Anesthesiology* **64**: 43-53.

FLEETWOOD-WALKER SM, HOPE PJ AND MITCHELL R (1987). Delta opioids exert antinociceptive effects in lamina I, but not lamina III-V of rat dorsal horn. *Journal of Physiology* **382**: 152P.

GREEN CJ (1982). *Animal Anaesthesia* Laboratory Animals Ltd, London.

HAYES AG, SHEEHAN MJ AND TYERS MB (1987). Differential sensitivity of models of antinociception in the rat, mouse and guinea-pig to μ- and κ-opioid receptor agonists. *British Journal of Pharmacology* **91**: 823-832.

HEADLEY PM, PARSONS CG AND WEST DC (1984). Comparison of mu, kappa and sigma preferring agonists for effects on spinal nociceptive and other responses in rats. *Neuropeptides* **5**: 249-252.

HEADLEY PM, PARSONS CG AND WEST DC (1987a). The role of *N*-methylaspartate receptors in mediating responses of rat and cat spinal neurones to defined sensory stimuli. *Journal of Physiology* **385**: 169-188.

HEADLEY PM, IVORRA MI, PARSONS CG AND WEST DC (1987b). The effects of several general anaesthetics on nociceptive spinal reflexes of the rat. *Journal of Physiology* **391**: 42P.

HEADLEY PM, PARSONS CG AND WEST DC (1987c). Opioid receptor-mediated effects on spinal responses to controlled noxious natural peripheral stimuli: technical considerations. In: *Fine Afferent Nerve Fibres and Pain*. Eds. R.F. Schmidt, H.G. Schaible and C. Vahle-Hinz. VCH Press, Weinheim, FRG. pp 225-235.

JANSSEN PAJ, NIEMEGEERS CJE AND DONY JGH (1963). The inhibitory effect of fentanyl and other morphine-like analgesics on the warm water induced withdrawal reflex in rats. *Arzneimittel Forschung* **13**: 502-507.

KNOX RJ AND DICKENSON AH (1987). Effects of selective and non-selective κ-opioid receptor agonists on cutaneous C-fibre evoked responses of rat dorsal horn neurones. *Brain Research* **415**: 21-29.

LAHTI RA, MICKELSON MM, McCALL JM AND VONVOIGTLANDER PF (1985). [^{3}H]U-69593 A highly selective ligand for the opioid κ receptor. *European Journal of*

Pharmacology **109**: 281-284.

LEIGHTON GE, RODRIGUEZ RE, HILL RG AND HUGHES J (1988). κ -opioid agonists produce antinociception after i.v. and i.c.v. but not intrathecal administration in the rat. *British Journal of Pharmacology* **93**: 553-560.

LODGE D, ANIS NA, BERRY SC AND BURTON NR (1983). Arylcyclohexylamines selectively reduce excitation of mammalian neurones by aspartate-like amino acids. In: *Phencyclidine and Related Arylcyclohexylamines: Present and Future Applications.* Eds: Kamenka JM Domino E F and Geneste P. NPP Books, Ann Arbor. pp 595-616.

PARSONS CG, WEST DC AND HEADLEY PM (1986). Similar actions of kappa and mu agonists on spinal nociceptive reflexes in rats and their reversibility by naloxone. *N.I.D.A. Research Monographs* **75**: 461-464.

PARSONS CG AND HEADLEY PM (1988). Have current concepts of spinal opioid receptor function been influenced by the routes of drug administration used? In: *Pain Research and Clinical Management.* **3**. Eds. Dubner R, Gebhart GF and Bond MR. Elsevier. pp 449-453.

PEKOE GM AND SMITH DJ (1982). The involvement of opiate and monoaminergic neuronal systems in the analgesic effects of ketamine. *Pain* **12**: 57-73.

RUBIN J, MANKOWITZ E, BROCK-UTNE JG AND DOWNING JW (1983). Ketamine and postoperative pain. *South African Medical Journal* **63**: 433.

SLATER P AND PATEL S (1983). Autoradiographic localization of opiate κ receptors in the rat spinal cord. *European Journal of Pharmacology* **92**: 159-160.

TRAYNOR JR, KELLY PD AND RANCE MJ (1982). Multiple opiate binding sites in rat spinal cord. *Life Sciences* **31**: 1377-1380.

TUNG AS AND YAKSH TL (1981). Analgesic effect of intrathecal ketamine in the rat. *Regional Anesthesia* **6**: 91-94.

WHITE PF, WAY WL AND TREVOR AJ (1982). Ketamine - its pharmacology and therapeutic uses. *Anesthesiology* **56**: 119-136.

YAKSH TL AND NOUEIHED R (1985). The physiology and pharmacology of spinal opiates. *Annual Review of Pharmacology and Toxicology* **25**: 433-462.

YAKSH TL, NOUEIHED RY AND DURANT PAC (1986). Studies of the pharmacology and pathology of intrathecally administered 4-anilinopiperidine analogues and morphine in the rat and cat. *Anesthesiology* **64**: 54-66.

DISCUSSION ON SECTION VII

Rapporteur: V. Molony

Department of Preclinical Veterinary Sciences, Royal (Dick) School of Veterinary
Studies, University of Edinburgh, Summerhall, Edinburgh EH9 1QH, U.K.

The Chairman, R. Dubner, introduced the session. He expressed the hope that the
reliability of various techniques could be discussed so that workers, particularly in other
disciplines, could assess the quality of results obtained from the various approaches. He
briefly outlined some of the main technical problems which affect opinions about the
superficial dorsal horn.

With reference to physiological studies, he emphasised problems arising from the
general physiological state of the animal preparation, the quality of homeostatic control
and the effects of anaesthesia. He commented on the need for clear definition of the
region of the stimulus-response curve of the population(s) of sensory receptors being
stimulated and on the problems which occur when the intensity or frequency of
stimulation is too high or too low. He reminded everyone of the difficulties involved in
restricting stimulation to a single population of receptors. He emphasised the problem
of defining a population of dorsal horn neurones for study and pointed out that
considerable variation existed between laboratories in the working definitions used to
define such populations of neurones. The particular example he chose was that of wide
dynamic range or multireceptive neurones; he concluded that efforts to define such
neurones with precision have been relatively unsuccessful.

Referring to anatomical studies his main point was that the intensity of staining
could vary greatly even within a laboratory. The sensitivity of some methods can be
very high and the functional significance of some positive results should be viewed with
caution. He suggested that the main safeguards are the reproducibility of results and
their confirmation in independent laboratories.

J.G. Collins addressed the problem of misinterpretation of experimental data as a
result of the use of those animal preparations which involve extensive surgery and
anaesthesia and in which the animal is not in a well defined physiological, metabolic or
neurobiological state. He described experiments on unanaesthetised restrained cats in
which extracellular recordings were made from neurones in the dorsal horn. His results
indicated that anaesthetic doses of barbiturate could greatly increase both the numbers
of wide dynamic range neurones recorded and that intravenous methysergide increased
the number of wide dynamic range neurones and their receptive field size.

It did not appear to be generally accepted by participants that the results obtained so
far from unanaesthetised conscious animals were sufficiently different to those
predicted to demand radical reinterpretation of results obtained from *acute*

preparations. It did, however, appear that participants acknowledged the need for such experiments to permit the results obtained in *acute* experiments to be more correctly interpreted.

Collins acknowledged that quantitative control of stimuli presented a problem and reminded participants that regard for the welfare of the conscious animal ruled out the use of repeated noxious stimuli in searching for populations of nocireceptive neurones.

In discussion participants were concerned with the results obtained with methysergide. J.M. Besson raised the problems of dosage and G.J. Gebhart the peripheral effects of this agent. Collins reminded participants that he was concerned, at this stage, to show that it was possible to work on unanaesthetised conscious cats in a humane way. He suggested that his main finding was that there was evidence of tonic inhibition of dorsal horn neurones. He indicated that further control experiments were planned, as were investigations of other antagonists. Most concern was expressed about the dependence of any tonic inhibition on the response of the cats to restraint for the purposes of recording. Collins described the behaviour of the cats under restraint as calm and co-operative, but acknowledged that training to accept restraint may result in modifications to dorsal horn activity. This point was further pursued by M. Devor and J.M. Besson who asked about changes in tonic activity with different states of attention such as distraction by mice or during sleep.

There was discussion of the stability and repeatability of responses to noxious stimulation and F. Cervero asked if he had found nocispecific neurones. Collins again stated that he did not consider it humane to use repeated noxious stimulation to search for nocireceptive specific neurones and that he had not therefore been able to study such neurones.

Concern was expressed by P.M. Headley and D. Le Bars over the detailed results describing the stimulus-response characteristics of the neurones. They were particularly concerned that the quality and intensity of stimulation used and the detailed analysis of responses should permit clear comparison with data obtained from *acute* preparations.

P.M. Headley reviewed problems highlighted by mismatches between the potency with which various opioid and other agents affect the responses of multireceptive dorsal horn neurones to natural stimulation and their potency as analgesics or anaesthetics in behavioural testing procedures. He made it clear that the mechanisms of action of such agents when used on unanaesthetised freely behaving animals and man can only be studied in *acute* experiments if appropriate quantitative allowance can be made for various experimental problems.

He emphasised the importance of the anaesthetic being used and the effects of the surgery. He advocated the use of several different types of anaesthetic in different doses as well as unanaesthetised, decerebrate and spinalised preparations to confirm the general applicability of results.

He showed that it was necessary to match the intensity and frequency of natural stimulation so that the same level of excitability of the dorsal horn neurones was obtained with noxious heat, pinch and non-noxious stimulation.

He stressed the importance of ensuring that the amounts of the test agent reaching and remaining at active sites in or on the neurones being studied, is similar under the conditions of the behavioural tests and those in the *acute* experiments.

Some of the discussion was concerned with details of the results used for illustration of points. A.I. Basbaum recalled positive effects of U 50,488H administered by intracerebroventricular injection and of low doses applied to the surface of the spinal cord. J.M. Besson also commented upon the access of opioids and asked Headley about the relative potency of α_2 adrenergic agents. Headley said that he had no detailed results for α_2 agonists.

E.R. Perl raised the problem of differential effects of anaesthetic agents on polysynaptic and monosynaptic pathways and suggested that powerful excitatory inputs to neurones, in particular monosynaptic inputs, are much less affected by anaesthetics than are inhibitory inputs. He referred particularly to the direct inputs of high threshold mechanoreceptors to neurones in lamina I. Although Headley accepted this as a general view for some anaesthetics he suggested that not all types of anaesthetic act at the same sites within the spinal cord.

F. Cervero pointed out the potential mechanisms which might be expected to result in progressive changes in response characteristics, but Headley affirmed that it was possible to obtain very stable responses to stimulation of peripheral receptors if suitable precautions are taken. G.F. Gebhart supported this view and quoted a variability of $\pm 10\%$ for responses to noxious stimulation obtained from dorsal horn neurones in the rat. Cervero re-emphasised the problem of supramaximal stimulation of peripheral receptors and its ability to obscure important effects.

R. Dubner commented upon the stability of responses obtained from primary afferents provided the stimulus-response characteristics of the receptors were respected and sufficient time permitted for recovery.

Both Perl and Dubner again emphasised the importance of the quality of the preparation and the need for careful monitoring and control of its physiological state.

A general discussion on the value of *in vitro* and *in vivo* preparations was introduced with three short presentations. P.M. Headley reviewed problems of the immaturity of spinal cord tissue used in most slice preparations from young animals and discussed the development of neurotransmitter systems such as those involving opioids. Some aspects of the histochemistry of the spinal cord of rats have been shown to continue changing for up to 30 days postnatally and subdivisions of the opioid systems can begin development and reach maturity at different times.

He suggested that these difficulties may be overcome by the use of spinal cord slices obtained from adult rats. He briefly described some results including some from superficial dorsal horn neurones. He described how it was possible to recognise three groups of neurones from a) the shape of their after hyperpolarisations and b) their responses to intracellular depolarising currents. These properties were correlated with their response to afferent volleys. He suggested that with this preparation it should also be possible to correlate post synaptic responses with cell morphology and the distribution of synaptic inputs.

C.J. Woolf also reviewed the value of spinal cord slice preparations and concluded that for some questions it was no better than *in vivo* studies. He suggested that, whatever the question being attacked in such preparations, it is necessary to show that the state of maturity of the neurones and their connections does not matter. He supported the use of slices for developmental studies but emphasised that the problem of producing an appropriate afferent input to spinal neurones in such slices can be insuperable. To offer a possible solution to some of these problems he briefly described an intact hind limb and isolated spinal cord preparation from which it was possible to obtain prolonged intracellular recordings. In this preparation flexor reflexes had been demonstrated and motoneurones had been labelled retrogradely with horseradish peroxidase. He was optimistic that although it is still in the development stage, such a preparation would provide an adequate model for investigation of the superficial dorsal horn and spinal cord. In particular he suggested it would be useful for investigating cellular mechanisms including those of genetic expression involved in the persistent responses to afferent inputs carried by C fibres.

Schneider discussed the need for practical ways of identifying monosynaptic responses produced by stimulation of peripheral receptors with C fibre afferent connections to neurones in the spinal cord. The problem was of particular concern to him in his attempts to identify transmitters and modulators released by such afferents. Traditional tests for monosynaptic connections such as *security* and the ability to follow relatively high frequency inputs, he considered inadequate. Inhibitory post-synaptic potentials could show such characteristics and yet monosynaptic inhibitory inputs from primary afferents were not known to be present in these mammalian preparations. He asked for discussion of methods which could be used routinely in *in vitro* preparations of spinal cord and skin such as described by Perl and himself.

Discussion was directed at the problem of confirming monosynaptic C fibre afferent connections. It was generally acknowledged that distance measurements are not accurate enough and that conduction times are too variable to confirm that only one synapse is involved. It was suggested that it might be possible to demonstrate the existence of a presynaptic action potential in the intracellularly recorded potential if averaging techniques were used and if the membrane conductance was increased. By using low Ca^{++} and high Mg^{++} bathing solutions to block synaptic transmission it might then be confirmed that this presynaptic action potential was in a primary afferent.

Further formal discussion was adjourned when participants retired to the Mesón de Cándido, Segovia, where serial sectioning of roast suckling pig was demonstrated by the patron using a blunt dinner plate, and excellent hospitality was enjoyed by all!

It was clear to this rapporteur that during the workshop all participants were not only prepared to remind each other of the problems that technical approaches brought to the interpretation of results but they were also prepared to be diplomatically persuaded to look again at their methods and interpretation of results.

The problems which have the greatest effect on opinions about the superficial dorsal horn are those of sampling and the physiological state of the preparation from which the sample is obtained. Ideally results should describe a truly random sample of a well defined population. Most of the problems referred to above lead to bias and such bias can only be overcome if it is clearly described and where possible quantified.

The physiological state of the preparation can also bias sampling away from biological normality, to an unquantified extent. To reduce variability between laboratories new quantitative measures of the state of the superficial dorsal horn need to be sought, and clearly defined limits agreed. This might be attempted, for example, by using a quantitative monitor of polysynaptic responses obtained from a ventral root recording, since a significant part of such responses are dependent on the integrity of the superficial dorsal horn.

If all possible surgical precautions, surgical skill, monitoring, control and supplementation of physiological parameters are carried out it should be possible to maintain animal preparations for several days longer than is required for any acute experiment. In this way it should not only be possible to reduce interlaboratory variability but also to increase the average yield of results from each animal.

LIST OF PARTICIPANTS

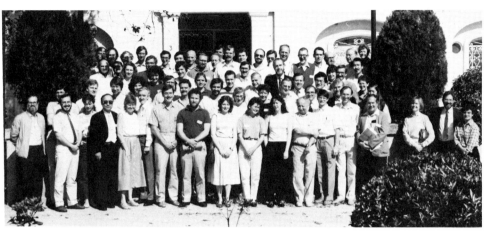

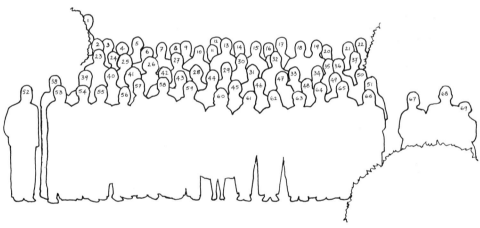

1. Leah	11. Grant	21. Sinclair *	31. Kruger	41. Lima	51. Hylden	61. Boissonade
2. Light	12. Giesler	22. Pubols L.	32. Molony	42. Le Bars	52. Sobrino	62. Hope
3. Snow	13. Mense	23. Dubner	33. Beal	43. Plenderleith	53. Cervero	63. Abrahams
4. Devor	14. Molander	24. Coimbra	34. Wakisaka	44. Parsons	54. El-Yassir	64. Cliffer
5. Schneider	15. Woolf	25. Ruda	35. Rausell	45. Steedman	55. Sugiura	65. Dostrovsky
6. Besson	16. Schaible	26. Laird	36. Foreman	46. Lumb	56. Lawson	66. Willis
7. Cruz	17. Kniffki	27. Wilson	37. Sugimoto	47. Iggo	57. Duggan	67. Alexander[+]
8. Castro-Lopes	18. Pubols B.	28. Hunt	38. Headley	48. Matthews	58. Gebhart	68. Bennett
9. Perl	19. Gonzalez	29. Kajander	39. Sandkuhler	49. Collins	59. Basbaum	69. Rodriguez
10. Anton	20. Wall	30. Traub	40. Schouenborg	50. Seybold	60. Allerton	

* NATO   [+] Secretary

V. C. Abrahams
Department of Physiology
Queen's University
Botterell Hall
Kingston K7L 3N6
Canada

C. Allerton
Parke-Davis Research Unit
Addenbrookes Hospital Site
Hills Road
Cambridge CB2 2QB
U.K.

F. Anton
Institut für Physiologie und Biokybernetik
Universität Erlangen-Nürnberg
Universitätstrasse 17
D-8520 Erlangen
F.R.G.

A. I. Basbaum
Department of Anatomy
School of Medicine
University of California
San Francisco CA 94143
U.S.A.

J. A. Beal
Department of Anatomy
School of Medicine
Louisiana State University
1501 Kings Highway PO Box 33932
Shreveport LA 71130-3932
U.S.A.

G. J. Bennett
Neurobiology and Anesthesiology Branch
National Institute of Dental Research
National Institutes of Health
Building 30 Rm B-20
Bethesda MD 20892
U.S.A.

J. M. Besson
INSERM
Unité 161
2 rue d'Alésia
Paris 75014
France

F. Boissonade
Department of Physiology
University of Bristol
Medical School
University Walk
Bristol BS8 1TD
U.K.

J. Castro-Lopes
Instituto de Histologia e Embriologia
     Abel Salazar
Faculdade de Medicina
Oporto 4200
Portugal

F. Cervero
Department of Physiology
University of Bristol
Medical School
University Walk
Bristol BS8 1TD
U.K.

K. Cliffer
The Marine Biomedical Institute
University of Texas
Medical Branch
200 University Boulevard
Galveston TX 77550-2772
U.S.A.

A. Coimbra
Instituto de Histologia e Embriologia
     Abel Salazar
Faculdade de Medicina
Oporto 4200
Portugal

J. G. Collins
Department of Anesthesiology
Yale University
School of Medicine
333 Cedar Street PO Box 3333
New Haven CT 06510
U.S.A.

F. Cruz
Instituto de Histologia e Embriologia
     Abel Salazar
Faculdade de Medicina
Oporto 4200
Portugal

M. Devor
Life Sciences Institute
Hebrew University of Jerusalem
Jerusalem 91904
Israel

J.O. Dostrovsky
Physiology Department
University of Toronto
Toronto M5S 1A8
Canada

R. Dubner
Neurobiology and Anesthesiology Branch
National Institute of Dental Research
National Institutes of Health
Building 30 Rm B-20
Bethesda MD 20892
U.S.A.

A. W. Duggan
Dept. of Pre-Clinical Vet. Studies
University of Edinburgh
Royal (Dick) School of Vet. Studies
Summerhall
Edinburgh EH9 1QH
U.K.

N. El Jassir
Dept. of Pre-Clinical Vet. Studies
University of Edinburgh
Royal (Dick) School of Vet. Studies
Summerhall
Edinburgh EH9 1QH
U.K.

R.D. Foreman
Department of Physiology & Biophysics
University of Oklahoma
Health Sciences Center
PO Box 26901
Oklahoma City OK 73190
U.S.A.

G.F. Gebhart
Department of Pharmacology
University of Iowa
Iowa City IA 52242
U.S.A.

G. J. Giesler
Dept. of Cell Biology and Neuroanatomy
University of Minnesota
4-135 Jackson Hall
321 Church Street S.E.
Minneapolis MN 55455
U.S.A.

A. González
Departamento de Biología Celular
Facultad de Biología
Universidad Complutense
Ciudad Universitaria
28040 Madrid
Spain

G. Grant
Karolinska Institute
Department of Anatomy
Box 60400
10401 Stockholm
Sweden

P. M. Headley
Department of Physiology
University of Bristol
Medical School
University Walk
Bristol BS8 1TD
U.K.

P. Hope
Dept. of Pre-Clinical Vet. Studies
University of Edinburgh
Royal (Dick) School of Vet. Studies
Summerhall
Edinburgh EH9 1QH
U.K.

S.P. Hunt
MRC Molecular Neurobiology Unit
University of Cambridge
Medical School
Hills Road
Cambridge CB2 2QH
U.K.

J.L.K. Hylden
Neurobiology and Anesthesiology Branch
National Institute of Dental Research
National Institutes of Health
Building 30 Rm B-20
Bethesda MD 20892
U.S.A.

A. Iggo
Dept. of Pre-Clinical Vet. Studies
University of Edinburgh
Royal (Dick) School of Vet. Studies
Summerhall
Edinburgh EH9 1QH
U.K.

K. Kajander
Neurobiology and Anesthesiology Branch
National Institute of Dental Research
National Institutes of Health
Building 30 Rm B-20
Bethesda MD 20892
U.S.A.

K. D. Kniffki
Physiologisches Institut
Universität Würzburg
Röentgenring 9
D-8700 Würzburg
F.R.G.

L. Kruger
Department of Anatomy
UCLA Center for Health Sciences
Los Angeles CA 90024
U.S.A

J.M.A. Laird
Department of Physiology
University of Bristol
Medical School
University Walk
Bristol BS8 1TD
U.K.

S.N. Lawson
Department of Physiology
University of Bristol
Medical School
University Walk
Bristol BS8 1TD
U.K.

J.D. Leah
II Physiologisches Institut
University of Heidelberg
Im Neuenheimer Feld 326
D-6900 Heidelberg 1
F.R.G.

D. Le Bars
INSERM
Unité 161
2 rue d'Alésia
Paris 75014
France

A. R. Light
Department of Physiology
School of Medicine
University of North Carolina
79 Medical Research Building 206H
Chapel Hill NC 27599-7545
U.S.A.

D. Lima
Instituto de Histologia e Embriologia
        Abel Salazar
Faculdade de Medicina
Oporto 4200
Portugal

B.M. Lumb
Department of Physiology
University of Bristol
Medical School
University Walk
Bristol BS8 1TD
U.K.

B. Matthews
Department of Physiology
University of Bristol
Medical School
University Walk
Bristol BS8 1TD
U.K.

S. Mense
Anatomisches Institut III
Universität Heidelberg
Im Neuenheimer Feld 307
6900 Heidelberg
F.R.G.

C. Molander
Department of Anatomy
University College London
Gower Street
London WC1E 6BT
U.K.

V. Molony
Dept. of Pre-Clinical Vet. Studies
University of Edinburgh
Royal (Dick) School of Vet. Studies
Summerhall
Edinburgh EH9 1QH
U.K.

C. Parsons
Department of Physiology
University of Bristol
Medical School
University Walk
Bristol BS8 1TD
U.K.

E. R. Perl
Department of Physiology
School of Medicine
University of North Carolina
79 Medical Research Building 206H
Chapel Hill NC 27514
U.S.A.

M. B. Plenderleith
Department of Anatomy
University of Queensland
St Lucia QLD 4067
Australia

B.H. Pubols
Neurological Science Institute
Good Samaritan Hospital
        and Medical Center
1120 NW Twentieth Avenue
Portland OR 97209
U.S.A.

L.M. Pubols
Neurological Science Institute
Good Samaritan Hospital
        and Medical Center
1120 NW Twentieth Avenue
Portland OR 97209
U.S.A.

E. Raussell
Departamento de Morfología
Facultad de Medicina
Universidad Autónoma de Madrid
calle Arzobispo Morcillo s/n
28029 Madrid
Spain

R. E. Rodríguez
Departamento de Bioquímica
Facultad de Medicina
calle Espejo 12
37007 Salamanca
Spain

M. A. Ruda
Neurobiology and Anesthesiology Branch
National Institute of Dental Research
National Institutes of Health
Building 30 Rm B-20
Bethesda MD 20892
U.S.A.

J. Sandkühler
II Physiologisches Institut
University of Heidelberg
Im Neuenheimer Feld 326
D-6900 Heidelberg 1
F.R.G.

H.G. Schaible
Physiologisches Institut
Universität Würzburg
Röentgenring 9
D-8700 Würzburg
F.R.G.

S. Schneider
Department of Physiology
School of Medicine
University of North Carolina
79 Medical Research Building 206H
Chapel Hill NC 27514
U.S.A.

J. Schouenborg
Department of Physiology
University of Lund
Sölvegatan 19
S-223 62 Lund
Sweden

V. Seybold
Dept. of Cell Biology and Neuroanatomy
University of Minnesota
4-135 Jackson Hall
321 Church Street S.E.
Minneapolis MN 55455
U.S.A.

P. J. Snow
Department of Anatomy
University of Queensland
St Lucia QLD 4067
Australia

J. A. Sobrino
Departamento de Fisiologia
Universidad Computense de Madrid
Facultad de Medicina
Ciudad Universitaria
Madrid 28040
Spain

W. Steedman
Dept. of Pre-Clinical Vet. Studies
University of Edinburgh
Royal (Dick) School of Vet. Studies
Summerhall
Edinburgh EH9 1QH
U.K.

T. Sugimoto
2nd Department of Oral Anatomy
Osaka University
Faculty of Dentistry
1-8 Yamadaoka
Suita, Osaka 565
Japan

Y. Sugiura
Institut of Basic Medical Sciences
University of Tsukuba
Tsukuba, Ibaraki 305
Japan

R. Traub
Neurobiology and Anesthesiology Branch
National Institute of Dental Research
National Institutes of Health
Building 30 Rm B-20
Bethesda MD 20892
U.S.A.

S. Wakisaka
Neurobiology and Anesthesiology Branch
National Institute of Dental Research
National Institutes of Health
Building 30 Rm B-20
Bethesda MD 20892
U.S.A.

P. D. Wall
Department of Anatomy
University College London
Gower Street
London WC1E 6BT
U.K.

W. D. Willis
The Marine Biomedical Institute
University of Texas
Medical Branch
200 University Boulevard
Galveston TX 77550-2772
U.S.A.

P. Wilson
Department of Anatomy
University of Queensland
St Lucia QLD 4067
Australia

C. Woolf
Department of Anatomy
University College London
Gower Street
London WC1E 6BT
U.K.

AUTHOR INDEX

SUBJECT INDEX